HANDBOOK OF
COGNITIVE-BEHAVIORAL THERAPIES

HANDBOOK OF COGNITIVE-BEHAVIORAL THERAPIES

THIRD EDITION

Edited by
Keith S. Dobson

THE GUILFORD PRESS
New York   London

© 2010 The Guilford Press
A Division of Guilford Publications, Inc.
72 Spring Street, New York, NY 10012
www.guilford.com

Printed in the United States of America

This book is printed on acid-free paper.

Last digit is print number: 9 8 7 6 5 4 3

Library of Congress Cataloging-in-Publication Data

Handbook of cognitive-behavioral therapies / editor Keith S. Dobson. — 3rd ed.
   p. cm.
  Includes bibliographical references and index.
  ISBN 978-1-60623-437-2 (alk. paper)
  1. Cognitive therapy—Handbooks, manuals, etc. 2. Behavior therapy—
Handbooks, manuals, etc. I. Dobson, Keith S.
  RC489.C63H36 2010
  616.89′1425—dc22

2009031648

About the Editor

Keith S. Dobson, PhD, is Professor of Clinical Psychology at the University of Calgary, in Calgary, Alberta, Canada, where he has served in various roles, including past Director of Clinical Psychology and current Head of Psychology and Co-Leader of the Hotchkiss Brain Institute Depression Research Program. Dr. Dobson's research has focused on cognitive models and mechanisms in depression and the treatment of depression, particularly using cognitive-behavioral therapies. His research has resulted in over 150 published articles and chapters, eight books, and numerous conference and workshop presentations in many countries. In addition to his research on depression, Dr. Dobson has written about developments in professional psychology and ethics, and he has been actively involved in psychology organizations, including a term as President of the Canadian Psychological Association. He was a member of the University of Calgary Research Ethics Board for many years and is President of the Academy of Cognitive Therapy as well as President-Elect of the International Association for Cognitive Psychotherapy. Dr. Dobson is a recipient of the Canadian Psychological Association's Award for Distinguished Contributions to the Profession of Psychology.

IN MEMORIAM
Albert Ellis, PhD (1913–2007)

Albert Ellis, PhD, was a titan in the field of psychotherapy. His collected works include more than 70 books and 700 articles in the areas of psychotherapy, sex, love and relationships, religion, and research in psychotherapy, among a wide range of other topics. Notably, he was the originator of rational emotive therapy, which he later renamed as rational emotive behavior therapy (REBT), and he was certainly a sustained luminary in the field of cognitive-behavioral therapy. Dr. Ellis was also a key contributor to this volume; from its inception he supported the book and he wanted REBT represented within its pages.

Dr. Ellis died on July 24, 2007, of natural causes. His death has left an enormous void in the field. The loss of his humor, wit, and intelligence, as well as his candid and direct character, will be missed by all whose lives he had touched.

Contributors

Donald H. Baucom, PhD, Department of Psychology, University of North Carolina at Chapel Hill, Chapel Hill, North Carolina

Aaron T. Beck, MD, Department of Psychology, University of Pennsylvania, Philadelphia, Pennsylvania

Rinad S. Beidas, MA, Department of Psychology, Temple University, Philadelphia, Pennsylvania

Larry E. Beutler, PhD, Pacific Graduate School of Psychology, Palo Alto, California

Kirk R. Blankstein, PhD, Department of Psychology, University of Toronto at Mississauga, Mississauga, Ontario, Canada

Lauren Braswell, PhD, Department of Psychology, University of St. Thomas, St. Paul, Minnesota

Mylea Charvat, MS, Pacific Graduate School of Psychology, Palo Alto, California

Sarah A. Crawley, MA, Department of Psychology, Temple University, Philadelphia, Pennsylvania

Daniel David, PhD, Faculty of Psychology and Educational Sciences, Babes-Bolyai University, Cluj-Napoca, Cluj, Romania

Joan Davidson, PhD, San Francisco Bay Area Center for Cognitive Therapy, Oakland, California

Robert J. DeRubeis, PhD, Department of Psychology, University of Pennsylvania, Philadelphia, Pennsylvania

Keith S. Dobson, PhD, Department of Psychology, University of Calgary, Calgary, Alberta, Canada

David J. A. Dozois, PhD, Department of Psychology, University of Western Ontario, London, Ontario, Canada

Windy Dryden, PhD, Professional and Community Education, Goldsmiths College, London, United Kingdom

David M. Dunkley, PhD, Department of Psychiatry, Sir Mortimer B. Davis Jewish General Hospital and McGill University, Montreal, Quebec, Canada

Thomas J. D'Zurilla, PhD, Department of Psychology, Stony Brook University, Stony Brook, New York

Albert Ellis, PhD, (deceased) The Albert Ellis Institute, New York, New York

Amanda M. Epp, MSc, Department of Psychology, University of Calgary, Calgary, Alberta, Canada

Norman B. Epstein, PhD, Department of Family Science, University of Maryland, College Park, Maryland

Karen R. Erikson, MS, Department of Psychology, University of Nevada, Reno, Reno, Nevada

Alan E. Fruzzetti, PhD, Department of Psychology, University of Nevada, Reno, Reno, Nevada

T. Mark Harwood, PhD, Department of Psychology, Wheaton College, Wheaton, Illinois

Rick E. Ingram, PhD, Department of Psychology, University of Kansas, Lawrence, Kansas

Gayle Y. Iwamasa, PhD, Department of Psychology, Logansport State Hospital, Logansport, Indiana

Philip C. Kendall, PhD, ABPP, Department of Psychology, Temple University, Philadelphia, Pennsylvania

Jennifer S. Kirby, PhD, Department of Psychology, University of North Carolina at Chapel Hill, Chapel Hill, North Carolina

Jaslean J. LaTaillade, PhD, Department of Family Science, University of Maryland, College Park, Maryland

Christopher R. Martell, PhD, ABPP, Department of Psychiatry and Behavioral Sciences, University of Washington, Seattle, Washington

Rachel Martin, MSc, Department of Psychology, University of Calgary, Calgary, Alberta, Canada

Arthur M. Nezu, PhD, Department of Psychology, Drexel University, Philadelphia, Pennsylvania

David W. Pantalone, PhD, Department of Psychology, Suffolk University, Boston, Massachusetts

Jacqueline B. Persons, PhD, San Francisco Bay Area Center for Cognitive Therapy, Oakland, California

Jennifer L. Podell, MA, Department of Psychology, Temple University, Philadelphia, Pennsylvania

Zindel V. Segal, PhD, Departments of Psychiatry and Psychology, University of Toronto, Toronto, Ontario, Canada

Greg J. Siegle, PhD, Department of Psychiatry, Western Psychiatric Institute and Clinic, Pittsburgh, Pennsylvania

Tony Z. Tang, PhD, Department of Psychology, Northwestern University, Evanston, Illinois

Christian A. Webb, MA, Department of Psychology, University of Pennsylvania, Philadelphia, Pennsylvania

Jeffrey Young, PhD, Schema Therapy Institute, New York, New York

Preface

When the first edition of the *Handbook of Cognitive-Behavioral Therapies* was published in 1988, I would not have guessed that it would become a mainstay in the field of cognitive-behavioral therapy (CBT). More than 20 years later, though, this volume is regularly used in training programs and has been translated into Italian and Portuguese. It has been gratifying to see that the breadth and depth of CBT have increased and to have been a part of that process.

The third edition reflects a continuing belief in the importance of CBT. As I noted in the preface to the first edition, at that time there really was no comprehensive book, written by the best experts in the field, that covered the broad domain of CBT. The completion of this edition reflects the belief that the publisher and I continue to have that it fills an important place in the CBT literature. The intended audience remains one that is learning about psychotherapy and wishes to explore the growth in the cognitive-behavioral models.

This edition contains several important changes. While some of the core chapters discussing conceptual issues in CBT are retained, as are chapters on fundamental CBT therapies, some of the chapters in the second edition have been replaced or supplemented here. In addition to critical chapters on problem-solving therapy, rational emotive behavior therapy, and cognitive therapy, the therapy chapters now include a discussion of schema-focused cognitive therapy and acceptance-based interventions, as these approaches have continued to gain prominence in the field. A new chapter focuses on the application of CBT to diverse populations, which is particularly important as CBT principles and practices become further disseminated.

One of the important new chapters in this edition is that on the evidence base for CBT. In the preface to the second edition I wrote about the empirically supported treatment movement and my belief that "the field of psychotherapy must move to a transparent, common-sense, evidence-based set of practices as soon as possible, in order to fulfill the mission of providing a human service that is worthy of the public's investment of trust, confidence, time, energy, and money." This chapter does much to reveal that the evidence base for CBT has grown dramatically in a fairly short period of time, and that the public generally can invest its trust in CBT.

In the second edition preface, I also wrote: "Although the field of cognitive-behavioral therapies has advanced a long distance in the period of time between the first edition of this book and the current one, there remains much to be done. There are questions about the models that underlie these treatments, their conceptual relations, the mechanisms of action, which treatments are efficacious, which treatments are most efficacious, which treatments are most efficacious for which client groups, the acceptability of these treatments to patients, how best to train and disseminate these treatments, the age specificity of these treatments, the transportability of these treatments among various cultural and language groups, and many other issues as well." These words still ring true today. Even while important efficacy data are needed for some treatment models and areas of practice and the mechanisms of action in CBT require ongoing study, the field now desperately needs to explore issues related to the *effectiveness* of CBT, with respect to both specific client groups and diverse cultures and language groups.

In closing, I want to thank a number of people who have shaped, and who continue to shape, my own thinking and work. These include my family, and in particular my wife, Debbie, and children, Kit, Aubrey, and Beth, but also my "extended family" in CBT. I owe a debt of gratitude to so many people, but notably to Tim Beck, Judy Beck, Bob Leahy, Jackie Persons, Neil Jacobson, Steve Hollon, Sona Dimidjian, Chris Martell, Leslie Sokol, Brian Shaw, Zindel Segal, John Teasdale, Ed Watkins, Willem Kuyken, Rob DeRubeis, Nik Kazantzis, and David Dozois. It has been my distinct pleasure to work among such thoughtful and caring people, as well as the great many other "CBT people" I have had the good fortune to meet around the world. I also want to acknowledge the support and assistance from the staff at The Guilford Press; in particular Senior Editor Jim Nageotte, but also Assistant Editor Jane Keislar and, of course, Editor-in-Chief Seymour Weingarten. The Guilford Press has become the world's leader in the publication of CBT books and materials, and in so doing has also had a significant positive effect on the growth of the field.

Contents

PART IV. APPLICATIONS TO SPECIFIC POPULATIONS

PART I

HISTORICAL, PHILOSOPHICAL, AND SCIENTIFIC FOUNDATIONS

CHAPTER 1

Historical and Philosophical Bases of the Cognitive-Behavioral Therapies

Keith S. Dobson
David J. A. Dozois

Although the earliest of the cognitive-behavioral therapies (CBTs) emerged in the early 1960s (Ellis, 1962), not until the 1970s did the first major texts on "cognitive-behavior modification" appear (Kendall & Hollon, 1979; Mahoney, 1974; Meichenbaum, 1977). The intervening period was one of considerable interest in cognition and in the application of cognitive theory to behavior change. Mahoney (1977), for example, noted that while psychology had generally undergone a "cognitive revolution" in the 1960s, the same theoretical focus was being brought to bear upon clinical psychology only somewhat later. As part the cognitive revolution in clinical psychology, different theorists and practitioners created a number of models for cognitive and behavior change, and a veritable armamentarium of clinical techniques.

This chapter reviews the major developments in the history of CBTs, with a focus on the period from the early 1960s to the present. After briefly defining the current scope of CBTs and the essential nature of the model, CBTs, we review the historical bases of CBT. Six major reasons for the development of CBTs are proposed and discussed. The chapter then summarizes the major philosophical underpinnings of the various forms of CBTs, with a view to both the principles that all of these therapies share and those that vary from approach to approach. The last section of the chapter presents a formal chronology of the major CBT approaches. This section also describes unique contemporary approaches within the overall field of CBT in terms of the historical developments for each approach and the behavior change principles each approach encourages.

DEFINING COGNITIVE-BEHAVIORAL THERAPY

At their core, CBTs share three fundamental propositions:

1. Cognitive activity affects behavior.
2. Cognitive activity may be monitored and altered.
3. Desired behavior change may be effected through cognitive change.

Although using a slightly different title, Kazdin (1978) argued for a similar implicit set of propositions in his definition of cognitive-behavior modification: "The term 'cognitive-behavior modification' encompasses treatments that attempt to change overt behavior by altering thoughts, interpretations, assumptions, and strategies of responding" (p. 337). Cognitive-behavior modification and CBT are thus nearly identical in their assumptions and treatment methods. Perhaps the one area where the two labels identify divergent therapies is with respect to treatment outcomes. While cognitive-behavior modification seeks overt behavior change as an end result (Kazdin, 1978; Mahoney, 1974), some contemporary forms of CBT focus their treatment effects on cognitions per se, in the belief that behavior change will follow. Ellis's (1962, 1979a; Dryden, David, & Ellis, Chapter 8, this volume) efforts relative to belief change, for example, constitute a type of therapy that Kazdin's (1978) definition would not incorporate as a form of cognitive-behavior modification. The term "cognitive-behavior therapy," therefore, is broader than *cognitive-behavior modification,* and subsumes the latter within it (see also Dobson, Backs-Dermott, & Dozois, 2000).

The first of the three fundamental propositions of CBT, that cognitive activity affects behavior, is a restatement of the basic mediational model (Mahoney, 1974). Although early cognitive-behavioral theorists had to document the theoretical and empirical legitimacy of the mediational proposition (e.g., Mahoney, 1974), there is now overwhelming evidence that cognitive appraisals of events can affect the response to those events, and that there is clinical value in modifying the content of these appraisals (e.g., Dobson et al., 2000; Dozois & Beck, 2008; Granvold, 1994; Hollon & Beck, 1994). While debate continues about the degree and exact nature of the appraisals an individual makes in different contexts (cf. Coyne, 1999; Held, 1995), the fact of mediation is no longer strongly contested.

The second CBT proposition states that cognitive activity may be monitored and altered. Implicit in this statement is the assumption that we may gain access to cognitive activity, and that cognitions are knowable and assessable. There is, however, reason to believe that access to cognitions is not perfect, and that people may report cognitive activities on the basis of their likelihood of occurrence rather than actual occurrence (Nisbett & Wilson, 1977). Most researchers in the area of cognitive assessment, however, continue to attempt to document reliable and valid cognitive assessment strategies, usually with behavior as the source of validational data (Merluzzi, Glass, & Genest, 1981;

Segal & Shaw, 1988; Dunkley, Blankstein, & Segal, Chapter 5, this volume). Thus, while reports of cognition are often taken at face value, there is reason to believe that in some cases there are biases in cognitive reports, and that further validation of cognitive reports is required (Dunkley et al., Chapter 5, this volume).

Another corollary stemming from the second CBT proposition is that assessment of cognitive activity is a prelude to the alteration of cognitive activity. However, although it makes conceptual sense that once we measure a construct we may then begin to manipulate it, one action does not *necessarily* follow the other. In the area of human change, the measurement of cognition does not necessarily assist change efforts. As has been written elsewhere (Dunkley et al, Chapter 5, this volume; Mischel, 1981; Segal & Cloitre, 1993; Shaw & Dobson, 1981), most cognitive assessment strategies emphasize the content of cognitions and the assessment of cognitive results rather than the cognitive process. Examining the process of cognition, as well as the interdependence among cognitive, behavioral, and affective systems, will most likely advance our understanding of change. This form of cognitive monitoring remains relatively underdeveloped compared to the assessment of cognitive content.

The third CBT proposition is a direct result of the adoption of the mediational model. It states that desired behavior change may be effected through cognitive change. Thus, while cognitive-behavioral theorists accept that overt reinforcement contingencies can alter behavior, they are likely to emphasize that there are alternative methods for behavior change, one in particular being cognitive change.

Due to the statement that cognitive change may influence behavior, a lot of the early effort of cognitive-behavioral researchers was to document the effects of cognitive mediation. In one of the earliest demonstrations of this type, Nomikos, Opton, Averill, and Lazarus (1968) demonstrated that the same loud noise created different degrees of physiological disturbance, based upon the research participant's expectancy for the noise. In a similar vein, Bandura (1977, 1997) employed the construct of self-efficacy to document that a participant's perceived ability to approach a fearful object strongly predicts actual behavior. Many studies have documented the role of cognitive appraisal processes in a variety of laboratory and clinical settings (Bandura, 1986, 1997).

Although the inference of cognitive activity has been generally accepted, it is still extremely difficult to document the further assumption that changes in cognition mediate behavior change. To do so, the assessment of cognitive change must occur, independent of behavior. For example, if a phobic person approaches within 10 feet of a feared object, is treated through a standard type of systematic desensitization (including a graduated approach), and is then able to predict and demonstrate a closer approach to the feared object, making the inference that cognitive mediation of the behavior change is difficult at best and unnecessary or superfluous at worst. On the other hand, if the same phobic person is treated with some form of cognitive intervention (e.g., imagined approach of the feared object), and then demonstrates the same behavior change, then cognitive mediation of that behavior change is much more plausible. Moreover, if that same phobic person demonstrates changes in his or her behavior toward objects previously feared but not specifically treated, then the cognitive mediation of that behavior change is essential, in that there must be some cognitive "matching" between the treated object and the other object of generalization. Unfortunately, tests of cognitive mediation are often less than methodologically adequate, and many fail to produce compelling results (DeRubeis et al., 1990; Longmore & Worrell, 2007), which renders these models subject to ongoing debate.

WHAT CONSTITUTES COGNITIVE-BEHAVIORAL THERAPY?

A number of treatment approaches exist within the scope of CBT as it was defined earlier. These approaches share the theoretical perspective that assumes internal covert processes called "thinking" or "cognition" occur, and that cognitive events mediate behavior change. In fact, many cognitive-behavioral theorists explicitly state that because of the mediational hypothesis, not only is cognition able to alter behavior, but it must alter behavior, so that behavior change may thus be used as an indirect index of cognitive change. At the same time, these approaches argue that behavioral change does not have to involve elaborate cognitive mechanisms. In some forms of therapy the interventions may have very little to do with cognitive appraisals and evaluations but be heavily dependent on client action and behavior change. The actual outcomes of CBT will naturally vary from client to client, but in general the two main indices used for change are cognition and behavior. To a lesser extent, emotional and physiological changes are also used as indicators of change in CBT, particularly if emotional or physiological disturbance is a major aspect of the presenting problem in therapy (e.g., anxiety disorders, psychophysiological disorders). One of the trends in the development of the CBTs has been a growing interest in how cognitive mediation affects behavioral, emotional, *and* physiological processes, and how these various systems can reinforce each other in practice.

Three major classes of CBTs have been recognized, as each has a slightly different class of change goals (Mahoney & Arnkoff, 1978). These classes are coping skills therapies, problem-solving therapies, and cognitive restructuring methods. Since a later section of this chapter details the specific therapies that fall within these categories of CBTs, this topic is not reviewed here. What is important to note, however, is that the different classes of therapy orient themselves toward different degrees of cognitive versus behavioral change. For example, coping skills therapies are primarily used for problems that are external to the client. In this case, therapy focuses on the identification and alteration of the ways the person may exacerbate the influence of negative events (e.g., engaging in anxiety-provoking thoughts and images; using avoidance) or employ strategies to lessen the impact of the negative events (e.g., learning relaxation skills). Thus, the primary markers of success within this form of therapy involve behavioral signs of improved coping abilities, and the concomitant reductions in the consequences of negative events (e.g., less demonstrated anxiety). In contrast, cognitive restructuring techniques are used more when the disturbance is created from within the person him- or herself. Such approaches focus on the long-term beliefs and situation-specific automatic thoughts that engender negative outcomes.

Although CBT targets both cognition and behavior as primary change areas, certain types of desired change clearly fall outside of the realm of CBT. For example, a therapist who adopts a classical conditioning approach to the treatment of self-destructive behavior in an autistic child is not employing a cognitive-behavioral framework; such an approach might instead be called "behavioral analysis" or "applied behavioral therapy." In fact, any therapeutic regimen that adopts a stimulus–response model is not a CBT. Only in instances where cognitive mediation can be demonstrated, and where cognitive mediation is an important component of the treatment plan, can the label "cognitive-behavioral" be applied.

Just as strictly behavioral therapies are not cognitive-behavioral, strictly cognitive therapies also are not cognitive-behavioral. For example, a therapeutic model that states memories of a long-past traumatic event cause current emotional disturbance and consequently targets those memories for change is not a CBT. It should be noted that this example carries the provision that no association between the current disturbance and past trauma is possible. In a case where a past trauma has occurred and a recent event is highly similar to that past event, and the client is experiencing distress as a function of both the past trauma and the current event, cognitive mediation is much more likely, and the therapy may be cognitive-behavioral in nature. Certainly, there do exist CBTs for trauma and its consequences (Resick et al., 2008).

Finally, therapies that base their theories in the expression of excessive emotions, as may be seen in cathartic models of therapy (Janov, 1970), are not cognitive-behavioral. Thus, although these therapies may posit that the emotions derive from extreme or negative cognitive mediational processes, the lack of a clear mediational model of change places them outside the field of CBT.

HISTORICAL BASES
OF THE COGNITIVE-BEHAVIORAL THERAPIES

Two historical strands serve as historical bases for the CBTs. The dominant strand relates to behavioral therapies, which is often seen as the primary precursor to CBTs. To a lesser extent, CBTs also have grown out of psychodynamic models of therapy. These two historical themes are discussed in turn in this section.

Behavior therapy was an innovation from the radical behavioral approach to human problems (Bandura, 1986). It drew on the classical and operant conditioning principles of behaviorism, and developed a set of interventions focused on behavior change. In the 1960s and 1970s, however, a shift that began to occur in behavior therapy made the development of cognitive-behavior theory possible, and CBT, more broadly, a logical necessity. First, although the behavioral perspective had been a dominant force for some time, it was becoming apparent by the end of the 1960s that a nonmediational approach was not expansive enough to account for all of human behavior (Breger & McGaugh, 1965; Mahoney, 1974). Bandura's (1965, 1971) accounts of vicarious learning defied traditional behavioral explanation, as did the work on delay of gratification by Mischel, Ebbesen, and Zeiss (1972). Similarly, children were learning grammatical rules well outside the ability of most parents and educators to reinforce discriminatively (Vygotsky, 1962), and behavioral models of language learning were under serious attack. Yet another sign of dissatisfaction with behavioral models was the attempt to expand these models to incorporate "covert" behaviors (i.e., thought; Homme, 1965). Although this approach met with some limited optimism, criticisms from behavioral quarters made it apparent that extensions of this sort were not consistent with the behavioral emphasis on overt phenomena.

A second factor that facilitated the development of CBT was that the very nature of some problems, such as obsessional thinking, made noncognitive interventions irrelevant. As was appropriate, behavior therapy was applied to disorders that were primarily demarcated by their behavioral correlates. Also, for multifaceted disorders, behavioral therapists targeted the behavioral symptoms for change (e.g., Ferster, 1974). This focus on behavior provided a significant increase in therapeutic potential over past efforts but was not fully satisfying to therapists who recognized that entire problems, or major components of problems, were going untreated. The development of cognitive-behavioral treatment interventions helped to fill a void in the clinician's treatment techniques.

Third, the field of psychology was changing in general, and cognitivism, or what has been called the "cognitive revolution," was a major part of that change. A number of mediational concepts were being developed, researched, and established within experimental psychology (Neisser, 1967; Paivio, 1971). These models, the most influential of which was perhaps the information-processing model of cognition, were explicitly mediational and were receiving considerable support from cognition laboratories. One of the natural developments was the extension of information-processing models to clinical constructs (e.g., Hamilton, 1979, 1980; Ingram & Kendall, 1986).

Even beyond the development of general cognitive models, a number of researchers in the 1960s and 1970s conducted basic research into the cognitive mediation of clinically relevant constructs. Lazarus and associates, for example, documented that anxiety involves cognitive mediation in a number of studies during this time period (Lazarus, 1966; Lazarus & Averill, 1972;

Lazarus & Folkman, 1984; Monat, Averill, & Lazarus, 1972; Nomikos et al., 1968). Taken together, the two research areas of general cognitive psychology and what may be termed "applied cognitive psychology" challenged behavioral theorists to account for the accumulating data. In essence, the challenge amounted to a need for behavioral models to redefine their limits and incorporate cognitive phenomena into the models of behavioral mechanisms. Perhaps one of the earliest signs of this attempt at incorporation can be seen in the self-regulation and self-control literature, which developed during the early part of the 1970s (Cautela, 1969; Goldfried & Merbaum, 1973; Mahoney & Thoresen, 1974; Stuart, 1972). All of these various attempts to delineate self-control perspectives on behavioral modification shared the idea that the individual has some capacity to monitor his or her behavior, to set internally generated goals for behavior, and to orchestrate both environmental and personal variables to achieve some form of regulation in the behavior of interest. To develop these self-control models, several cognitive processes had to be hypothesized, including attempts to define self-control strategies largely in terms of internal "cybernetic" components of functioning (e.g., Jeffrey & Berger, 1982).

In addition to behaviorism, the second historical strand that conspired to lead to the cognitive-behavioral field was that of psychodynamic theory and therapy. Just as there was growing dissatisfaction with strict behaviorism, there continued to be a rejection of the strongest alternative perspective, the psychodynamic model of personality and therapy. Early work in the area of CBT (e.g., Beck, 1967, pp. 7–9; Ellis, 1973, 1979a, p. 2) included statements that summarily rejected psychoanalytic emphases on unconscious processes, review of historical material, and the need for long-term therapy that relied on the development of insight regarding the transference–countertransference relationship. It remains an interesting fact, however, that the work of Aaron Beck and Albert Ellis, the two principal figures in the field, whose early training had been psychodynamic in nature, both later develop variants of CBT that emphasized cognitive restructuring, and the need for analysis and potential change of more trait-like and persistent beliefs or schemas.

Beyond the philosophical disagreements with some of the basic tenets of psychodynamic models, reviews of the outcome literature suggested that the efficacy of traditional psychotherapy was not particularly impressive (Eysenck, 1969; Luborsky, Singer, & Luborsky, 1975; Rachman & Wilson, 1971, 1980). Perhaps the boldest evaluative comment about the demonstrated efficacy of psychodynamic therapies comes from Rachman and Wilson (1980), who stated that "there still is no acceptable evidence to support the view that psychoanalysis is an effective treatment" (p. 76). An emphasis on short-term symptom relief and problem solution was one of the themes seen in the early cognitive-behavioral therapists whose work derived from psychodynamic bases.

As is true for any social movement, a critical aspect of the early formation of the CBTs was the development and identification of a number of theorists and therapists who identified themselves as joining this movement. Some of the people who explicitly began this process were Beck (1967, 1970), Cautela (1967, 1969), Ellis (1962, 1970), Mahoney (1974), Mahoney and Thoresen (1974), and Meichenbaum (1973, 1977). The establishment of several key proponents of a cognitive-behavioral perspective clearly had the effect of creating a *zeitgeist* that drew the attention of others in the field. In addition, the creation of a journal specifically tailored to the emerging cognitive-behavioral field helped to further this trend. Thus, the establishment in 1977 of *Cognitive Therapy and Research,* with Michael Mahoney as the inaugural editor, provided a forum "to stimulate and communicate research and theory on the role of cognitive processes in human adaptation and adjustment" (from the cover of the journal). The existence of a regular publication in the area of cognitive-behavior theory and modification allowed researchers and therapists to present provocative ideas and research findings to a wide audience.

A final important historical factor that has contributed to continued interest in the cognitive-behavioral perspective has been the publication of research studies that have found cognitive-behavioral treatment outcomes to be equally or more effective than strictly behavioral approaches. In a critical review of cognitive-behavior modification, Ledgewidge (1978) reviewed 13 studies that contrasted cognitive-behavioral versus behavioral therapies and found no demonstrated superiority for either, although he noted that the studies he reviewed were based upon analogue populations, and that clinical trials were required for a more summative judgment. Ledgewidge's largely critical review prompted a reply that largely dismissed his criticisms as "premature" (Mahoney & Kazdin, 1979). After this early controversy about the efficacy of CBTs, a number of reviews clearly demonstrated that CBTs have a clinical impact (Berman, Miller, & Massman, 1985; Dobson & Craig, 1996; Dush, Hirt, & Schroeder, 1983; Miller & Berman, 1983; Shapiro & Shapiro, 1982). Indeed, the CBTs are notable for their presence among the list of empirically supported therapies (Chambless et al., 1996; Chambless & Hollon, 1998; Chambless & Ollendick, 2001). It is important to note, however, that meta-analyses of therapeutic effectiveness question the extent to which cognitive-behavioral treatments are superior to strictly behavioral treatments (Berman et al., 1985; Glogcuen, Cottraux, Cucherat, & Blackburn, 1998; Miller & Berman, 1983). As the database is further enlarged, more definitive statements about the effectiveness of these types of therapy will be possible (Epp & Dobson, Chapter 2, this volume). What we hope will emerge from continued research is specific conclusions about not only the overall efficacy of CBTs but also specific statements about the relative efficacy of different types of CBTs with specific types of clinical problems.

It becomes apparent from this review that a number of compelling reasons have existed and continue to exist for the development of cognitive-behavioral models of dysfunction and therapy. These reasons include dissatisfaction with previous models of therapy, clinical problems that emphasize the need for a cognitive-behavioral perspective, the research conducted into cognitive aspects of human functioning, the *zeitgeist* phenomenon that has led to an identified group of cognitive-behavioral theorists and therapists, and the growing body of research that supports the clinical efficacy of cognitive-behavioral interventions. With this general trend in mind, we now provide more in-depth summaries of the historical developments behind the large number of specific CBTs that have evolved over the past 40 or so years.

MAJOR COGNITIVE-BEHAVIORAL THERAPIES

CBTs represent the convergence of behavioral strategies and cognitive processes, with the goal of achieving behavioral and cognitive change. However, even a brief review of the therapeutic procedures subsumed under the heading of CBT reveals a diversity of principles and procedures. The diversification in the development and implementation of the cognitive-behavioral approach may be explained in part by the differing theoretical orientations of those who generated intervention strategies based on this perspective. For example, Ellis and Beck, authors of rational emotive behavior therapy and cognitive therapy, respectively, came from psychoanalytic backgrounds. In contrast, Goldfried, Meichenbaum, and Mahoney were trained originally in the principles of behavior modification.

Mahoney and Arnkoff (1978) organized the CBTs into three major divisions: (1) cognitive restructuring, (2) coping skills therapies, and (3) problem-solving therapies. Therapies included under the heading of "cognitive restructuring" assume that emotional distress is the consequence of maladaptive thoughts. Thus, the goal of these clinical interventions is to examine and challenge maladaptive thought patterns, and to establish more adaptive thought patterns. In contrast, "coping skills therapies" focus on the development of a repertoire of skills designed to assist the client in coping with a variety of stressful situations. The "problem-solving therapies" may be characterized as a combination of cognitive restructuring techniques and coping skills training procedures. Problem-solving therapies emphasize the development of general strategies for dealing with a broad range of personal problems, and stress the importance of an active collaboration between client and therapist in the planning of the treatment program. In the sections that follow, we describe the evolution of the major therapies associated with the cognitive-behavioral tradition. This review is not intended to be exhaustive and therefore excludes a number of therapies that have not stimulated a significant amount of research or clinical application.

Rational Emotive Behavior Therapy

Rational emotive behavior therapy (REBT) is regarded by many as the premiere example of the cognitive-behavioral approach. The basic theory and practice of REBT was formulated by Albert Ellis almost 50 years ago. Following extensive training and experience in psychoanalysis, Ellis began to question the efficacy and efficiency of the classical analytic method. He observed that patients tended to remain in therapy for considerable periods of time and frequently resisted psychoanalytic techniques, such as free association and dream analysis. Moreover, Ellis questioned whether the personal insight that psychoanalytic theory assumed led to therapeutic change resulted in durable changes in behavior:

> Still, however, I was not satisfied with the results I was getting. For, again, a great many patients improved considerably in a fairly short length of time, and felt much better after getting certain seemingly crucial insights. But few of them were really cured, in the sense of being minimally assailed with anxiety or hostility. And, as before, patient after patient would say to me: "Yes, I see exactly what bothers me now and why I am bothered by it; but I nevertheless still am bothered. Now what can I do about that?" (Ellis, 1962, p. 9)

Discouraged by the limitations of the analytic method, Ellis began to experiment with more active and directive treatment techniques. Through a process of clinical trial and error, he formulated a theory of emotional disturbance and a set of treatment methods that emphasized a practical approach to dealing with life problems. Although advocates of analytic theory considered Ellis's methods heretical, the advent of behavior therapy in the 1960s and the growing acceptance of the role of cognitions in understanding human behavior eventually fostered the acceptance of REBT (formerly called rational emotive therapy [RET]) as a potentially valid alternative to the more traditional models of psychotherapy.

At the core of REBT is the assumption that human thinking and emotion are significantly interrelated. According to Ellis's ABC model, symptoms are the consequences (C) of a person's irrational belief systems (B) regarding particular activating experiences or events (A). The goal of therapy is to identify and challenge the irrational beliefs at the root of emotional disturbance. REBT assumed that individuals possess innate and acquired tendencies to think and to behave irrationally. Thus, to maintain a state of emotional health, individuals must constantly monitor and challenge their basic belief systems.

Ellis (1970) identified 12 basic irrational beliefs that take the general form of unrealistic or absolutistic expectations. REBT assumes that by substituting unrealistic, overgeneralized demands with realistic desires, preferences, or wishes, major changes in emotions and behaviors can occur. However, since individuals tend forcefully to preserve their irrational thought patterns, significant and durable changes require forceful methods of intervention.

REBT employs a multidimensional approach that incorporates cognitive, emotive, and behavioral techniques. Nevertheless, the major therapeutic tool remains a "logico-empirical method of scientific questioning, challenging, and debating" (Ellis, 1979a, p. 20) designed to assist individuals in surrendering irrational beliefs. In addition to disputation, REBT therapists selectively employ a broad variety of techniques, including self-monitoring of thoughts, bibliotherapy, role playing, modeling, rational emotive imagery, shame-attacking exercises, relaxation methods, operant conditioning, and skills training (Ellis, 1979b). The theory and practice of REBT are largely the same as when the approach was first introduced. Thus, Ellis's original conceptualization of RET as outlined in his book *Reason and Emotion in Psychotherapy* (1962) remains a primary reference for this approach. Renaming of RET to become REBT did not represent a change in philosophy or emphasis, so much as it reflected Ellis's desire to reflect more accurately the broad interests of REBT therapists.

One of the major differences between REBT and other cognitive-behavioral approaches lies in its philosophical emphasis. Ellis's (1980) distinctly philosophical outlook is reflected in what he identified as the major goals of REBT: self-interest, social interest, self-direction, tolerance of self and others, flexibility, acceptance of uncertainty, commitment to vital interests, self-acceptance, scientific thinking, and a nonutopian perspective on life. REBT assumes that individuals who adopt this type of rational philosophy will experience a minimum of emotional disturbance.

REBT has generated a large body of literature (see Dryden et al., Chapter 8, this volume) and is being applied to areas as diverse as leadership and business (Criddle, 2007; Greiger & Fralick, 2007), and schools (Vernon & Bernard, 2006). Unfortunately, the majority of published articles have been authored by REBT advocates rather than researchers concerned with collecting objective data concerning their validity and utility (Mahoney, 1979). Other publications suggest, however, that REBT is beginning to receive the objective empirical scrutiny that has been absent in the past (Haaga & Davison, 1993; Dryden et al., Chapter 8, this volume).

Cognitive Therapy

Aaron Beck, the developer of cognitive therapy, was originally trained in psychoanalysis. Like Ellis, Beck began to question psychoanalytic formulations of the neuroses, and particularly with respect to depression. In 1963, Beck observed that cognitive factors associated with depression were largely ignored in favor of the psychoanalytic emphasis on motivational–affective conceptualizations. However, based on an investigation of the thematic content of the cognitions of psychiatric patients, Beck was able to distinguish consistent differences in the ideational content associated with common neurotic disorders, including depression. He also found that patients exhibited systematic distortions in their thinking patterns. Consequently, he generated a typology of cognitive distortions to describe these systematic errors, which included the now well-known concepts of arbitrary inference, selective abstraction, over-generalization, magnification, and minimization.

A 5-year research project at the University of Pennsylvania culminated in the 1967 publication of *Depression: Causes and Treatment*. In this volume,

Beck outlined his cognitive model and therapy of depression and other neuroses. A second book, *Cognitive Therapy and the Emotional Disorders* (Beck, 1976), presented in more detail the specific cognitive distortions associated with each of the neuroses and described the principles of cognitive therapy, with special reference to depression. In 1979, Beck coauthored a comprehensive treatment manual for depression that presented cognitive interventions developed over the previous decade of clinical work and inquiry (Beck, Rush, Shaw, & Emery, 1979). This book, *Cognitive Therapy of Depression*, remains a key reference in the field and has served as the treatment manual for a considerable body of outcome research.

From the early emphasis on depression, Beck's model (1970) was extended to other disorders and difficulties, including anxiety (Beck & Emery, 1985), bipolar disorder (Basco & Rush, 2005), marital problems (Beck, 1988), personality disorders (Beck, Freeman, & Associates, 2003; Layden, Newman, Freeman, & Morse, 1993; Linehan, 1993), substance use problems (Beck, Wright, Newman, & Liese, 1993), crisis management (Dattilio & Freeman, 1994), anger (Beck, 1999), and psychosis (Beck, Grant, Rector, & Stolar, 2008). Throughout these developments, the cognitive model has maintained an emphasis on the way distorted thinking and unrealistic cognitive appraisals of events can negatively affect one's feelings and behavior. Therefore, it is assumed that the way an individual structures reality determines his or her affective state. Furthermore, the cognitive model proposes that a reciprocal relation exists between affect and cognition, such that one tends to reinforce the other, resulting in a possible escalation of emotional and cognitive impairment (Beck, 1971).

"Schemas" are defined as cognitive structures that organize and process incoming information. Schemas are proposed to represent the organized thought patterns that are acquired early in an individual's development and develop over the lifespan with accumulated experiences. Whereas the schemas of well-adjusted individuals allow for the realistic appraisal of life events, those of maladjusted individuals result in distorted perceptions, faulty problem-solving, and psychological disorders (Beck, 1976; Dozois & Beck, 2008). For example, the schematic processes of depressed individuals can be characterized by a negative cognitive triad, in which views of the self (the self as a "loser"), the world (the world is harsh and demanding, and leads to helplessness) and the future (the future is bleak and hopeless) are disturbed (Hollon & Beck, 1979).

The principal goal of cognitive therapy is to replace the client's presumed distorted appraisals of life events with more realistic and adaptive appraisals. Treatment is based on a collaborative, psychoeducational approach that involves designing specific learning experiences to teach clients to (1) monitor automatic thoughts; (2) recognize the relations among cognition, affect, and behavior; (3) test the validity of automatic thoughts; (4) substitute more realistic cognitions for distorted thoughts; and (5) identify and alter underlying beliefs, assumptions, or schemas that predispose individuals to engage in faulty thinking patterns (Kendall & Bemis, 1983).

Unlike REBT, Beck's cognitive theory of psychopathology and cognitive techniques have been subjected to a substantial degree of empirical scrutiny (Clark, Beck, & Alford, 1999; Ingram, Miranda, & Segal, 1998). Cognitive therapy of depression is now considered to be a viable alternative to behavioral and biochemical interventions (Hollon & Beck, 1979; Hollon, DeRubeis, & Evans, 1996; Hollon, Stewart, & Strunk, 2006). Cognitive therapy for anxiety disorders, in fact, has superior efficacy to pharmacotherapy. The generalizability of Beck's model and therapy, and treatment efficacy with respect to other mental disorders, requires further research (Clark et al., 1999). Nonetheless, the contributions of Beck and his associates have significantly impacted researchers and clinicians alike, and will in all probability continue to stimulate research for many years to come (Dobson & Khatri, 2000).

Self-Instructional Training

Donald Meichenbaum's clinical interests developed during a period when behavior therapy was flourishing and the then-radical ideas of Ellis (1962), Beck (1970), and other advocates of cognitive treatment approaches were beginning to attract the attention of a new generation of clinicians. In this climate, Meichenbaum (1969) carried out a doctoral research program that investigated the effects of an operant treatment procedure for hospitalized patients with schizophrenia trained to emit "healthy talk." He observed that patients who engaged in spontaneous self-instruction to "talk healthy" were less distracted and demonstrated superior task performance on a variety of measures. This observation provided impetus for a research program that focused on the role of cognitive factors in behavior modification (Meichenbaum, 1973, 1977).

Meichenbaum's research was heavily influenced by two Soviet psychologists, Luria (1961) and Vygotsky (1962), who studied the developmental relation among language, thought, and behavior. They suggested that the development of voluntary control over one's behavior involves a gradual progression from external regulation by significant others (e.g., parental instructions) to self-regulation as a result of the internalization of verbal commands. Consequently, the relation between verbal self-instruction and behavior became the major focus of Meichenbaum's research. He proposed that covert behaviors operate according to the same principles as do overt behaviors, and that covert behaviors are thus subject to modification using the same behavioral strategies employed to modify overt behaviors (Homme, 1965; Meichenbaum, 1973).

Meichenbaum's early attempts to explore the validity of this proposal involved the development of a self-instructional training (SIT) program designed to treat the mediational deficiencies of impulsive children (Meichenbaum & Goodman, 1971). The goals of the treatment program were fourfold:

(1) to train impulsive children to generate verbal self-commands and respond to them appropriately; (2) to strengthen the mediational properties of children's inner speech to bring their behavior under their own verbal control; (3) to overcome any comprehension, production, or mediational deficiencies; and (4) to encourage children to self-regulate their behavior appropriately. The specific procedures were designed to replicate the developmental sequence outlined by Luria (1961) and Vygotsky (1962): (1) A model performed a task of talking aloud, while a child observed; (2) the child performed the same task, while the model gave verbal instructions; (3) the child performed the task, while instructing him- or herself aloud; (4) the child performed the task, while whispering the instructions; and (5) the child performed the task covertly. The self-instructions employed in the program included (1) questions about the nature and demands of the task, (2) answers to these questions in the form of cognitive rehearsal, (3) self-instructions in the form of self-guidance while performing the task, and (4) self-reinforcement. Meichenbaum and Goodman (1971) found that self-instructional training significantly improved the task performance of impulsive children across a number of measures relative to attentional and control groups.

Encouraged by the results of their initial studies, Meichenbaum and his associates sought to expand and refine SIT. Additional investigations were designed to examine the ability of SIT to generalize in the treatment of a variety of psychological disorders, including schizophrenia, speech anxiety, test anxiety, and phobias (Mahoney, 1974).

The behavioral background of Meichenbaum is evident in the procedural emphasis that SIT places on graduated tasks, cognitive modeling, directed mediational training, and self-reinforcement. SIT provides a basic treatment paradigm that may be modified to suit the special requirements of a particular clinical population. In general, clients are trained in six global skills related to self-instruction: (1) problem definition, (2) problem approach, (3) attention focusing, (4) coping statements, (5) error-correcting options, and (6) self-reinforcement (Kendall & Bemis, 1983). The flexibility of SIT is perhaps one of its most attractive features, and not surprisingly, a large literature has accumulated on the utility of SIT for a variety of psychological disorders (Meichenbaum, 1985).

In recent years, the primary use of SIT appears to be in the treatment of youth, mentally handicapped individuals, and in some areas where specific skills training is needed, such as athletics. It does not appear to serve often as a stand-alone therapy, but SIT is often employed in the context of a broader set of methods to develop and foster a broader sense of self-efficacy and capability. An interesting side note is that Meichenbaum's clinical interests have shifted since the development of SIT. He developed a constructive, narrative approach to the problem of posttraumatic stress disorder (Meichenbaum, 1994), in which more traditional SIT methods do not figure largely. He also maintains an interest and involvement in stress inoculation training (see below).

Self-Control Treatments

A series of interventions have developed within the broad field of CBT that focus on the self and its regulation in various settings. These approaches have employed terms such as "self-efficacy," "self-control," and "self-regulation" to emphasize that these broad interventions can hypothetically be deployed in many different contexts (Kanfer, 1970, 1971).

Marvin Goldfried was among the growing number of clinicians in the early 1970s who challenged the adequacy of learning theory and advocated the incorporation of cognitive processes into conceptualizations of human behavior. He supported the shift in emphasis from discrete, situation-specific responses and problem-specific procedures to a focus on coping skills that could be applied across response modalities, situations, and problems (Mahoney, 1974). In 1971, Goldfried proposed that systematic desensitization be conceptualized in terms of a general mediational model, in contrast to Wolpe's (1958) counterconditioning model. Goldfried interpreted "systematic desensitization" as a means of teaching clients a general self-relaxation skill. In the attempt to transform desensitization into a more comprehensive coping skills training program, emphasis was placed on four components: (1) the description of the therapeutic rationale in terms of skills training, (2) the use of relaxation as a generalized or multipurpose coping strategy, (3) the use of multiple-theme hierarchies, and (4) training in "relaxing away" scene-induced anxiety as opposed to the traditional method of terminating the imaginal scene at the first indication of subjective distress (Goldfried, 1973, 1979).

Goldfried's coping skills orientation eventually led to the development of a technique called "systematic rational restructuring" (SRR; Goldfried, Decenteceo, & Weinberg, 1974). Borrowing from the work of Dollard and Miller (1950) on the development of symbolic thinking processes, Goldfried and Sobocinski (1975) suggested that early social learning experiences teach individuals to label situations in different ways. They argued that emotional reactions may be understood as a response to the way an individual labels situations as opposed to a response to the situation per se. The extent to which individuals inappropriately distinguish situational cues as personally threatening determines their subsequent maladaptive emotional and behavioral responses. Goldfried assumed that individuals can acquire more effective coping repertoires by learning to modify the maladaptive cognitive sets that engage automatically when they face anxiety-provoking situations. Thus, the goal of SRR is to train clients to perceive situational cues more accurately in a series of five discrete stages: (1) exposure to anxiety-provoking situations, using imaginal presentation or role playing; (2) self-evaluation of subjective anxiety level; (3) monitoring of anxiety-provoking cognitions; (4) rational reevaluation of these maladaptive cognitions; and (5) observing one's subjective anxiety level following the rational reevaluation. Techniques include relaxation methods, behavioral rehearsal, *in vivo* assignments, modeling, and bibliotherapy (Goldfried & Davison, 1976). As a coping skills approach, the ultimate goal of SRR is to provide clients with the personal resources to cope independently with future life stresses.

SRR is one of several coping skills training approaches designed and tested by behavioral researchers. Some of these treatment packages have received more research attention than others; many are similar in terms of their underlying rationale and therapeutic strategies, and although SSR has conceptual integrity, it has not been investigated as extensively as other coping skills training programs. Nevertheless, it represents one of the first attempts to design an operational self-control treatment model to enhance treatment generalization through the use of training in the general coping skills that we believe are applicable in a variety of stress-provoking situations.

Suinn and Richardson's (1971) anxiety management training (AMT) program represents another effort at self-control, applied to the problem of anxiety. AMT, a nonspecific approach for anxiety control, was designed to provide clients with a short-term coping skills training program applicable to a wide range of problem areas. The premise of the model that underlies AMT is that anxiety is an acquired drive that has stimulus generalization properties. Autonomic responses associated with anxiety act as cues that facilitate and maintain avoidance behavior. Clients can be conditioned to respond to these discriminative cues with responses that eliminate the anxiety through the process of reciprocal inhibition. Thus, the goal of AMT is to teach clients to use relaxation and competency skills to control their feelings of anxiety.

AMT emphasizes the elimination of anxiety without specific attention to the particular anxiety-provoking stimulus. In the first stage of treatment, clients receive training in deep muscle relaxation. Following this, clients are instructed to visualize anxiety-arousing scenes, then practice their relaxation skills and/or imagine responding to stimuli in a competent fashion (Suinn, 1972). A variety of anxiety-arousing scenes that may be unrelated to clients' specific problems are incorporated into the treatment program.

Empirical data regarding AMT have emerged slowly. AMT has been shown to be superior to a defined control group in a randomized clinical trial (Suinn, 1995). Other data, however, are sparse. Given the lack of research, AMT has remained a less well-developed cognitive-behavioral approach than it might otherwise be.

The trend toward treatment models that promote a philosophy of self-control influenced Rehm's (1977) development of a self-control model of depression. The work of Rehm was guided, to a great extent, by the general model of self-regulation proposed by Kanfer (1970, 1971), which explains the persistence of certain behaviors in the absence of reinforcement in terms of a closed-loop feedback system of adaptive self-control. Kanfer suggested that three interconnected processes are involved in self-regulation: self-monitoring, self-evaluation, and self-reinforcement. Rehm adapted this model to conceptualize the symptoms of depression as the consequence of one or some combination of six deficits in self-control behavior. In the self-monitoring phase, potential deficits include the selective monitoring of negative events and of immediate versus delayed consequences of behavior. Self-evaluative deficits comprise stringent self-evaluative criteria and inaccurate attributions of responsibility. In the self-reinforcement phase, deficits involving insufficient self-reward and excessive self-punishment may be observed in depressed individuals. According to Rehm (1981), the varied symptom profile in clinical depression is a function of different subsets of these deficits. The occurrence of a depressive episode is postulated to be a joint function of the degree of stress experienced and the self-control skills available for coping with the stressful situation.

Fuchs and Rehm (1977) developed the original treatment package based on Rehm's (1977) model of depression. "Self-control therapy" involves the sequential application of Kanfer's (1970, 1971) three self-regulatory processes as adapted by Rehm: "The assumption is that each may be conceptualized as a therapy module and that self-evaluation builds on self-monitoring, and that self-reinforcement builds on self-evaluation" (O'Hara & Rehm, 1983, p. 69). Each of the six self-control deficits is described over the course of treatment, with an emphasis on how a particular deficit is causally related to depression and what can be done to remedy the deficit. A variety of clinical strategies are employed to teach self-control skills to clients, including therapist-directed group discussion, overt and covert reinforcement, behavioral assignments, self-monitoring, and modeling.

The appeal of Rehm's (1977) self-control model lies in its integration of a range of cognitive and behavioral variables on which other models of depression focus exclusively. In addition, Rehm's framework provides a logical analysis of the manner in which each of the various symptoms of depression is associated with a particular aspect of self-control. From a broader perspective, this self-control model appears to have potential as a general model of psychopathology. Unfortunately, the ability of Rehm's theoretical approach to generalize to other clinical disorders has not been researched (Rehm & Rokke, 1988). However, efforts to develop a comprehensive self-control therapy would seem a worthwhile endeavor.

Stress Inoculation Training

Like many of his contemporaries in the 1970s, Meichenbaum developed an interest in the multicomponent coping skills approach as a potentially effective therapeutic strategy. Following a review of the stress literature, Meichenbaum, Turk, and Burstein (1975) incorporated several guidelines into the development of a coping skills treatment program. These included the need for flexibility, sensitivity to individual differences, the need to use provocative stimuli to encourage the use of the skills, and progressive exposure to threatening situations (Meichenbaum, 1977). Meichenbaum emphasized the systematic acquisition of coping skills, and highlighted the importance of learning to cope with small, manageable amounts of stress as a means of facilitating treatment maintenance and generalization. Stress inoculation training, the behavioral analogue of Orne's (1965) immunization model, incorporated the guidelines that Meichenbaum and his associates gleaned from their review of the stress literature. The rationale underlying this approach assumes that clients who learn ways of coping with mild levels of stress are "inoculated" against uncontrollable levels of stress.

Meichenbaum and Cameron (1973) operationalized stress inoculation training in three stages. The first stage is educational and involves didactic training about the nature of stressful reactions. The second stage involves the presentation of a number of behavioral and cognitive coping skills, including relaxation exercises, coping self-statements, and self-reinforcement. In the final stage of application training, the client is exposed to a variety of stressors to rehearse his or her newly acquired coping skills.

Since its introduction in 1973, researchers have applied the stress inoculation training approach to a variety of problems, including anxiety, anger, and pain (Meichenbaum & Deffenbacher, 1988; Meichenbaum & Jaremko, 1983; Meichenbaum & Turk, 1976). These studies led to a detailed clinical guidebook (Meichenbaum, 1985) and a large body of studies (for reviews, see Meichenbaum, 1993, 2007). However, as Jaremko (1979) has observed, investigations into stress inoculation training have introduced a considerable degree of procedural variation. In this regard, Jaremko proposed a revised procedural model intended to add greater uniformity to the current research, as well as to increase the "usability" of this approach as a therapeutic procedure. As is the case with other multicomponent treatment programs, there remains a need for further empirical investigations to demonstrate the utility of the individual treatment components employed in stress inoculation training. Nonetheless, stress inoculation training has been widely employed as a therapeutic approach for the development of generalized coping skills (Meichenbaum, 2007).

Problem-Solving Therapy

In 1971, D'Zurilla and Goldfried published an article that proposed the application of problem-solving theory and research in behavior modification. With the goal of facilitating "generalized" behavior change, D'Zurilla and Goldfried conceptualized problem-solving therapy as a form of self-control training, emphasizing the importance of training the client to function as his or her own therapist. Its authors summarize the rationale underlying this approach as follows:

> Ineffectiveness in coping with problematic situations, along with its personal and social consequences, is often a necessary and sufficient condition for an emotional or behavior disorder requiring psychological treatment; ... general effectiveness may be most efficiently facilitated by training individuals in general pro-

cedures or skills which would allow them to deal independently with the critical problematic situations that confront them in day-to-day living. (p. 109)

According to D'Zurilla and Goldfried (1971) "problem solving" refers to an overt or cognitive process that makes available a variety of effective response alternatives for coping with a problem situation and increases the likelihood of selecting the most effective response available. Drawing on a large body of research regarding the fundamental operations involved in effective problem solving, D'Zurilla and Goldfried identified five overlapping stages as representative of the problem-solving process: (1) general orientation or "set," (2) problem definition and formulation, (3) generation of alternatives, (4) decision making, and (5) verification. Training in problem solving involves teaching clients these basic skills and guiding their application in actual problem situations.

Spivack and Shure (1974) initiated the systematic investigation into the efficacy of a problem-solving treatment approach. The interpersonal cognitive problem-solving (ICPS) model proposed by these researchers involves essentially the same skills outlined by D'Zurilla and Goldfried (1971). According to Spivack, Platt, and Shure (1976), effective interpersonal problem solving involves the ability (1) to recognize the range of possible problem situations in the social environment; (2) to generate multiple, alternative solutions to interpersonal problems; (3) to plan a series of steps necessary to achieve a given goal; (4) to foresee the short-term and long-term consequences of a given alternative; and (5) to identify the motivational elements related to one's actions and those of others. ICPS training has been most commonly used with preschoolers and emotionally disturbed children. In general, ICPS training programs include discussion and structured activities involving hypothetical and actual interpersonal problem situations designed to teach problem-solving skills. Despite numerous methodological problems, the work of Spivack and his colleagues has resulted in the development of a growing interest in the potential of problem-solving therapies.

D'Zurilla and Nezu (1982) conducted an early review of the applications of D'Zurilla and Goldfried's (1971) original model of problem solving in adult clinical populations, and concluded that there is a relation between problem-solving skills and psychopathology.

The clinical intervention objectives recommended by D'Zurilla and Goldfried (1971) stimulated the development of a number of problem-solving therapies (Mahoney & Arnkoff, 1978). Problem-solving therapies have now been developed in several areas, including stress management and prevention (D'Zurilla, 1990), depression (Nezu, 1986), anger management (Crick & Dodge, 1994), and coping with cancer (Nezu, Nezu, Friedman, Faddis, & Houts, 1998). An excellent addition to the list of available clinical procedures was a general problem-solving approach (D'Zurilla & Nezu, 1999). It is likely that the flexibility and pragmatism of these approaches will continue to attract the attention of clinicians in search of comprehensive treatment programs.

Structural and Constructivist Psychotherapy

Guidano and Liotti (1983) introduced a structural approach to psychotherapy. Following an extensive study of numerous literatures, including behavior therapy, social learning theory, evolutionary epistemology, cognitive psychology, psychodynamic theory, and cognitive therapy, Guidano and Liotti concluded that to understand the full complexity of emotional disorder and subsequently develop an adequate model of psychotherapy, an appreciation of the development and the active role of an individual's knowledge of self and the world is critical: "Only a consideration of the structure within which the single elements of an individual's knowledge are placed allows us to understand how these elements rule and coordinate that individual's emotions and actions" (p. 34).

Guidano and Liotti's (1983) structural model of cognitive dysfunction borrowed heavily from Bowlby's (1977) attachment theory. They suggested that relationships with significant others (i.e., parents) determine the development of a child's self-image and provide continuous confirmation and reinforcement of this self-image. The definition of "self" is assumed to coordinate and integrate cognitive growth and emotional differentiation. If the self-concept is distorted or rigid, the individual is unable to assimilate life experiences effectively, which leads to maladjustment and emotional distress, the final product being cognitive dysfunction. Different abnormal patterns of attachment are assumed to correspond to different clinical syndromes.

Guidano and Liotti's original formulation was expanded in subsequent writings by Guidano (1987, 1991). These writings expanded the idea that problem behaviors are believed to be the consequence of an individual's cognitive organization (i.e., the causal theories, basic assumptions, and tacit rules of inference that determine thought content). The patient is perceived as struggling to maintain a particular dysfunctional cognitive organization in the face of a continuously challenging environment. Thus, the ultimate goal of psychotherapy is to modify these cognitive structures. For therapy to be effective, the therapist begins by identifying and modifying superficial cognitive structures that lead in turn to the identification and modification of deeper cognitive structures (i.e., the implicit causal theories held by the patient). This therapeutic strategy bears close resemblance to Beck's cognitive therapy (Beck et al., 1979) that begins with the assessment of the patient's automatic thoughts and subsequently leads to the specification of basic assumptions underlying these thoughts. A major difference between the authors of structural psychotherapy and Beck, however, is the former writers' emphasis on a postrationalist philosophy. Whereas Beck and related authors make a philosophical assumption that there is an external world that can be perceived accurately or distorted, Guidano's later writings in particular make it clear that he was increasingly less concerned with the "truth value" of cognitive structures than with the "validity value" or coherence of these structures:

Adaptation, therefore, is the ability to transform perturbation arising from interaction with the world into information meaningful to one's experiential order.
Maintaining an adaptive adequacy essentially means reserving one's sense of
self by continuously transforming the perceived world rather than merely corresponding to it. This explains why the notion of the *viability* of knowing processes
has become much more important in recent evolutionary epistemology than that
of their *validity*. (Guidano, 1991, p. 9, emphasis in original)

In discussing psychotherapy as a strategic process, structural therapists
refer to the analogy between the empirical problem-solving approach of the
scientist and that of the patient: "Therapists should enable patients to disen-
gage themselves from certain engrained beliefs and judgments, and to consider
them as hypotheses and theories, subject to disproof, confirmation, and logical challenge" (Guidano & Liotti, 1983, p. 144). This analogy is similar to
that drawn by Mahoney (1977) in his personal science approach. A variety
of behavioral experiments and cognitive techniques comprise the therapeutic
armory from which the therapist selects a range of suitable tactics for a particular patient. They include techniques such as imaginal flooding, systematic
desensitization, assertiveness training, coping skills training, problem-solving
procedures, and rational restructuring. The final stage of the therapeutic process is conceptualized in terms of a "personal revolution" (Mahoney, 1980;
Guidano, 1991) during which the patient, having rejected his or her old view
of self and the world, is in a state of transformation and is establishing a new,
more adaptive belief system.

Those who are familiar with the work of Beck et al. (1979), Ellis (1962),
Mahoney (1977), and other advocates of the cognitive-behavioral perspective will recognize the many parallels between their writings and the structural approach to therapy. The distinction between rational and postrational
approaches, however, is important and has been further amplified in the
work of individuals who refer to their work as constructivist psychotherapy
(Mahoney, 1991; 1995; Neimeyer, 1993, 1995; Neimeyer & Mahoney, 1995).
Constructivist therapy takes the view of the individual as an imperfect personal scientist, who uses cognitive constructs to make sense out of experiences and to order choices in the world. From this perspective, a key feature
of treatment involves identifying preferences in behavior, and understanding
how meaning is attached to experience. There is less focus on the *content* of
what is being thought about (e.g., as opposed to Beck's [1976] work, in which
a typology of cognitions is associated with different emotional states), and
more focus on the *process* of making meaning and connections among experiences. Consequently, therapy is less involved with corrective exercises about
what is being thought, and more about facilitative exercises that emphasis the
process of thinking and the generation of meaning.

Constructivist therapy has a close affinity to the philosophical schools of
hermeneutics, and narrative and discourse approaches to psychology. Nonetheless, there are more or less "radical" approaches within constructivism (see

Neimeyer & Mahoney, 1995). At the extreme perspective in constructivist therapy, which has been referred to as discursive critique or "radical constructivism" (Efran & Fauber, 1995), the epistemological position that reality exists *only* in the mind of the individual, and that its only criterion for mental health is the coherence of that mind-set. Individuals are viewed as contextual, and as temporally, culturally, sexually, and otherwise positioned with respect to other persons. As such, predetermined concepts of health and illness, such as the diagnostic nomenclature traditionally associated with mental disorders, lose their meaning, and treatment is no longer a process of helping people to recover from their diagnosed disorders. At this extreme, the relationship between constructivist therapies and other CBTs begins to break down. Some have even questioned the extent to which constructivist therapies are conceptually compatible with CBTs: "We suspect that the full integration of cognitive and constructivist models advocated by some authors ... will encounter conceptual obstacles" (Neimeyer & Raskin, 2001, p. 421). Other authors (e.g., Held, 1995) who have critiqued the movement toward constructivist schools of thought in psychotherapy have suggested that therapies need to turn "back to reality."

Clearly, the final chapter of the constructivist approaches to psychotherapy has yet to be written. It is not lost upon us, however, that many former advocates of traditional cognitive and CBTs have later advocated, in whole or in part, the use of treatments that draw on constructivist principles (Mahoney, 1991; Meichenbaum, 1994; Young, 1994). The extent to which these therapies will be considered a part of the cognitive-behavioral movement, or will move off into antithetical and alternative approaches to therapy, remains to be seen.

"Third-Wave" Cognitive-Behavioral Therapy

A recent trend within the field of CBT has been that of the "third wave." This group of therapies is most often associated with acceptance and commitment therapy (ACT; Hayes & Strosahl, 2004). ACT and related models focus not so much on the accuracy of perception as on the functional utility of different ways to think and behave. As in the structural psychotherapies, the emphasis is on the process of interacting with the world rather than on the content of what is being thought about or done. That said, the originator of ACT, Steven Hayes would argue that this approach is radically behavioral, in that it emphasizes taking action to maximize mental health and adaption in the world (Hayes, 2004a). Thus, there is a focus on both thought and action, as is true for the other CBTs.

One of the ways in which ACT differs from many of the other CBTs is that the cognitive focus is not only on specific situations, or the appraisal and meaning attached to different experiences, but also the process of appraisal itself. There is thus a focus on the "metacognitive" processes, such as worry about worry, or distress about depression. Associated with this focus on metacognition is a concomitant focus on "mindfulness," being aware of the process of appraisal for events, emotions, and other thoughts (Hayes, 2004b; Roemer & Orsillo, 2003).

Another aspect of the model that underlies some of the third-wave models is that the process of change can take place in different ways. Thus, whereas problem-solving, self-control and cognitive restructuring approaches to CBT emphasize the need to assess cognition and behavior, and to correct these phenomena when they are associated with emotional distress or problems, the third-wave approach suggests that sometimes the "change" that is needed is to recognize that the metacognitive processes are at fault; thus, there is no need for direct cognitive or behavioral change; rather, the focus shifts to acceptance of the current distress or situation, and a change in the metacogition from something like "This experience is intolerable; I must do something about this problem" to "This experience is a part of life; I can watch this experience, but I do not have to try to change it directly." This latter way of thinking about experience, it is argued, reduces the pressure on patients to try to solve chronic or repetitive problems, and frees them to make purposeful and creative choices in their lives. The ACT therapist explicitly reinforces the processes of acceptance of difficult situations, even while making a commitment to do what the patient wants to fulfill his or her life. A common question is "What would you do if you were not _____?", followed by the therapist's assistance to help the patient do just that. It is further argued that the positive and adaptive behavior that is encouraged will be positively reinforced by the patient's experience, and that the need to change "the problem" is eliminated through this process.

As described by Hayes (2004a) and others (e.g., Fruzzetti & Murphy, Chapter 11, this volume), the third-wave therapies are a part of the cognitive-behavioral tradition due to their emphases on cognitive appraisal and behavioral change. It is clear, however, that the approach these treatments take to symptoms, distress, and problems is radically different than that of other CBTs, and so their relationship to "mainstream" CBT remains to be discerned. Furthermore, the evidence base related to outcome for these treatments, while encouraging, is relatively sparse. It will be interesting to see whether the evidence substantiates the interest in this approach (see Fruzzetti & Murphy, Chapter 11, this volume; Öst, 2008).

SIMILARITY AND DIVERSITY
AMONG THE COGNITIVE-BEHAVIORAL THERAPIES

As the preceding chronology of cognitive-behavioral models of psychopathology and therapy suggest, there are a large number of cognitive-behavioral approaches. The bases of all these approaches share the three fundamental assumptions we discussed earlier in this chapter related to the mediational position. Briefly stated, the "mediational position" is that cognitive activity mediates the responses the individual has to his or her environment, and to some extent dictates the degree of adjustment or maladjustment of the individual. As a direct result of the mediational assumption, the CBTs share a belief that therapeutic change can be effected through an alteration of idiosyncratic, dysfunctional modes of thinking. Additionally, due to the behavioral heritage, many of the cognitive-behavioral methods draw upon behavioral principles and techniques in the conduct of therapy, and many of the cognitive-behavioral models rely to some extent upon behavioral assessment of change to document therapeutic progress.

Beyond these central assumptions regarding the mediated nature of therapeutic change, a number of commonalities occur between limited sets of CBTs. Kendall and Kriss (1983), for example, have suggested that five dimensions can be employed to characterize CBTs: the theoretical orientation of the therapeutic approach and the theoretical target of change, various aspects of the client–therapist relationship, the cognitive target for change, the type of evidence used for cognitive assessment, and the degree of emphasis on self-control on the part of the client. The scheme that they have proposed is a useful one for the identification of both similarities and differences between the various CBTs. Notwithstanding the coverage of the topic by Kendall and Kriss, it also appears that other commonalities between the approaches that are not theoretically central can be identified. For example, one commonality among the various CBTs is their time-limited nature. In clear distinction from longer-term psychoanalytic therapy, CBTs attempt to effect change rapidly, and often with specific, preset lengths of therapeutic contact. Many of the treatment manuals written for CBTs recommend treatment in the range of 12–16 sessions (Chambless et al., 1996).

Related to the time-limited nature of CBT is the fact almost all applications of this general therapeutic approach are to specific problems. While this commonality is in no way a criticism of the various CBTs, and although there has also been some recent interest in transdiagnostic approaches to psychopathology and treatment (Allen, McHugh, & Barlow, 2008; Dozois, Seeds, & Collins, in press), the problem-focused nature of cognitive-behavioral interventions does in part explain the time limitations that are commonly set in these approaches to therapy. Indeed, the use of these therapies for specific disorders and problems is a heritage from behavior therapy's emphasis on the collection of outcome data, and the focus on the remediation of specific, predefined problems. Thus, rather than being a limitation of CBTs, the application of these therapies to specific problems serves as a further demonstration of the continuing desire for the complete documentation of therapeutic effects. Also, the focus on specific problems allows for the measurement of the therapeutic limits of these various approaches, and the potential to select the most efficacious therapy for a given patient's problem.

A third commonality among cognitive-behavioral approaches is the belief that clients are, in a sense, the architects of their own misfortune, and that they therefore have control over their thoughts and actions. This assumption is clearly reflected in the type of patient problems that have been identified for cognitive-behavioral interventions. The most frequently cited appropriate problems include the "neurotic" conditions (e.g., anxiety, depression, and anger problems), self-control problems (e.g., overeating, behavioral management difficulties, child dysfunction), and general problem-solving abilities. These types of problems make the assumption of patient control tenable. Even in general approaches to treatment, such as the constructivist models, the emphasis on the individual as the active agent in his or her own life is a predominant focus.

Related to the assumption of patient control is another element shared by a number of CBTs. This commonality has to do with the fact that many CBTs are by nature either explicitly or implicitly educative. Many of the therapeutic approaches include the therapist teaching the therapeutic model to the patient, and many also involve the explication of the rationale for any interventions that are undertaken (Dobson & Dobson, 2009). This type of educative interaction between the therapist and patient is one facet that the various CBTs share, and that, again, sets them apart from other schools of therapy. Compare traditional psychoanalytic therapy, in which the therapist offers interpretations to the client (Blanck, 1976; Kohut, 1971), or strategic family therapy, in which the therapist may even dictate that the client do the opposite of what the therapeutic goal is in a "paradoxical" intervention (Minuchin & Fishman, 1981).

Directly related to the educative process often seen in CBTs is the implicit goal set by many cognitive-behavioral therapists: that the patient will not only overcome the referral problem during the course of therapy but also learn something about the process of therapy. In the event that the patient suffers a recurrence of the problem, he or she will therefore have some therapeutic skills to deal with the problem themselves. In some of the CBTs the desire to have patients learn about the process of therapy is taken to its logical conclusion, and time in therapy is spent reviewing the therapeutic concepts and skills that patients have learned over the course of therapy, so that they may later employ them in a maintenance or preventive manner (Beck et al., 1979; Dobson & Dobson, 2009).

It may appear that CBTs have so many commonalities that distinctions between them are more illusory than real. In fact, however, Kendall and Kriss (1983) have provided an excellent framework for the identification of differences between the specific approaches. Furthermore, even the brief overview of the various CBTs provided in this chapter demonstrates a very real diversity of models and techniques developed by cognitive-behavioral therapists. It is thus no more appropriate to state that there is really a single cognitive-behavioral approach than to state that there is one monolithic psychoanalytic therapy. As the chapters in this volume demonstrate, many different facets of the cognition-behavioral processes may be attended to, identified, and altered within the overarching definition of the cognitive-behavioral approach. The diversity of the CBTs, while undeniably present, does argue for further definitional and technical discussion between the proponents of the various approaches. There are at least two areas where further theory and research are required to further differentiate the different therapies labeled as "cognitive-behavioral" the targets of therapeutic change, and the modality specificity of intervention techniques.

Although CBTs share the mediational approach and therefore all target "cognitions" for change the variety of different specific labels and descriptions of cognitions seen in the cognitive-behavioral literature is truly overwhelming. A partial list of the various terms that have applied to cognitive constructs and processes includes "cognitions," "thoughts," "beliefs," "attitudes," "ideas," "assumptions," "attributions," "rules for living," "self-statements," "cognitive distortions," "expectancies," "notions," "stream of consciousness," "script," "narratives," "ideation," "private meanings," "illusions," "self-efficacy predictions," "cognitive prototypes," and "schemas." Adding further to the confusion is that a number of these constructs have been developed in a purely clinical context (e.g., self-efficacy predictions) and therefore have relatively clear definitions, but many other terms are employed in other areas of psychology. Where terms are shared across disciplines of psychology the usage may not be identical, and semantic confusion may be the end result. The use of the "schema" notion, for example, is fraught with potential difficulty, since the concept was first developed within cognitive psychology (Neisser, 1967) and later applied to social cognition (Markus, 1977), then also applied to clinical problems (Clark et al., 1999; Dobson, 1986; Dozois & Dobson, 2001; Goldfried & Robins, 1983; Ingram et al., 1998; Turk & Speers, 1983). Even a quick reading of the various applications of the term reveals that while the essence of the "schema" concept is intact throughout its various uses, there are several idiosyncratic applications. Thus, while the elaboration of various specific cognitive processes and constructs is useful, it is important for theorists to define constructs precisely, and for others in the field to subscribe to these definitions. This increase in precision would help to clarify the terrain of cognitive-behavioral theory and may also assist the efforts of researchers whose interest is cognitive assessment (Meichenbaum & Cameron, 1981; Merluzzi et al., 1981). In this latter regard, it is clear that cognitive assessment is severely hampered by a lack of clear definitions of cognitive phenomena (e.g., Genest & Turk, 1981; Glass & Merluzzi, 1981; Shaw & Dobson, 1981), and it is equally clear that further efforts in the area of cognitive assessment are required to fully document the nature and process of change during CBT (Clark, 1997; Segal & Shaw, 1988; Sutton-Simon, 1981).

A second area where the further delineation of different approaches to CBT may be possible is with respect to modality-specific techniques. Cognitive-behavioral therapists have been extremely innovative in the development of techniques, and have thereby added to the clinical armamentarium in numerous ways. In doing so, however, it is not always clear what manner of technique is being developed (i.e., whether it is a generic and nonspecific technique or a modality-specific method). While it may be reasonably argued that such distinctions are not important at a practical level, from a theoretical perspective it is important to know what limits different theorists place upon their models of therapy. Process research that actually records and analyzes therapeutic interventions espoused by various therapeutic models, while often suggested (DeRubeis, Hollon, Evans, & Bemis, 1982; Mahoney & Arnkoff, 1978; Prochaska, 2000), has not yet become well advanced. This type of research has the potential of adding greatly to our knowledge of the extent to which different descriptions of therapies translate themselves in different clinical practice.

Finally, another area of research that may profitably be expanded is that which investigates applications of various modes of CBT to different presenting problems (Harwood, Beutler, & Chervat, Chapter 4, this volume). By contrasting different approaches in the context of different problems, it may become possible to suggest preferred treatment methods for specific patient problems. This matching of problems to therapies would not only represent a practical advantage over current clinical practice, but it would also enable a better understanding of the mechanisms of change within each type of intervention, and within different types of patient problems.

Clearly, the field of CBT has developed dramatically since its inception in the 1960s and 1970s. There are now a number of identifiable models of a cognitive-behavioral nature, and the demonstrated efficacy of these methods is generally strong (Chambless et al., 1996; Dobson et al., 2000; Epp & Dobson, Chapter 2, this volume). The continuing emphasis on the outcome research has enabled cognitive-behavioral theorists and therapists to make steady progress in research and practice, and will certainly lead to continued improvements in the future. Some of the most pressing areas that require further conceptualization and research include the definition of cognitive phenomena (both at construct and process levels), and the procedural overlap among the variety of CBTs that currently exist. Another emerging area for the field is that of dissemination. The next decade is likely to see considerable advances in the field.

REFERENCES

Allen, L. B., McHugh, R. K., & Barlow, D. H. (2008). Emotional disorders: A unified protocal. In D. H. Barlow (Ed.), *Clinical handbook of psychological disorders: A step-by-step treatment manual* (4th ed., pp. 216–249). New York: Guilford Press.

Bandura, A. (1965). Vicarious processes: A case of no-trial learning. In L. Berkowitz (Ed.), *Advances in experimental social psychology* (Vol. 2, pp. 3–57). New York: Academic Press.

Bandura, A. (1971). Vicarious and self-reinforcement processes. In R. Glaser (Ed.), *The nature of reinforcement* (pp. 51–130). New York: Academic Press.

Bandura, A. (1977). Self-efficacy: Toward a unifying theory of behavioral change. *Psychological Review, 84,* 191–215.

Bandura, A. (1986). *Social foundations of thought and action: A social cognitive therapy*. Englewood Cliffs, NJ: Prentice-Hall.

Bandura, A. (1997). *Self-efficacy: The exercise of control*. New York: Freeman.

Basco, M. R., & Rush, A. J. (2005). *Cognitive-behavioral therapy for bipolar disorder* (2nd ed.). New York: Guilford Press.

Beck, A. T. (1967). *Depression: Causes and treatment*. Philadelphia: University of Pennsylvania Press.

Beck, A. T. (1970). Cognitive therapy: Nature and relation to behavior therapy. *Behavior Therapy, 1*, 184–200.

Beck, A. T. (1971). Cognition, affect, and psychopathology. *Archives of General Psychiatry, 24*, 495–500.

Beck, A. T. (1976). *Cognitive therapy and the emotional disorders*. New York: International Universities Press.

Beck, A. T. (1988). *Love is never enough*. New York: Harper & Row.

Beck, A. T. (1999). *Prisoners of hate: The cognitive bases of anger, hostility and violence*. New York: HarperCollins.

Beck, A. T., & Emery, G. (1985). *Anxiety disorders and phobias: A cognitive perspective*. New York: Basic Books.

Beck, A. T., Freeman, A., & Associates. (2003). *Cognitive therapy of personality disorders* (2nd ed.). New York: Guilford Press.

Beck, A. T., Grant, P., Rector, N. A., & Stolar, N. (2008). *Schizophrenia: Cognitive theory, research, and therapy*. New York: Guilford Press.

Beck, A. T., Rush, A. J., Shaw, B. F., & Emery, G. (1979). *Cognitive therapy of depression*. New York: Guilford Press.

Beck, A. T., Wright, F. D., Newman, C. F., & Liese, B. S. (1993). *Cognitive therapy of substance abuse*. New York: Guilford Press.

Berman, J. S., Miller, R. C., & Massman, P. J. (1985). Cognitive therapy versus systematic desensitization: Is one treatment superior? *Psychological Bulletin, 97*, 451–461.

Blanck, G. (1976). Psychoanalytic technique. In B. J. Wolman (Ed.), *The therapist's handbook* (pp. 61–86). New York: Van Nostrand Reinhold.

Bowlby, J. (1977). The making and breaking of affectional bonds: 1. Etiology and psychopathology in the light of attachment theory. *British Journal of Psychiatry, 130*, 201–210.

Breger, L., & McGaugh, J. L. (1965). Critique and reformulation of "learning theory" approaches to psychotherapy and neurosis. *Psychological Bulletin, 63*, 338–358.

Cautela, J. R. (1967). Covert sensitization. *Psychological Reports, 20*, 459–468.

Cautela, J. R. (1969). Behavior therapy and self-control: Techniques and implications. In C. M. Franks (Ed.), *Behavior therapy: Appraisal and status* (pp. 323–340). New York: McGraw-Hill.

Chambless, D. L., & Hollon, S. D. (1998). Defining empirically supported therapies. *Journal of Consulting and Clinical Psychology, 66*, 7–18.

Chambless, D. L., & Ollendick, T. H. (2001). Empirically supported psychological interventions: Controversies and evidence. *Annual Review of Psychology, 52*, 685–716.

Chambless, D. L., Sanderson, W. C., Shoham, V., Bennett-Johnson, S., Pope, K. S., Crits-Cristoph, P., et al. (1996). An update on empirically validated therapies. *Clinical Psychologist, 49*, 5–18.

Clark, D. A. (1997). Twenty years of cognitive assessment: Current status and future directions. *Journal of Consulting and Clinical Psychology, 65,* 996–1000.

Clark, D. A., Beck, A. T., & Alford, B. A. (1999). *Scientific foundations of cognitive theory and therapy of depression.* New York: Wiley.

Coyne, J. C. (1999). Thinking interactionally about depression: A radical restatement. In T. Joiner & J. C. Coyne (Eds.), *The interactional nature of depression* (pp. 365–392). Washington, DC: American Psychological Association.

Crick, N. R., & Dodge, K. A. (1994). A review and reformulation of social information-processing mechanisms in children's social adjustment. *Psychological Bulletin, 115,* 73–101.

Criddle, W. D. (2007). Adapting REBT to the world of business. *Journal of Rational-Emotive and Cognitive-Behavior Therapy, 25,* 87–106.

Dattilio, F. M., & Freeman, A. (Eds.). (1994). *Cognitive-behavioral strategies in crisis intervention.* New York: Guilford Press.

DeRubeis, R., Hollon, S. D., Evans, M., & Bemis, K. (1982). Can psychotherapies be discriminated?: A systematic investigation of cognitive therapy and interpersonal therapy. *Journal of Consulting and Clinical Psychology, 50,* 744–756.

DeRubeis, R. J., Hollon, S. D., Grove, W. M., Evans, M. D., Garvey, M. J., Tuason, V. B., et al. (1990). How does cognitive therapy work?: Cognitive change and symptom change in cognitive therapy and pharmacotherapy for depression. *Journal of Consulting and Clinical Psychology, 58,* 862–869.

Dobson, D. J. G., & Dobson, K. S. (2009). *Evidence-based practice of cognitive-behavioral therapy.* New York: Guilford Press.

Dobson, K. S. (1986). The self-schema in depression. In L. M. Hartman & K. R. Blankstein (Eds.), *Perception of self in emotional disorders and psychotherapy* (pp. 187–217). New York: Plenum Press.

Dobson, K. S., Backs-Dermott, B. J., & Dozois, D. (2000). Cognitive and cognitive-behavioral therapies. In C. R. Snyder & R. E. Ingram (Eds.), *Handbook of psychological change: Psychotherapy processes and practices for the 21st century* (pp. 409–428). New York: Wiley.

Dobson, K. S., & Craig, K. S. (Eds.). (1996). *Advances in cognitive-behavioral therapy.* Thousand Oaks, CA: Sage.

Dobson, K. S., & Khatri, N. (2000). Cognitive therapy: Looking forward, looking back. *Clinical Psychology: Science and Practice, 56,* 907–923.

Dollard, J., & Miller, N. E. (1950). *Personality and psychotherapy.* New York: McGraw-Hill.

Dozois, D. J. A., & Beck, A. T. (2008). Cognitive schemas, beliefs and assumptions. In K. S. Dobson & D. J. A. Dozois (Eds.), *Risk factors in depression* (pp. 121–143). Oxford, UK: Elsevier/Academic Press.

Dozois, D. J. A., & Dobson, K. S. (2001). A longitudinal investigation of information processing and cognitive organization in clinical depression: Stability of schematic interconnectedness. *Journal of Consulting and Clinical Psychology, 69,* 914–925.

Dozois, D. J. A., Seeds, P. M., & Collins, K. A. (in press). Transdiagnostic approaches to the prevention of depression and anxiety. *International Journal of Cognitive Psychotherapy: An International Quarterly.*

Dush, D. M., Hirt, M. L., & Schroeder, H. (1983). Self-statement modification with adults: A meta-analysis. *Psychological Bulletin, 94,* 408–422.

D'Zurilla, T. J. (1990). Problem-solving training for effective stress management and prevention. *Journal of Cognitive Psychotherapy: An International Quarterly, 4,* 327–355.

D'Zurilla, T. J., & Goldfried, M. R. (1971). Problem-solving and behavior modification. *Journal of Abnormal Psychology, 78,* 107–126.

D'Zurilla, T. J., & Nezu, A. (1982). Social problem solving in adults. In A. C. Kendall (Ed.), *Advances in cognitive-behavioral research and therapy* (pp. 281–294). New York: Academic Press.

D'Zurilla, T. J., & Nezu, A. (1999). *Problem-solving therapy: A social competence approach to clinical intervention* (2nd ed.). New York: Springer.

Efran, J. S., & Fauber, R. L. (1995). Radical constructivism: Questions and answers. In R. A. Neimeyer & M. J. Mahoney (Eds.), *Constructivism in psychotherapy* (pp. 275–304). Washington, DC: American Psychological Association Press.

Ellis, A. (1962). *Reason and emotion in psychotherapy.* New York: Stuart.

Ellis, A. (1970). *The essence of rational psychotherapy: A comprehensive approach to treatment.* New York: Institute for Rational Living.

Ellis, A. (1973). *Humanistic psychotherapy.* New York: McGraw-Hill.

Ellis, A. (1979a). The basic clinical theory of rational emotive therapy. In A. Ellis & M. M. Whiteley (Eds.), *Theoretical and empirical foundations of rational-emotive therapy.* Monterey, CA: Brooks/Cole.

Ellis, A. (1979b). The practice of rational emotive therapy. In A. Ellis & J. M. Whiteley (Eds.), *Theoretical and empirical foundations of rational-emotive therapy.* Monterey, CA: Brooks/Cole.

Ellis, A. (1980). Rational-emotive therapy and cognitive-behavior therapy: Similarities and differences. *Cognitive Research and Therapy, 4,* 325–340.

Eysenck, H. (1969). *The effects of psychotherapy.* New York: Science House.

Ferster, C. G. (1974). Behavior approaches to depression. In R. J. Friedman & M. M. Katz (Eds.), *The psychology of depression: Contemporary theory and research* (pp. 29–54). New York: Wiley.

Fuchs, C. Z., & Rehm, L. P. (1977). A self-control behavior therapy program for depression. *Journal of Consulting and Clinical Psychology, 45,* 206–215.

Genest, M., & Turk, D. C. (1981). Think-aloud approaches to cognitive assessment. In T. Merluzzi, C. R. Glass, & M. Genest (Eds.), *Cognitive assessment* (pp. 233–269) New York: Guilford Press.

Glass, C., & Merluzzi, T. (1981). Cognitive assessment of social-evaluative anxiety. In T. Merluzzi, C. R. Glass, & M. Genest (Eds.), *Cognitive assessment* (pp. 388–438). New York: Guilford Press.

Glogcuen, V., Cottraux, J., Cucherat, M., & Blackburn, I. (1998). A meta-analysis of the effects of cognitive therapy in major depression. *Journal of Affective Disorders, 49,* 59–72.

Goldfried, M. R. (1971). Systematic desensitization as training in self-control. *Journal of Consulting and Clinical Psychology, 37,* 228–234.

Goldfried, M. R. (1973). Reduction of generalized anxiety through a variant of systematic desensitization. In M. R. Goldfreid & M. Merbaum (Eds.), *Behavior change through self-control* (pp. 297–304). New York: Holt, Rinehart & Winston.

Goldfried, M. R. (1979). Anxiety reduction through cognitive-behavioral intervention. In P. C. Kendall & S. D. Hollon (Eds.), *Cognitive-behavioral interventions: Theory, research, and procedures* (pp. 117–152). New York: Academic Press.

Goldfried, M. R., & Davison, G. C. (1976). *Clinical behavior therapy.* New York: Holt, Rinehart & Winston.

Goldfried, M. R., Decenteceo, E. T., & Weinberg, L. (1974). Systematic rational restructuring as a self-control technique. *Behavior Therapy, 5,* 247–254.

Goldfried, M. R., & Merbaum, M. (Eds.). (1973). *Behavior change through self-control.* New York: Holt, Rinehart & Winston.

Goldfried, M. R., & Robins, C. (1983). Self-schema, cognitive bias, and the processing of therapeutic experiences. In P. C. Kendall (Ed.), *Advances in cognitive-behavioral research and therapy* (Vol. 2, pp. 330–380). New York: Academic Press.

Goldfried, M. R., & Sobocinski, D. (1975). Effect of irrational beliefs on emotional arousal. *Journal of Consulting and Clinical Psychology, 43,* 504–510.

Granvold, D. K. (Ed.). (1994). *Cognitive and behavioral treatment: Methods and applications.* Belmont, CA: Wadsworth.

Grieger, R., & Fralick, F. (2007). The use of REBT principles and practices in leadership training and development. *Journal of Rational-Emotive and Cognitive-Behavior Therapy, 25,* 143–154.

Guidano, V. F. (1987). *Complexity of the self: A developmental approach to psychopathology and therapy.* New York: Guilford Press.

Guidano, V. F. (1991). *The self in process.* New York: Guilford Press.

Guidano, V. F., & Liotti, G. (1983). *Cognitive processes and emotional disorders: A structural approach to psychotherapy.* New York: Guilford Press.

Haaga, D. A. F., & Davison, G. C. (1993). An appraisal of rational-emotive therapy. *Journal of Consulting and Clinical Psychology, 61,* 215–220.

Hamilton, V. (1979). An information processing approach to neurotic anxiety and the schizophrenias. In V. Hamilton & D. M. Warburton (Eds.), *Human stress and cognition: An information processing approach* (pp. 383–430). Chichester, UK: Wiley.

Hamilton, V. (1980). An information processing analysis of environmental stress and life crises. In I. G. Sarason & C. D. Spielberger (Eds.), *Stress and anxiety* (Vol. 7, pp. 13–30). Washington, DC: Hemisphere.

Hayes, S. C. (2004a). Acceptance and commitment therapy, relational frame theory, and the third wave of behavioral and cognitive therapies. *Behavior Therapy, 35,* 639–665.

Hayes, S. (2004b). Acceptance and commitment therapy and the new behavior therapies: Mindfulness, acceptance, and relationship. In S. C. Hayes, V. M. Follette, & M. M. Linehan (Eds.), *Mindfulness and acceptance: Expanding the cognitive-behavioral tradition* (pp. 1–29). New York: Guilford Press.

Hayes, S. C., & Strosahl, K. D. (Eds.). (2004). *A practical guide to acceptance and commitment therapy.* New York: Springer.

Held, B. S. (1995). *Back to reality: A critique of postmodern theory in psychotherapy.* New York: Norton.

Hollon, S. D., & Beck, A. T. (1979). Cognitive therapy of depression. In P. C. Kendall & S. D. Hollon (Eds.), *Cognitive-behavioral interventions* (pp. 153–204). New York: Academic Press.

Hollon, S. D., & Beck, A. T. (1994). Cognitive and cognitive-behavioral therapies. In A. E. Bergin & S. L. Garfield (Eds.), *Handbook of psychotherapy and behavior change* (4th ed., pp. 428–466). New York: Wiley.

Hollon, S. D., DeRubeis, R. J., & Evans, M. D. (1996). Cognitive therapy in the treatment and prevention of depression. In P. M. Salkovskis (Ed.), *Frontiers of cognitive therapy* (pp. 293–317). New York: Guilford Press.

Hollon, S. D., Stewart, M. O., & Strunk, D. (2006). Enduring effects for cognitive behavior therapy in the treatment of depression and anxiety. *Annual Review of Psychology, 57,* 285–315.

Homme, L. E. (1965). Perspectives in psychology: XXIV. Control of coverants, the operants of the mind. *Psychological Reports, 15,* 501–511.

Ingram, R. E., & Kendall, P. C. (1986). Cognitive clinical psychology: Implications of an information processing perspective. In R. E. Ingram (Ed.), *Information processing approaches to clinical psychology* (pp. 3–21). London: Academic Press.

Ingram, R. E., Miranda, J., & Segal, Z. V. (1998). *Cognitive vulnerability to depression.* New York: Guilford Press.

Janov, A. (1970). *The primal scream.* New York: Dell Books.

Jaremko, M. E. (1979). A component analysis of stress inoculation: Review and prospectus. *Cognitive Therapy and Research, 3,* 35–48.

Jeffrey, D. B., & Berger, L. H. (1982). A self–environmental systems model and its implications for behavior change. In K. R. Blankstein & J. Polivy (Eds.), *Self-control and self-modification of emotional behavior* (pp. 29–70). New York: Plenum Press.

Kanfer, F. H. (1970). Self-regulation: Research issues and speculations. In C. Neuringer & L. L. Michael (Eds.), *Behavior modification in clinical psychology* (pp. 178–220). New York: Appleton-Century-Crofts.

Kanfer, F. H. (1971). The maintenance of behavior by self-generated stimuli and reinforcement. In A. Jacobs & L. B. Sachs (Eds.), *The psychology of private events: Perspectives on covert response systems* (pp. 39–61). New York: Academic Press.

Kazdin, A. E. (1978). *History of behavior modification: Experimental foundations of contemporary research.* Baltimore: University Park Press.

Kendall, P. C., & Bemis, K. M. (1983). Thought and action in psychotherapy: The cognitive- behavioral approaches. In M. Hersen, A. E. Kazdin, & A. S. Bellack (Eds.), *The clinical psychology handbook* (565–592). New York: Pergamon.

Kendall, P. C., & Hollon, S. D. (Eds.). (1979). *Cognitive-behavioral interventions.* New York: Academic Press.

Kendall, P. C., & Kriss, M. R. (1983). Cognitive-behavioral interventions. In C. E. Walker (Ed.), *The handbook of clinical psychology: Theory, research, and practice* (pp. 770–819). Homewood, IL: Dow Jones–Irwin.

Kohut, H. (1971). *The analysis of the self.* New York: International Universities Press.

Layden, M., Newman, C. F., Freeman, A., & Morse, S. (1993). *Cognitive therapy of borderline personality disorder.* Needham Heights, MA: Allyn & Bacon.

Lazarus, R. S. (1966). *Psychological stress and the coping process.* New York: McGraw-Hill.

Lazarus, R. S., & Averill, J. R. (1972). Emotion and cognition: With special reference to anxiety. In C. D. Spielberger (Ed.), *Anxiety:Current trends in theory and research* (Vol. 2, pp. 242–284). New York: Academic Press.

Lazarus, R. S., & Folkman, C. (1984). *Stress, appraisal and coping.* New York: Springer.

Ledgewidge, B. (1978). Cognitive behavior modification: A step in the wrong direction? *Psychological Bulletin, 85,* 353–375.

Linehan, M. M. (1993). *Cognitive-behavioral treatment of borderline personality disorder.* New York: Guilford Press.

Longmore, R. J., & Worrell, M. (2007). Do we need to challenge thoughts in cognitive behavior therapy? *Clinical Psychology Review, 27,* 173–187.

Luborsky, L., Singer, G., & Luborsky, L. (1975). Comparative studies of psychothera-pies: Is it true that everyone has one and that all must have prizes? *Archives of General Psychiatry, 32,* 995–1008.

Luria, A. R. (1961). *The role of speech in the regulation of normal and abnormal behavior.* New York: Liveright.

Mahoney, M. J. (1974). *Cognition and behavior modification.* Cambridge, MA: Ball-inger.

Mahoney, M. J. (1977). Personal science: A cognitive learning therapy. In A. Ellis & R. Grieger (Eds.), *Handbook of rational psychotherapy* (pp. 352–368). New York: Springer.

Mahoney, M. (1979). A critical analysis of rational-emotive theory and therapy. In A. Ellis & J. M. Whiteley (Eds.), *Theoretical and empirical foundations of rational-emotive therapy* (pp. 167–180). Monterey, CA: Brooks/Cole.

Mahoney, M. J. (1980). Psychotherapy and the structure of personal revolution. In M. H. Mahoney (Ed.), *Psychotherapy process* (pp. 157–180). New York: Plenum Press.

Mahoney, M. J. (1991). *Human change processes.* New York: Basic Books.

Mahoney, M. J. (1995). The continuing evolution of the cognitive sciences and psycho-therapies. In R. A. Neimeyer & M. J. Mahoney (Eds.), *Constructivism in psycho-therapy* (pp. 39–65). Washington, DC: American Psychological Association.

Mahoney, M. J., & Arnkoff, D. B. (1978). Cognitive and self-control therapies. In S. L. Garfield & A. E. Bergin (Eds.), *Handbook of psychotherapy and behavior change: An empirical analysis* (pp. 689–722). New York: Wiley.

Mahoney, M. J., & Kazdin, A. E. (1979). Cognitive-behavior modification: Miscon-ceptions and premature evacuation. *Psychological Bulletin, 86,* 1044–1049.

Mahoney, M. J., & Thoresen, C. E. (1974). *Self-control: Power to the person.* Monterey, CA: Brooks/Cole.

Markus, H. (1977). Self-schemata and processing information about the self. *Journal of Personality and Social Psychology, 35,* 63–78.

Meichenbaum, D. (1969). The effects of instructions and reinforcement on thinking and language behaviors of schizophrenics. *Behaviour Research and Therapy, 7,* 101–114.

Meichenbaum, D. H. (1973). Cognitive factors in behavior modification: Modifying what clients say to themselves. In C. M. Franks & G. T. Wilson (Eds.), *Annual review of behavior therapy, theory, and practice* (pp. 416–432). New York: Brunner/Mazel.

Meichenbaum, D. H. (1977). *Cognitive behavior modification.* New York: Plenum Press.

Meichenbaum, D. H. (1985). *Stress inoculation training: A clinical guidebook.* New York: Pergamon.

Meichenbaum, D. H. (1993). Stress inoculation training: A twenty-year update. In R. L. Woolfolk & P. M. Lehrer (eds.) *Principles and practice of stress management* (pp. 152–174). New York: Guilford Press.

Meichenbaum, D. H. (1994). *A clinical handbook/practical therapist manual for assessing and treating adults with post-traumatic stress disorder.* Waterloo, Ontario: Institute Press.

Meichenbaum, D. H. (2007). Stress inoculation training: A preventative and treat-ment approach. In P. M. Lehrer, R. L. Woolfolk, & W. E. Sime (Eds.), *Principles and practice of stress management* (3rd ed., pp. 497–516). New York: Guilford Press.

Meichenbaum, D. H., & Cameron, R. (1973). Training schizophrenics to talk to themselves. *Behavior Therapy, 4,* 515–535.

Meichenbaum, D. H., & Cameron, R. (1981). Issues in cognitive assessment: An overview. In T. Merluzzi, C. R. Glass, & M. Genest (Eds.), *Cognitive assessment* (pp. 3–15). New York: Guilford Press.

Meichenbaum, D. H., & Deffenbacher, J. L. (1988). Stress inoculation training. *Counseling Psychologist, 16,* 69–90.

Meichenbaum, D. H., & Goodman, J. (1971). Training impulsive children to talk to themselves. *Journal of Abnormal Psychology, 77,* 127–132.

Meichenbaum, D., & Jaremko, M. (Eds.). (1983). *Stress management and prevention: A cognitive-behavioral perspective.* New York: Plenum Press.

Meichenbaum, D., & Turk, D. (1976). The cognitive-behavioral management of anxiety, anger, and pain. In P. O. Davidson (Ed.), *The behavioral management of anxiety, depression, and pain* (pp. 1–34). New York: Brunner/Mazel.

Meichenbaum, D., Turk, D., & Burstein, S. (1975). The nature of coping with stress. In I. G. Sarason & C. D. Spielberger (Eds.), *Stress and anxiety: Vol. II* (pp. 337–360). New York: Wiley.

Merluzzi, T., Glass, C., & Genest, M. (1981). *Cognitive assessment.* New York: Guilford Press.

Miller, R. C., & Berman, J. S. (1983). The efficacy of cognitive behavior therapists: A quantitative review of the research evidence. *Psychological Bulletin, 94,* 39–53.

Minuchin, S., & Fishman, H. C. (1981). *Family therapy techniques.* Cambridge, MA: Harvard University Press.

Mischel, W. (1981). A cognitive-social learning approach to assessment. In T. Merluzzi, C. Glass, & M. Genest (Eds.), *Cognitive assessment* (pp. 479–502). New York: Guilford Press.

Mischel, W., Ebbesen, E. B., & Zeiss, A. (1972). Cognitive and attentional mechanisms in delay of gratification. *Journal of Personality and Social Psychology, 21,* 204–218.

Monat, A., Averill, J. R., & Lazarus, R. S. (1972). Anticipating stress and coping reactions under various conditions of uncertainty. *Journal of Personality and Social Psychology, 24,* 237–253.

Neimeyer, R. A. (1993). Constructivism and the problem of psychotherapy integration. *Journal of Psychotherapy Integration, 3,* 133–157.

Neimeyer, R. A. (1995). Constructivist psychotherapies: Features, foundations and future directions. In R. A. Neimeyer & M. J. Mahoney (Eds.), *Constructivism in psychotherapy* (pp. 231–246). Washington, DC: American Psychological Association.

Neimeyer, R. A., & Mahoney, M. J. (Eds.) (1995). *Constructivism in psychotherapy.* Washington, DC: American Psychological Association.

Neimeyer, R. A., & Raskin, J. D. (2001). Varieties of constructivism in psychotherapy. In K. S. Dobson (Ed.), *Handbook of cognitive-behavioral therapies, second edition* (pp. 393–430). New York: Guilford Press.

Neisser, U. (1967). *Cognitive psychology.* New York: Appleton-Century-Crofts.

Nezu, A. M. (1986). Efficacy of a social problem solving therapy approach for unipolar depression. *Journal of Consulting and Clinical Psychology, 54,* 196–202.

Nezu, A. M., Nezu., C. M., Friedman, S. H., Faddis, S., & Houts, P. S. (1998). *Helping cancer patients cope: A problem-solving approach.* Washington, DC: American Psychological Association.

Nisbett, R. E., & Wilson, T. D. (1977). Telling more than we can know: Verbal reports on mental processes. *Psychological Review, 84,* 231–259.

Nomikos, M. S., Opton, E. M., Jr., Averill, J. R., & Lazarus, R. S. (1968). Surprise versus suspense in the production of stress reaction. *Journal of Personality and Social Psychology, 8,* 204–208.

O'Hara, M. W., & Rehm, L. P. (1983). *Self-control group therapy of depression.* New York: Plenum Press.

Orne, M. (1965). Psychological factors maximizing resistance to stress with special reference to hypnosis. In S. Klausner (Ed.), *The quest for self-control* (pp. 286–328). New York: Free Press.

Öst, L. (2008). Efficacy of the third wave of behavioral therapies: A systematic review and meta-analysis. *Behaviour Research and Therapy, 46,* 296–321.

Paivio, A. (1971). *Imagery and verbal processes.* New York: Holt, Rinehart, & Winston.

Prochaska, J. O. (2000). Change at differing stages. In C. R. Snyder & R. E. Ingram (Eds.), *Handbook of psychological change: Psychotherapy processes and practices for the 21st century* (pp. 109–127). New York: Wiley.

Rachman, S. J., & Wilson, G. T. (1971). *The effects of psychological therapy.* Oxford, UK: Pergamon.

Rachman, S. J., & Wilson, G. T. (1980). *The effects of psychological therapy, second edition.* Oxford, UK: Pergamon.

Rehm, L. (1977). A self-control model of depression. *Behavior Therapy, 8,* 787–804.

Rehm, L. (1981). A self-control therapy program for treatment of depression. In J. F. Clarkin & H. Glazer (Eds.), *Depression: Behavioral and directive intervention strategies.* New York: Garland STPM Press.

Rehm, L. P., & Rokke, P. (1988). Self-management therapies. In K. S. Dobson (Ed.), *Handbook of cognitive-behavioral therapies* (pp. 136–166). New York: Guilford Press.

Resick, P. A.,Galovski, T. E., Uhlmansiek, M. O., Scher, C. D., Clum, G. A., & Young-Xu, Y. (2008). A randomized clinical trial to dismantle components of cognitive processing therapy for posttraumatic stress disorder in female victims of interpersonal violence. *Journal of Consulting and Clinical Psychology, 76,* 243–258.

Roemer, L., & Orsillo, S. (2003). Mindfulness: A promising intervention strategy in need of further study. *Clinical Psychology: Science and Practice, 10,* 172–178.

Segal, Z. V., & Cloitre, M. (1993). Methodologies for studying cognitive features of emotional disorder. In K. S. Dobson & P. C. Kendall (Eds.), *Psychopathology and cognition* (pp. 19–50). San Diego, CA: Academic Press.

Segal, Z. V., & Shaw, B. F. (1988). Cognitive assessment: Issues and methods. In K. S. Dobson (Ed.), *Handbook of cognitive-behavioral therapies* (pp. 39–84). New York: Guilford Press.

Shapiro, D. A., & Shapiro, D. (1982). Meta-analysis of comparative therapy outcome studies: A replication and refinement. *Psychological Bulletin, 92,* 581–604.

Shaw, B. F., & Dobson, K. S. (1981). Cognitive assessment of depression. In T. Merluzzi, C. Glass, & M. Genest (Eds.), *Cognitive assessment* (pp. 361–387). New York: Guilford Press.

Spivack, G., Platt, J. J., & Shure, M. B. (1976). *The problem-solving approach to adjustment.* San Francisco: Jossey-Bass.

Spivack, G., & Shure, M. B. (1974). *Social adjustment of young children.* San Francisco: Jossey-Bass.

Stuart, R. B. (1972). Situational versus self-control. In R. D. Rubin, H. Fensterheim, J. D. Henderson, & L. P. Ullmann (Eds.), *Advances in behavior therapy* (pp. 67–91). New York: Academic Press.

Suinn, R. M. (1972). Removing emotional obstacles to learning and performance by visuomotor behavior rehearsal. *Behavior Therapy, 3,* 308–310.

Suinn, R. M. (1995). Anxiety management training. In K. D. Craig & K. S. Dobson (Eds.), *Anxiety and depression in adults and children* (pp. 159–179). Thousand Oaks, CA: Sage.

Suinn, R. M., & Richardson, F. (1971). Anxiety management training: A nonspecific behavior therapy program for anxiety control. *Behavior Therapy, 2,* 498–510.

Sutton-Simon, K. (1981). Assessing belief systems: Concepts and strategies. In P. C. Kendall & S. D. Hollon (Eds.), *Assessment strategies for cognitive-behavioral interventions* (pp. 59–84). New York: Academic Press.

Turk, D. C., & Speers, M. A. (1983). Cognitive schemata and cognitive processes in cognitive behavioral interventions: Going beyond the information given. In P. C. Kendall (Ed.), *Advances in cognitive-behavioral research and therapy* (Vol. 2, pp. 112–140). New York: Academic Press.

Vernon, A., & Bernard, M. E. (2006). Applications of REBT in schools: Prevention, promotion, intervention. In A. Ellis & M. E. Bernard (Eds.), *Rational emotive behavioral approaches to childhood disorders: Theory, practice and research* (pp. 415–460). New York: Springer Science+Business Media.

Vygotsky, L. S. (1962). *Thought and language.* Cambridge, MA: MIT Press.

Wolpe, J. (1958). *Psychotherapy by reciprocal inhibition.* Stanford, CA: Stanford University Press.

Young, J. (1994). *Cognitive therapy for personality disorders: A schema-focused approach.* Sarasota, FL: Professional Resource Press.

CHAPTER 2

The Evidence Base
for Cognitive-Behavioral Therapy

Amanda M. Epp
Keith S. Dobson

Cognitive-behavioral therapy (CBT) has received an incredible amount of research attention and considerable support (Butler, Chapman, Forman, & Beck, 2006). CBT is the most frequently endorsed empirically supported treatment (EST) on the list compiled by the Task Force on Promotion and Dissemination of Psychological Procedures, across disorders and age groups (for the comprehensive list, see Chambless et al., 1998). Despite debate surrounding the movement toward the identification and dissemination of ESTs (see Elliott [1998] and the special section of *Psychotherapy Research*), CBT has been widely adopted as a primary treatment approach. In fact, it is one of the most commonly used psychotherapeutic treatments in adults (Leichensring, Hiller, Weissberg, & Leibing, 2006), and its importance in the field of psychotherapy is predicted to increase (Norcross, Hedges, & Prochaska, 2002). In this chapter we review the empirical literature regarding the efficacy of CBT. We begin with a description of the nature of the evidence and end with a discussion of the limitations and knowledge gaps in the current literature, and provide suggestions for future research.

THE NATURE OF THE EVIDENCE

The "gold standard" in psychotherapy research to determine the clinical efficacy of a given treatment is the randomized controlled trial (RCT). RCTs are advantageous in that they are well controlled and conducive to comparisons across studies. Due to their controlled nature, RCTs address the "efficacy," or the outcomes within an experimental setting of a particular treatment, as opposed to its "effectiveness," or the outcomes in actual clinical practice (Kazdin, 2003). Several types of efficacy can be investigated. The "absolute efficacy" of a treatment indicates whether it has any impact at all, as determined by either a comparison with a no-treatment control condition (e.g., waiting-list control condition, placebo drug condition), or by a within-subjects comparison of target measures from pretreatment to posttreatment. The former method is referred to as "controlled absolute efficacy," whereas the latter is referred to as "uncontrolled absolute efficacy." Controlled absolute efficacy is generally considered to be a methodologically stronger approach, although uncontrolled absolute efficacy may be necessary and more appropriate given certain research questions. The "relative efficacy" of a treatment indicates whether the treatment under investigation outperforms an active comparison treatment (e.g., CBT compared with pharmacotherapy). Relative efficacy studies of psychological treatments can involve comparisons among psychotherapies, or between a psychotherapy and a pharmacotherapy. "Combined efficacy" studies, in the context of CBT treatment outcome research, generally investigate whether a combination of CBT and medication (or CBT plus treatment as usual, which typically comprises medication and case management) is superior to medication or to CBT alone. Combined efficacy studies are common with disorders such as schizophrenia, which are managed predominantly by pharmacotherapy but may also benefit from additional psychotherapy. The "long-term efficacy" of a treatment simply refers to whether the gains obtained through an acute phase of treatment are maintained over a follow-up period.

A meta-analysis is a data aggregation method that allows for a quantitative summation across studies (Kazdin, 2003). It is based on effect sizes that reflect standardized differences between the treatment of interest (CBT in this case) and a comparison condition (Cohen, 1988). Conventions are used to determine the strength of an effect size: A small effect size is around 0.2, a medium effect size is around 0.5, and a large effect size is around 0.8. One of the strong advantages to a meta-analysis is that it takes into account sample size and the magnitude of the effect size for the interventions compared in each study. In addition, the meta-analysis removes effects of individual studies, such as reviewer bias (Rodebaugh, Holaway, & Heimberg, 2004).

Given the wealth of efficacy literature for CBT, many meta-analyses of RCTs have been conducted to summarize the data efficiently. The following review relies primarily on the results of these meta-analyses, though findings from recent, single RCTs are also reported where appropriate. Controlled outcome studies (nonrandomized designs) are described when RCTs are insufficient or not available, and qualitative reviews are recapitulated when they provide an efficient summary of the quantitative data or important additional information.

The following review examines the CBT outcome literature for 20 disorders, or problems, in adults. For each disorder, or problem, we examined six content areas regarding the efficacy of CBT: (1) the specific components of CBT investigated in the studies, (2) controlled and/or uncontrolled absolute efficacy, (3) relative efficacy compared with other psychotherapies, (4) relative efficacy compared with pharmacotherapy, (5) relative efficacy compared with a combination of CBT and pharmacotherapy, and (6) long-term efficacy. In this review, we recognize that CBT is a set of techniques that targets both a change in cognition and behavior. CBT models adhere to the theory that cognition mediates behavioral and emotional responses to the environment, and determines the individual's level of adjustment (Dobson, 2001). CBT thus refers to both Beck's standard cognitive therapy (CT; Beck, Rush, Shaw, & Emery, 1979), and any combination of cognitive and behavioral therapeutic techniques. Hence, standard CT and the various forms of CBT are all considered under the rubric of CBT for the purposes of this review.

EFFICACY OF COGNITIVE-BEHAVIORAL THERAPY

Mood Disorders

Unipolar Depression

Unipolar depression has received considerable attention in the CBT treatment outcome literature, and several meta-analyses have been published on the subject (e.g., Dobson, 1989; Gloaguen, Cottraux, Cucherat, & Blackburn, 1998). Gloaguen et al. included in their analyses studies that contained at least one CT group and one comparison group; the CT treatments had to either follow Beck's CT manual or refer explicitly to Beck's model. They also required random assignment of participants. Comparison groups included untreated controls; waiting-list, pharmacotherapy, and behavior therapy conditions; and a heterogeneous group of "other therapies" in the 48 studies that they considered. Gloaguen et al. found strong evidence for the absolute efficacy of CT, and superiority of CT over other therapies, although they warned that these latter findings should be interpreted with caution because they did not meet between-trial homogeneity. Their results also provided evidence for the superiority of CT over antidepressants, and the equivalence of behavior therapy (BT) and CT, this time with high between-trial homogeneity. They also found that the relapse rates for antidepressants exceeded CT at 1- to 2-year follow-up, although this result was obtained simply by comparing the percentage of relapses (see Hollon, Stewart, & Strunk [2006] for a similar conclusion). Gloaguen et al. (1998) failed to find significance for any of their postulated moderators (initial Beck Depression Inventory [BDI] score, sex, age). They concluded that CT demonstrates absolute efficacy in individuals with mild or moderate depression, equivalence to BT, and superiority to antidepressants.

Wampold, Minami, Baskin, and Tierney (2002) were dissatisfied with the classification of "other therapies" by Gloaguen et al. (1998). They asserted that the merger of bona fide and non–bona fide psychotherapies into the "other therapies" category potentially explained their outcomes relative to CT. They investigated this hypothesis by reanalyzing the Gloaguen et al. (1998) data. They found that CT was approximately as efficacious as bona fide other treatments, but superior to non–bona fide treatments. They concluded that all bona fide psychological treatments for depression are equally efficacious.

DeRubeis et al. (2005) conducted an RCT comparing CT and pharmacotherapy in patients with moderate to severe depression, and found that 24 sessions of CT delivered by experienced therapists was as efficacious as pharmacotherapy. Long-term results indicated that participants who had received CT were significantly less likely to relapse over a period of 12 months than those who discontinued medication, and had relapse rates comparable to those who continued medication (Hollon et al., 2005; for comparable results, see also Dimidjian et al., 2006).

Segal, Vincent, and Levitt (2002) concluded that combining antidepressant medications with CT may be more effective than either treatment modality alone, particularly for individuals with more severe depression. This question may become moot, however, because a recent meta-analysis found virtually no difference in treatment outcome between patients with moderate levels of initial depression who received a pill-placebo and those who received antidepressants, and relatively small effects for initially severely depressed patients (Kirsch et al., 2008).

Bipolar Disorder

Several review articles have examined the treatment efficacy for bipolar disorder, but no meta-analyses have yet been conducted. Medications remain the first line of treatment for bipolar disorder, but due to the limitations inherent in pharmacotherapy, such as poor adherence, frequent symptom recurrences, subsyndromal exacerbations, and maintenance of significant functional impairments, psychotherapy may be an important adjunctive treatment in bipolar disorder (Miklowitz & Otto, 2006). Psychotherapy may enhance early intervention strategies, adjustment, quality of life, and the protective effects of family and social support systems; increase patient understanding of and motivation to control episodes; encourage the regulation of daily routines and sleep–wake cycles; and increase medication adherence (Miklowitz & Otto, 2006).

Zaretsky, Rizvi, and Parikh (2007) reviewed RCTs of psychoeducation, family-focused therapy, brief CBT interventions (e.g., psychoeducation, homework, and self-monitoring), CBT for bipolar disorder, CBT for relapse prevention (e.g., psychoeducation, CT for depression, identification of prodromes of relapse and prevention, and stabilizing routines), interpersonal therapy, and social rhythm therapy (i.e., stabilizing social and circadian rhythms) for bipolar disorder. They concluded that manualized, short-term, specifically targeted psychotherapies offer consistent benefits as adjuncts to medication. The most robust relapse prevention effects were demonstrated by CBT, family-focused therapy, and psychoeducation, whereas residual depressive symptoms were most effectively treated with interpersonal therapy and CBT (Zaretsky et al., 2007).

Miklowitz and Otto (2006), Gonzalez-Pinto et al. (2004), and Colom and Vieta (2004) generally agree that psychotherapy is an effective adjunct to medication in the treatment of bipolar disorder. Jones (2004) noted that the effectiveness of psychosocial interventions may be overestimated due to the uncontrolled nature and poor quality of much of the treatment efficacy research, though he agreed that progress has been made in the development of adjunctive psychological approaches. He also commented that different interventions impact differently on depression and mania, and that some approaches may be more effective for one or another phase of the disorder. Gonzalez-Pinto et al. (2004) also warned that otherwise beneficial interventions for residual depressive symptoms and bipolar depression may be detrimental in the early phase of manic symptoms. Colom and Vieta (2004) observed that most psychosocial interventions are similar, in that they include a psychoeducational component, and that most have demonstrated similarly positive results. CBT has demonstrated efficacy on some measures up to 9 years posttreatment, but heterogeneity across studies does not permit conclusive long-term statements.

Anxiety Disorders

Specific Phobia

Whereas the anxiety disorders are generally represented strongly in the treatment outcome literature, the literature for specific phobias is relatively sparse. Data that exist are largely of poor quality due to studies being conducted in nonclinical settings, and due to methodological limitations, such as small sample sizes, uncontrolled designs, and confusion between purely behavioral and CBT treatments (Choy, Fyer, & Lipsitz, 2006). No meta-analysis has been conducted on the subject, although Choy et al. wrote a comprehensive narrative review of treatment studies. They employed a "best evidence" approach and concluded that treatments are not equally effective, and that they have differential efficacy among phobia subtypes. The BTs were most widely supported, with robust acute results for *in vivo* exposure across the majority of phobia subtypes. *In vivo* exposure, however, was associated with relatively high dropout rates and low treatment acceptance. Systematic desensitization demonstrated more moderate efficacy, and virtual reality exposure was found to be a potentially acceptable alternative to *in vivo* exposure given comparable results for height phobia and flying phobia.

Choy et al. (2006) found that the use of cognitive restructuring, either alone or in combination with *in vivo* exposure, was efficacious in the treatment of claustrophobia. In fact, they suggested that CT may be a good alternative to *in vivo* exposure for claustrophobia. Although CT was not found to improve outcomes of *in vivo* exposure for animal or flying phobias, the authors speculated that this may have been due to ceiling effects given the high level of efficacy of *in vivo* exposure. CT has also demonstrated beneficial effects as a solo treatment for dental and flying phobias, and gains have been maintained at 12 months for CT combined with *in vivo* exposure for the one animal study (spiders). Also, the effects of CT alone were found to be long-lasting for claustrophobia but less so for flying or dental phobias. Two other studies found that participants rated treatments that incorporated cognitive components and behavioral components as less aversive and/or less intrusive than treatments based solely on exposure (Hunt et al., 2006; Koch, Spates, & Himle, 2004).

Social Anxiety Disorder

"Social anxiety disorder" (SAD), otherwise referred to as social phobia, has received considerable attention in the CBT treatment literature. To our knowledge, six meta-analyses and several review papers (e.g., Fresco & Heimberg, 2001; Heimberg, 2002; Rodebaugh et al., 2004; Rowa & Antony, 2005) have been published on the subject. The most recent meta-analysis directly compared pharmacotherapy, CBT, or a combination of the two in 16 studies on panic disorder, six studies on SAD, and two studies on generalized anxiety disorder (Bandelow, Seidler-Brandler, Becker, Wedekind, & Rüther, 2007). CBT included cognitive techniques, exposure, and anxiety management techniques delivered in a group or individual format. All treatments for SAD led to large pre- and posttreatment effect sizes; clinicians rated the greatest changes from pre- to posttreatment in pharmacotherapy, whereas patients rated the combined treatment as most efficacious. At posttreatment, there was a minimal advantage for pharmacotherapy alone over CBT alone. There was also preliminary support for CBT combined with pharmacotherapy based on two studies. Bandelow et al. found mixed results for follow-up data examining the stability of CBT and pharmacotherapy.

Rodebaugh et al. (2004) summarized the results of five meta-analyses (Chambless & Hope, 1996; Fedoroff & Taylor, 2001; Feske & Chambless, 1995; Gould, Buckmeister, Pollack, Otto, & Yap, 1997; Taylor, 1996), and reported moderate to large controlled effect sizes for CBT at posttreatment in all meta-analyses. They also found that moderate to large within-group uncontrolled effect sizes were reported for CBT, similar to Bandelow et al.'s (2007) findings. Furthermore, they found that all studies demonstrated maintenance of CBT gains at follow-up, if not modest further improvements. Although the majority of meta-analyses included studies with follow-up assessments of 2–6 months, Feske and Chambless (1995) and Chambless and Hope (1996) included studies with follow-up assessments of up to 12 months. The absolute efficacy of CBT for social phobia has been well established.

The relative efficacy of CBT for social phobia is somewhat difficult to discern. Federoff and Taylor (2001) examined medications, exposure, cognitive restructuring, exposure plus cognitive restructuring, social skills training, and applied relaxation, and found that the most consistently efficacious treatments were medications. On the other hand, Gould et al. (1997) reported that CBT, pharmacotherapy, and their combination were all nonsignificantly different from one another. Exposure, cognitive restructuring, cognitive restructuring plus exposure, and social skills training also appear to be nonsignificantly different in efficacy (Taylor, 1996).

Differences among variants of cognitive-behavioral treatments are difficult to ascertain based on these meta-analyses. As reviewed in Rodebaugh et al. (2004), the only significant difference among treatments favored exposure plus cognitive restructuring over placebo (Taylor, 1996), although only by clinician rating, not by client self-report. Gould et al. (1997) found that exposure resulted in the largest effect sizes among their conditions, whether alone or combined with cognitive restructuring. Unlike the previous researchers, Feske and Chambless (1995) differentiated between CBT and exposure, defining CBT as cognitive restructuring plus exposure. They determined that exposure and CBT were equally effective. Rodebaugh et al. (2004) noted that if one considers nonsignificant differences between effect sizes, CBT that incorporates cognitive restructuring and exposure may be the best supported.

Most of the meta-analyses examined dropout rates. Although Gould et al. (1997) found no statistically significant difference in dropout rates between pharmacotherapy, the combined condition, and CBT, the respective attrition rates of 13.7, 6.7, and 10.7% suggested that the presence of CBT moderates the attrition from medications alone. Fedoroff and Taylor (2001) also found nonsignificant differences among their 11 conditions. However, attrition rates varied considerably, from approximately 6% for waiting-list control to approximately 23% for benzodiazepines and monoamine oxidase inhibitors, with cognitive restructuring plus exposure falling to almost 19%. Taylor (1996) found similarly nonsignificant differences in dropout rates, ranging from 5.7% for waiting-list control to 18% for cognitive restructuring plus exposure.

Finally, Rodebaugh et al. (2004) found no differences between individual and group formats of CBT (Federoff & Taylor, 2001; Gould et al., 1997). Gould et al. computed cost projections and determined that group CBT was the most cost-effective choice among treatment options. Feske and Chambless (1995) also examined the "dose–response" issue for CBT, and explored whether treatment gains increased with an increasing number of sessions for CBT compared with exposure. They found that length of treatment only affected treatment outcomes for exposure, in that a greater number of sessions resulted in improved outcomes.

Obsessive–Compulsive Disorder

According to a review article (Allen, 2006), CBT and pharmacotherapy have been established as the two treatments of choice for obsessive–compulsive disorder (OCD), with exposure and ritual, or response, prevention (ERP) being the most efficacious form of CBT. Although exposure-based treatments are considered behavioral, they are almost always combined with cognitive techniques, because cognitive techniques are included to motivate clients and help them manage the exposure (Abramowitz, Taylor, & McKay, 2005; Allen, 2006). Allen thus refers to ERP and CBT interchangeably (see also Abramowitz et al., 2005). Abramowitz et al. examined dropout rates and determined that the inclusion of cognitive techniques with behavioral experiments reduces treatment dropout, suggesting that CBT is more acceptable to patients with OCD than ERP.

Among the psychotherapies, Allen (2006) contended that CBT (with ERP) is the only treatment that has proven effective. He further concluded that the combination of pharmacotherapy and CBT is more efficacious than CBT alone in individuals with comorbid depression and OCD. However, he also maintained that preliminary evidence suggests that CBT is superior to pharmacotherapy in relapse prevention, particularly following medication discontinuation. Last, Allen warned that many individuals with OCD remain symptomatic posttreatment, and that many individuals do not even experience improvements as a result of treatment, often because they are unable to meet the terms of treatment.

At least three meta-analyses have been conducted on the use of CBT in treating OCD. The overall pattern of these meta-analyses is consistent with the previous synopsis. Eddy, Dutra, Bradley, and Westen (2004) recently separately examined ERP, CBT, and CT, and a range of pharmacological interventions. They determined that psychotherapy and pharmacotherapy both result in significant decreases in OCD symptoms, as reflected by unstandardized effect sizes, considerable percentages of patients who improve with treatment, and significant declines in symptoms from pre- to posttreatment. They specified that the behaviorally based treatments were more efficacious than the cognitively based interventions. They analyzed a small number of studies that included psychotherapy plus pharmacotherapy and found a robust effect that was greater than for either treatment alone. Despite the paucity of such trials, they tentatively concluded that combined psychotherapy and pharmacotherapy may be the treatment of choice for OCD. They noted that there were insufficient data to make any conclusive statements about the sustained efficacy of psychotherapy, and that their findings suggested that continued pharmacotherapy is needed to maintain treatment gains in the long term. Last, and somewhat disappointingly, they reported that one-third of those who complete a course of therapy, and nearly one-half of those who begin but do not complete treatment, will not make expected gains.

Abramowitz (1997) found that cognitive and exposure-based approaches to the treatment of OCD are equally efficacious, which he attributed to procedural overlap between the two approaches and the hypothesis that they result in similar mechanisms of change. Abramowitz calculated effect size as the standardized difference between treatments at posttest (unlike Eddy et al., 2004), thus providing more substantial support for the absolute efficacy of

CBT. A direct comparison between pharmacotherapy and psychotherapy was not conducted, but several types of pharmacotherapy were compared. The most support was found for serotonergic medications (compared with other classes of antidepressants), which substantially reduced OCD symptoms at posttest. Abramowitz (1997), due to insufficient data, did not report follow-up results. Although van Balkom et al. (1994) did not directly compare CT with BT in their meta-analysis, their results did not support equal efficacy between CT and BT. They found that serotonergic antidepressants, BT, and their combination were the only active treatments that were significantly superior to placebo treatment. They also reported that upon visual inspection, it appeared that effect sizes remained stable up to 6 years posttest.

Panic Disorder with or without Agoraphobia

The most recent meta-analysis to directly compare pharmacological, psychological, and combined interventions for the treatment of panic disorder with (PDA) or without (PD) agoraphobia was conducted by Bandelow et al. (2007). They found that pharmacological treatment or CBT alone, and their combination, yielded large effect sizes from pre- to posttreatment on both clinician and self-report ratings. Interestingly, patients reported higher pre–post differences for CBT alone than for drug treatment alone, whereas clinicians reported the opposite pattern. However, the only statistically significant difference among treatments for pre- and posttreatment effect sizes was between combined CBT and pharmacotherapy, and pharmacotherapy alone. Bandelow et al. reported few follow-up studies, which yielded inconsistent results.

A large meta-analysis of 124 studies also examined the relative and absolute efficacies of CBT (exposure and cognitive restructuring), pharmacotherapy, and their combination in the treatment of PD (Mitte, 2005a). Controlled absolute efficacy was found for both treatments. There was no incremental value from the addition of cognitive elements to BT when examining anxiety outcome measures, but the inclusion of cognitive elements led to enhanced reduction of depressive symptoms. CBT was also associated with lower rates of attrition compared with BT. This meta-analysis also suggested that CBT is at least as effective as pharmacotherapy. In fact, Mitte reported that while there are some situations in which CBT is more appropriate and others in which pharmacotherapy is more appropriate, there were no important differences between CBT, BT, and pharmacotherapy in terms of treatment outcome. Contrary to the results by Bandelow et al. (2007), this study found that a combination of CBT and pharmacotherapy was not significantly more effective than CBT alone, either in the short or the long term (average 16.8 months). In an older study by Gould, Otto, and Pollack (1995), a similar meta-analysis found slightly divergent results. They used pill-placebo controls as opposed to waiting-list controls, which likely affected their outcomes.

Siev and Chambless (2007) conducted a focused meta-analysis of the relative efficacy of CT (incorporating interoceptive exposure) and relaxation therapy (RT) in the treatment of PD to examine the differential efficacy of different forms of CBT. They found that CT was superior to RT on all panic-related measures and on indices of clinically significant change. Oei, Llamas, and Devilly (1999) also conducted a more specific analysis of the available data on PDA. Through a different meta-analytic technique they compared a CBT for PDA treatment group's pretreatment, posttreatment, and follow-up scores on the Fear Questionnaire (FQ), with normative scores obtained from a community sample and a college sample. They concluded that CBT is effective, as demonstrated by the fact that the treatment group's scores on the FQ fell within 2 standard deviations of a normal population's mean at post-treatment and follow-up (1 to 16 months posttreatment). They argued that treatment for PDA should incorporate *in vivo* exposure, because avoidance is a distinctive characteristic of the disorder. In contrast, they contended that PD is amenable to CT or RT, because it is associated with calamitous misinterpretations of neutral stimuli.

Landon and Barlow (2004) reviewed the literature and, in addition to examining the absolute and relative efficacy of CBT for the treatment of PD/PDA, they discussed the treatment efficacy for individuals with multiple diagnoses, effectiveness, cost-effectiveness, barriers to treatment dissemination, recent innovations in CBT, and predictors of outcome for CBT. They found that brief forms of CBT are superior to other forms of psychotherapy, and that lengthy CBT is not necessary for successful treatment. They determined that individual or group therapy CBT can be effectively used by trained clinicians in a variety of settings. They also observed that when the cost of treatment sessions and medications is taken into account, pharmacotherapy is the most costly of treatment modalities, and CBT has the most favorable cost profile.

Posttraumatic Stress Disorder

Since the National Institute for Clinical Excellence (NICE; National Collaborating Centre for Mental Health, 2005) guidelines were published, at least two meta-analyses have been published that synthesize the treatment outcome research for posttraumatic stress disorder (PTSD). The most recent publication (Bisson et al., 2007) examined the absolute and relative efficacies of trauma-focused CBT (TFCBT), stress management (SM), other therapies (supportive therapy, nondirective counseling, psychodynamic therapy, and hypnotherapy), group CBT, and eye movement desensitization and reprocessing (EMDR). The National Collaborating Centre for Mental Health included exposure and various cognitive techniques (e.g., cognitive reprocessing therapy, cognitive restructuring) under the rubric of TFCBT. Thirty-eight studies were included in the analyses, and results were reported in terms of both statistical and clinical significance. Bisson et al. found that TFCBT showed clinically important benefits over waiting-list and usual care on all measures of PTSD symptoms, and limited evidence for efficacy with comorbid depression and anxiety. EMDR also demonstrated efficacy over waiting-list and usual care. Although

TFCBT and EMDR were not significantly different, there was limited evidence that both TFCBT and EMDR were superior to other therapies. Bisson et al. did not find evidence to support the use of "other therapies" for PTSD, but they did find limited evidence for the use of SM and group CBT. Seidler and Wagner (2006) sought to clarify the relative efficacy of TFCBT and EMDR through a meta-analysis of seven studies. They found no clear evidence for the superiority of one over the other, and concluded that observed differences are probably not clinically important. Long-term results were not reported.

The National Collaborating Centre for Mental Health (2005) also conducted a meta-analysis of pharmacological and physical interventions for adult PTSD, as part of the review for the NICE guidelines. Although some drug treatments demonstrated statistical significance over placebo, they performed disappointingly when considering an a priori criterion for a clinically important effect. In one small study, TFCBT was superior to paroxetine for the reduction of PTSD severity on a self-rated measure, for reduced depression symptoms on a self-rated measure, and in terms of patient attrition. The evidence was inconclusive as to which treatment modality was more efficacious in terms of depression symptoms as rated by a clinician, and PTSD severity as assessed by self-report. Long-term results were not reported.

These results are all in the context of chronic PTSD, not as early interventions employed directly after the trauma, or for acute stress disorder. The National Collaborating Centre for Mental Health (2005) systematically reviewed the literature on early interventions, which focused on (1) treatments delivered to all trauma survivors within the first month after the incident; (2) treatments delivered to people at high risk of chronic PTSD, initiated within 3 months of the incident; and (3) drug treatments for people in the acute phase of the disorder. These results indicate that single-session debriefing (sometimes referred to as "critical incident debriefing") immediately after the traumatic incident may be at best ineffective, and may actually increase the risk of later traumatic symptoms. TFCBT, when delivered 1 to 6 months postincident, reduced rates of diagnosis posttreatment, as well as self-reported PTSD severity, anxiety, quality of life, and clinician-rated PTSD severity. Whereas TFCBT was also more efficacious than waiting-list control in terms of PTSD diagnosis at 9- to 13-month follow-up, further evidence was inconclusive, because there was no clinically important difference for clinician-assessed PTSD severity. TFCBT was also more efficacious than self-help booklets, relaxation, or supportive counseling. Last, there were insufficient data available on early intervention drug treatments to provide any conclusive statements about their efficacy.

Generalized Anxiety Disorder

Three meta-analyses on treatments for generalized anxiety disorder (GAD) were published in 2007. Bandelow et al. (2007) included only two studies in their review, and the studies had small sample sizes; thus, their results are not discussed here. Siev and Chambless (2007) included five studies in their analysis, and found that the uncontrolled posttreatment effect sizes comparing CT and RT on anxiety, anxiety-related cognitions, and depression were small and nonsignificant. In addition, the relative odds of achieving clinically significant change at posttreatment were modest for both treatment groups and did not differ. Last, dropout rates were approximately equivalent.

Hunot, Churchill, Teixeira, and Silva de Lima (2007) conducted the largest (22 studies) and most comprehensive meta-analysis with an exclusive focus on GAD, published in the Cochrane Library. The Cochrane Collaboration is a group of entities that uses and advances systematic reviews of health research (Davidson, Trudeau, Ockene, Orleans, & Kaplan, 2004). It has its own set of stringent guidelines for study selection and data analysis, including peer review. Once approved, the reviews are published in the Cochrane Library. Based on new evidence and feedback from library users, reviews are updated regularly (Davidson et al., 2004). Hunot et al. (2007) compared CBT, psychodynamic, and supportive therapies with control conditions and with each other. Within the CBT therapies they included anxiety management training, cognitive restructuring, situational exposure, self-controlled desensitization, RT/training, CT alone, and BT alone. As opposed to effect sizes, they reported weighted mean differences, standardized mean differences, 95% confidence intervals, pooled relative risks, and the number they needed to treat to produce a clinically meaningful outcome.

Hunot et al. (2007) determined that patients assigned to CBT were more likely to achieve clinical response at posttreatment than those assigned to treatment as usual or waiting-list control. CBT also had greater absolute efficacy in anxiety, worry, and depression symptoms at posttreatment than treatment as usual or waiting-list control. There was insufficient data to determine the long-term absolute efficacy of CBT. The comparative efficacy of CBT and psychodynamic therapy was limited to a single, though relatively large, study, which found that patients who received CBT were more likely to show a clinical response and a reduction in anxiety and depression symptoms than those who received psychodynamic therapy, both at posttreatment and at 6-month follow-up. The difference between CBT and supportive therapy was not statistically significant in terms of clinical response at posttreatment or at 6-month follow-up, although patients who received CBT were more likely than those who received supportive therapy to achieve clinical response. CBT also demonstrated a greater reduction in anxiety and depressive symptoms at posttreatment, and anxiety at 6-month follow-up than did supportive therapy. Hunot et al. found mixed results between CT and BT; CT was more likely to result in clinical response and was more efficacious in reducing depression symptoms than BT, but there was a nonsignificant difference in anxiety symptoms.

Although Gould, Otto, Pollack, and Yap (1997) conducted the most frequently cited meta-analysis on treatment outcomes for GAD, Mitte (2005b) conducted a more recent meta-analysis, including 65 studies. She found support for the controlled absolute efficacy of CBT at reducing symptoms of anxiety and depression, and at improving quality of life, but she did not specifically identify which techniques were considered under the rubric of CBT. Many of the patients who dropped out were excluded from the analyses, so the reported effect sizes may have overestimated the real effects. When direct comparisons of CBT and pharmacotherapy were analyzed, Mitte found that CBT demonstrated superiority over pharmacotherapy. However, when the study population was modified in the sensitivity analyses, this effect disappeared. Thus, CBT was determined to be at least as effective as pharmacotherapy. Overall, Mitte concluded that the relative efficacy of CBT and pharmacotherapy remains questionable, but that CBT appears to be better tolerated than pharmacotherapy. She also found that there was a high impact of specific treatment factors for CBT and a strong impact of common factors for pharmacotherapy.

Eating Disorders

Bulimia Nervosa

Bulimia nervosa (BN) has received the most attention in the treatment outcome literature related to eating disorders, with at least two meta-analyses (Whittal, Agras, & Gould, 1999; Lewandowski, Gebing, Anthony, & O'Brien, 1997), and one review (Shapiro et al., 2007) published to date. Shapiro et al. conducted the most recent, comprehensive, and systematic review (including 37 RCTs); thus, only their results are reported. They found strong supportive evidence for the absolute efficacy of CBT and specific evidence for the importance of the cognitive component of CBT in the production of favorable outcomes. They found that CT was superior to support only on certain measures, and CBT was superior to nutritional counseling alone, supportive–expressive therapy, behavioral therapy components alone, ERP, and self-monitoring only. However, exercise therapy was superior to CBT at 18-month follow-up on certain measures. They did not find evidence of added benefit in augmenting CBT with ERP. When administered in a group format, interpersonal therapy (IPT) and CBT were found to be equal to each other and more efficacious than waiting-list control in terms of decreases on days binged, psychological features of BN, disinhibition, and restraint. However, individually administered CBT was associated with a significantly greater probability of remission, and greater decreases in vomiting and restraint than individually administered IPT. Based on a range of findings, with a variety of drugs employed and outcome measures examined, Shapiro et al. concluded that there is preliminary evidence for the incremental efficacy of psychotherapy combined with medication for BN.

Hay, Bacaltchuk, and Stefano (2004) reviewed the psychotherapy literature for BN, binge-eating disorder (BED), and eating disorder not otherwise specified (EDNOS). They computed relative risks for binary outcome data and standardized mean differences for continuous variable outcome data. Forty

RCTs were included in the analyses of effects for BN, which investigated the efficacy of CBT, CBT tailored specifically for bulimia nervosa (CBT-BN), IPT, hypnobehavioral therapy, supportive psychotherapy, and self-monitoring. They found that all psychotherapies demonstrated absolute efficacy on measures of bulimic symptoms and abstinence rates at posttreatment compared with waiting-list control. CBT demonstrated significantly greater improvements in binge-eating abstinence rates than other psychotherapies, but not other bulimic and psychiatric symptoms. There were insufficient data to compare guided CBT versus self-help CBT, and there were no changes in comparisons of CBT versus CBT augmented by ERP or CBT versus "dismantled" CBT. Hay et al. found that CBT-BN was associated with significantly greater improvements in bulimic symptoms and binge-eating abstinence rates than the other psychotherapies, but not a greater reduction in depression scores. The authors concluded that their findings support the efficacy of CBT, particularly CBT-BN for BN. They also asserted that other psychotherapies were efficacious, particularly IPT in the longer-term, and that highly structured self-help CBT is promising, though less so without guidance, and the results are inconclusive with regard to BN specifically. Finally, they deduced that CBT plus ERP does not demonstrate incremental value over and above CBT alone.

Binge-Eating Disorder

Although BED was included in the Hay et al. (2004) study, analyses were performed on BN, BED, and EDNOS as a group, and only for BN as a separate disorder. Brownley, Berkman, Sedway, Lohr, and Bulik (2007) conducted a systematic review of 26 RCTs that addressed treatment efficacy solely for BED, however. One of the studies that they reviewed confirmed the controlled absolute efficacy of CBT in terms of reduced days binged, body mass index (BMI), disinhibition, hunger, depression, self-esteem, and increased odds of being abstinent posttreatment relative to waiting-list controls. However, they reported minimal weight change from baseline to follow-up. Another study reviewed by Brownley et al. demonstrated equal efficacy between group CBT and group IPT in terms of reduction in the number of days binged (at posttreatment and 4-month follow-up), although neither treatment significantly reduced BMI. At 12-month follow-up, illness severity and depression levels were equally reduced for both groups, and abstinence and dropout rates did not differ between groups. The latter study also demonstrated that CBT resulted in greater improvements in Eating Disorders Examination Restraint scores at all time points. Brownley et al. also found that a combination of CBT and medication may improve both eating and weight loss outcomes, although they were unable to determine which medications would produce the most favorable results. They noted that most studies found marked dropout for both CBT and medication trials. Bowers and Andersen (2007) determined that evidence supports the efficacy of CBT combined with medications, but treatment recommendations cannot be made due to limitations in the available literature.

Anorexia Nervosa

Bulik, Berkman, Brownley, Sedway, and Lohr (2007) conducted a systematic review of 19 RCTs on treatment efficacy for anorexia nervosa (AN). They found serious flaws in the literature base, and were of the opinion that it is meager and uncertain. Despite these limitations, they found tentative supportive evidence for CBT in the reduction of relapse risk for adults after weight restoration. Long-term outcomes were only reported for one study, where a combination of CBT and BT resulted in greater improvements than those for a control group on some measures, but not others, at 12-month follow-up. They did not find superiority of CBT over IPT and nonspecific supportive clinical management in the acutely underweight state. In one study, CBT resulted in reduced relapse risk and increased positive outcomes compared with nutritional counseling. However, a large number of studies that demonstrated positive outcomes included participants who were also taking antidepressant medications. That said, Bulik et al. asserted that medication is inappropriate for individuals with AN, because medication was associated with high rates of attrition and was not associated with significant changes in weight or psychological features of AN. Bowers and Andersen (2007) agreed with Bulik et al. (2007), and stated that there is little evidence to support the use of antidepressants during and after inpatient treatment.

Other Disorders

Schizophrenia

Psychotherapy for schizophrenia is used as an adjunctive treatment to pharmacotherapy to improve the management of positive symptoms and encourage medication compliance. Zimmermann, Favrod, Trieu, and Pomini (2005) included 14 studies in their examination of treatment outcomes on positive psychotic symptoms (e.g., hallucinations and delusions) in schizophrenia spectrum disorders. Overall, CBT demonstrated promising moderate positive effects compared with other adjunctive measures (i.e., treatment as usual, waiting-list, supportive psychotherapy, and recreation). In addition, these effects increased slightly at early follow-up (3 to 12 months) and were maintained at longer-term follow-up (more than 12 months). However, Zimmermann et al. cautioned that although the studies included in their analyses were controlled, they were not all blinded. When they analyzed the blinded trials only, the effect size decreased from 0.37 to 0.29 at posttreatment. Further analyses revealed that the effects of CBT were greater when compared with waiting list than compared with supportive psychotherapy or treatment as usual. CBT also demonstrated greater efficacy for patients in an acute psychotic episode than for those stabilized chronic patients with enduring psychotic symptoms.

Pilling et al. (2002) conducted a meta-analysis on the data from RCTs of 18 family therapy and eight CBT trials. They included a range of strategies under the rubric of CBT, including challenging and testing key beliefs, modifying dysfunctional beliefs, coping skills enhancement, environmental and emotional monitoring, and psychoeducation. Depending on the availability of comparison interventions, they compared both family therapy and CBT to either standard care or to other treatments, but not directly with each other. They found a clear and positive effect for CBT up to 9 months posttreatment on continuous measures of mental state. Although they did not find evidence for increased effectiveness of CBT during treatment, CBT showed superiority over all other treatments in terms of important improvements in mental state during treatment and up to 18 months posttreatment. CBT also had a lower rate of attrition than did standard care, and some evidence for improvement of global functioning at posttreatment, but not positive effects in terms of prevention of relapse or readmission during or after treatment.

Rector and Beck (2001) performed a meta-analysis on treatment outcome data for seven RCTs that tested the efficacy of CBT for schizophrenia. They found that CBT resulted in large effect sizes on measures of both positive and negative psychotic symptoms, above and beyond routine care. Both groups demonstrated maintenance of gains at 6-month follow-up, and CBT showed a greater reduction of negative symptoms compared with routine care. At 9-month follow-up, CBT demonstrated continued gains on measures of overall symptomatology. CBT also demonstrated greater change on both positive and negative symptoms than supportive therapy. Gould, Mueser, Bolton, Mays, and Goff (2001) performed a meta-analysis of seven controlled studies and found a relatively large positive effect size for change in psychotic symptoms from pre- to posttreatment, and that treatment gains increased at 6-month follow-up.

Marital Distress

Dunn and Schwebel (1995) examined the efficacy of cognitive-behavioral marital therapy (CBMT; see Wood, Crane, Schaalje, & Law [2005] for a meta-analysis of behavioral marital therapy [BMT] and emotion-focused marital therapy) for marital distress. Treatments were defined as CBMT if they incorporated both behavioral interventions and an emphasis on "overt attempts to identify and change partners' maladaptive cognitions concerning themselves, their partner, or the relationship" (Dunn & Schwebel, 1995; p. 60). They found significant effects for changes in behavior for CBMT, BMT, and interpersonally oriented marital therapy (IOMT) at posttreatment and at follow-up (1 to 48 months posttreatment), but no significant differences among the treatment modalities. Only CBMT produced a significant controlled effect size on relationship-related cognitions at posttreatment, though the effect sizes for BMT and CBMT did not differ significantly, and neither produced significant effects at follow-up. Posttreatment affect was only examined by one study for each treatment modality; significant treatment effects were produced at posttreatment, and long-term effects were not significant, though they were only reported for the IOMT study. All three treatment approaches resulted in significant controlled effect sizes on general measures of the relationship and its quality. Post hoc comparisons indicated that IOMT was significantly more efficacious than BMT and CBMT in eliciting change in the relationship and relationship quality, but this superiority was attenuated at follow-up, because all three approaches differed significantly from no treatment, but not from one another.

Anger and Violent Offending

Beck and Fernandez (1998) conducted the first meta-analysis of 50 studies in the anger treatment literature that specifically examined CBT, defined as a combination of various techniques that may include relaxation, cognitive restructuring, problem solving, and stress inoculation. They reported that CBT was associated with a relatively large controlled effect size, and that CBT patients did better than 76% of untreated patients on reduction of anger. The majority of the subjects included in their analyses were in programs for violent offenders. No long-term results were reported.

Landenberger and Lipsey (2005) reviewed several meta-analyses, with 58 experimental and quasi-experimental trials, and concluded that the efficacy of CBT for violent offender recidivism has been established, but not which variants of CBT are most effective, or for which offenders. Specifically, they found a 25% decrease in rates of recidivism in the 12 months posttreatment for the treated group compared with the untreated group. They failed to find a difference in efficacy for different brand-name CBT programs or generic forms of CBT, when they accounbted for variables such as high-risk offenders and high-quality treatment implementation. These variables were independently associated with larger recidivism reductions.

Sexual Offending

Lösel and Schmucker (2005) reviewed psychological and biological treatments for sex offenders published in five languages. They computed odds ratios on data from 69 studies of varied research design and found that offenders who were treated with CBT had a 37% lower rate of sexual recidivism, and similar rates for violent and general recidivism to controls, over an average follow-up period of more than 5 years. In terms of relative efficacy, physical treatments had greater effects than the psychosocial interventions. Specifically, surgical castration resulted in the largest effect, followed by hormonal treatment, CBT, and BT. The latter two were the only psychosocial treatments found to have a significant impact on sexual recidivism. However, Lösel and Schmucker noted that the difference in effect size between physical and psychosocial treatments was partially confounded by methodological and offender variables. Specifically, the control groups often refused castration or were not accepted for surgery by expert consensus; thus, they differed markedly from the highly selected and motivated group that voluntarily chose surgery. Given this consideration, the authors concluded that the individuals in the treatment group were probably less likely to reoffend than those in the control group in any event, and that these results might not be found in a truly randomized clinical trial. Lösel and Schmucker designated CBT and hormonal treatments as the most promising treatment options because of the previously mentioned confounds in the findings and the ethical, legal, and medical implications of surgical castration. The specific components of CBT were not identified. Comparisons between group and individual treatments did not yield significantly different outcomes, and only interventions that were designed specifically for sex offenders had a significant effect; in fact, others demonstrated negative outcomes. Last, there were no significant differences in outcome between randomized and other research designs.

Hanson et al. (2002) conducted a similar study to that of Lösel and Schmucker (2005), except that they computed odds ratios in 43 studies and focused solely on psychological treatments. Overall, they found a small advantage for the treated offenders compared with the untreated offenders on sexual and general recidivism rates (over an average 46-month follow-up period). Treatments employed prior to 1980 did not demonstrate much of an effect on rates of recidivism, whereas current treatments, such as CBT and systemic treatment, were associated with reductions in sexual and general recidivism. Hall (1995) conducted a smaller meta-analysis of only 12 studies and also found a small overall effect size for treated versus untreated sexual offenders by computing Pearson product–moment correlations. Hall's findings differed somewhat from those of Lösel and Schmucker's (2005) in that they found hormonal treatments and CBT (not defined) to be approximately equally efficacious in reducing recidivism rates, and significantly more effective than behavioral treatments (average 6.85-year follow-up period).

Chronic Pain

Morley, Eccleston, and Williams (1999) conducted a meta-analysis of 25 studies for chronic pain, excluding headache. Outcomes were related to pain experience, mood/affect, cognitive coping and appraisal, pain behavior, biology/physical fitness, social role functioning, use of health care system, and other measures. CBT-based therapies were classified as (1) CBT, with a primary focus on changing cognitive activity to achieve changes in behavior, thought and emotion; (2) BT; and (3) biofeedback. CBT-based therapies were superior to waiting-list controls on all domains, with the exception of expression of pain behavior. Although the different treatments were not directly compared with one another, the reported effect sizes were larger for CBT than for BT in all domains except mood/affect, negative cognitive coping and appraisal, and behavior activity. Interestingly, biofeedback demonstrated large effect sizes for several domains and was superior to both CBT and BT in pain experience, mood/affect expression, behavior expression, and social role functioning. Morley et al. noted that there were fewer BT and biofeedback trials than strictly CBT trials. Also, when compared with a heterogeneous sample of other active treatments, CBT was superior in terms of reduced pain experience and expression, and increased positive coping, but not for other domains. Long-term outcomes were not reported.

Personality Disorders

No narrative or meta-analytic review of the treatment outcome literature on personality disorders has been conducted. However, several recent RCTs have been published related to borderline personality disorder (BPD), which has received the most research attention. Linehan et al. (2006) and Bohus et al. (2004) examined the efficacy of dialectical behavior therapy (DBT; Linehan, 1993), a form of CBT developed specifically for the treatment of BPD. Bohus et al. (2004) found that DBT resulted in several significant positive reductions and improvements in a sample of female inpatients 1-month postdischarge. Compared with waiting-list controls, the also had greater clinical improvements on all but two outcome measures. Linehan et al. (2006) found similarly positive results; DBT was superior to community treatment in terms of reductions on several clinically important outcomes.

Also regarding BPD, Davidson et al. (2006) did not find significant differences between a CBT plus treatment as usual group and a treatment as usual (only) group, at 12- or 24-month follow-up, but results favored the former group at 1- and 2-year follow-ups. Although the Brown, Newman, Charlesworth, Crits-Christoph, and Beck (2004) study was a smaller, uncontrolled trial, they found that CT for BPD was associated with significant improvements on several measures at posttreatment and at 6-month follow-up. Giesen-Bloo et al. (2006) also found that significantly more patients who received Young's schema-focused CT (SFCT; Young, Klosko, & Weishaar, 2003) recovered or showed more reliable clinical improvements on measures of BPD severity, psychopathological dysfunction, and quality of life than those who received psychodynamic transference-focused psychotherapy (TFP) over a 3-year period. There was also a higher rate of attrition for the TFP group. Finally, Svartberg, Stiles, and Seltzer (2004) found that short-term dynamic psychotherapy and CT demonstrated equally significant patient improvements on all measures during and after treatment. The only significant difference between groups was change in symptom distress at posttreatment that favored the dynamic psychotherapy group.

Substance Use Disorders

The treatment efficacy of CBT has yet to be subjected to meta-analyses in the areas of substance use disorders, sleep disorders, and somatoform disorders. However, review papers exist for all three disorders. Morgenstern and McKay (2007) recently found consistent empirical support for motivational interviewing, behavioral couple treatment, CBT (i.e., cognitive or behavioral coping skills geared towards substance dependence disorders), and 12-step treatment in the area of substance use. They concluded that these interventions have specific effects, but they did not find any of them superior to the others, although motivational interviewing produced equivalent results with fewer sessions. Denis, Lavie, Fatseas, and Auriacombe (2007) conducted a review of the literature that was recently published in the Cochrane Library.

Due to heterogeneity, they chose to review rather than meta-analyze six studies on the treatment of cannabis use. No clear conclusion was evident, but they asserted that cannabis dependence is not easily treated by psychotherapies in outpatient settings, based on low observed abstinence rates. Hesse (2004) conducted a focused study on the comparative effects of antidepressants and antidepressants combined with psychotherapy (CBT or manualized, broadly focused counseling) in the treatment of depressive symptoms in individuals with comorbid drug or alcohol dependence. They found no incremental benefit to the combination treatment for substance-dependent depressed patients. In fact, they found that CBT combined with antidepressants did not reveal a significant effect, and that manualized counseling combined with antidepressants resulted in a smaller effect size than that for medications alone. However, Hesse determined that the combination may be useful for individuals who do not experience success with a single treatment. Long-term results were not reported for any of these studies.

Somatoform Disorders

Somatoform disorders have been the subject of at least two reviews. Looper and Kirmayer (2002) reviewed the evidence for CBT in the treatment of hypochondriasis, body dysmorphic disorder (BDD), and undifferentiated somatoform disorders. They calculated the possible effect sizes for RCTs and found positive results for the efficacy of individual CBT for the treatment of hypochondriasis, BDD, medically unexplained symptoms, and functional somatic syndromes. They also found supportive evidence for the efficacy of group CBT for the treatment of BDD and somatization disorder. Long-term results differed by disorder and study. Mai (2004) reviewed the etiology, prevalence, diagnosis, and treatment of somatization disorder, and found that while somatization disorder is common, few patients seek mental health treatment. Although CBT appears to be the most efficacious treatment, both antidepressants and supportive therapy may be effective for some patients.

Sleep Difficulties

Wang, Wang, and Tsai (2005) conducted a systematic review of the literature on the efficacy of CBT for persistent primary insomnia (PI). They focused exclusively on studies that included adult participants, citing the fact that because circadian rhythms change with age, the mechanism that maintains insomnia is different in older populations. They reviewed seven RCTs and found that CBT produced statistically significant changes compared with placebo or waiting list on outcomes such as improvement of sleep efficacy, sleep onset latency, waking after sleep onset, and reductions in sleep medication use. CBT also outperformed less complete treatments, such as stimulus control, relaxation training, and educational programs. One study found that CBT and CBT combined with pharmacotherapy outperformed pharmacotherapy alone, and there were no significant differences in outcomes between CBT and the combination intervention. The beneficial effects of CBT endured over time (3 months to 2 years, depending on the study), whereas those for pharmacotherapy were more time-limited. Wang et al. noted that the components of CBT varied across studies, which led to difficulties in the comparison of findings. Behavioral techniques such as stimulus control and sleep hygiene education were commonly incorporated, but other components, such as relaxation training, differed.

Edinger and Means (2005) also reviewed the efficacy of CBT for treating PI. However, they only reviewed four RCTs that were not specific to a certain age group, and covered two of the same studies as Wang et al. (2005; see also Smith & Neubauer, 2003). Montgomery and Dennis (2003, 2004) reviewed the outcome literature of CBT interventions for improving sleep quality, duration, and efficiency among adults age 60 and up. They found that CBT resulted in a mild effect, best demonstrated for sleep maintenance insomnia. They were unable to make conclusive statements about the efficacy of bright light and exercise for this population due to the lack of data to date. They also indicated that booster sessions of CBT may improve maintenance of gains over the long term.

SUMMARY OF EFFICACY FINDINGS

Given the volume of information provided, a synopsis of the efficacy literature is warranted. Table 2.1 provides a succinct overview, although it does not summarize information regarding the efficacy of CBT relative to a combination of CBT and pharmacotherapy, or the long-term efficacy of CBT, because that evidence was too variable and inconsistent. The following sections summarize the information in Table 2.1 in more detail, directly addressing the six content areas delineated at the beginning of the chapter.

Mood Disorders

There is ample and strong evidence for the controlled absolute efficacy of CBT for unipolar depression. Most of the efficacy studies for unipolar depression did not describe the components included in their definition of CBT. The evidence with regard to the relative efficacy of CBT is equivocal; CBT has been found to be superior to other psychotherapies (e.g., strictly behavioral therapies and non–bona fide treatments) in some studies, and equivalent to some psychotherapies in others (e.g., BT and other bona fide treatments). CBT and pharmacotherapy are equally efficacious in the acute treatment of depression, but CBT has an enduring effect beyond the end of treatment, greater than that observed for pharmacotherapy. A combination of CBT and pharmacotherapy may be more effective than either treatment alone. However, the absolute efficacy of antidepressants relative to pill-placebo has recently been called

TABLE 2.1. Summary of Efficacy Findings by Disorder or Problem

Disorder	Treatment	Absolute efficacy	Efficacy relative to medications	Efficacy relative to other psychotherapies
Unipolar depression	CBT	+	+	≈
Bipolar disorder*	CBT	+		=
Specific phobia	Exposure and cognitive restructuring	++	+	+
Social phobia	Exposure and cognitive restructuring	++	≈	≈
Obsessive–compulsive disorder	Exposure and response prevention and cognitive restructuring	+		+
Panic disorder	Exposure and cognitive restructuring	++	≈	+
Chronic posttraumatic stress disorder	Exposure and cognitive techniques	+		=
Generalized anxiety disorder	CBT	+	+	+
Bulimia nervosa	CBT	+	+	+
Binge-eating disorder	CBT	+		=
Anorexia nervosa	CBT	+	+	=
Schizophrenia*	CBT	+		+ ≈
Marital distress	CBT	+		
Anger and violent offending	CBT	+		
Sexual offending	CBT	+	–**	+ ≈
Chronic pain	CBT	+		≈
Borderline personality disorder	CBT	+		≈
Substance use disorders	CBT	+	+	=
Somatoform disorders	CBT	+	+	+
Sleep difficulties	CBT	+	+	+

Note. A blank space indicates insufficient or no evidence; – indicates negative evidence; + indicates positive evidence; = indicates approximate equivalence; ++ indicates treatment of choice; ≈ indicates equivocal evidence; "CBT" indicates efficacy of specific components unknown; * indicates that CBT is typically used as an adjunct to medication in these disorders; ** indicates efficacy relative to physical treatments (i.e., surgical castration and hormonal treatments).

into question. The long-term efficacy of CBT has been demonstrated up to 2 years.

As an adjunct to pharmacotherapy, CBT can reduce relapse rates for bipolar disorder in the short-term and up to 9 years posttreatment on some measures, although there is significant heterogeneity in long-term findings across studies. CBT combined with pharmacotherapy is equivalent to several other psychotherapy–medication combinations in relapse prevention and in treating depressive symptoms. CBT alone has not been investigated as a treatment for BPD; thus, conclusions cannot be made regarding the relative efficacy of CBT compared with medications or a combination intervention.

Anxiety Disorders

The most robust results for the treatment of specific phobias are obtained by BT, *in vivo* exposure in particular, but it is associated with high dropout rates and low treatment acceptance. Thus, a combination of cognitive and behavioral components may be desirable. Cognitive restructuring alone and in combination with *in vivo* exposure is efficacious in the treatment of claustrophobia, and cognitive restructuring alone is efficacious in the treatment of dental and flying phobias. CBT demonstrates more positive results than hypnotherapy and medication for the treatment of specific phobias. CBT has demonstrated long-term maintenance of gains from 12.0 to 13.8 months for some phobias. CBT demonstrates moderate to large absolute efficacy for the treatment of social phobia. The most frequent combination of CBT components is cognitive restructuring plus exposure, although the superiority of this combination over other combinations, or solo elements, is questionable due to variable findings. One study found that CBT alone and CBT plus pharmacotherapy were equally efficacious. Complicating the data is the fact that CBT and exposure are defined differently across studies. However, group CBT is the most cost-effective and tolerable treatment, and may thus be considered the treatment of choice for social phobia. The long-term efficacy of CBT for social phobia has been demonstrated for up to 12 months.

The absolute efficacy of CBT for OCD is positive and well-supported. Cognitive restructuring and ERP are two frequently combined components of well-defined CBT interventions. The incremental benefit of adding cognitive techniques to BT is not supported; BT typically outperforms CBT. However, cognitive techniques increase the tolerability of the intervention, motivate clients, and help them manage the exposure-based components. CBT has not been compared with other psychotherapies, aside from BT. A direct comparison between pharmacotherapy and CBT has not been conducted, so conclusive statements cannot be made. A small amount of data indicates that a combination of pharmacotherapy and CBT may be superior to either intervention alone. There are insufficient data to comment on the sustained efficacy of CBT, and to differentiate between the results for PD and for PDA.

The controlled and uncontrolled absolute efficacy of CBT for PD/PDA has been amply demonstrated. The typical components of CBT for PD/PDA are exposure and cognitive restructuring. The addition of cognitive components to behavioral components for the treatment of PD/PDA does not result in incremental value in terms of reduced anxiety, but it does in terms of reduced depressive symptoms and attrition rates. CT is superior to RT, but no other comparisons between psychotherapies and CBT have been reviewed. The evidence for the relative efficacy of pharmacotherapy and CBT is mixed; some studies have found that the two are equally efficacious; others have found divergent results depending on the outcome measures examined, and still others have found evidence for the superiority of CBT over pharmacotherapy. There are also mixed results regarding the relative efficacy of CBT alone and a combined CBT–pharmacotherapy intervention. Last, CBT has the best cost profile of the interventions, and the long-term efficacy of CBT has been demonstrated up to an average of 16.8 months.

Chronic PTSD has received the most research attention, but immediate posttrauma experiences and acute PTSD have also been examined in the CBT treatment efficacy literature. TFCBT (i.e., exposure and cognitive techniques focused on the trauma) is the form of CBT most widely studied. For chronic PTSD, TFCBT and EMDR have both demonstrated controlled absolute efficacy, are superior to "other therapies," and are not significantly different from one another. Due to limited and inconclusive evidence, TFCBT can only tentatively be considered superior to pharmacotherapy (i.e., paroxetine) for the treatment of chronic PTSD. The controlled absolute efficacy of CBT for the treatment of GAD is well-established for the short-term; however, long-term results are indeterminate due to insufficient data. The relative efficacy of pharmacotherapy compared with CBT is less clear; the evidence is mixed, depending on the specific effects calculated. However, researchers in at least one review surmised that CBT is better tolerated than pharmacotherapy. CBT has demonstrated superiority over psychodynamic therapy (at posttreatment and 6-month follow-up), partial superiority over supportive therapy, mixed results compared with BT, and equivalent efficacy compared with RT. The relative efficacy of CBT compared with combined CBT and pharmacotherapy was not reported in the meta-analyses we reviewed. The treatment literature on CBT for GAD includes many components under the rubric of CBT, including anxiety management training, cognitive restructuring, situational exposure, self-controlled desensitization, RT/training, CT alone, and BT alone.

Eating Disorders

Among several other psychotherapies, CBT has demonstrated waiting-list controlled absolute efficacy for the treatment of BN. A variety of procedures are considered CBT or CBT-BN. On some outcome measures, CBT is superior to support, nutritional counseling, supportive–expressive therapy, BT components alone, ERP, self-monitoring, and hypnobehavioral therapy. Group CBT and IPT are equal and more efficacious than waiting-list on certain measures; however, individually administered CBT is superior to individually administered IPT on others. CBT augmented by ERP is not superior to CBT alone, but there is some evidence for an incremental benefit of psychotherapy combined with medication over either intervention alone. CBT alone is also superior to pharmacotherapy alone, and although dropout rates are higher in the medication trials than in the CBT trials, the difference is not significant. Most studies do not report long-term findings due to insufficient data and heterogeneity in outcome measures and follow-up time spans. CBT has demonstrated controlled absolute efficacy on several outcome measures for BED, although weight was not significantly reduced from baseline to follow-up (4 months). CBT and IPT are equally efficacious on several measures, but CBT is superior to IPT on others. There is some evidence to suggest that a combination of CBT and medication is efficacious, but the efficacy of either measure alone is unknown.

The treatment outcome literature regarding CBT for AN is sparse and flawed. However, there is some evidence to support CBT in reducing risk of relapse after weight restoration. One study found superiority for CBT over nutritional counseling, but these results were confounded by a large percentage of participants with positive outcomes, who were also taking medications. Otherwise, CBT has not been found to demonstrate superiority over other psychotherapies. It is generally agreed that the use of medications, antidepressants in particular, is not warranted for the treatment of AN due to lack of supportive evidence and high rates of attrition. Long-term results were not reported frequently enough to make any conclusive statements.

Other Disorders

CBT for schizophrenia is an adjunctive treatment to pharmacotherapy and comprises a range of techniques. Both the controlled and uncontrolled absolute efficacy of CBT for schizophrenia has been demonstrated at posttreatment, with maintenance of gains for more than 12 months, and increased improvements in gains at early follow-up. The efficacy of CBT for schizophrenia is greater for patients with an acute psychotic episode than those suffering from chronic symptoms, and has been demonstrated for both positive and negative symptoms. CBT has demonstrated superiority over problem solving, recreation and support, supportive therapy, a befriending intervention, and psychoeducation, with gains persisting up to 18 months posttreatment. CBT for schizophrenia has demonstrated lower rates of attrition than those for standard care. Comparisons between CBT alone and medication alone, and combinations of the two compared with the solo therapies, were not found, presumably due to the fact that CBT is always administered in conjunction with pharmacotherapy for schizophrenia.

CBMT for couple distress incorporates behavioral interventions and an emphasis on changing maladaptive cognitions regarding individuals, their partners, or the relationship. CBMT, BMT, and IOMT are all associated with significant changes in behavior from pre- to posttreatment, and over follow-up. Comparisons of CBMT with pharmacotherapy and with a combination intervention were not reported.

CBT is often considered the treatment of choice for anger management, incorporating techniques such as relaxation, cognitive restructuring, problem solving, and stress inoculation. In terms of absolute efficacy, CBT has demonstrated a large controlled effect size, but no long-term results were reported. Positive controlled absolute efficacy for CBT in the reduction of criminal offenses posttreatment and up to 12 months posttreatment has also been demonstrated. No differences in efficacy between brand-name and generic forms of CBT were found when researchers controlled for certain variables. The relative efficacy of CBT compared with other psychotherapies and with pharmacotherapy was not reported.

Treated sexual offenders have lower rates of recidivism than untreated offenders, up to 5 years posttreatment. That said, only those treatments specific to the treatment of sex offenders are efficacious; others have demonstrated negative outcomes. One study found that surgical castration resulted in the largest effects, followed by hormonal treatments, CBT, and then BT. The components of CBT were not defined. However, CBT and hormonal treatments were deemed the most promising due to the methodological confounds inherent in the findings associated with physical treatments, and the ethical, legal, and medical implications for surgical castration. Another study found that hormonal treatments and CBT were equally efficacious and superior to behavioral treatments. In the studies reviewed, comparisons were made between psychotherapies and physical therapies, but not pharmacotherapies.

CBT for chronic pain has demonstrated moderately large, controlled absolute effect sizes. Although the studies reviewed did not directly compare treatments, the effect sizes for CBT were larger than those for BT on most domains, and biofeedback was superior to both on several domains. When compared with a heterogeneous sample of other active treatments, not including BT or biofeedback, CBT was found to be superior on some domains but not on others. Long-term outcomes and comparisons with pharmacotherapy were not reported. DBT is the most frequently studied form of CBT for use in treating BPD, which is the most studied of the personality disorders. DBT has demonstrated significant pre- to posttest changes on several measures, as well as controlled absolute efficacy on some measures. CBT plus treatment as usual was not significantly different from treatment as usual at posttreatment, but it did demonstrate superiority on some measures at 1- and 2-year follow-up. Young's SFCT for BPD demonstrated superiority over TFP over a 3-year period. In contrast, short-term dynamic psychotherapy and CT demonstrated equally significant patient improvements for the treatment of one or more Cluster C personality disorders, with the exception of one outcome measure, on which the former outperformed the latter.

Motivational interviewing, behavioral couple treatment, CBT (i.e., cognitive or behavioral coping skills geared towards substance dependence disorders), and 12-step treatments have consistently demonstrated efficacy and specific effects for the treatment of substance use disorders, without significant differences among the interventions. However, motivational interviewing produced equivalent results with fewer sessions. The data are not forthcoming with regard to the treatment for cannabis use, although, based on low abstinence rates, a tentative conclusion can be made that cannabis use is not easily treated by psychotherapies in outpatient settings. One review found no incremental benefit to combining antidepressants with psychotherapy for the treatment of substance-dependent depressed patients, although reviewers estimated that the combination may be useful for those individuals who do not experience success with one treatment or the other. Long-term results, and the comparative efficacy of CBT and pharmacotherapy alone were not reported.

The components of CBT for the treatment of somatoform disorders vary widely. One review found positive results supporting the efficacy of individual CBT for the treatment of hypochondriasis, BDD, medically unexplained symptoms, and functional somatic syndromes, such as noncardiac chest pain and chronic fatigue syndrome, and supportive evidence for the efficacy of group CBT for the treatment of BDD and somatization disorder. Long-term results differed by disorder and by study. Another review found that although both antidepressants and supportive therapy may be effective for some individuals, CBT is the most efficacious treatment for somatization disorder. The components of CBT for sleep difficulties differ widely across studies, though they have demonstrated positive benefits singularly and in combination. Multifaceted CBT has demonstrated significant changes compared with waiting-list or placebo and other programs. CBT alone and in combination with pharmacotherapy has outperformed pharmacotherapy alone, but the combination has not outperformed CBT alone. CBT has enduring positive effects up to 2 years posttreatment.

LIMITATIONS OF THE LITERATURE
AND ISSUES FOR FUTURE RESEARCH

CBT has been applied to a wide variety of disorders and problems, and has shown positive treatment gains across the board in terms of absolute efficacy. CBT has also demonstrated strengths such as lower dropout rates than pharmacotherapy (e.g., PD, Gould et al., 1995; BN, Whittal et al., 1999), lower dropout rates than ERP in the treatment of OCD (Abramowitz et al., 2005), and greater acceptability (i.e., perceived as less aversive or intrusive) than exposure for the treatment of specific phobias (Hunt et al., 2006; Koch et al., 2004). Despite these significant positive findings, there remain several areas in which the literature on the efficacy of CBT is lacking or equivocal, requiring further study: insufficient research comparing the efficacy of CBT with that of pharmacotherapy; insufficient research on the comparison of other psychotherapies with CBT; insufficient empirical evaluation of treatments for use with diverse populations; insufficient research investigating the efficacy of CBT in the prevention of relapse; insufficient research on CBT for use with comorbid disorder presentations; insufficient research on the efficacy of specific forms of CBT for specific disorders; and insufficient research on long-term evidence. Follow-up time points are not consistently reported; some studies only assess short-term outcomes, but no long-term outcomes at all.

The assessment of long-term outcome is not easy due to concerns about the randomization of participants to certain control conditions. Some studies resolve this issue by incorporating waiting-list conditions in which participants receive therapy after a certain period of time. However, the length of wait time cannot be protracted for the same ethical concerns. Another means of circumventing this difficulty is to conduct within-group analyses. Literature on the efficacy of CBT for use with diverse populations is increasing, and there are now recommendations for adaptations of CBT for use with minority populations (e.g., Hays & Iwamasa, 2006), as well as research on the efficacy of culturally adapted CBT for use with minority populations (e.g., Muñoz et al., 1995). However, the suitability and efficacy of CBT for use with diverse populations remains an empirical question given the paucity of data.

Other criticisms pertain to research methodology. It has been argued that amalgamating placebo and waiting-list controls into a composite control condition confounds results (Parker, Roy, & Eyers, 2003). Specifically, Parker et al. asserted that participants assigned to a placebo condition are hopeful, because they assume that they are being treated, whereas participants assigned to a waiting-list control condition are discouraged, because they are not undergoing any treatment. They recommended that future research compare active treatments to different control conditions to disentangle potentially differing results. In the same vein, Gould et al. (1995; Gould, Buckminster, et al., 1997; Gould, Otto, et al., 1997) have argued that because CBT is frequently compared with a waiting-list control condition, whereas drug trials typically involve pill-placebo controls, CBT is favored in comparisons with pharmacotherapy, so the difference in treatment gains would be greater in a CBT versus waiting-list comparison than in a pharmacotherapy versus placebo comparison. Gould and colleagues have recommended nondirective therapy as an alternative control to waiting-list control given its greater similarity to a placebo control in terms of resulting positive treatment effects.

Another concern involves the issue of treatment labeling. Therapies using similar treatment elements are sometimes classified as "behavioral" and sometimes as "cognitive-behavioral," thereby confounding comparisons between studies. Moreover, the comparison between CBT and other psychotherapies may be distorted in some studies. Analysis of the videotaped therapy sessions of the National Institute of Mental Health collaborative project, which compared IPT, CT, placebo, and pharmacotherapy, found that therapists in the

IPT group adhered more to the CT protocol than to the interpersonal therapy protocol, thus providing a salient example of confounded treatment comparisons (Ablon & Jones, 2002). This result reinforces the importance of adherence to treatment manuals and the assessment of therapist fidelity to treatment conditions in research trials, to ensure a reasonable test of the treatment under investigation (McGlinchey & Dobson, 2003).

In addition to limitations to the research base on the efficacy of CBT, there are limitations to efficacy research in general. Although RCTs are highly utilized and respected in efficacy research, the reelvance of their results to routine clinical practice has been questioned (Leichsenring et al., 2006). For example, the restrictive exclusion criteria of many RCTs may undermine the representativeness of the participants to the general population of people with the disorder. Also, comorbidities are common among disorders but are controlled for in RCTs through exclusionary criteria, or are simply not addressed. Also, researcher allegiance, or the tendency of the authors of a comparative treatment study to prefer one treatment over another, may introduce bias into the study design that results in findings supportive of the preferred treatment (Butler et al., 2006). There has been a call for more treatment effectiveness studies to complement the wealth of treatment efficacy studies in the literature, because effectiveness studies are conducted in clinical practice and their findings are considered more generalizable than efficacy findings to actual clinical practice. Some studies have addressed this issue. Wade, Treat, and Stuart (1998) compared treatment outcome data collected in a community mental health setting with results from two controlled efficacy trials. They found comparably positive results for CBT across both study designs, in the acute treatment of PD, and at 1-year follow-up (Stuart, Treat, & Wade, 2000). Merrill, Tolbert, and Wade (2003) also demonstrated the comparability of results across designs when they found that CBT delivered in a community outpatient setting produced similar treatment gains for depression as those treatment gains observed in two RCTs.

Meta-analysis has also been criticized on several grounds. It minimizes methodological differences across studies, such as variable outcome measures (Rosenthal, 1998). The choice of outcome measures can bias the relative strength of a treatment effect, as can the number of treatment sessions and length per session, but meta-analysis masks these variable details across studies. Interactions among treatment and patient characteristics are also concealed, because meta-analysis collapses treatment effects across divergent samples. Last, the conclusions of different meta-analyses within a given treatment area differ as a result of the use of different computational formulae and procedures (e.g., weighted vs. unweighted effect size estimates, within-study vs. control comparisons). Further research is indicated to clarify the comparative efficacy of different active treatments and the long-term efficacy of CBT.

In summary, a large body of evidence indicates that CBT is an efficacious treatment for a wide variety of disorders. Gaps in the knowledge base, however, require further research on the relative efficacy of CBT compared with pharmacotherapy, and with other psychotherapies. Further research is also required to determine the efficacy of CBT for use with diverse populations, for the prevention of relapse, and for use with comorbid disorder presentations. Future research determining the efficacy of specific forms of CBT for specific disorders and the long-term efficacy of CBT would also contribute to the treatment outcome literature on CBT. Researchers should consider their use of control conditions and be careful to define specifically the treatment approaches included in their studies.

REFERENCES

Ablon, J., & Jones, E. (2002). Validity of controlled clinical trials of psychotherapy: Findings from the NIMH Treatment of Depression Collaborative Research Program. *American Journal of Psychiatry, 159*, 775–783.

Abramowitz, J. (1997). Effectiveness of psychological and pharmacological treatments for obsessive–compulsive disorder: A quantitative review. *Journal of Consulting and Clinical Psychology, 65*, 44–52.

Abramowitz, J. S., Taylor, S., & McKay, D. (2005). Potentials and limitations of cognitive treatments for obsessive–compulsive disorder. *Cognitive Behaviour Therapy, 34*(3), 140–147.

Allen, A. (2006). Cognitive-behavior therapy and other psychosocial interventions in the treatment of obsessive–compulsive disorder. *Psychiatric Annals, 36*(7), 474–479.

Bandelow, B., Seidler-Brandler, U., Becker, A., Wedekind, D., & Rüther, E. (2007). Meta-analysis of randomized controlled comparisons of psychopharmacological and psychological treatments for anxiety disorders. *World Journal of Biological Psychiatry, 8*(3), 175–187.

Beck, R., & Fernandez, E. (1998). Cognitive-behavioral therapy in the treatment of anger: A meta-analysis. *Cognitive Therapy and Research, 22*(1), 63–74.

Beck, A. T., Rush, A. J., Shaw, B. F., & Emery, G. (1979). *Cognitive therapy of depression*. New York: Guilford Press.

Bisson, J., Ehlers, A., Matthews, R., Pilling, S., Richards, D., & Turner, S. (2007). Psychological treatments for chronic post-traumatic stress disorder: Systematic review and analysis. *British Journal of Psychiatry, 190*, 97–104.

Bohus, M., Haaf, B., Simms, T., Limberger, M. F., Schumahl, C., & Unckel, C. (2004). Effectiveness of inpatient dialectical behavior therapy for borderline personality disorder: A controlled trial. *Behaviour Research and Therapy, 42*, 487–499.

Bowers, W. A., & Andersen, A. E. (2007). Cognitive-behavior therapy with eating disorders: The role of medications in treatment. *Journal of Cognitive Psychotherapy: An International Quarterly, 21*(1), 16–27.

Brown, G. K., Newman, C. F., Charlesworth, S. E., Crits-Christoph, P., & Beck, A. T. (2004). An open clinical trial of cognitive therapy for borderline personality disorder. *Journal of Personality Disorders, 18*(3), 257–271.

Brownley, K. A., Berkman, N D., Sedway, J. A., Lohr, K. N., & Bulik, C. M. (2007). Binge eating disorder treatment: A systematic review of randomized controlled trials. *International Journal of Eating Disorders, 40*(4), 337–348.

Bulik, C. M., Berkman, N. D., Brownley, K. A., Sedway, J. A., & Lohr, K. N. (2007).

Anorexia nervosa treatment: A systematic review and randomized controlled trials. *International Journal of Eating Disorders, 40*(4), 310–320.

Butler, A. C., Chapman, J. E., Forman, E. M., & Beck, A. T. (2006). The empirical status of cognitive-behavioral therapy: A review of meta-analyses. *Clinical Psychology Review, 26,* 17–31.

Chambless, D. L., Baker, M. J., Baucom, D. H., Beutler, L. E., Calhoun, K. S., Crits-Christoph, P., et al. (1998). Update on empirically validated therapies, II. *The Clinical Psychologist, 51,* 3–16.

Chambless, D. L., & Hope, D. A. (1996). Cognitive approaches to the psychopathology and treatment of social phobia. In P. M. Salkovskis (Ed.), *Frontiers of cognitive therapy* (pp. 345–382. New York: Guilford Press.

Choy, Y., Fyer, A. J., Lipsitz, J. D. (2006). Treatment of specific phobia in adults. *Clinical Psychology Review, 27*(3), 266–286.

Cohen, J. (1988). *Statistical power analysis for the behavioral sciences* (2nd ed.). Mahwah, NJ: Erlbaum.

Colom, F., & Vieta, E. (2004). A perspective on the use of psychoeducation, cognitive-behavioral therapy and interpersonal therapy for bipolar patients. *Bipolar Disorders, 6,* 480–486.

Davidson, K., Norrie, J., Tyrer, P., Gumley, A., Tata, P, Murray, H., et al. (2006). The effectiveness of cognitive behavior therapy for borderline personality disorder: Results from the borderline personality disorder study of cognitive therapy (BOSCOT) trial. *Journal of Personality Disorders, 20*(5), 450–465.

Davidson, K. W., Trudeau, K. J., Ockene, J. K., Orleans, C. T., & Kaplan, R. M. (2004). A primer on current evidence-based review systems and their implications for behavioral medicine. *Annals of Behavioral Medicine, 28*(3), 226–238.

Denis, C., Lavie, E., Fatseas, M., & Auriacombe, M. (2007). Psychotherapeutic interventions for cannabis abuse and/or dependence in outpatient settings. *Cochrane Database of Systematic Reviews, 3.*

DeRubeis, R. J., Hollon, S. D., Amsterdam, J. D., Shelton, R. C., Young, P. R., Salomon, R. M., et al. (2005). Cognitive therapy vs. medications in the treatment of moderate to severe depression. *Archives of General Psychiatry, 62,* 409–416.

Dimidjian, S., Hollon, S. D., Dobson, K. S., Kohlenberg, R. J., Gallop, R., Markley, D. K., et al. (2006). Randomized trial of behavioral activation, cognitive therapy, and antidepressant medication in the acute treatment of adults with major depression. *Journal of Consulting and Clinical Psychology, 74,* 658–670.

Dobson, K. S. (1989). A meta-analysis of the efficacy of cognitive therapy for depression. *Journal of Consulting and Clinical Psychology, 57*(3), 414–419.

Dobson, K. S. (Ed.). (2001). *Handbook of cognitive-behavioral therapies* (2nd ed.). New York: Guilford Press.

Dunn, R. L., & Schwebel, A. I. (1995). Meta-analytic review of martial therapy outcome research. *Journal of Family Psychology, 9*(1), 58–68.

Eddy, K. T., Dutra, L., Bradley, R., & Westen, D. (2004). A multidimensional meta-analysis of psychotherapy and pharmacotherapy for obsessive–compulsive disorder. *Clinical Psychology Review, 24,* 1011–1030.

Edinger, J. D., & Means, M. K. (2005). Cognitive-behavioral therapy for primary insomnia. *Clinical Psychology Review, 25,* 539–558.

Elliott, R. (1998). Editor's introduction: A guide to the empirically supported treatments controversy. *Psychotherapy Research, 8,* 115–125.

Fedoroff, I. C., & Taylor, S. (2001). Psychological and pharmacological treatments of social phobia: A meta-analysis. *Journal of Clinical Psychopharmacology, 21*(3), 311–324.

Feske, U., & Chambless, D. L. (1995). Cognitive behavioral versus exposure only treatment for social phobia: A meta-analysis. *Behavior Therapy, 26,* 695–720.

Fresco, D. M., & Heimberg, R. G. (2001). Empirically supported psychological treatments for social phobia. *Psychiatric Annals, 31*(8), 489–496.

Giesen-Bloo, J., van Dyck, R., Spinhoven, P., van Tilburg, W., Dirksen, C., van Asselt, T., et al. (2006). Outpatient psychotherapy for borderline personality disorder: A randomized trial of schema-focused therapy vs transference-focused psychotherapy. *Archives of General Psychiatry, 63,* 649–658.

Gloaguen, V., Cottraux, J., Cucherat, M., & Blackburn, I. (1998). A meta-analysis of the effects of cognitive therapy in depressed patients. *Journal of Affective Disorders, 49,* 59–72.

Gonzalez-Pinto, A., Gonzalez, C., Enjuto, S., Fernandez de Corres, B., Lopez, P., Palomo, J., et al. (2004). Psychoeducation and cognitive-behavioral therapy in bipolar disorder: An update. *Acta Psychiatrica Scandinavica, 109,* 83–90.

Gould, R. A., Buckminster, S., Pollack, M. H., Otto, M. W., & Yap, L. (1997). Cognitive-behavioral and pharmacological treatment for social phobia: A meta-analysis. *Clinical Psychology: Science and Practice, 4,* 291–306.

Gould, R. A., Mueser, K. T., Bolton, E., Mays, V., & Goff, D. (2001). Cognitive therapy for psychosis in schizophrenia: An effect size analysis. *Schizophrenia Research, 48,* 335–342.

Gould, R. A., Otto, M. W., & Pollack, M. M. (1995). A meta-analysis of treatment outcome for panic disorder. *Clinical Psychology Review, 15*(8), 819–844.

Gould, R. A., Otto, M. W., Pollack, M. H., & Yap, L. (1997). Cognitive behavioral and pharmacological treatment of generalized anxiety disorder: A preliminary meta-analysis. *Behavior Therapy, 28,* 285–305.

Hall, G. C. N. (1995). Sexual offender recidivism revisited: A meta-analysis of recent treatment studies. *Journal of Consulting and Clinical Psychology, 63*(5), 802–809.

Hanson, R. K., Gordon, A., Harris, A. J. R., Marques, J. K., Murphy, W., Quinsey, V. L., et al. (2002). First report of the collaborative outcome data project on the effectiveness of psychological treatment for sex offenders. *Sexual Abuse: A Journal of Research and Treatment, 14*(2), 169–194.

Hay, P. J., Bacaltchuk, J., & Stefano, S. (2004). Psychotherapy for bulimia nervosa and binging. *Cochrane Database of Systematic Reviews, 3,* 1–122.

Hays, P. A., & Iwamasa, G. Y. (2006). *Culturally responsive cognitive-behavioral therapy.* Washington, DC: American Psychological Association.

Heimberg, R. G. (2002). Cognitive-behavioral therapy for social anxiety disorder: Current status and future directions. *Biological Psychiatry, 51,* 101–108.

Hesse, M. (2004). Achieving abstinence by treating depression in the presence of substance-use disorders. *Addictive Behaviors, 29,* 1137–1141.

Hollon, S. D., DeRubeis, R. J., Shelton, R. C., Amsterdam, J. D., Salomon, R. M., O'Reardon, J. P., et al. (2005). Prevention of relapse following cognitive therapy vs. medications in moderate to severe depression. *Archives of General Psychiatry, 62,* 417–422.

Hollon, S.D., Stewart, M. O., & Strunk, D. (2006). Enduring effects for cognitive behavior therapy in the treatment of depression and anxiety. *Annual Review of Psychology, 57,* 285–315.

Hunot, V., Churchill, R., Teixeira, V., & Silva de Lima, M. (2007). Psychological therapies for generalized anxiety disorder. *Cochrane Database of Systematic Reviews, 1,* 1–75.

Hunt, M., Bylsma, L., Brock, J., Fenton, M., Goldberg, A., Miller, R., et al. (2006). The role of imagery in the maintenance and treatment of snake fear. *Journal of Behavior Therapy and Experimental Psychiatry, 37,* 283–298.

Jones, S. (2004). Psychotherapy of bipolar disorder: A review. *Journal of Affective Disorders, 80,* 101–114.

Kazdin, A. E. (2003). *Research design in clinical psychology* (4th ed.). Boston: Allyn & Bacon.

Kirsch, I., Deacon, B. J., Huedo-Medina, T. B., Scoboria, A., Moore, T. J., et al. (2008). Initial severity and antidepressant benefits: A meta-analysis of data submitted to the Food and Drug Administration. *PLoS Medicine, 5,* 0260–0268.

Koch, E. I., Spates, C. R., & Himle, J. A. (2004). Comparison of behavioral and cognitive-behavioral one-session exposure treatments for small animal phobias. *Behaviour Research and Therapy, 42,* 1483–1504.

Landenberger, N. A., & Lipsey, M. W. (2005). The positive effects of cognitive-behavioral programs for violent offenders: A meta-analysis of factors associated with effective treatment. *Journal of Experimental Criminology, 1,* 451–476.

Landon, T. M., & Barlow, D. H. (2004). Cognitive-behavioral treatment for panic disorder: Current status. *Journal of Psychiatric Practice, 10*(4), 211–226.

Leichensring, F., Hiller, W., Weissberg, M., & Leibing, E. (2006). Cognitive-behavioral therapy and psychodynamic psychotherapy: Techniques, efficacy, and indications. *American Journal of Psychotherapy, 60,* 233–259.

Lewandowski, L., Gebing, T. Anthony, J., & O'Brien, W. (1997). Meta-analysis of cognitive- behavioral treatment studies for bulimia. *Clinical Psychology Review, 17*(7), 703–718.

Linehan, M. M. (1993). *Cognitive-behavioral treatment of borderline personality disorder.* New York: Guilford Press.

Linehan, M. M., Comtois, K. A., Murray, A. M., Brown, M. Z., Gallop, R. J., Heard, H. L., et al. (2006). Two-year randomized controlled trial and follow-up of dialectical behavior therapy vs therapy by experts for suicidal behaviors and borderline personality disorder. *Archives of General Psychiatry, 63,* 757–766.

Looper, K. J., & Kirmayer, L. J. (2002). Behavioral medicine approaches to somatoform disorders. *Journal of Consulting and Clinical Psychiatry, 70*(3), 810–827.

Lösel, F., & Schmucker, M. (2005). The effectiveness of treatment for sexual offenders: A comprehensive meta-analysis. *Journal of Experimental Criminology, 1,* 117–146.

Mai, F. (2004). Somatization disorder: A practical review. *Canadian Journal of Psychiatry, 49*(10), 652–662.

McGlinchey, J., & Dobson, K. S. (2003). Treatment integrity concerns in cognitive therapy for depression. *Journal of Cognitive Psychotherapy: An International Quarterly, 17,* 299–318.

Merrill, K. A., Tolbert, V. E., & Wade, W. A. (2003). Effectiveness of cognitive therapy for depression in a community mental health center: A benchmarking strategy. *Journal of Consulting and Clinical Psychology, 71,* 404–409.

Miklowitz, D. J., & Otto, M. W. (2006). New psychosocial intervention for bipolar disorder: A review of literature and introduction of the systematic treatment enhancement program. *Journal of Cognitive Psychotherapy: An International Quarterly, 20*(2), 215–230.

Mitte, K. (2005a). A meta-analysis of the efficacy of psycho- and pharmacotherapy in panic disorder with and without agoraphobia. *Journal of Affective Disorders, 88*, 27–45.

Mitte, K. (2005b). Meta-analysis of cognitive-behavioral treatments for generalized anxiety disorder: A comparison with pharmacotherapy. *Psychological Bulletin, 131*(5), 785–795.

Montgomery, P., & Dennis, J. (2003). Cognitive behavioral interventions for sleep problems in adults aged 60+. *Cochrane Database of Systematic Reviews, 1,* 1–32.

Montgomery, P., & Dennis, J. (2004). A systematic review of non-pharmacological therapies for sleep problems in later life. *Sleep Medicine Reviews, 8*, 47–62.

Morgenstern, J., & McKay, J. R. (2007). Rethinking the paradigms that inform behavioral treatment research for substance use disorders. *Addiction, 102,* 1377–1389.

Morley, S., Eccleston, C., & Williams, A. (1999). Systematic review and meta-analysis of randomized controlled trials of cognitive behavior therapy and behavior therapy for chronic pain in adults, excluding headache. *Pain, 80*, 1–13.

Muñoz, R. F., Ying, Y. W., Bernal, G., Pérez-Stable, E. J., Sorensen, J. L., Hargreaves, W. A., et al. (1995). Prevention of depression with primary care patients: A randomized controlled trial. *American Journal of Community Psychology, 23,* 199–222.

Norcross, J. C., Hedges, M., & Prochaska, J. O. (2002). The face of 2010: A Delphi poll on the future of psychotherapy. *Professional Psychology: Research and Practice, 33*, 316–322.

National Collaborating Centre for Mental Health. (2005). *Clinical Guideline 26: Post-traumatic stress disorder: The management of PTSD in adults and children in primary and secondary care.* London: National Institute for Clinical Excellence.

Oei, T. P. S., Llamas, M., & Devilly, G. J. (1999). The efficacy and cognitive processes of cognitive behaviour therapy in the treatment of panic disorder with agoraphobia. *Behavioral and Cognitive Psychotherapy, 27*, 63–88.

Parker, G., Roy, K., & Eyers, K. (2003). Cognitive behavior therapy for depression?: Choose horses for courses. *American Journal of Psychiatry, 160*, 825–834.

Pilling, S., Bebbington, P., Kuipers, E., Garety, P., Geddes, J., Orbach, G., et al. (2002). Psychological treatments in schizophrenia: I. Meta-analysis of family intervention and cognitive behaviour therapy. *Psychological Medicine, 32*, 763–782.

Rector, N. A., & Beck, A. T. (2001). Cognitive behavioral therapy for schizophrenia: An empirical review. *Journal of Nervous and Mental Disease, 189*(5), 278–287.

Rodebaugh, T. L., Holaway, R. M., & Heimberg, R. G. (2004). The treatment of social anxiety disorder. *Clinical Psychology Review, 24*, 883–908.

Rosenthal, R. (1998). Meta-analysis: Concepts, corollaries and controversies. In J. G. Adair & D. Belanger (Eds.), *Advances in psychological science, Vol. 1: Social, personal, and cultural aspects* (pp. 371–384). Hove, UK: Psychology Press.

Rowa, K., & Antony, M. M. (2005). Psychological treatments for social phobia. *Canadian Journal of Psychiatry, 50*(6), 308–316.

Segal, Z., Vincent, P., & Levitt, A. (2002). Efficacy of combined, sequential and crossover psychotherapy and pharmacotherapy in improving outcomes in depression. *Journal of Psychiatry and Neuroscience, 27*(4), 281–290.

Seidler, G. H., & Wagner, F. E. (2006). Comparing the efficacy of EMDR and trauma-focused cognitive-behavioral therapy in the treatment of PTSD: A meta-analytic study. *Psychological Medicine, 36*, 1515–1522.

Shapiro, J. R., Berkman, N. D., Brownley, K. A., Sedway, J. A., Lohr, K. N., & Bulik, C. M. (2007). Bulimia nervosa treatment: A systematic review of randomized controlled trials. *International Journal of Eating Disorders, 40*(4), 321–336.

Siev, J., & Chambless, D. L. (2007). Specificity of treatment effects: Cognitive therapy and relaxation for generalized anxiety and panic disorders. *Journal of Consulting and Clinical Psychology, 75*(4), 513–522.

Smith, M.T., & Neubauer, D.N. (2003). Cognitive behavior therapy for chronic insomnia. *Clinical Cornerstone, 5*(3), 28–40.

Stuart, G. L., Treat, T. A., & Wade, W. A. (2000). Effectiveness of an empirically based treatment for panic disorder delivered in a service clinic setting: 1–year follow-up. *Journal of Consulting and Clinical Psychology, 68*, 506–512.

Svartberg, M., Stiles, T. C., & Seltzer, M. H. (2004). Randomized, controlled trial of the effectiveness of short-term dynamic psychotherapy and cognitive therapy for cluster C personality disorders. *American Journal of Psychiatry, 161*, 810–817.

Taylor, S. (1996). Meta-analysis of cognitive-behavioral treatments for social phobia. *Journal of Behavior Therapy and Experimental Psychiatry, 27*, 1–9.

van Balkom, A. J. L. M., van Oppen, P., Vermeulen, A. W. A., van Dyck, R., Nauta, N. C. E., & Vorst, H. C. H. (1994). A meta-analysis on the treatment of obsessive–compulsive disorder: A comparison of antidepressants, behavior, and cognitive therapy. *Clinical Psychology Review, 14*(5), 359–381.

Wade, W. A., Treat, T. A., & Stuart, G. L. (1998). Transporting an empirically supported treatment for panic disorder to a service clinic setting: A benchmarking strategy. *Journal of Consulting and Clinical Psychology, 66*, 231–239.

Wang, M., Wang, S., & Tsai, P. (2005). Cognitive behavioral therapy for primary insomnia: A systematic review. *Journal of Advanced Nursing, 50*(5), 553–564.

Whittal, M. L., Agras, W. S., & Gould. R. A. (1999). Bulimia nervosa: A meta-analysis of psychosocial and pharmacological treatments. *Behavior Therapy, 30*, 117–135.

Wampold, B. E., Minami, T., Baskin. T. W., & Tierney, S. C. (2002). A meta-(re) analysis of the effects of cognitive therapy versus "other therapies" for depression. *Journal of Affective Disorders, 68*, 159–165.

Wood, N. D., Crane, D. R., Schaalje, G. B., & Law, D. D. (2005). What works for whom: A meta-analytic review of marital and couples therapy in reference to marital distress. *American Journal of Family Therapy, 33*, 273–287.

Young, J. E., Klosko, J. S., & Weishaar, M. E. (2003). *Schema therapy: A practitioner's guide.* New York: Guilford Press.

Zaretsky, A. E., Rizvi, P., & Parikh, V. (2007). How well do psychosocial interventions work in bipolar disorder? *Canadian Journal of Psychiatry, 52*, 14–21.

Zimmermann, G., Favrod, T. J., Trieu, V. H., & Pomini, V. (2005). The effect of cognitive behavioral treatment on the positive symptoms of schizophrenia spectrum disorders: A meta-analysis. *Schizophrenia Research, 77*, 1–9.

CHAPTER 3

Cognitive Science and the Conceptual Foundations of Cognitive-Behavioral Therapy

Viva la Evolution!

Rick E. Ingram
Greg J. Siegle

Our goal in this chapter is to discuss the conceptual underpinnings of cognitive-behavioral therapy (CBT). We discuss the theoretical antecedents and assumptions that underlie information-processing ideas that inform our understanding of psychopathology, as well as ideas about how to treat psychopathology through changes in information processing. To appreciate these ideas, we briefly note the history of the cognitive concepts in clinical psychology, then examine the antecedents and assumptions of basic cognitive science.

Our focus is on cognitive science for two reasons. First, although CBT was not originally based on cognitive science as it is currently understood, the ideas and assumptions of cognitive science nonetheless can be seen as the foundation of contemporary CBT. Hence, we believe that to truly understand CBT, it is essential to understand the conceptualization, measurement, and methods to study cognition. Second, the understanding that cognitive science brings to the practice of CBT can also suggest treatment innovations, novel methods, and new ways to measure treatment effects. Thus, we examine not only some of the concepts and methods of cognitive science but also ideas about how these concepts and methods can be, and have been, applied to CBT. We start with an examination of how ideas about cognition became blended with clinical psychological science.

FROM REVOLUTION TO EVOLUTION

The version of this chapter for the second edition of the *Handbook of Cognitive-Behavioral Therapies* was titled "Cognition and Clinical Science: From Revolution to Evolution." We started the chapter with a quote from 1986, noting that the "cognitive revolution" was over, and that "cognitive psychology has become mainstream psychology" (Ingram & Kendall, 1986, p. 3). Now, over 20 years since the end of the revolution was declared, students and even some professionals new to the field may wonder about this revolution; what was it and why was it needed, and was cognitive psychology ever not mainstream? Such questions are refreshing in that the field no longer debates the scientific legitimacy of cognitive concepts, and we can get on with the design, testing, and refinement of effective methods of behavior change, without concerns over their scientific appropriateness. However, these questions remain critical, in that it is not possible to comprehend fully the conceptual underpinnings and assumptions of CBT without at least some knowledge and appreciation of the historical context of this approach.

To start, then, what was the cognitive revolution? Michael Mahoney's (1974) *Cognition and Behavior Modification* volume arguably launched the cognitive revolution in clinical psychology. Fourteen years later, in the inaugural edition of the *Handbook of Cognitive-Behavioral Therapies*, Mahoney (1988) reexamined many of the issues about the role of cognition in the understanding and treatment of psychopathology. Ingram, Kendall and Chen (1991) traced these issues to the lack of parallel development between the CBTs and cognitive psychology. For example, as behaviorism was taking hold in experimental psychology, clinical psychology was in the process of shifting from an emphasis on Freudian constructs to an emphasis on humanistic concepts, such as those pioneered by Carl Rogers. The preeminence of humanistic ideas was, however, short-lived, and the behavioristic approach soon took root in clinical psychology. Indeed, there was much excitement as research suggested that behavioral interventions might be effective in alleviating behavioral problems. Clinical application of behavioral concepts thus promised, and delivered, substantial success.

Buoyed by early applied successes and the mantle of scientific status that behaviorism had claimed, behavioral researchers sought to uncover the stimulus–response links that would fully explicate behavior, particularly disordered behavior, thus pointing the way toward the effective modification of problematic behavior. It was in this milieu that journals devoted to behavioral concepts, interventions, and applied behavioral analysis arose, as did organizations such as the Association for the Advancement of Behavior Therapy (Mahoney, 1974), which were designed to promote behaviorism. Part of behaviorism at that time, however, was repudiation of cognitive constructs, because what was not directly observable was viewed as unscientific.

Although the behavioral paradigm had been instrumental in basic experimental psychology and clinical psychology (Kanfer & Hagerman, 1985), and despite success the treatment of some "simple" problems (e.g., phobias), disenchantment grew over the explanatory limits of behavioral concepts and treatment of complex problems. Fueled by the limits of a purely behavioral approach, basic psychological scientists began to revisit the role of cognition as a meaningful factor in human behavior. Perhaps because of the treatment success that behaviorists had enjoyed in some clinical areas, however, the acknowledgment and incorporation of cognition into mainstream clinical psychology proceeded at a significantly slower pace than it did in other areas of psychology.

It is impossible to pinpoint all of the factors that propelled cognition into the clinical enterprise, although there appear to be at least two discernible stages in the gradual unification of cognitive and clinical perspectives. First was the development of social learning theory and the emphasis on vicarious learning processes emphasized by theorists such as Bandura (1969) and Mischel (1973). They argued that cognitive variables were important as "covert behaviors," and that they operated according to behavioral principles. Given current knowledge about the functioning and structure of cognition, it may be difficult to appreciate this subtle introduction of cognitive variables into clinical psychology. At that time, however, behavioral approaches not only dominated clinical psychology and applied journals but also openly eschewed as unscientific concepts that incorporated cognition or other phenomena that were not directly observable. Shifts to a cognitive perspective were, of necessity, quite subtle and had to be couched in the dominant vernacular of the times (e.g., "cognitive behaviors," "covert events"). The placement of cognition within a behavioral model provided a mantle of scientific legitimacy. Social learning approaches that relied on vicarious learning and covert behavior thus constituted perhaps the earliest clinical predecessors of current cognitive approaches to clinical problems.

The incremental inclusion of cognitive perspectives into scientific respectability stimulated what can be considered a second phase in the linkage between cognition and practice, which was an explicit move toward the incorporation of cognition into clinical assessment and treatment paradigms. This move is evident in the work of pioneering researchers whose primary interest was in developing effective treatment procedures. Because most of these researchers had emerged from a behavioral background, they adopted the term "cognitive-behavioral" to describe the explicit focus on cognition as an appropriate and important focus of treatment efforts. This group included Kendall and Hollon (1979, 1981), Mahoney (1974) and Meichenbaum (1977). Similar pioneering perspectives on cognitive treatment processes also appeared in the work of Beck (1976; Beck, Rush, Shaw, & Emery, 1979) and Ellis (1962). Although these latter approaches emerged from humanistic and psychodynamic traditions, they coalesced with other work to bring legitimacy to a focus on cognition in the context of treatment efforts.

The emphasis at this stage of development in cognitive-behavioral treatment was on creating effective treatment strategies rather than on developing a conceptual understanding of the cognitive system as a whole. Nevertheless, this work moved away from the notion that cognitions were best represented as a covert class of behaviors, suggesting that cognition warranted causal status in its own right. Thus, cognitive systems could not only be thought of as causal in terms of dysfunction and mediators of behavior, but it could be argued that they also operated according to a set of principles that were different in important respects than those espoused by learning theory and behaviorist conceptions. The theoretical premise of much of this work was a relatively straightforward assumption that dysfunctional thoughts are causal precursors to dysfunctional behavior. The development of this relatively simple premise has done much to clarify the complexity of cognitive functioning in both normal and abnormal behavior.

Beyond the factors that legitimized a cognitive view of psychopathology and its treatment, many other theoretical and empirical developments took place. Two areas stand out in this body of work. The first was not specific to the cognitive context but has had a great deal of relevance for medical and mental health therapies. In particular, ideas related to evidence-based medicine and empirically supported treatments infused much of the work on the development of treatments, as well as on established interventions. To be viable, CBTs were compelled to show efficacy, and in fact there has been good, and increasing, evidence of treatment efficacy for the CBTs (Ingram, Hayes, & Scott, 2000).

A second emphasis was and is in neuroscience. There has been a great deal of excitement about the potential identification of the neural substrates of cognitive constructs in both normal and abnormal behavior. Perhaps more important, neuroscience might suggest treatment innovations that may either stand alone or be incorporated into established treatments. Such treatment approaches are explicitly cognitive in nature, even if they originate from a different perspective than existing cognitive approaches. A "traditional" intervention might target cognition, with the idea that neurological functioning would be associated with therapeutic change, which evidence thus far appears to support (Eddington & Strauman, 2009). In this view, "experience changes the brain" (e.g., Lilienfeld, 2007). On the other hand, a neuroscience approach might assert that changes in neural functioning are reflected in changes in cognition; that the "brain changes experience." A critical mass of such work is still in the distance, but some early data have suggested promise for these latter ideas (Siegle, Ghinassi, & Thase, 2007).

The "cognitive revolution" has thus come a long way. As cognition research now proceeds at a rapid pace, we can think of this process as evolution rather than revolution. Indeed, clinical psychology has evolved to a remarkable extent, particularly with respect to the development and refinement of cognitive components of effective treatments. The evolution in basic cognitive psychology has been even more remarkable as cognitive psychology has evolved into a distinct yet diverse cognitive science that incorporates basic psychological concepts and empirical methods, as well as concepts and empirical methods from physiology and neuroanatomy, computer science, artificial intelligence, linguistics and language research, anthropology, and philosophy

(Gardener, 1987). We turn now to an examination of some current trends and developments in cognitive science, starting with a brief historical précis.

A BRIEF HISTORY OF COGNITIVE SCIENCE

"Cognitive science" is an inherently integrative discipline that encompasses aspects of cognitive psychology, artificial intelligence, neuroanatomy, philosophy of knowledge, linguistics, and anthropology (Gardener, 1987). This integration has provided a rich theoretical foundation on which the effects of CBT can be understood and perhaps enhanced. A number of factors led to the integration of these separate fields into the discipline of cognitive science.

The decline of behaviorism as a basic science enabled psychologists to consider theory and research from other disciplines. Among the goals of these psychologists was to understand aspects of complex cognitive events, such as how long chains of actions, or planning and organization, occur (Gardener, 1985). Without denying the importance of stimuli and responses, this pursuit often centered on the question of what cognitive events occurred between a stimulus and a response. There were many possible answers from a variety of sources.

As summarized by Stein (1992), several disciplines had much to offer to the nascent field of cognitive science. For instance, philosophers had long addressed the question of cognition from the perspective of what is "knowable," and it was natural that "philosophy of mind" was incorporated into developing cognitive-psychological models. The advent of computers led to computer metaphors of mind and information-processing models of cognition (Newell & Simon, 1972). Computer science and neuroscience could be integrated as well, as luminaries such as Von Neumann and McCullogh equated the same logic circuits used in building computers to the functioning of biological neurons (Jeffress, 1951). As linguists had long-held clinical interests in disorders such as dyslexia, the insights from this field were incorporated into a developing cognitive science (Stein, 1992). Thus, the disciplines of computer science, artificial intelligence, neuroscience, linguistics, and philosophy of knowledge were closely enough tied to the questions posed by cognitive psychology that an integrated field of cognitive science was born.

FOUNDATIONS OF COGNITIVE SCIENCE

As noted, several disciplines of philosophy, neuroscience, and artificial intelligence contributed to cognitive science. Although linguistics and anthropology have contribute to cognitive science, their implications are not as well articulated for CBT as for some other disciplines, so we limit our discussion here to the developments of philosophical and neuroscience foundations, and artificial intelligence that are relevant to models and methods of CBT.

Philosophical Foundations

"Epistemology," or the philosophy of what can be known, has been linked to models of mental disorder since the advent of recorded history. Zoroastrian philosophers from Persia had a developed theory of consciousness and a model of mind–body relations as early as 500 B.C. Aristotle believed in interactions among the bodily humors and mental faculties. As early as the 12th century A.D., Maimonides used Aristotelian theory to suggest that changes in thoughts could be associated with changes in mood (Pies, 1997), a concept that is fundamental to CBT. As noted by Mahoney (1988), most of the philosophical foundations of CBT can be seen in "constructivism," which holds that reality is a socially constructed phenomenon that exists as a function of the observer who creates it, and is embodied in dynamic and subjective knowledge. Although not all versions of CBT were developed explicitly from these philosophical perspectives, these perspectives are the basis of Beck's approach to treatment (see Beck, 1967, 1996; Beck et al., 1979), which arguably forms the core of all contemporary CBT. Bedrosian and Beck (1980) noted that the philosophical roots of Beck's work can be seen in the arguments of individuals such as Kant and Marcus Aurelius, to whom the statement "If thou are pained by any external thing, it is not this thing that disturbs thee, but thine own judgment about it" is widely attributed. The modification of thought as a way to modify behavior is the natural consequence of this view.

Neuroscience Foundations

"Neuroscience" is the study of the brain and brain–behavior relationships, and it has fueled the emerging interest in the biological basis of psychopathology. Neuroscience has been concerned with the building blocks of cognition; how individual neurons operate and interact in concert to perform cognitive functions. Development of precise measurement of the central nervous system *in situ* and of correlates of cognitive processes may eventually pave the way for understanding the biological basis of change in therapy. Indeed, although the empirical study of changes in brain structure and chemistry during cognitive therapy is relatively recent, it has been suggested that advances in cognitive neuroscience may lead to better understanding of change processes in therapy (Tataryn, Nadel, & Jacobs, 1989). We thus describe the focus of much of the contemporary work in neuroscience and speculate about the possible roles that neuroscience may play in the induction of cognitive change.

Brain Structure

Cognitive-behavioral treatment of any given disorder should assume some knowledge of the factors that underlie the disorder. Brain imaging techniques, such as magnetic resonance imagining (MRI), allow identification of brain structures associated with a disorder to be identified. For example, research has shown that depression is associated with volume changes in a number of different structures, including frontal and basal ganglia lesions. Furthermore, ventricle-to-brain ratio anomalies (Videbech, 1997), and temporal lobe asymmetries (Amsterdam & Mozley, 1992) have been reported. As information is gained about structures that actively maintain affective disorders, and upon what structures CBTs seem to act, more precise treatments might be geared to target functions that are assumed to be disrupted by physiological anomalies. For example, the amygdala is thought to be responsible for the assignment of emotional valences to information, and for the mediation of ruminative processes (Siegle, Steinhauer, Thase, Stenger, & Carter, 2002). Emerging evidence suggests that the right amygdala responds to positive and negative information, whereas the left amygdala only responds to negative information (Davidson, 1998). Functional asymmetries in these structures could lead to an understanding of the perception of positive and negative stimuli in affective disorder. Preliminary studies have further suggested that some of these structural abnormalities correlate with treatment response to antidepressants (e.g., Pillay et al., 1997), which might then potentially be used to predict response to cognitive-behavioral treatment.

Brain Activation

Brain imaging techniques, such as positron emission tomography (PET) and functional MRI (fMRI), as well as traditional physiological measurement techniques (e.g., EEG), and neuropsychological assessment techniques, allow localization of brain activity. PET scanners measure the amount of a radioactive isotope present in brain tissue. By using an isotope that binds to the same places as substances found in the brain, the rate at which these quantities are being used can be determined. PET scanning has been used to understand the rate of glucose and oxygen metabolism and cerebral blood flow, and the degree to which quantities such as neurotransmitters are used (Powledge, 1997). fMRI examines proton radio signal generation, a factor that has been observed to correlate with brain activity. Thus, fMRI can be used to examine relative amounts of brain activation during cognitive tasks.

Localization may be important to understand the mechanisms behind the symptom remission during cognitive-behavioral treatment, and may be useful to target procedures that target functionally relevant brain areas. For example, fMRI data reported by Schwartz (1998) suggest that obsessive–compulsive disorder is characterized by abnormal activation in the orbitofrontal complex. After CBT, changes were found in left orbitofrontal activation in treatment responders, which suggests that cognitive therapy may operate directly on the parts of the brain most affected by the disorder. Schwartz has used this information to inform CBT in two ways. First, compliance with particularly difficult aspects of therapy is improved by showing patients changes in brain activation as they practice the therapeutic techniques. Second, Schwartz modified some of the techniques of CBT to address specifically the caudate–

orbitofrontal brain areas. In particular, he helps patients change behaviors while uncomfortable urges are still present, a technique that appears to allow adaptation in the caudate–orbitofrontal circuits.

Results are similarly promising for other disorders. For example, depression has been associated with left frontal lobe hypoactivation (e.g., Henriques & Davidson, 1991). Because the dorsolateral prefrontal cortex seems to be responsible for the inhibition of emotional reactions, research suggests that emotional responses may become especially uninhibited in depression. Using neuropsychological tasks, Bruder et al. (1997) have shown that CBT is associated with a disappearance of these hemispheric asymmetries, so perhaps CBT could increase emotional inhibition processes to reverse the effects of depression. Through this type of analysis, models might be developed to understand the mechanisms of CBT.

The correlates of brain activity can also be evaluated using physiological assessment techniques. For example, event-related-potentials (ERPs) can indicate brain activity milliseconds after a stimulus is presented, thus allowing investigation of the time course of variables relevant to cognitive therapy (e.g., shifts in attentional allocation). Dipole localization techniques (e.g., Wood, 1982) are mathematical interpolation techniques to find where brain activity associated with ERPs originates, and to allow approximate identification of the sources of brain activity. Similarly, general cognitive activity can be measured physiologically by other indices derived from activity in structures innervated by multiple brain areas of interest. For example, pupil dilation has long been used as an index of overall cognitive load (Beatty, 1982).

The ways in which variables targeted in therapy, such as attentional style or stress, contribute to the onset and maintenance of disorder can be gauged by measuring physiological variables in response to the presentation of affective or feared stimuli. Consequently, theoretically derived physiological response profiles might be used to predict who will be more or less amenable to therapy. Moreover, because these techniques are often noninvasive and inexpensive, physiological measurement could be incorporated during therapy to gauge aspects of cognition during techniques such as role playing and thought challenging.

Neurochemistry

In addition to structural and localization information, knowledge about the roles that diffuse hormones and neurotransmitters play in the brain helps us to understand psychopathology. For example, McEwen, DeKloet, and Rostene (1986) have shown that although the hippocampal system is responsible for memory formation, it is populated with stress hormone receptors. Jacobs and Nadel (1985) speculate that the hippocampal system may allow stress to be associated with particular stimuli and lead to phobias. They suggest the development of psychological treatments for phobias based on presumed hippocampal activity.

Similarly, diffuse neurotransmitters, such as dopamine, norepinephrine, and serotonin, have been implicated in the maintenance of a number of disorders, including depression (e.g., Klimek et al., 1997; Stockmeier, 1997), schizophrenia (e.g., Cohen & Servan-Schreiber, 1993), and anxiety (e.g., McCann et al., 1995). To understand the role of these neurochemicals in therapeutic change it will be useful to examine relationships among affective state, cognitive function, and neurochemical metabolism. To this end, a great deal of recent interest has been directed toward techniques that allow real-time measurement of the rate at which neurochemicals are metabolized, such as magnetic resonance spectroscopy (MRS; e.g., Frangou & Williams, 1996). MRS, a noninvasive method to measure neurochemical concentrations using the same tools as used for fMRI, has been used to implicate changes in chemical quantities in depression, including membrane phospholipid metabolism, high-energy phosphate metabolism, and intracelluar pH (Kato, Inubushi, & Kato, 1998). Such methodologies have been applied to understand the role that drugs can play in changing neurochemical quantities (e.g., Kato et al., 1998; Renshaw et al., 1997). MRS has also been applied to understanding diffuse metabolism and pharmacotherapy response in disorders such as social phobia (Tupler, Davidson, Smith, & Lazeyras, 1997). Although studies have yet to be published using MRS to understand the effects of CBT on neurochemical concentrations, this work in pharmacotherapy suggests a number of promising possibilities.

Comparing Cognitive and Pharmacological Therapies

Research has suggested that similar efficacy rates for disorders such as depression can be achieved through either cognitive or pharmacological therapies (e.g., Hollon, De Rubeis, Evans, & Wierner, 1992). Yet it is unclear whether the mechanisms behind these treatments are the same and, consequently, whether there are relative trade-offs in long-term effects of each type of treatment. Neuroimaging data, physiological measurements, or spectrographic analysis of neurochemical metabolism may help to elucidate the mechanisms behind any differential treatment effects of cognitive and pharmacological therapies. In this regard, Eddington and Strauman (2009) have noted that neural changes may mediate the response to different types of treatment. For example, changes in the dorsolateral and ventromedial prefrontal cortex, and changes in resting glucose metabolism in the anterior cingulate cortex have been found following CBT, but not following pharmacotherapy (Goldapple et al., 2004; Kennedy et al., 2007). The mechanisms that underlie different treatments may thus be derived from similarities and differences in measured physiological indices.

Creation of Pharmacological Mood Primes

One method to evaluate aspects of change and subsequent vulnerability to disorder recurrence after therapy involves the use of priming (e.g., Segal &

Ingram, 1994). When individuals are induced into a state reminiscent of their disorder, their responses to aspects of that state can be determined. Although psychological procedures have been used effectively to create such states, pharmacological challenges have also been created as a way to simulate brain conditions involved in states associated with various disorders. For example, tryptophan depletion modifies serotonin availability; it is associated with lowered mood and other psychological phenomena associated with serotonin (Reilly, McTavish, & Young, 1998). The continued exploration of neurological correlates of psychopathology may reveal new and useful ways to prime aspects of disorder to evaluate vulnerability after cognitive or pharmacological challenges, and the mechanisms that underlie the efficacy of CBT may be further understood.

Artificial Intelligence

Artificial intelligence (AI) involves the programming of computers to perform tasks that model human behavior. Often the goal is to make the computer's performance indistinguishable from that of a human (e.g., Jaquette, 1993; Turing, 1936, 1950). Two aspects of this pursuit have been applied to the evolution of CBT. The first is from AI researchers who consider humans to be analogous to extraordinarily efficient computers, and who try to program computers to perform tasks in the ways that people perform them. By understanding the performance in computer models of aspects of disorder, it may be possible to learn about ways to remediate a disorder cognitively. The second aspect involves using computers actively to perform therapy with people. Each of these areas is discussed in turn.

Computers as Analogues of Psychopathology

As greater understanding is gained of mechanisms behind psychopathology, analogues of these mechanisms can be formalized as computer programs. Such computer programs behave in accordance with their programmer's directions about mechanisms of disorder but can produce responses to inputs that were not anticipated by the programmer. The procedure is similar to understanding a statistical formula but not knowing the result of the application of a formula on a particular dataset until the analysis is performed. Computers may thus reveal some of the implications of theories about cognition in disorder, as well as contradictions that had not been considered before the theories were formalized (e.g., Cohen & Servan-Schreiber, 1992; Siegle, 1997).

AI modeling of cognitive variables relevant to CBT can serve as a heuristic mechanism to test aspects of cognitive theories (Siegle, 1997). If a program can generate behaviors (i.e., outputs) similar to those of people with a disorder, then the incorporation of analogues of therapy change processes can be used to see whether specific interventions produce reliable changes in behaviors. This technique has an advantage over pure theory, in that because as many of the systems underlying cognition are quite complex and nonlinear, they are hard to predict without simulating them in a computer program. Additionally, models of disorder implemented as AI systems can be used to refine cognitive-behavioral treatment through modifications to simulate cognitive change processes that affect a program's simulated behaviors.

AI researchers may add unique perspectives to concepts central to CBT through modeled aspects of cognition and emotion. For example, CBT is often concerned with problem solving. AI modeling has long dealt with problems of planning sequences of events and solving problems (e.g., Charniak & McDermott, 1985). Through computer programs that solve problems, often as simple as mathematical equations or arranging blocks in specified sequences, AI researchers have learned a great deal about how people solve problems (Newell & Simon, 1972). Webster (1995) has used both simulations and traditional computational problem solvers to demonstrate that techniques such as storing and examining past problem-solving failures lead to especially effective problem solution. He suggests that such processes are like adaptive aspects of negative thinking and rumination in a disorder such as affective disorder, but that taking adaptive strategies to extremes might lead to nonadaptive problem-solving deficits. There are many potential implications of this research for cognitive-behavioral therapists, such as understanding that rumination may sometime be adaptive, and that finding a client's optimal level of rumination may be a useful pursuit.

AI models of reasoning can also be applied to understanding change in CBT. A central goal of many AI programs involves reasoning about situations that an artificially intelligent agent (e.g., a robot) could experience in the world. The notion of schemas, on which CBTs are often based, has been formalized in this literature (e.g., Schank & Abelson, 1977). Schemas were traditionally useful to AI researchers as an efficient concept to represent collections of information typically associated with a behavioral context. It is noteworthy that Beck's cognitive therapy is based on the notion that depressed individuals have negative schemas about themselves.

A final area in which traditional AI can help to model the substrates of therapy is that of theoretical logic. A frequent goal of CBT is to help individuals to reconcile inconsistent beliefs (e.g., the belief that one is guilty of something over which one also believes he or she had no control). The discipline of logic programming addresses questions of how a system should behave when it holds inconsistent beliefs. Grant and Subrahmanian (1995a) have shown that when inconsistent beliefs are central to a network of beliefs forming a database, few conclusions can be drawn from the database. By implication, the more central an individual's inconsistent beliefs are, the less the individual is able to make decisions (Dombeck, Siegle, & Ingram, 1996). Because so many beliefs depend on these central beliefs, they are difficult to change without disruption to the entire network. Subrahmanian (Grant & Subrahmanian, 1995a, 1995b; Pradhan, Minker, & Subrahmanian, 1995) has shown that when a database is constrained, so that inconsistent beliefs cannot be considered together, the database can again be used to draw conclusions. Based on this logic, if individuals can be helped to consider pockets of mutually consistent beliefs, and to prioritize which beliefs are held in which situations, this strategy may be used by cognitive therapists in cases in which patients' inconsistent beliefs are so central to their cognitive network that they cannot easily be changed.

A SYNTHESIS OF COGNITIVE PSYCHOLOGY, ARTIFICIAL INTELLIGENCE, AND NEUROSCIENCE

"Connectionism" is a term given to theoretical models arising from cognitive psychology and AI, in which cognition is assumed to involve activation that spreads among nodes. For example, the nodes could represent propositions or beliefs, and activation could represent memory processes that associate beliefs with each other. For example, Bower (1981) used semantic networks to understand the relationship between emotion and cognition by suggesting that they could be represented as connected nodes in such a system. Depression might involve strong connections among certain thoughts and emotions in semantic networks. In this way, many thoughts could lead to the experience of a sad emotion, and as such, could be used to argue that cognitive therapies change the connections within semantic networks.

Connectionist models have been created within a parallel distributed processing framework, in which patterns of information processing are theorized to result from networks of simple, connected neuron-like units. These so-called "neural network" models have advantages over other connectionist models, because they can be designed as analogues of biological systems. Such physiologically informed models bridge a gap between cognitive and neuroscientific research. Possible mechanisms of disorder derived from neuroscientific research can be embodied in neural networks designed to mimic known brain circuits. Knowledge in a neural network is acquired through learning mechanisms developed in cognitive psychology. Because the networks are constructed of individually meaningless units that perform simple computations, they can be readily implemented on a computer. This process allows a computational network to process inputs to simulated systems, and to generate outputs that represent behavior. Mechanisms that underlie disorders and cognitive change can be simulated in such systems (Siegle, 1997, 1999). Conclusions about therapy derived from neural network models are integrative, because they unite behavioral, cognitive, and physiological views of change (Tryon, 1993a).

Neural network models preserve a number of other advantages over other modeling techniques that do not have interdisciplinary appeal. For example, many processes in nature are chaotic, because future states of a system cannot be predicted from its current state. Neural network models allow observation of the effects of theoretically chaotic processes (Movellan & McClelland, 1994). Specific advantages of neural networks to understand psychopathology, over other more symbolic AI models, include the ability to represent gradations of phenomena, and to capture aspects of variable change (Caspar, Rosenfluh, & Segal, 1992).

Tryon (1993b) proposed that the principles of neural networks can be incorporated into CBTs as a way to bridge gaps between cognitive and behavioral perspectives. Tryon suggested that therapy can be thought of as affecting connection weights, so that stimuli (represented as activations of inputs to a network) are associated with different consequent responses (represented as functions of activations of a network's outputs). The role of cognition in such behavioral change can be understood through the examination of changes inside the network associated with changes in stimulus–response pairings.

Neural network models of aspects of psychopathologies have been created. For example, Siegle (1999; Siegle & Ingram, 1997) developed a model of the cognitive processes involved in the recognition of emotional (e.g., sad) and nonemotional features (e.g., knowledge that the birthday is the day on which a person is born) of environmental (e.g., the word *birthday*) stimuli. This model also incorporated rumination, operationalized as excessive feedback among brain areas responsible for representing emotional and nonemotional aspects of information. Computer simulations with this model suggest that once individuals are depressed, excessive rumination interferes with the ability to learn positive information. An implication of this result is that it may be necessary to address depressive rumination in therapy before helping an individual to experience positive thoughts.

Casper et al. (1992) show that theories about neural network models can lead to advances in therapy for other clinical phenomena, such as "repetition compulsion," which is a debilitating condition characterized by repetition of actions. They reason that neural network models could learn nonoptimal associations. Under certain conditions, relevant connections could become strong and lead to a state in which such associations are hard to unlearn. Stimuli could be repeatedly associated with responses, without attainment of desirable goals. They generalize techniques used to break neural networks out of such nonoptimal learning to propose mechanisms for change in cognitive therapy for repetition compulsion.

The preceding discussion suggests that connectionism can play an important role in the emerging role of cognitive science in cognitive therapy. Although basic cognitive science integrates research from cognitive psychology, AI, and neuroscience, the contributions from these disciplines to advancing cognitive therapy have largely been separate. By combining these intuitions from these disciplines using connectionist modeling techniques, the integrated field of cognitive science can be appealed to en masse for advancement of cognitive therapy.

SUMMARY AND CONCLUSIONS

Concepts from cognitive science provide a solid link to the theoretical ideas that underlie CBT. Such a link can also benefit the evolution of cognitive science. For example, cognitive science has often focused on cognition as if it were a static phenomenon, such as in investigations of attentional "style." CBT, in contrast, is devoted to affective and behavioral modification created by changes in cognition. For example, a number of authors have sought to clarify the role of cognitive variables, such as schemas (e.g., Goldfried & Robins, 1983; Hollon & Kriss, 1984), encoding (Greenberg & Safran, 1980, 1981), and the integration of multiple data streams in the production of a cognition (Teasdale & Barnard, 1993). Research on CBT may thus contribute to basic cognitive science research through the elucidation of the role of dynamic cognitive variables in ongoing cognitive processes.

Another example of how research on CBT might provide insights about change processes involves Safran and Segal's (1990) analysis of interpersonal processes in CBT. Although many proponents of cognitive science analyze the role of individuals, Safran and Segal use evidence from experiments in traditional cognitive psychology to suggest that alliances with other people (e.g., therapists) may be involved in cognitive change processes. They suggest that it is likely that individuals who have interpersonal deficits develop schemas related to the self, as well as toward others (see also Ingram, Miranda, & Segal, 1998). Safran and Segal suggest that an interpersonal schema could serve as "a program for maintaining relatedness" (1990, p. 68). Because clinical disorders often involve disrupted interpersonal relationships, the authors suggest that the interpersonal schema could be targeted for cognitive interventions. The understanding of interpersonal relationships is still in its infancy in cognitive science.

A noteworthy idea about change processes involves efforts to understand the role of therapies derived from other cultures (e.g., mindfulness meditation) in changes to the biological substrates of cognitions (e.g., Davidson, 1998) and the prevention of depressive relapse (e.g., Teasdale, Segal, & Williams, 1996). Both Teasdale's and Davidson's cross-cultural research programs started from the idea that processing is parallel and distributed, and use concepts from cognitive science to understand ideas such as awareness of self. For example, Teasdale et al. employed Teasdale and Barnard's (1993) integrative model to suggest that meditative techniques could be used to interrupt cyclic activations that link negative thoughts and emotions; indeed, research has begun to support this contention (Teasdale et al., 2002). Although this research is conducted to help solve clinical problems, it opens cognitive science to integration with an entirely novel discipline.

Cognitive and behavioral change may be induced by methods that target neural functioning rather than cognitive functioning. Siegle et al. (2007) have reported a novel way to treat depression by teaching cognitive control. Cognitive control training specifically targets the amygdala and prefrontal cortex, with the goal of prefrontal cortex activation to inhibit increased amygdala activity. This treatment initially uses Wells's (2000) attention training. Patients direct their attention to a sound that occurs in a naturalistic environment, then switch between attending to and counting the sounds. Once this task is completed, patients perform a serial digit task in which they keep a running sum for a series of numbers. These tasks require attention that is mediated by prefrontal activity, and the idea is that the performance of prefrontally mediated tasks over a period of time will reinstate the prefrontal function of amygdala inhibition. Results reported by Siegle et al. (2007) showed considerable promise for decreasing depression, and how methods that specifically target brain functioning might be useful in affecting therapeutic change. CBT may work because cognition is altered; in this case, cognition is altered not by psychotherapy but by "resetting" brain structures. Efforts such as this offer to both CBT and cognitive science the promise of better understanding how change can take place.

In conclusion, we note that Beck's original (1967) cognitive therapy was based on the best cognitive science of its day. Advances in cognitive science have begun to articulate better the foundations of contemporary CBT, however, and have presumably provided new insights into change processes. This chapter illustrates the power of cognitive science to elucidate mechanisms that drive cognitive phenomena associated with psychopathology and its treatment. As noted by MacLeod (1987):

> Our ultimate ability to refine cognitive treatment approaches such that they comprise the most useful therapeutic techniques, will therefore depend upon our ability to identify the precise nature of the actual processing biases which underlie any particular disorder, or indeed any specific patient, and our ability to sensitively measure the effectiveness of those techniques in overcoming such biases. (p. 180)

We contend that cognitive science models represent especially useful tools to clarify the flow of information through cognitive systems and, as such, provide a conceptual foundation for the improvement of CBT; that is, the incorporation of an explicit cognitive science perspective into CBT can provide a theoretically driven platform for understanding the nature of clinical change in a multitude of disorders. Likewise, by using neuroscience data about brain mechanisms underlying disorder, some approaches to therapy can target specific brain areas and patterns of activation. In short, the full appreciation of the links between cognitive science and CBT, as well as the subdisciplines of cognitive science, might make CBT stronger, more rigorous, broader, and thus more useful in the treatment of human suffering.

REFERENCES

Amsterdam, J. D., & Mozley, P. D. (1992). Temporal lobe asymmetry with iofetamine (IMP) SPECT imaging in patients with major depression. *Journal of Affective Disorders, 24,* 43–53.

Baldwin, M. W. (1992). Relational schemas and the processing of social information. *Psychological Bulletin, 112,* 461–484.

Bandura, A. (1969). *Principles of behavior modification.* New York: Holt, Rinehart & Winston.

Beatty, J. (1982). Task-evoked pupillary responses, processing load, and the structure of processing resources. *Psychological Bulletin, 91,* 276–292.

Beck, A. T. (1967). *Depression: Clinical, experimental, and theoretical aspects.* New York: Hoeber.

Beck, A. T. (1976). *Cognitive therapy and the emotional disorders.* New York: International Universities Press.

Beck, A. T. (1996). Beyond belief: A theory of modes, personality, and psychopathology. In P. M. Salovskis (Ed.), *Frontiers of cognitive therapy* (pp. 1–25). New York: Guilford Press.

Beck, A. T., Rush, A. J., Shaw, B. F., & Emery, G. (1979). *Cognitive therapy of depression.* New York: Guilford Press.

Bedrosian, R. C., & Beck, A. T. (1980). Principles of cognitive therapy. In M. J. Mahoney (Ed.), *Psychotherapy process* (pp. 127–152). New York: Plenum Press.

Bower, G. (1981). Mood and memory. *American Psychologist, 36,* 129–148.

Bruder, G. E., Stewart, J. W., Mercier, M. A., Agosti, V., Leslie, P., Donovan, S., et al. (1997). Outcome of cognitive-behavioral therapy for depression: Relation to hemispheric dominance for verbal processing. *Journal of Abnormal Psychology, 106,* 138–144.

Caspar, F., Rosenfluh, T., & Segal, Z. (1992). The appeal of connectionism for clinical psychology. *Clinical Psychology Review, 12,* 719–762.

Charniak, E., & McDermott, D. (1985). *Introduction to artificial intelligence.* Reading, MA: Addison-Wesley.

Cohen, J. D., & Servan-Schreiber, D. (1992). Introduction to neural network models in psychiatry, *Psychiatric Annals, 22,* 113–118.

Cohen, J. D., Servan-Schreiber, D. (1993). A theory of dopamine function and its role in cognitive deficits in schizophrenia. *Schizophrenia Bulletin, 19,* 85–104.

Davidson, R. J. (1998). Affective style and affective disorders: Perspectives from affective neuroscience. *Cognition and Emotion, 12,* 307–330.

Dombeck, M., Siegle, G., & Ingram, R. E. (1996). Cognitive interference and coping strategies in vulnerability to negative affect: The threats to identity model. In I. G. Sarason, B. Sarason, & G. Pierce (Eds.), *Cognitive interference: Theories, methods, and findings* (pp. 299–323). Hillsdale, NJ: Erlbaum.

Eddington, K. M., & Strauman, T. J. (2009). Neuroimaging and psychosocial treatments for depression. In R. E. Ingram (Ed.), *International encyclopedia of depression* (pp. 410–412). New York: Springer.

Ellis, A. (1962). *Reason and emotion in psychotherapy.* New York: Lyle Stuart.

Frangou, S., & Williams, S. C. (1996). Magnetic resonance spectroscopy in psychiatry: Basic principles and applications. *British Medical Bulletin, 52,* 474–485.

Gardener, H. (1985). *The mind's new science: A history of the cognitive revolution.* New York: Basic Books.

Gardener, H. (1987). Cognitive science characterized. In P. K. Moser & A. vander Nat (Eds.), *Human knowledge: Classical and contemporary approaches* (pp. 375–393). New York: Oxford University Press.

Goldapple, K., Segal, Z., Garson, C., Lau, M., Bieling, P., Kennedy, S., et al. (2004). *Archives of General Psychiatry, 61,* 34–41.

Goldfried, M. R., & Robins, C. (1983). Self-schema, cognitive bias, and the processing of therapeutic experiences. In P. C. Kendall (Ed.), *Advances in cognitive-behavioral research and therapy* (Vol. 2, pp. 330–380). New York: Academic Press.

Grant, J., & Subrahmanian, V. S. (1995a). Reasoning in inconsistent knowledge bases. *Transactions on Knowledge and Data Engineering, 7,* 177–189.

Grant, J., & Subrahmanian, V. S. (1995b). The optimistic and cautious semantics for inconsistent knowledge bases. *Acta Cybernetica, 12,* 37–55.

Greenberg, L. S., & Safran, J. D. (1980). Encoding, information processing and the cognitive behavioural therapies. *Canadian Psychology, 21,* 59–66.

Greenberg, L. S., & Safran, J. D. (1981). Encoding and cognitive therapy: Changing what clients attend to. *Psychotherapy: Theory, Research and Practice, 18,* 163–169.

Henriques, J. B., & Davidson, R. (1991). Left frontal hypoactivation in depression. *Journal of Abnormal Psychology, 100,* 535–545.

Hollon, S. D., DeRubeis, R. J., Evans, M. D., & Wiemer, M. J. (1992). Cognitive therapy and pharmacotherapy for depression: Singly and in combination. *Archives of General Psychiatry, 49,* 774–781.

Hollon, S. D., & Kriss, M. R. (1984). Cognitive factors in clinical research and practice. *Clinical Psychology Review, 4,* 35–76.

Ingram, R. E., Hayes, A., & Scott, W. (2000). Empirically supported treatments: A critical analysis. In C. R. Snyder & R. E. Ingram (Eds.), *Handbook of psychological change: Psychology processes and practices for the 21st century* (pp. 40–60). New York: Wiley.

Ingram, R. E., & Kendall, P. C. (1986). Cognitive clinical psychology: Implications of an information processing perspective. In R. E. Ingram (Ed.), *Information processing approaches to clinical psychology* (pp. 3–21). Orlando, FL: Academic Press.

Ingram, R. E., Kendall, P. C., & Chen, A. H. (1991). Cognitive-behavioral interventions. In C. R. Snyder & D. R. Forsyth (Eds.), *Handbook of social and clinical psychology: The health perspective* (pp. 509–522). New York: Pergamon Press.

Ingram, R. E., Miranda, J., & Segal, Z. V. (1998). *Cognitive vulnerability to depression.* New York: Guilford Press.

Jacobs, W. J., & Nadel, L. (1985). Stress-induced recovery of fears and phobias. *Psychological Review, 92,* 512–531.

Jacquette, D. (1993). Who's afraid of the Turing Test? *Behavior and Philosophy, 20,* 63–74.

Jeffress, L. A. (1951). *Cerebral mechanisms in behavior: The Hixon Symposium.* New York: Wiley.

Kanfer, F. H., & Hagerman, S. M. (1985). Behavior therapy and the information processing paradigm. In S. Reiss & R. R. Bootzin (Eds.), *Theoretical issues in behavior therapy* (pp. 3–35). New York: Academic Press.

Kato, T., Inubushi, T., & Kato, N. (1998). Magnetic resonance spectroscopy in affective disorders. *Journal of Neuropsychiatry and Clinical Neurosciences, 10,* 133–147.

Kendall, P. C., & Hollon, S. D. (1979). *Cognitive-behavioral interventions: Theory, research, and procedures.* New York: Academic Press.

Kendall, P. C., & Hollon, S. D. (1981). *Assessment strategies for cognitive-behavioral interventions.* New York: Academic Press.

Kennedy, S. H., Kornarski, J. Z., Segal, Z. V., Lau, M., Bieling, P. J., McIntyre, R. S., et al. (2007). Differences in brain glucose metabolism between responders to CBT and venlafaxine in a 16-week randomized controlled trial. *American Journal of Psychiatry, 164,* 778–788.

Klimek, V., Stockmeier, C., Overholser, J., Meltzer, H. Y., Kalka, S., Dilley, G., et al. (1997). Reduced levels of norepinephrine transporters in the locus coeruleus in major depression. *Journal of Neuroscience, 17,* 8451–8459.

Lilienfeld, S. O. (2007). Cognitive neuroscience and depression: Legitimate versus illegitimate reductionism and five challenges. *Cognitive Therapy and Research, 31,* 263–272.

MacLeod, C. (1987). Cognitive psychology and cognitive therapy. In H. Dent (Ed.), *Clinical psychology: Research and developments* (pp. 175–181). London: Croom Helm.

Mahoney, M. J. (1974). *Cognition and behavior modification.* Cambridge, MA: Ballinger.

Mahoney, M. J. (1988). The cognitive sciences and psychotherapy: Patterns in a developing relationship. In K. S. Dobson (Ed.), *Handbook of cognitive-behavioral therapies* (pp. 357–386). New York: Guilford Press.

Mahoney, M. J. (1990). *Human change processes.* New York: Basic Books.

McCann, U. D., Thorne, D., Hall, M., Popp, K., Avery, W., Sing H., et al. (1995). The effects of L-dihydroxyphenylalanine on alertness and mood in alpha-methyl-para-tyrosine-treated healthy humans: Further evidence for the role of catecholamines in arousal and anxiety. *Neuropsychopharmacology, 13,* 41–52.

McEwen, B. S., DeKloet, E. R., & Rostene, W. (1986). Adrenal steroid receptors and actions in the nervous system. *Physiological Reviews, 66,* 1121–1188.

Meichenbaum, D. (1977). *Cognitive behavior modification.* New York: Plenum Press.

Mischel, W. (1973). Toward a cognitive social learning conceptualization of personality. *Psychological Review, 80,* 252–283.

Movellan, J. R., & McClelland, J. L. (1994). *Stochastic interactive processing, channel separability, and optimal perceptual interference: An examination of Morton's law* [Technical report]. Department of Psychology, Carnegie Mellon University, Pittsburgh.

Newell, A., & Simon, H. A. (1972). *Human problem solving.* Englewood Cliffs, NJ: Prentice-Hall.

Pies, R. (1997). Maimonides and the origins of cognitive-behavioral therapy. *Journal of Cognitive Psychotherapy, 11,* 21–36.

Pillay, S. S., Yurgelun-Todd, D. A., Bonello, C. M., Lafer, B., Fava, M., & Renshaw, P. F. (1997). A quantitative magnetic resonance imaging study of cerebral and cerebellar gray matter volume in primary unipolar major depression: Relationship to treatment response and clinical severity. *Biological Psychiatry, 42,* 79–84.

Powledge, T. M. (1997). Unlocking the secrets of the brain. *Bioscience, 47,* 403–409.

Pradhan, S., Minker, J., & Subrahmanian, V. S. (1995). Combining databases with prioritized information. *Journal of Intelligent Information Systems, 4,* 231–260.

Reilly, J. G., McTavish, S. F. B., & Young, A. H. (1998). Rapid depletion of plasma tryptophan: A review of studies and experimental methodology. *Journal of Psychopharmacology, 11,* 381–392.

Renshaw, P. F., Lafer, B., Babb, S. M., Fava, M., Stoll, A. L., Christensen, J. D., et al. (1997). Basal ganglia choline levels in depression and response to fluoxetine treatment: An *in vivo* proton magnetic resonance spectroscopy study. *Biological Psychiatry, 41,* 837–843.

Safran, J. D., & Segal, Z. V. (1990). *Interpersonal processes in cognitive therapy.* New York: Basic Books.

Schank, R. C., & Abelson, R. P. (1977). *Scripts, plans, goals, and understanding.* Hillsdale, NJ: Erlbaum.

Schwartz, J. M. (1998). Neuroanatomical aspects of cognitive-behavior therapy response in obsessive–compulsive disorder. *British Journal of Psychiatry, 173,* 38–44.

Segal, Z. V., & Ingram, R. E. (1994). Mood priming and construct activation in tests of cognitive vulnerability to unipolar depression. *Clinical Psychology Review, 14,* 663–695.

Siegle, G. J. (1997). Why I make models (or what I learned in graduate school about validating clinical causal theories with computational models). *Behavior Therapist, 20,* 179–184.

Siegle, G. J. (1999). A neural network mode of attention biases in depression. In J. Reggia & E. Ruppin (Eds.), *Neural network models of brain and cognitive disorders* (Vol. 2, pp. 415–441). Amsterdam: Elsevier.

Siegle, G. J., Ghinassi, F., & Thase, M. (2007). Neurobehavioral therapies in the 21st century: Summary of an emerging field and an extended example of cognitive control training for depression. *Cognitive Therapy and Research, 31,* 235–262.

Siegle, G. J., & Ingram, R. E. (1997). Modeling individual differences in negative information processing biases. In G. Matthews (Ed.), *Cognitive science perspectives on personality and emotion* (pp. 302–353). Amsterdam: Elsevier.

Siegle, G. J., Steinhauer, S. R., Thase, M. E., Stenger, V. A., & Carter, C. S. (2002). Can't shake that feeling: Event-related fMRI assessment of sustained amygdala activity in response to emotional information in depressed individuals. *Biological Psychiatry, 51,* 693–707.

Stein, D. J. (1992). Clinical cognitive science: Possibilities and limitations. In D. Stein & J. Young (Eds.), *Cognitive science and clinical disorders* (pp. 3–17). San Diego: Academic Press.

Stockmeier, C. A. (1997). Neurobiology of serotonin in depression and suicide. *Annals of the New York Academy of Sciences, 836,* 220–232.

Tataryn, D. J., Nadel, L., & Jacobs, W. J. (1989). Cognitive therapy and cognitive science. In A. Freeman, K. M Simon, L. E. Beutler, & H. Arkowitz (Eds). *Comprehensive handbook of cognitive therapy* (pp. 83–98). New York: Plenum Press.

Teasdale, J. D., & Barnard, P. (1993). *Affect, cognition, and change: Remodeling depressive thought.* Hillsdale, NJ: Erlbaum.

Teasdale, J. D., Moore, R. G., Hayhurst, H., Pope, M., Williams, S., & Segal, Z. V. (2002). Metacognitive awareness and prevention of relapse in depression: Empirical evidence. *Journal of Consulting and Clinical Psychology, 70,* 275–287.

Teasdale, J. D., Segal, Z., & Williams, M. G. (1996). How does cognitive therapy prevent depressive relapse and why should attentional control (mindfulness) training help? *Behaviour Research and Therapy, 33,* 25–39.

Tryon, W. W. (1993a). Neural networks: I. Theoretical unification through connectionism. *Clinical Psychology Review, 13,* 341–352.

Tryon, W. W. (1993b). Neural networks: II. Unified learning theory and behavioral psychotherapy. *Clinical Psychology Review, 13,* 353–371.

Tupler, L. A., Davidson, J. R. T., Smith, R. D., & Lazeyras, F. (1997). A repeat proton magnetic resonance spectroscopy study in social phobia. *Biological Psychiatry, 42,* 419–424.

Turing, A. M. (1936). On computable numbers, with an application to the Entscheidungs problem. *Proceedings of the London Mathematical Society, 42,* 230–265.

Turing, A. M. (1950). Computing machinery and intelligence. *Mind, 59,* 433–460.

Videbech P. (1997). MRI findings in patients with affective disorder: A meta-analysis. *Acta Psychiatrica Scandinavica, 96,* 157–168.

Webster, C. (1995). Computer modeling of adaptive depression, *Behavioral Science, 40,* 314–330.

Wells, A. (2000). *Emotional disorders and metacognition: Innovative cognitive therapy.* New York: Wiley.

Wood, C. C. (1982). Application of dipole localization methods to source identification of human evoked potentials. *Annals of the New York Academy of Sciences, 388,* 139–155.

CHAPTER 4

Cognitive-Behavioral Therapy and Psychotherapy Integration

T. Mark Harwood
Larry E. Beutler
Mylea Charvat

The history of psychotherapy is one of conflict and change. The evolution of theory and practice has been both the product and the precipitator of rivalry and discord, between those who would instigate change and those who espouse the accepted theory of the day (Freedheim, Freudenberger, Kessler, & Messer, 1992). Early theories evolved largely through disagreements among the practitioners of the "talking cure." Freud's disciples broke with him because of disagreements regarding both the nature of psychopathology and the techniques of treatment. Such disjunctive progress is understandable in any new field. When scientific findings are sparse and the major means of discovery (as in early psychotherapy) is through uncontrolled observations (e.g., individual case analysis), changes in the field are inevitably stimulated by personal disagreements and differences in interpretation.

Particularly in psychotherapy's early development, the disagreements that occurred among theorists and practitioners were founded inextricably in the fundamental question of what constitutes evidence of truth. Theoretical positions about psychotherapy became sacrosanct, and scientific findings were rejected because they did not fit the canons of one or another theoretical position (Beutler & Harwood, 2001). This situation created a virtual tower of Babel, and theories developed with unchecked abandon during the 1970s. When the proliferation of different theoretical viewpoints reached its zenith in the 1980s, it would have been hard to find any position about the nature or effectiveness of psychotherapy that would earn majority, let alone consensual, agreement.

While remnants of this discord remain, there is more acceptance of scientific findings than previously, and "evidence-based practice" has become the norm in medicine and other health professions (Harwood & Beutler, 2008; Roth & Fonagy, 1996). Scientific inquiry and evidence derived via the scientific method have gained ground as change agents for the field. The arguments that arise among practitioners, and between academic and practitioner communities, less frequently address the value of scientific evidence as the basis of knowledge than what constitutes "good" science. Most psychotherapists accept, at least in principle, the value of scientific inquiry, even while they differ widely in what they consider to be acceptable scientific methods. Despite this development, however, there has been a decided lag in the acceptance of scientific findings as the basis for setting new directions or for deciding what is factual among practicing therapists. Indeed for many practitioners, the true test of a given psychotherapy rests in both its theoretical logic and evidence from clinicians' observations rather than data from sound scientific methods, even when the latter are available (Beutler & Harwood, 2001; Beutler, Williams, & Wakefield, 1993; Beutler, Williams, Wakefield, & Entwistle, 1995).

What practitioners accept as valid hinges on both the methods used to derive results and the strength of their opinions. Practitioners prefer naturalistic research over randomized clinical trials, $N = 1$ or single-case studies over group designs, and individualized over group measures of outcome (Heppner & Anderson, 1985; Fava, 1986; Morrow-Bradley & Elliott, 1986). They also tend to believe research favoring the brand that they practice over research that supports alternative psychotherapy approaches or equivalency among approaches. Since most psychotherapy research fails to comply with these values, psychotherapists often are quick to reject scientific findings that disagree with their own theoretical systems. Thus, while the reasons given for rejecting scientific evidence may be more sophisticated today than in the past, it may be no less likely to occur.

THE EMERGENCE OF ECLECTIC AND INTEGRATIONIST VIEWS

Theorists who depart from the views of a mentor have frequently been treated as pariahs. As a consequence, it was not unusual to find that a practitioner of a particular theoretical orientation was quite ignorant of the principles and practices of other theoretical schools. While this theoretical isolation may have motivated therapists and clinicians to refine and enhance the skills and techniques espoused by their respective theoretical orientations, it also severely limited their horizons and perspectives (Safran & Messer, 1997).

Since the 1980s, the field of psychotherapy has changed in response to the emergence of integrationist and eclectic views. This change was stimulated in part by the diversity of opinion in the field and the status of scientific evidence.

With over 400 different theories on the psychotherapy landscape, the inescapable conclusion was that there existed no single truth about psychopathology or psychotherapy. Practitioners became suspicious of theory and developed a profound disaffection for narrow theoretical orientations. Dissatisfaction was compounded by the failure of scientific studies firmly to indicate clear superiority of any psychotherapy relative to the others. Indeed, evidence indicated that none of the psychotherapies successfully generated the comprehensive interventions that would result in the effective treatment of patients who presented with complex and serious problems (Goldfried, 1995). In recent years, practitioners have incorporated theories, techniques, and interventions from diverse schools of thought in an effort to enhance their own overall clinical efficacy (Safran & Messer, 1997).

While the eclectic and integrationist movement caught on during the 1980s, its nucleus was in the early work of Thorne (1962) and Goldstein and Stein (1976). Thorne's "eclectic" psychotherapy arose from a relationship perspective in counseling theory. He argued that training doomed therapists to a single-method perspective that was ill-suited to the variety of conditions, personalities, and needs of different patients, in much the same way that a carpenter who had only a screwdriver would be poorly equipped to build a house. Thorne offered a conceptual argument for eclecticism but few direct procedural guidelines. In contrast, Goldstein and Stein suggested that the procedures selected should be based on scientific evidence of efficacy, and they presented examples of evidence-based treatments. Given their scientific bent, these latter recommendations were largely drawn from the behavior therapy literature, since behaviorism was the dominant research approach at that point in time. Modern eclecticism has become more broad ranging but has retained some of the values inherent in Thorne's acceptance of procedures from a variety of perspectives, and in Goldstein and Stein's admonition to let scientific evidence, rather than theory, dictate the methods of application.

Surveys indicate that most mental health professionals in North America identify with some form of eclecticism (Lambert, Garfield, & Bergin, 2004), or what is more commonly called "integration," as the term implies a systematic application of concepts and techniques spawned by a variety of psychotherapies and theories of pathology (Lambert & Ogles, 2004). The growth in the integrationist movement is international in scope, as documented by the membership of the Society for Exploration of Psychotherapy Integration (SEPI).

At least four perspectives can be identified within the integrationist movement (Goldfried, 1995; Norcross & Goldfried, 1992; Norcross, Martin, Omer, & Pinsoff, 1996): (1) common factors eclecticism, (2) theoretical integrationism, (3) technical eclecticism, and (4) strategic eclecticism. These approaches exist in addition to the unsystematic form of "haphazard eclecticism" to which many practitioners adhere (e.g., Norcross et al., 1996). Haphazard eclecticism is based on some of the general beliefs and scientific "facts" that characterize the more systematic movements within the eclectic tradition, most notably the empirical observation that different approaches seem to be best suited for different people. However, unsystematic eclecticism fails to define the principles that govern the merging of viewpoints or a replicable procedure for selecting and applying treatments. This approach to eclecticism is widespread, but its effectiveness is hard to evaluate, as it varies both among and within therapists. Its effectiveness is inextricably bound to the judgment and skills of the particular therapist who applies it.

Among the more systematic approaches, "common factors eclecticism" relies on the factors that are common or similar across approaches. The common factors approach to psychotherapy is distinct from the way one usually thinks of eclecticism. Common factors eclecticism accepts that all effective psychotherapies rely on a core of basic ingredients, beyond which their distinctive effects are inconsequential or unpredictable. This approach attempts to identify techniques or interventions that appear in all successful treatments, and proposes that research ought to evaluate the interventions and psychotherapeutic interactions that promote or contain these common factors or qualities (Arkowitz, 1995). This posture proposes that an effective psychotherapy will comprise these common interventions.

The therapist who works within the common factors approach is seldom concerned with specific techniques or strategies, beyond those that result in a congenial and caring relationship. Common factors therapists, like most relationship-oriented therapists, create an accepting and nonthreatening atmosphere in which the patient may explore problems. But unlike relationship-oriented therapies that are driven by particular theories of psychopathology and change, a certain type of relationship in therapy is considered to be necessary and sufficient, and no more specific techniques or procedures are thought to be useful (e.g., Garfield, 1981).

Although common factors are important elements of change, a growing body of research supports the contribution of specific classes of treatment interventions (Beutler et al., 2004; Lambert, Garfield, & Bergin, 2004). For example, recent research with manualized cognitive-behavioral and family systems treatments for alcoholism delivered in a couple format has suggested that both common treatment elements and specific interventions contribute to change. More specifically, treatment components appear to operate independently and/or in interaction, in a complex manner. Moreover, the balance of common to specific treatment elements exerts positive or attenuating effects depending on the phase of treatment, type of treatment administered, and time at posttreatment follow-up (Harwood, Beutler, Castillo, & Karno, 2006).

The preponderance of systematic eclectic theories addresses patient and treatment complexity and variability (aptitude x treatment interactions, or ATIs) through structure and systematization of recommended therapeutic procedures, because maximization of exposure to this unique combination of therapeutic factors best reduces patients' problems (Stricker & Gold, 1996). These efforts are anchored at one end by what is referred to as "theoretical integrationism" and at the other by "technical eclecticism." Between these extremes are the strategic eclectics, who integrate both theoretical concepts and techniques at the level of intervention strategies and principles of therapeutic influence (Beutler & Clarkin, 1990; Beutler, Clarkin, & Bongar, 2000; Beutler & Harwood, 2000; Harwood & Beutler, 2008). All three of these approaches are more systematic than either haphazard eclecticism or common factors eclecticism. They share a common aim of directing the therapist through decisions about what procedures to apply, to whom, and when. They identify both the range of procedures to be used, and the patient or temporal and situational cues that index the point of their maximal impact. At the broadest level, the theoretical integration movement attempts to amalgamate at least two theoretical viewpoints but leaves the specific techniques and procedures to the clinician's judgement. These approaches view good theory as the avenue to develop good techniques; they contrast those approaches often referred to as either "eclectic" or "strategic" in nature (Goldfried, 1995; Stricker & Gold, 1996).

The term "integration" has a set of meanings beyond the interdigitation of psychotherapy theories. It can refer to the quality of one's personality, for example, when one refers to an integrated personality in which the component traits, needs, wants, perceptions, values, emotions, and impulses are in a stable state of harmony and communication. An integrated person is someone who is whole with regard to overall functioning and well-being. Psychotherapy integration includes harmonious efforts to connect affective, cognitive, behavioral, and systems approaches to psychotherapy under a single theory, and the application of this theory to the treatment of individuals, couples, and families. This notion goes beyond any single theory or set of techniques and integrates diverse models of human functioning (Goldfried, 1995).

At least superficially, theoretical integration requires the translation of concepts and methods from one psychotherapeutic system into the language and procedures of another (Stricker & Gold, 1996). What often emerges is a new theory that embodies parts of each of the former ones. This theory encompasses the identification and standardization of effective concepts, terms, and methods, and includes the application of the resulting theoretical concepts to the grist mill of research and application. Using a framework of integration, theoretical linkages have been made among psychodynamic, behavioral, and cognitive approaches (Arkowitz & Messer, 1984; Safran & Messer, 1997; Stricker & Gold, 1996; Wachtel, 1978).

Theoretical integration is the most theoretically abstract of the various systematic approaches. Theoretical integration attempts to bring various theories together through the development of a theoretical framework that can explain the environmental, motivational, cognitive, and affective domains of an individual that influence or are influenced by change efforts; that is, theoretical integrative approaches blend two or more traditional theoretical orientations to yield a new model of personality functioning, psychopathology, and psychological change. Such new forms of therapies ideally capitalize on the strengths of each of the therapeutic elements (Safran & Messer, 1997).

In contrast to theoretical integration, technical and strategic eclecticism are often considered to be more clinically oriented and practical. Strategic and technical eclectic approaches to therapy are less abstract than models of theoretical integration, and rely more on the use of specific techniques, procedures, or principles. They define a variety of strategies (strategic eclecticism) or develop menus of psychotherapeutic interventions (technical eclecticism) that are independent of the theory that gave birth to these procedures. These types of integration are accomplished through a neutral perspective relative to theories of change, or the adoption of a superordinate theory to replace or supplant the originals.

Technical and strategic eclectics are concerned primarily with the clinical efficacy of treatment procedures, and do not attend much to the validity of theories of psychopathology and personality that give rise to these procedures. These eclectics employ interventions from two or more psychotherapeutic systems, and apply them systematically and successively to patients who have indicated qualities, using guidelines or heuristics based either on demonstrated or presumed clinical efficacy (Beutler, 1983; Lazarus, 1996; Harwood & Beutler, 2008; Safran & Messer, 1997; Stricker & Gold, 1996). This is not to say that the approaches within the technical eclectic tradition are devoid of theory; however, to the degree that theories are used, they are theories that link numerous empirical observations, and they seldom require the level of abstractness that is inherent in most traditional theories of therapeutic change.

The first and best known of the technical eclectic approaches is multimodal therapy (MMT; Lazarus, 1996). MMT therapists apply different theoretical approaches and models at the same time, or in a coordinated sequence, dependent on the relative importance of the patient's symptoms. In other forms of technical eclecticism, prescriptive matching is devoted to an integration of a host of specific procedures, selected from a wide variety of menus, into a coherent and seamless treatment (e.g., Beutler, 1983).

The major distinction between technical eclecticism and strategic eclecticism is in the specificity of recommended procedures and techniques. Technical eclecticism offers a menu of procedures to fit a given person or problem (Beutler, 1983; Harwood & Williams, 2003; Lazarus, 1996). In contrast, strategic eclecticism identifies principles and goals but leaves technique selection to the proclivities of the individual therapist (Beutler & Harwood, 2000). The implicit or working assumption of technical eclecticism is that all techniques have a finite range of applicability and use, whereas strategic eclecticism assumes that all techniques can be used in different ways and toward different ends, depending on how and by whom they are applied.

Strategic therapy offers a middle ground between the technique focus of technical eclecticism and the abstractness of theoretical integrationism. These approaches articulate principles of therapeutic change that lead to general strategies of intervention. The strategies are designed to implement the guiding principles, but an objective is to remain true to the principles rather than focus only on the specific techniques (Beutler & Clarkin, 1990; Beutler et al., 2000; Beutler & Harwood, 2000; Harwood & Beutler, 2008; Norcross et al., 1996). As such, these approaches preserve the flexibility of the individual therapist to select specific techniques. They also maximize the use of techniques with which the therapist is both familiar and skilled, without forsaking the use of patient factors as reliable cues for the selective application of different interventions. These approaches usually include an explicit definition of guiding principles that facilitate relationship qualities, and evoke symptomatic and structural changes. Thus, of the various approaches to integration, they are probably the most flexible and practical: not as complex and elaborate as integrationist approaches, and not as simplistic as technical eclecticism.

Although prescriptive psychotherapy (Beutler & Harwood, 2000) at times resembles technical eclecticism, it goes beyond the latter by constructing *principles* of change. The objective is a coherent treatment based on a comprehensive view of the patient's presentation (Stricker, 1994). Treatments based on explicit principles of change, like those based on elaborate theories of psychopathology, are most usefully integrated if they are researchable, do not rely on abstract concepts for which no measurement exists, and place few theory-driven proscriptions on the use of various therapeutic techniques.

While most systematic eclectic psychotherapies span multiple theories, others employ principles to guide the use of specific theories. For example, cognitive therapy (CT) is amenable to the use of eclectic principles because it relies on research findings rather than abstract theories of causation, and it values sound measurement of patient characteristics, change, and treatment processes. CT does not depend on the validity of insights into the nature of psychopathology for effectiveness in the therapeutic arena. First and foremost, cognitive theory emphasizes reliable observation and measurement in the assessment of the effects of treatment.

Thus, cognitive theory offers a platform from which one might begin to integrate principles of change and the definition of strategies that includes, but is not limited by, an already known array of technical interventions. For example, Hollon and Beck (2004) discuss the expansion of cognitive-behavioral therapy (CBT) to include elements of psychodynamic and experiential therapies. Stricker and Gold's *Casebook of Psychotherapy Integration* (2006) provides numerous examples of integration between cognitive-behavioral techniques and myriad forms of psychotherapy. Beitman, Soth, and Good (2006) describe a three-tier psychosocial treatment with an assimilative psychodynamic therapy (first tier) that integrates cognitive (second tier) and behavioral (third tier) interventions. Ryle and McCutcheon (2006) describe a cognitive analytic therapy that integrates psychoanalytic, cognitive, constructivist, behavioral, and Vygotskian sources. McCullough (2000) describes a cognitive-behavioral analysis system of psychotherapy that integrates Bandura's (1977) social learning theory, Piaget's conceptualization of cognitive-emotive development (1954/1981), interpersonal procedures à la Kiesler (1996), and situational analysis, which is a problem-solving approach for real-life situations

(McCullough, 2000). Finally, Goldfried (2006) provides an excellent description of a CBT that incorporates experiential and relational interventions.

EXAMPLES OF RECENT DEVELOPMENTS
IN RESEARCH AND THEORY

As alluded to earlier, the past decade has seen the emergence of many therapies that are heavily influenced by the CT model. Dialectical behavior therapy (DBT), acceptance and commitment therapy (ACT), and mindfulness-based cognitive therapy (MBCT) are recent examples of CT-influenced therapies. Fincucane and Mercer (2006) define MBCT as a semistructured model that integrates mindfulness meditation practices with traditional CT approaches. They found that in a sample of 13 patients with a history of relapsing depression, mindfulness training was both acceptable and beneficial to the majority of patients. More than half the patients continued to incorporate mindfulness techniques into their lives 3 months after they finished the 8-week course. Overall significant reductions in mean depression and anxiety scores were observed in this study. Kenny and Williams (2007) found that MBCT resulted in improved depression scores for a set of patients who had failed to respond fully to standard CT and CBT approaches to treating depression. A tenet of CT is that mediation by cognitive processes is linked to the successful treatment of depression. In a review of the extant literature, Garratt, Ingram, Rand, and Sawalani (2007) found that while this principle is generally supported by the evidence, findings with regard to cognitive specificity are mixed. In other words, evidence supports the principle that cognitive changes support therapeutic improvement, but the specificity of cognitive changes to CT remains unclear.

Whitfield (2006) hypothesized that the integration of mindfulness interventions with rational emotive behavior therapy (REBT), a variant of CBT, should render a more patient-tailored treatment. He recommended the application of an integrated clinical practice. In a randomized clinical trial, Gaudiano and Herbert (2006) combined CBT with ACT and compared integrated treatment and an enhanced treatment-as-usual (ETAU) condition in the treatment of psychotic inpatients. These investigators provided preliminary support for the clinical utility of mindfulness- and acceptance-based CBT approaches in the treatment of psychosis. More specifically, the CBT/ACT group had better outcomes than ETAU group on measures of affect severity, global improvement, distress associated with hallucinations, and social functioning. Moreover, the CBT/ACT group had greater overall clinically significant symptom reduction (Gaudiano & Herbert, 2006). In a similar vein, Barrowclough, Haddock, Fitzsimmons, and Johnson (2006) described an in-process randomized controlled trial (RCT) that evaluated motivational interviewing combined with CBT in the treatment of comorbid psychosis and substance misuse.

Dialectical behavioral therapy (DBT) is part of the new generation of CT- and CBT-based therapies designed to move beyond the traditional focus solely on cognitions yet maintain some aspects of CT and CBT approaches. Marsha Linehan and Linda Dimeff (2001) describe DBT as largely based in behaviorist theory yet incorporating aspects of CT, with an additional focus on mindfulness. Although DBT is based in the biosocial theory of personality, it utilizes hallmarks of CBT such as self-monitoring and interpersonal skills training. According to Linehan and Dimeff, DBT uses mindfulness techniques to help patients get into their "wise mind," defined as a balance between the "rational mind" and the "emotional mind." The ability to tolerate distress and ambiguous situations is a specific goal set forth in DBT that also resonate with more traditional CBT approaches utilized by Aaron Beck, such as the development of alternatives to one's "automatic thoughts." Contrasts between traditional CBT and DBT reveal how well CBT is integrated with other treatment elements to create the DBT model.

ACT is recognized to have evolved from the basic tenets of CT and CBT, with the emphasis on cognitions and subjective experiences. ACT is sometimes grouped together with DBT, functional-analytic psychotherapy, and MBCT as the "third wave" of behavior therapy. In his Association for the Advancement of Behavior Therapy (AABT) presidential address, Hayes described ACT as grounded in an empirical, principle-focused approach. He then described the "third wave of behavioral and cognitive therapy" as being sensitive to the context and functions of psychological experiences, so that therapies such as ACT emphasize subjective experience and context-driven strategies, in addition to more direct and instructive approaches. These treatments help the patient to develop a set of broad, flexible, and effective repertoires rather than to adopt a symptom reduction approach focused on a certain diagnosis or disorder. ACT and DBT both synthesize and reconstruct previous concepts of behavioral and cognitive therapy, and propel these therapies into domains previously addressed primarily by other traditions (i.e., psychoanalytic, humanistic, and Gestalt therapy) in which therapy outcome has been elusive for more traditional CBT and CT therapies. ACT has similarities to many Eastern approaches, such as Buddhism, and the mystical aspects of most major spiritual and religious traditions. However, ACT is not a mystical or religious movement; it resulted from decades of development via Western science and philosophy. Even so, ACT has reached similar conclusions to many Eastern philosophies with respect to coping and healing, which is particularly relevant in a field that considers the cross-cultural relevance of many Western-designed psychotherapy interventions (Hayes & Smith, 2005; Hayes & Strosahl, 2004).

Rosner, Lyddon, and Freeman (2004) have integrated dream work into CBT based on the assertion that automatic thoughts and cognitive distortions will be evident in dream content. Working from this perspective, the clinician and patient can examine the veracity of recalled thoughts and beliefs, and ultimately displace distorted perceptions with more reality-based thinking. "The cognitive model sees the dreamer as idiosyncratic and the dream as a dramatization of the patient's view of self, world and future, subject to the same cognitive distortions as the waking state" (Brink, 2005, p. 85, quoting Freeman and White, 2004). Aspects of this approach are based on the constructivist model, and the chapter in Rosner et al. by Oscar Gonçalves and Joao Barbosa provides a detailed description of the cognitive-narrative approach to dream work. Brink (2005) characterizes this book as both practically and theoretically valuable.

The relationship between CBT and religion is poorly understood, controversial, and yet important, according to Taylor (2006). In his commentary on Andersson and Asmundson (2006), Taylor reiterates three major issues: (1) Many individuals hold firmly to their religious beliefs even though they have become sophisticated consumers of scientific knowledge; (2) psychology, as a means of change, has joined rather than replaced religious thinking; and (3) the majority of CBT descriptions fail to mention issues relevant to religion or spirituality; although third-wave behavior therapies do address these issues to varying degrees.

Attention to religious or spiritual issues is important in any therapeutic endeavor with a patient who holds religious or spiritual beliefs. For example, Hawkins, Tan, and Turk (1999) concluded that Christian cognitive-behavioral therapy (CCBT) was superior to traditional CBT with inpatient Christian adults. This study does not allow one to conclude that CCBT would be especially efficacious for all patients, but it does imply that patient–treatment matching along the dimension of religious values, compared with therapies that ignore this potentially important patient dimension, enhances outcomes. The importance of religious views and feelings in patient–treatment matching is supported by the finding from the Princeton Religious Research Center (1996) that approximately 96% of adults in America report that they believe in God (Ano & Vasconcelles, 2005). Relatedly, a meta-analysis involving 49 studies and 105 effect sizes found that positive and negative forms of religious coping were associated, respectively, with positive and negative psychological adjustment to stress (Ano & Vasconcelles, 2005). McMinn and Campbell (2007) developed a treatment model that integrates CBT with a Christian approach to psychotherapy.

CBT has incorporated aspects of psychodynamic treatments to produce a more comprehensive, and perhaps more effective, treatment. For example, Futterman, Lorente, and Silverman (2005) proposed a model of substance abuse treatment that integrates CBT, psychodynamic, and behavioral theories to render a novel harm reduction model. This integration incorporates Marlatt's (1998; Marlatt, Blume, & Parks, 2001) harm reduction philosophy and his relapse prevention focus (Marlatt & Gordon, 1985), which are primarily a set of CBT techniques. They describe how this unique blending or "assimilative integration" (Futterman et al., 2005) of theories has created a comprehensive cognitive-behavioral substance abuse theory/treatment, with a process focus that is hypothesized to foster insight, behavior change, and symptom relief.

Another recent example in which CBT incorporates other forms of psychosocial treatment involves a child- and family-focused CBT (CFF-CBT; West, Henry, & Pavuluri, 2007). In this model, both the acute treatment phase and the maintenance phase of treatment integrate interpersonal, CBT, and psychoeducational techniques into a multifaceted treatment program for pediatric bipolar disorder that ideally, also includes pharmacotherapy. In a similar vein, Parsons, Rosof, Punzalan, and Di Maria (2005) integrated motivational interviewing and CBT to enhance medication compliance and reduce substance abuse among HIV-positive men and women. Based on the results of a pilot study, the authors concluded that this form of integrated therapy may comprise an effective intervention that both improves HIV medication compliance and reduces substance use within the HIV-positive population.

Kushner et al. (2006) integrated CBT treatment for panic disorder with a component that focuses on the interaction of alcohol use and panic symptoms in a treatment for comorbid alcoholism and anxiety disorder. They report that the integrated treatment was well received by patients in alcoholism treatment, and that it offers advantages over alcoholism treatment alone. Kushner et al. concluded that this integrated CBT treatment appears to be a practical and efficacious alternative to standard alcoholism treatment.

Choi et al. (2005) compared the effects of the Panic Control Program, traditional CBT integrated with virtual reality technology, and an experiential CBT in the treatment of panic disorder with agoraphobia. They found comparable short-term effects between the two treatments; however, long-term effectiveness appeared to favor the Panic Control Program. In a similar type of study, Stiles, Barkham, Twigg, Mellor-Clark, and Cooper (2006) compared three enhanced therapies with their traditional variants. These authors concluded that the enhanced therapies (including CBT plus an integrative, supportive, or art component) produced a minimally significant benefit compared with the traditional variants. This ambitious study unfortunately had a number of limitations, including missing data, that made reaching clear conclusions tenuous.

A unique integration of psychotherapy technique with CBT involves the melding of psychodrama and CBT to treat depression (Hamamçi, 2006). The investigator concluded that CBT techniques enhance the application and efficiency of psychodrama. Kellogg (2004) reported on the Gestalt technique of "chairwork" and how this technique may be integrated with CBT. More specifically, Kellogg suggested that because gestalts are schemas, and chairwork is an effective method of cognitive restructuring, Gestalt therapy and CBT share a compatible platform for integration. In a qualitative study, DiGiorgio, Arnkoff, Glass, Lyhus, and Walter (2004) discuss how eye movement desensitization and reprocessing (EMDR) can be integrated with various theoretical orientations, including CBT. These authors suggest that qualitative studies similar to theirs can shed light on how practicing clinicians can contribute to the body of research on psychotherapy integration.

Temporomandibular disorders have been successfully treated with CBT integrated with biofeedback. Crider, Glaros, and Gevirtz (2005) found that surface electromyography (SEMG) training combined with CBT proved to be an efficacious treatment for temporomandibular disorders and outperformed biofeedback-assisted relaxation training or SEMG training alone. CBT has also been combined with mirror box therapy to facilitate the rehabilitation of patients with chronic complex regional pain syndrome type I (Tichelaar, Geertzen, Jan, Keizer, & van Wilgen, 2007).

Although they do not focus specifically on CBT and psychotherapy integration, Hwang, Wood, Lin, and Cheung (2006) discuss how theory, research, and clinical practice can be integrated to increase understanding with respect to how Chinese culture may influence the application and process of CBT for Chinese immigrants. Because cultural aspects are potentially interactive with the elements of psychosocial treatment, the level of cultural depth and the breadth of cultural attributes are important elements to consider in the application of various treatment strategies or techniques. In a clinical case study, Kenny (2006) utilized an integrative approach in the treatment of a Native American client with depression. Kenny describes how sensitivity to cultural factors was critical throughout the integrated, client-centered, behavioral, cognitive-behavioral, pharmacological, and support-group treatment.

In this section we have provided examples of CBT and psychotherapy integration. These examples do not represent concerted efforts to systematically and strategically fit a package of empirically supported treatment elements or strategies characteristic of CBT, nor do they show how these efficacious treatment elements may be integrated to meet the specific needs of the patient. We now focuses on CBT's potential as a foundation for prescriptive psychotherapy, and how a CBT-based patient–treatment matching model may increase the likelihood and magnitude of positive change (see Beutler et al. [2003] for the results of an RCT that involved a patient–treatment matching model that produced astonishing results when applied to a population of comorbid depressed and substance-abusing patients).

COGNITIVE THERAPY AS AN INTEGRATIVE FRAMEWORK

Behavior therapy became a formal approach for treating psychological disorders in the late 1950s (Wilson, 1989). Contemporary behavior therapy encompasses four main areas: (1) behavioral analysis, with a focus on observable behavior; (2) a neobehavioristic stimulus–response model, which employs classical and avoidant conditioning; (3) social learning theory, which examines the mediation of environmental events by cognitive processes; and (4) cognitive-behavioral modification, which focuses on how interpretation of events determines behavior.

CT is a specific form of the more general CBTs. CT was developed in the early 1960s by Beck and colleagues at the University of Pennsylvania. As a result of his research on the psychodynamic theory of depression (i.e., the hypothesis that depression is retroflected anger; Beck & Weishaar, 1989), Beck observed that depressed individuals have predictable cognitive patterns that negatively characterized their view of the self, the world, and the future. This observation led Beck to realize that faulty cognitive patterns, typically incorrect and untested assumptions, misperceptions, or dysfunctional belief systems, are responsible for many patients' difficulties. While rooted in a tradition of methodological behaviorism, CT has now extended beyond this perspective and is recognized as an approach in its own right.

Cognitive theory has been empirically based since its inception, in that it used findings from formal research to establish its theoretical principles. Likewise, it allows for a variety of viewpoints and applications. CT, like behavior therapy, has a commitment to the scientific method, and both emphasize the patient's ability to learn new and adaptive ways of functioning. CT may best be defined as the application of cognitive theory to a certain disorder and the use of techniques to modify the dysfunctional beliefs and maladaptive information-processing systems that are characteristic of the disorder (Beck, 1993). CT continues to evolve, partially due to the recognition that the integration of techniques that characterize other therapies' views often enhances the overall effectiveness of this treatment (Dowd, 2004; Robins & Hayes, 1993). Beck (1991) has argued that CT is the epitome of an integrative psychosocial treatment, because it addresses the common factor that cuts across all effective therapies, which is cognitive change. This integration allows a CT therapist to select interventions from a variety of theoretical viewpoints.

The collection of procedures and microtheories that comprise the CBT and CT traditions has also borrowed techniques and theoretical perspectives from other psychosocial orientations (Norcross & Halgin, 2005). Indeed, neither CBT nor the more specific CT is a closed system. As a general class of procedures, CBT has always evolved through the integration of techniques and theoretical concepts from other approaches (Hollon & Beck, 2004; McCullough, 2000; Robins & Hayes, 1993). For example, the schema concept allows for the influence of early developmental conflicts and their later manifestation in personality styles. Moreover, from its inception, CBT expanded on behavioral theory and recognized the need to consider patients' inner lives.

The refinements that have occurred through integration of diverse research and theoretical principles have allowed for the inclusion of concepts and techniques that are consistent with the application of relationship therapy, behavior therapy, interpersonal therapy, and others. The concepts of dysfunctional cognition–schemas–behaviors remain at the core of cognitive theory and serve as integrative principles for concepts from other theories that reflect on the roles of early experience and unconscious processes. Recently, integrated components of CT and CBT include the role of defense processes, an emphasis on the exploration of the therapeutic relationship and the patient's interpersonal dynamics, facilitative aspect of affective arousal, and the developmental experiences in the formation of maladaptive schemas (Safran & Muran, 2000; Robins & Hayes, 1993), which are constructs associated with psychodynamic theories. For example, defense processes are thought by some (e.g., Young, 1990) to help the patient avoid schema-related material through denial, repression of memories, or depersonalization. Emotional avoidance of painful schema-related material may appear as defensive numbing, dissociation, or minimization of negative experiences. Behavioral defenses may include physical avoidance of situations that activate dysfunctional or painful schemas.

Although CT has long recognized the importance of a sound therapeutic relationship, attention to the interpersonal processes within the broader array of CBTs has taken on a greater emphasis in recent years (Ellis, 2005; Liotti, 1991; Mahoney, 1991; Robins & Hayes, 1993; Safran & Segal, 1990). Interpersonal processes are now seen as important avenues to explore and ameliorate dysfunctional interpersonal schemas. Due to the early and important influence of interpersonal events in the development of schemas, attachment theory (Bowlby, 1977) has also been incorporated by some cognitive therapists to help them understand the dynamics of the therapeutic relationship (Robins & Hayes, 1993). Although not referred to as "countertransference" within the cognitive perspective, Safran and Segal (1990) argue that cognitive therapists need to attend to the feelings and behaviors elicited by their interactions with the patient, and to avoid involvement in the patient's dysfunctional interpersonal cycle. They also recommend that the thoughts and feelings uncovered in this type of interaction be thoroughly explored in therapy.

The eclecticism of cognitive treatments can be seen in their success with a wide variety of conditions, problems, and disorders (Hollon & Beck, 2004; Lambert & Ogles, 2004). Integrative therapies, such as CBT, may increase the likelihood and magnitude of positive outcomes, because they have more comprehensive effects and seem to reduce attrition (Lambert & Ogles, 2004). The range of effectiveness attests to the flexibility of the techniques and suggests that these procedures may be used within a prescriptive, strategic framework.

THE RANGE OF EFFECTIVENESS
ASSOCIATED WITH COGNITIVE THERAPY

Comparative outcome studies of psychotherapies for various psychological problems have generally led to the conclusion that treatments are broadly equivalent in effectiveness (Shapiro, Barkham, Rees, & Hardy, 1994; Robinson, Berman, & Neimeyer, 1990; Bowers, 1990; Hogg & Deffenbacher, 1988). However, in contrast to those who maintain that research reveals equivalent outcomes among therapies, disciples of CT have asserted that their treatment is more effective than others across a variety of conditions and disorders (Hollon & Beck, 2004; Lambert & Ogles, 2004; Brown, 1997; Blackburn, Jones, & Lewin, 1986).

Studies have illustrated that CT is effective in the treatment of various types of depression, such as unipolar, major, minor and acute depression (Dobson, 1989; Gitlin, 1995; Billings & Moos, 1984). Positive findings have also been obtained in samples of patients with endogenous depression, a subtype often thought to be refractory to psychotherapy (Simons & Thase, 1992; Thase & Simons, 1992). CT appears to be effective in reducing symptoms of depression and anxiety, and increasing assertiveness in both group and individual formats (Scogin, Hamblin, & Beutler, 1987; Steur, 1984; Shaffer, Shapiro, Sark, & Coghlan, 1981). A study by Ogles, Sawyer, and Lambert (1995) for the National Institute of Mental Health found that a substantial number of clients who completed cognitive treatment for depression showed reliable change on all measures of outcome. In addition, Brown and Barlow (1995) found that CT significantly reduced somatic depressive symptoms and depressed and anxious mood for patients with alcoholism. In addition to these studies, Scogin et al. (1987) found that cognitive bibliotherapy more effectively reduced depression than either a delayed-treatment control group or an attention–placebo–bibliotherapy condition. Although this latter finding has not uniformly been supported (Scogin, Bowman, Jamison, Beutler, & Machado, 1994), even studies that fail to replicate these findings report that patients who score relatively high on measures of cognitive dysfunction tend to have lower scores on posttreatment depression severity measures than those with low levels of cognitive impairment. These findings strongly implicate cognitive functions as important aspects of the change processes related to improvement, regardless of the model of treatment used to address them.

CT also does well in comparisons to pharmacotherapy. Most of the published trials have found CT to be at least equal, and sometimes superior, to pharmacotherapy (Blackburn, Jones, & Lewin, 1986, 1996). Specifically, studies have revealed that CT is equally or more efficacious than standard antidepressant medication (Beck & Emery, 1985) and tends to have lower rates of relapse (Hollon, 1996). Rush (1982), Rush, Beck, Kovacs, and Hollon (1977), Rush, Beck, Kovacs, Weissenburger, & Hollon (1982), and Murphy, Simons, Wetzel, and Lustman (1984) also found that CT was associated with more improvement and less attrition than pharmacotherapy. In fact, patients had a higher rate of dropout when researchers compared pharmacotherapy alone to CT. These studies also revealed that CT exceeded pharmacotherapy in improving depressive symptoms of hopelessness and low self-concept. Even when CT is combined with pharmacotherapy, patients tend to report significantly fewer depressive symptoms and negative cognitions at discharge than they report with pharmacotherapy alone (Bowers, 1990). It appears that CT has a significant impact on the cognitive and vegetative symptoms associated with moderate and severe depression, as well as the symptoms of mild and transitory depressive states.

CT has also been found to be more effective than behavioral- and interpersonally based therapies (Shapiro et al., 1994; Wilson, Goldin, & Charbourneau-Powis, 1983). Gaffan, Tsaousis, and Kemp-Wheeler (1995) replicated a study by Dobson (1989) comparing CT with other forms of treatment. Although their study focused primarily on allegiance effects, they also reported that CT was superior to other forms of treatment, including behavior therapy.

Clients who endorsed characterological and existential reasons for depression responded better to CT than to behavioral interventions (Addis & Jacobson, 1996). Overall, there is strong support for the value of CT in treating patients with depression, but researchers are still uncertain about the mechanisms through which this effect takes place (Jacobson, & Hollon, 1996).

CT also appears to be effective in treating other types of disorders. Thus, CT is effective in treating anxiety disorders, especially specific fears and phobias, and a host of other anxiety disorders and symptoms. Barlow, O'Brien, and Last (1984) and Lent, Russell, and Zamostry (1981) found that CT was superior to behavioral therapy in the treatment of patients who experienced anxiety. CT also fosters overall abstinence, both at the end of treatment and during follow-up periods, among patients with alcoholism (Brown & Barlow, 1995). Studies further suggest that CBT is effective in treating patients with eating disorders (Hollon & Beck, 1986). Fairburn, Jones, Paveler, Hope, and O'Connor (1993) used CT for patients with bulimia nervosa, and found substantial and well-maintained treatment effects reflected in all aspects of functioning. Moreover, Arntz and van den Hout (1996) found that among patients with panic disorder and a secondary diagnosis of either social or mood disorder, CT produced superior outcomes in comparison to applied relaxation by reducing the frequency of panic attacks. In addition, CT is effective in the treatment of patients with problems characterized by a lack of self-assertion (Safran, Alden, & Davidon, 1980), anger and aggression (Schlicter & Horan, 1981), and addictive disorders (Woody et al., 1984).

In addition to studies examining the effects of CT on a variety of patient problems and characteristics, an increasing number of studies in the literature have attested to the ability of CT interventions to lead to sustained reductions in problems. A 1-year follow-up study by Kovacs et al. (1981), for example, revealed that self-rated depression was significantly lower for those who had completed CT than for those treated with pharmacotherapy. Similarly, a 2-year follow-up study of patients treated with CT, pharmacotherapy, or their combination indicated that CT was associated with lower relapse rates (Blackburn et al., 1986). Moreover, patients in the pharmacotherapy group had the highest relapse rate at the 2-year follow-up. Thus, even though it remains unclear what aspects of CT produce improvement in various patient groups, it is certain that CT is effective, often more effective than other forms of treatment (Hollon & Beck, 2004; Lambert & Ogles, 2004).

CT has certain advantages over many other models by virtue of the variety of conditions for which it is effective, and in this sense has the makings of a flexible and eclectic intervention model. This is not to say, however, that the practice of CT is equally effective for all individuals. Research (e.g., Beutler, Mohr, Grawe, Engle, & MacDonald, 1991) reveals that the efficacy of CT is differentially influenced by a variety of qualities characteristic of the patient and problem. Qualities such as patient coping styles, reactance levels, and complexity and severity of problems, among others, may influence the way that CT is applied.

One patient characteristic that has proven to predict patients' response to CT is "coping style," the method that an individual adopts when confronted with anxiety-provoking situations, and that typically is viewed as a trait-like pattern. CT has been found to be most effective among patients who exhibit an extroverted, undercontrolled, externalizing coping style. For example, Kadden, Cooney, and Getter (1989) evaluated patients with alcoholism and implemented cognitive-based social skills training as a procedure to preventing relapse by remediating behavioral deficits in coping with interpersonal and intrapersonal antecedents to drinking. While CT was approximately as effective as other treatments overall, it was more effective than other approaches among patients who were relatively high on measures of sociopathy or impulsivity. This type of ATI was also found by Beutler, Engle, et al. (1991). Depressed patients who scored high on Minnesota Multiphasic Personality Inventory (MMPI) measures of externalization and impulsivity responded better to CT than to insight-oriented therapy. This pattern holds among both depressed inpatients and outpatients (Beutler & Mitchell, 1981; Beutler, Mohr, et al., 1991). Barber and Muenz (1996) also found that CT is more effective than treatment interventions for patients who avoid their problems through the externalization of blame. In addition, Beutler, Mohr, et al. (1991) and Beutler, Engle, et al. (1991) found that CT exerted substantially stronger effects on patients with externalizing coping styles than did client-centered therapy or supportive, self-directed therapy, respectively. On the other hand, internalizing patients did better with client-centered and self-directed therapy than with CT. Similarly, in the aforementioned studies, patient resistance traits and tendencies differentiated the level of benefit achieved from the therapist-guided procedures of CT and various patient-led or nondirective procedures.

A study by Tasca, Russell, and Busby (1994) examined patient characteristics, such as defensive style and psychological mindedness, as mediators of patient preferences for CT. Those patients who were expressive and externalized their anger by using projection and turning anger against others tended to choose activity-oriented therapy. Thus, it appears that CT is effective for clients who avoid their problems, perhaps because this treatment intervention tends to prompt clients to confront anxiety-provoking situations through symptom-focused homework and specific behavioral interventions and techniques.

Evidence supports the advantages of cognitive treatments among patients with complex or severe problems. Complexity and severity may be associated with factors such as comorbidity, enduring personality disturbances, and chronicity of the condition. As a result, patients with long-standing personality disturbances, or those whose problems and symptoms tend to recur and persist over a long period of time, tend to have specific treatment needs. Apparently, the initial severity of depression moderates the efficacy of treatment (Robinson et al., 1990), even while CT appears to be effective for patients exhibiting such symptom characteristics with varying degrees of complexity and severity. Woody et al. (1984) found that among persons addicted to opiates with low and moderate severity, those treated with CT made equal or greater progress than patients receiving other forms of psychotherapy. Knight-Law, Sugerman, and Pettinati (1988) found that the effectiveness of behavioral symptom–focused interventions was highest among those patients whose problems were reactional and situational, and more complex in nature. Similar patterns of interaction were observed by Beutler, Sandowicz, Fisher, and Albanese (1996); CT was more effective than emotion-focused treatments for patients with low levels of distress (acute indicators).

Brown and Barlow (1995) examined long-term effects of CBT in patients with panic disorder. Although the results did not support the notion that CT has long-term effects on reducing symptomatology, they did suggest that patients with more severe symptomatology were responsive to treatment in the short term. Moreover, patients were neither less able to maintain these treatment gains or more apt to experience marked fluctuations in symptoms over the longer term. This latter finding suggests that the long-term effects of CT are in part related to interactional matches between type of treatment and patient characteristics. This conclusion is supported by other research as well. For instance, Beutler, Mohr, et al. (1991; Beutler et al., 1993, 2003) found that patients whose personal characteristics indicated that they were poor candidates for CT (i.e., internalizers and those who were resistant to direction) had poorer long-term results than those who were better matched to the treatment demands. In contrast, good candidate patients were likely to maintain treatment gains and even to improve during the follow-up period. These findings underline the potential importance of external coping styles and low-resistance traits as indicators for CT. In addition, the evidence suggests that situation-specific problems respond better to cognitive-behavioral treatments than do chronic and recurrent problems among individuals with eating disorders (Sheppard et al., 1988), somatic symptoms (LaCroix, Clarke, Bock, & Doxey, 1986) and those with chronic back pain (Tref & Yuan, 1983).

It appears that change in CT is facilitated in a climate that fosters affective arousal. Robins and Hayes (1993) identified several affective arousal techniques that are advocated by cognitive therapists, including shame-attacking exercises, imagery dialogues, the use of dreams, repetition and exaggeration of key phrases, and focusing on physical cues/bodily sensations associated with currently experienced feelings. Affect-enhancing techniques have been integrated into CT by many therapists as a means to induce affect among those with low levels of arousal.

Finally, although CT is often conceptualized as present-focused, modifications have sought to make it more amenable to explorations of historical contributions to patient problems (Arnkoff, 1983; Kellogg, 2004; Robins & Hayes, 1993; Young, 1990). The examination of cognition within a developmental framework may help to induce affective arousal, and thereby enhance the opportunity for patient and therapist to identify and challenge maladaptive expectations, and to evaluate faulty assumptions associated with recalled events.

MAKING COGNITIVE THERAPY
SYSTEMATICALLY FIT HUMAN COMPLEXITY

The major impetus for psychotherapy integration comes from the evidence that no single school of psychotherapy has demonstrated consistent superiority over the others. Rather, psychotherapy research for specific problems, such as drug abuse or depression, has largely led to the conclusion that all approaches produce similar average effects (e.g., Lambert, Shapiro, & Bergin, 1986; Beutler, Crago, & Arizmendi, 1986; Smith, Glass, & Miller, 1980). Unfortunately, the nonsignificance of treatment main effects often draws more attention than the growing body of research that demonstrates meaningful differences in the types of patients for whom different aspects of treatment are effective (Beutler et al., 2003; Harwood & Beutler, 2008).

For example, research indicates that for patients with symptoms of anxiety and depression (1) experiential therapies are more effective than cognitive and dynamic therapies when initial distress about one's condition is insufficient to support movement (Beutler & Mitchell, 1981; Orlinsky & Howard, 1986); (2) nondirective and paradoxical interventions are more effective than directive treatments in patients with high levels of pretherapy resistance (i.e., "resistance potential"; Beutler et al., 2003; Beutler, Mohr, et al., 1991; Beutler, Engle, et al., 1991; Shoham-Salomon & Hannah, 1991; Forsyth & Forsyth, 1982); and (3) therapies that target cognitive and behavior changes through contingency management (e.g., Higgins, Budney, & Bickel, 1994) are more effective than insight-oriented therapies in impulsive or externalizing patients, but this effect is reversed in patients with less externalizing coping styles (Beutler et al., 2003; Beutler, Mohr, et al., 1991; Beutler, Engle, et al., 1991; Calvert, Beutler, & Crago, 1988; Sloane, Staples, Cristol, Yorkston, & Whipple, 1975).

CT may be adapted to meet the manifold needs and characteristics of patients with a wide array of problems and diagnoses. In a recent study at our Psychotherapy Research Lab at the University of California, Santa Barbara, several guiding principles and strategies informed the systematic application of tactics and techniques drawn from numerous theoretical perspectives. The techniques of CT may be used with virtually any patient; however, the greatest benefit is achieved when the strategies or techniques are employed differentially, depending on patient dimensions such as coping style, type of problem, subjective distress, functional and social impairment, and level of resistance.

For illustrative purposes, the remainder of this section addresses some of the techniques and strategies that guide the application of CT techniques for the internalizing or externalizing patient, the resistant patient, and for management of arousal level. A thorough discussion of patient–treatment matching dimensions (resistance/reactance level, styles of coping, severity of subjective distress, and functional impairment) and guiding principles, strategies, and technique selection can be found elsewhere (Beutler et al., 2000, 2003; Beutler & Harwood, 2000; Harwood & Beutler, 2008).

Patient resistance typically bodes poorly for treatment effectiveness, unless it is managed skillfully. It is generally assumed that some patients are more likely than others to resist therapeutic procedures. "Resistance" may be characterized as a dispositional trait and a transitory in-therapy state of oppositional (e.g., angry, irritable, and suspicious) behaviors. It involves both intrapsychic (image of self, safety, and psychological integrity) and interpersonal (loss of interpersonal freedom or power imposed by another) factors (Beutler et al., 1996). "Reactance," an extreme example of resistance, is manifested by oppositional and uncooperative behaviors.

A patient's level of resistance or reactance potential is determined by three hypothesized factors (Beutler et al., 1996). The first factor involves the subjective value placed by the patient on the particular freedom that is perceived to be threatened. For example, one patient may value the freedom associated with an unfixed schedule of time commitments, whereas another may be relatively comfortable with an imposed schedule or routine. The second factor involves the proportion of freedoms perceived to be threatened or eliminated. Introducing an element in treatment that eliminates or reduces a variety of freedoms (e.g., a homework assignment that proscribes substance use and requires social interaction at an event for a particular amount of time) will likely generate a high level of reactance among resistance-prone, substance-abusing, and socially withdrawn individuals. The third factor involves the magnitude of authority and power ascribed to the threatening force or individual. The resistance generated by this factor derives from a patient's preconceived notions and differential assignment of authority to various professional occupations (clinicians, law enforcement officials, etc.). Additionally, actual interactions with a mental health professional may operate to reduce or exaggerate these notions.

Resistance is easily identifiable, and differential treatment plans for patients with high and low resistance are easily crafted. The successful implementation of these plans, however, is often quite a different matter. Overcoming patient resistance to the clinician's efforts is difficult. It requires that the therapist set aside his or her own resistance to recognize that the patient's oppositional behavior may actually be iatrogenic. In a study of experienced and highly trained therapists in the Vanderbilt Study of Psychodynamic Psychotherapy, *none* were able to work effectively with patient resistance (Binder & Strupp, 1997). Rather, therapists often reacted to patient resistance by becoming angry, critical, and rejecting, which are reactions that tend to reduce the willingness of patients to explore problems.

In general, therapists should avoid open disagreement with highly resistant patients. The collaborative relationship of CT is an important antidote to resistance, and this component should be emphasized from the initiation of therapy. Socratic questioning or guided discovery, another common element of CT, must be handled carefully to minimize resistance tendencies. A clinician should introduce this technique as a collaborative effort and elicit feedback regarding the patient's willingness to participate. Comfort with direction and suggestions for exploration may also be elicited from the patient. Information regarding a patient's level of resistance potential may be gathered from the patient's history and behavior during recent stressful experiences or during the process of treatment itself. Table 4.1 provides examples of behaviors associated with high levels of *trait* or *state* resistance potential.

Research (Shoham-Salomon, Avner, & Neeman, 1989; Shoham-Salomon & Rosenthal, 1987; Horvath, 1989; Seltzer, 1986) suggests that nondirective, paradoxical, and self-directed procedures produce better outcomes among patients who exhibit high resistance behaviors. Patient-generated behavioral contracts and "suggested" homework assignments are nondirective interventions that help to manage resistant patients. For patients with extreme and persistent resistance, a "paradoxical intervention" in which the symptom is prescribed, or in which the patient is encouraged to avoid change for a period of time, might be considered. Simply put, paradoxical interventions induce change by discouraging it (Seltzer, 1986). A nondirective, paradoxical intervention could involve the *suggestion* that the patient continue or exaggerate the symptom/behavior. A classic example of such an intervention might be to prescribe wakefulness for the patient complaining of insomnia. An acceptable rationale should be provided for this type of intervention (e.g., "Your circadian rhythm is not properly set. Staying awake will help you reset your sleep cycle"). Non- or low-resistant behaviors indicate that patients are generally open to external direction or directive interventions and guidance from the therapist.

An example of how CT can be adapted to patient characteristics may be provided by briefly describing how homework can be applied to both

TABLE 4.1. Behaviors Characteristic of Resistance

Patient resistance level	
High *trait* resistance potential	High *state* resistance potential
1. Frequently expresses resentment of others.	1. Has trouble understanding or following instructions.
2. Seems to expect that others will take advantage of them.	2. Stubborn about accepting something that is obvious to the therapist.
3. Tends to be controlling and demanding in intimate relationships.	3. Seems closed to new experiences.
4. Is distrustful and suspicious of others' motives.	4. Responds to suggestions in a passive–aggressive way.
5. Expresses resentment over not having the advantages/opportunities of others.	5. Begins coming late or avoiding appointments.
6. Often has broken the "rules."	6. Expresses fear that the therapist is trying to take advantage of him or her.
7. Enjoys competition.	7. Begins to tenaciously hold a point of view and can't be argued out of a position once it is set.
8. Does the opposite when others try to control him or her.	8. Holds a grudge.
9. Resents those who make the rules.	9. Becomes overtly angry at the therapist.
10. Is happiest when in charge.	

high-resistant and low-resistant patients (see Table 4.2; Beutler & Harwood, 2000). Three guidelines distinguish between the use of homework with resistant patients and that assigned and utilized with low-resistant patients. First, homework for resistant patients should be of a self-directed nature, such as bibliotherapy selected by the patient from a predetermined list and accompanied by self-help workbooks. Second, the resistant patient should self-monitor success (e.g., recording self-control procedures or mood ratings). Third, the therapist should expend relatively little effort to check or collect homework assignments. On the other hand, homework for the nonresistant patient may be highly structured and can include assigned readings and exercises designed specifically to alter social behaviors and drug use patterns. With such patients, homework should be reviewed/checked regularly, and progress should be monitored on a weekly basis.

Another means to adapt CT to fit resistance levels involves therapist directiveness. Nondirective therapeutic interventions are effective with resistant patients; therefore, high levels of recurrent resistance suggest the need to reduce therapist directiveness, authoritarian stances, and confrontation. Nondirective interventions include reflection, clarification, questions, support, paradoxical interventions, and an approach–retreat method in which the therapist introduces difficult topics, followed by his or her withdrawal into relative silence. For patients who manifest few indicators of resistance, therapists can typically provide guidance and make interpretations, and direct suggestions and assignments. Research suggests that low-resistance patients may in fact do better with authoritative and directive roles compared with nondirective ones (Beutler et al., 2003; Beutler, Engle, et al., 1991). Therapists need to be vigilant for insession indicators of resistance and adapt interventions accordingly (see Table 4.3).

Empirical support for the role of patient resistance levels in treatment planning can be found in more than 30 investigations rendering a combined sample size of more than 8,000 inpatient and outpatient participants, and cov-

TABLE 4.2. General Guidelines for Treating High- and Low- Resistance Patients

Patient resistance level	
High resistance	Low resistance
1. Provide opportunities for self-directed improvement.	1. Increase relative reliance on procedures that invoke the therapists authority.
2. Increase reliance on nondirective interventions.	2. Therapists may provide direct guidance.
3. Consider using paradoxical interventions.	3. Suggestions and interpretation are typically well received.
4. Deemphasize the use of confrontive procedures.	4. Therapists may assign therapist-guided homework.
5. Deemphasize the use of procedures that invoke the therapist's authority.	5. Use behavioral strategies that structure and monitor therapeutic activities.

TABLE 4.3. Examples of Directive and Nondirective Interventions

Type of intervention	
Directive	Nondirective
1. Asking closed questions.	1. Asking open-ended questions.
2. Providing interpretations.	2. Reflection.
3. Confrontation.	3. Passive acceptance of feelings/thoughts.
4. Interrupting speech or behavior.	4. Self-monitored homework.
5. Providing information or instructions.	5. Self-directed therapy work.
6. Structured homework.	6. Paradoxical work.
7. Analysis of ABC relationships.	7. Low-percentage of incidences in which
8. Activity scheduling.	the therapist introduces topics.

ering myriad psychiatric diagnoses. Psychosocial treatment formats included individual, family, group, and parent training (Castonguay & Beutler, 2006a). A wide variety of psychotherapies and pharmacological agents were involved in these comparative outcome studies (Beutler et al., 2000; Harwood & Beutler, 2008).

Internalization and externalization represent opposite poles on the trait-like dimension of coping style. Both coping styles may be used to reduce uncomfortable experience (i.e., provide escape or avoidance). Some patients cope by activating externalizing behaviors that allow either direct escape or avoidance of the feared environment. Alternatively, other patients may prefer behaviors (i.e., self-blame, compartmentalization, sensitization) that control internal experiences such as anxiety. Internalizing patients are typically characterized by low impulsivity and overcontrol of impulses, whereas externalizers generally exhibit highly impulsive or exaggerated behaviors. Additionally, internalizers tend to be more insightful and self-reflective. Internalizers typically inhibit feelings, tolerate emotional distress better than externalizers, and frequently attribute difficulties they encounter to themselves. On the other hand, externalizers tend to deny personal responsibility for either the cause or the solution of their problems, experience negative emotions as intolerable, and seek external stimulation. It should be acknowledged, however, that some patients' complex styles include coping behaviors characteristic of both internalizers and externalizers.

Table 4.4 provides examples of patient characteristics that correspond to internalizing and externalizing coping styles. In the case of an excessively impulsive (externalizing) patient who, for example, may be a stimulation seeker (i.e., avoiding lack of stimulation), or who may avoid the anticipated consequences of social contact, the treatment might include learning to tolerate bland and nonstimulating environments. Therapeutic procedures to facilitate internal reattribution of responsibility (Beck, Wright, Newman, & Liese, 1993) may also help in the treatment of externalizers, who otherwise blame others or take a fatalistic view of problems. Daily thought records (DTRs) may help to identify impulsive behaviors and reactions. Activity schedules

TABLE 4.4. Characteristics of Externalizing and Internalizing Patients

Internalizers typically	Externalizers typically
1. Are more likely to feel hurt than anger.	1. Are gregarious and outgoing.
2. Are quiet in social gatherings.	2. Seek to impress others.
3. Worry and ruminate a lot before taking action.	3. Seek social status.
4. Feel more than passing guilt, remorse, or shame about minor things.	4. Avoid boredom by seeking novelty, activity, or stimulation.
5. Lack self-confidence.	5. Are insensitive to other's feelings.
6. Like to be alone.	6. Have and inflated sense of importance.
7. Are timid.	7. Are impulsive.
8. Are reluctant to express anger directly.	8. React to frustration with overt anger.
9. Are introverted.	9. Become easily frustrated.
10. Do not go to parties often.	10. Deny responsibility for problems that occur.
11. Do not let feelings show.	11. Have little empathy for others.

may be used to supplement the DTR to identify how the patient might prefer high-stimulation activities. Activity schedules can also be used to gauge behavioral change. Stimulus control strategies, such as identifying high-risk situations and developing adaptive coping responses, may be useful for impulsive individuals recovering from substance abuse or similar, impulse-related problems.

Internalizing individuals may avoid uncomfortable feelings, intimacy, or environmental stimulation and activity. In such cases, treatment might focus on the patient allowing emotional intensity to occur, or accepting an expression of love and intimacy. Although the principles of treatment are the same as those for externalizers, the treatment of internalizing individuals is more complex. Internalizing individuals' treatment cues are embedded within their unique history of conflict and feeling development. As such, the examination of patterns in the DTRs may be an efficient method to uncover cues that are indirectly associated with overt symptoms; that is, the DTR may help the patient and therapist to build a bridge between avoided knowledge and insight, or from feelings to awareness. The downward arrow technique (Beck et al., 1993) may also elicit hot cognitions, and encourage insight and increased focus on salient emotional states. Thus, a focus on schematic thoughts rather than automatic thoughts may be indicated. Cognitive skills and restructuring may be enhanced by uncovering the historical origins of the patient's dysfunctional negative schemas and relating them to present functioning. Activity schedules may identify withdrawal/lack of social contact or other deficiencies in the range of typical activity, and this information may help to identify social schemas.

Coping style was evaluated and identified as a participant factor by the APA Division 29 Task Force and is considered an empirically based principle of change due to "a preponderance of the available evidence" (Castonguay & Beutler, 2006b, p. 634). Empirical evidence comes in the form of at least

30 investigations involving both inpatient and outpatient populations. The combined sample size from these investigations totals to more than 5,600 participants with a wide range of disorders (Beutler et al., 2000; Harwood & Beutler, 2008).

The patient's level of subjective distress may help guide the therapist's differential use of cognitive techniques. A moderate but nondebilitating level of emotional intensity or distress may motivate therapy efforts; whereas a high level of distress can interfere with therapy, a low level of emotional intensity might be insufficient to motivate the patient to change. Therefore, evaluation and management of the patient's distress is an important aspect of most therapeutic endeavors (Orlinsky, Grawe, & Park, 1994; Frank & Frank, 1991).

Use of the downward arrow technique to pursue hot cognitions will likely increase emotional intensity. Table 4.5 illustrates a patient's completed DTR and the therapy interaction that may have ensued. The last statement from the patient contains hot cognitions that are characteristic of the core schema "I'm unlovable," which is often accompanied by emotional arousal. The structured analysis of dysfunctional thoughts/cognitive errors may be utilized after the identification of hot cognitions or core schemas, to reduce unduly high levels of emotional intensity. Direct relaxation (i.e., a focus on breathing and muscle relaxation) followed by suggestions for thought insertion, such as "I am relaxed and comfortable" or "I can control how I feel," can be particularly helpful to reduce arousal levels.

The patient–treatment matching dimension of subjective distress has received empirical support in at least 11 investigations, with a combined sample size of more than 1,250 participants. A variety of diagnoses and several different psychosocial and pharmacological treatments were represented in these studies.

Similarly, the patient's level of impairment may indicate the need for longer-term and more intensive therapies. Beutler et al. (2000) found that level of impairment is an indicator for the use of intensive treatments, including adjunctive medication, individual therapy, and alterations in the length and

---

TABLE 4.5. Example of the "Downward-Arrow" Technique

Situation: At home on a Saturday afternoon.

Emotions: Depressed (80%), anxious (60%).

Automatic thought: "I should have a date on Saturday night."

THERAPIST: What does it mean if you don't have a date on Saturday night?

PATIENT: It means that I'll be home by myself on Saturday night.

THERAPIST: What does being home alone on a Saturday night mean?

PATIENT: It means that I'm not out having fun like everybody else.

THERAPIST: And what does that mean to you?

PATIENT: That I'm a loser, nobody loves me, and I'll always be alone.

spacing of treatment among patients with depression, anxiety, alcohol abuse, and mixed diagnoses. Cognitive therapists can adapt the frequency and spacing of sessions to meet the needs presented by patients with high levels of social and interpersonal impairment; even patients with psychotic disorders may benefit from cognitive interventions (Haddock & Slade, 1996; Kingdon, & Turkington, 1994). Patients with low social support, low social functioning, and comorbidity may be the best candidates for long-term interventions, frequent sessions, and concomitant pharmacotherapy. Patients with adequate levels of social support, low impairment, and no Axis II comorbidity, on the other hand, may be successfully treated by a time-limited course of cognitive intervention.

"Functional impairment" (FI), both a level of care principle and a prognostic indicator, was identified as a participant factor by the Division 29 Task Force (Castonguay & Beutler, 2006b; Beutler, Blatt, Alahohamed, Levy, & Angtuaco, 2006) and it has also been identified by the Dysphoria Work Group on Empirically Based Principles of Therapeutic Change (Castonguay & Beutler, 2006a). Empirical support for the assessment of FI and application of this information in treatment planning can be found in more than 45 investigations rendering a combined sample size of more than 7,700 participants. Both inpatient and outpatient settings were involved, as were almost all of the major diagnostic categories. Moreover, myriad forms of psychosocial treatments were administered (Beutler et al., 2000; Harwood & Beutler, 2008).

Related to FI, social support was identified by the Dysphoria Work Group of the Task Force on Empirically Based Principles of Therapeutic Change (Castonguay & Beutler, 2006c). This patient–treatment matching dimension is well suited to CBT by virtue of the variety of techniques available to the cognitive-behavioral therapist to increase social support networks. The importance of social support has been demonstrated in at least 37 investigations, with a combined sample size of more than 7,700 inpatients and outpatients (Beutler et al., 2000; Harwood & Beutler, 2008). In a similar vein, the patient–treatment matching dimension of problem complexity and chronicity (PCC) has received empirical support in at least 23 investigations, with a combined sample size of nearly 2,300. Inpatients and outpatients with a variety of psychiatric diagnoses characterize the sample. PCC is related to FI and is a prognostic indicator, an indicator of treatment intensity, and an indicator of the need for multiperson or broadband treatment (Beutler et al., 2000; Harwood & Beutler, 2008).

Treatment may also be adjusted to fit patients who vary on the dimensions of sociotropy and autonomy. Individuals who are highly sociotropic are dependent on relationships with others for interpersonal needs. Sociotropic individuals place a high value on acceptance, intimacy, support, and guidance (Blackburn, 1998). Individuals who are highly autonomous value independence and freedom from external control, as well as mobility, superior levels of achievement, and choice. These individuals are predicted to be vulnerable to externally imposed constraints or personal limitations that result in a failure to attain goals (Moore & Blackburn, 1996). The Sociotropy–Autonomy Scale (SAS; Beck, Epstein, Harrison, & Emery, 1983) is a 60-item self-report measure that utilizes a 5-point scale format to assess these personality dimensions. Sociotropy has been shown to have stability over time (Blackburn, 1998) and the validity of the SAS has been demonstrated (Clark & Beck, 1991). The conceptual validity of autonomy as applied to differential treatment decisions has not been consistently demonstrated (Blackburn, 1998). The SAS is in the process of revision for further validation studies (Clark, Steer, Beck, & Ross, 1995).

Low resistance potential is characterized by avoidance of confrontation with others and acceptance of direction from those in authority, which appears to be similar to the sociotropic's need for acceptance, support, and guidance from others (Allen, Horne, & Trinder, 1996). Autonomous individuals also appear to share similarities with those scoring high on measures of resistance. Opposition to attempted or perceived control from others and a need to be in charge characterize high resistance. These characteristics seem to parallel the autonomous individual's need for independence and mobility. If a relationship between these patient dimensions can be discerned, then it may be that non-directive and patient-monitored interventions would produce better outcomes for autonomous/resistant patients, whereas sociotropic/low-resistant patients might respond best to directive interventions, frequent interpretations, and direct guidance from the therapist.

SUMMARY

Eclectic viewpoints have proliferated in recent years. Haphazard eclecticism is the most widely practiced but least systematic form of eclecticism. Theoretical integration is widely practiced but may be too abstract to provide clear and practical guidance to implement treatments. Systematic eclectic theories suffer from being too narrow and atheoretical. We have argued, however, that the theoretical and practical foundations of CT provide a framework and platform for the development of strategic eclectic interventions.

CT has traditions, such as adherence to empirical guidelines, a foundation in sound measurement, and an absence of confounding theoretical constructs, that provide a suitable environment to extend the use of cognitive interventions and to apply them more discriminatingly than is typically done. CT is applicable to a range of diverse problems, which provides the opportunity to increase the specificity of its procedures. This integration might be accomplished by the adaptation of procedures such as treatment frequency and length (associated with patient FI), degree of directiveness (associated with patient resistance), focus on symptoms or schematic thoughts (associated with patient coping style), and attention to hot cognitions (associated with the level of patient distress). Such adaptation may further increase the already powerful effects of CT.

We have summarized a number of articles and reviews related to CBT and psychotherapy integration. Collectively, and consistent with Lambert and Ogles (2004), these publications suggest that treatment outcome is enhanced when various strategies or techniques are integrated with CBT. We have outlined empirically supported general guidelines and patient dimensions that may assist the practitioner in adapting the procedures of CT to fit the unique needs of each patient, in an effort to increase the magnitude and likelihood of positive change.

REFERENCES

Addis, M. E., & Jacobson, N. S. (1996). Reasons for depression and the process and outcome of cognitive-behavioral psychotherapies. *Journal of Consulting and Clinical Psychology, 64*(6), 1417–1424.

Allen, N. B., Horne, D. J. L., & Trinder, J. (1996). Sociotropy, autonomy, and dysphoric emotional responses to specific classes of stress: A psychophysiological evaluation. *Journal of Abnormal Psychology, 105*, 25–33.

Andersson, G., & Asmundson, G. J. G. (2006). Editorial: CBT and religion. *Cognitive Behaviour Therapy, 35*, 1–2.

Ano, G. G., & Vasconcelles, E. B. (2005). Religious coping and psychological adjustment to stress: A meta-analysis. *Journal of Clinical Psychology, 61*, 461–480.

Arkowitz, H. (1995). Common factors or processes of change in psychotherapy? *American Psychological Association, 2*(1), 94–100.

Arkowitz, H., & Messer, S. B. (1984). *Psychoanalytic therapy and behavior therapy: Is integration possible?* New York: Plenum Press.

Arnkoff, D. B. (1983). Common and specific factors in cognitive therapy. In M. J. Lambert (Ed.), *Psychotherapy and patient relationships* (pp. 85–125). Homewood, IL: Dorsey.

Arntz, A., & van den Hout, M. (1996). Psychological treatments of panic disorder without agoraphobia: Cognitive therapy vs. applied relaxation. *Behaviour Research and Therapy, 34*, 113–121.

Bandura, A. (1977). *Social learning theory.* Englewood Cliffs, NJ: Prentice-Hall.

Barber, J. P., & Muenz, L. R. (1986). The role of avoidance and obsessiveness in matching patients to cognitive and interpersonal psychotherapy: Empirical findings from the Treatment of Depression Collaborative Research Project. *Journal of Consulting and Clinical Psychology, 64*, 951–958.

Barlow, D. H., O'Brien, G. T., & Last, C. G. (1984). Couples treatment of agoraphobia. *Behavior Therapy, 18*, 441–448.

Barrowclough, C., Haddock, G., Fitzsimmons, M., & Johnson, R. (2006). Treatment development for psychosis and co-occurring substance misuse: A descriptive review. *Journal of Mental Health, 15*, 619–632.

Beck, A. T. (1991). Cognitive therapy as *the* integrative therapy. *Journal of Psychotherapy Integration, 3*, 191–198.

Beck, A. T. (1993). Cognitive therapy: Nature and relation to behavior therapy. *Journal of Psychotherapy Practice and Research, 2*, 345–356.

Beck, A. T., & Emery, G. (1985). *Anxiety disorders and phobias: A cognitive perspective.* New York: Basic Books.

Beck, A. T., Epstein, N., Harrison, R. P., & Emery, G. (1983). *Development of the Sociotropy–Autonomy Scale: A measure of personality factors in psychopathology.* Unpublished manuscript, University of Pennsylvania, Philadelphia.

Beck, A. T., & Weishaar, M. E. (2008). Cognitive therapy. In R. J. Corsini & D. Wedding (Eds.), *Current psychotherapies* (8th ed., pp. 263–294). Belmont, CA: Thomson.

Beck, A. T., Wright, F. D., Newman, C. F., & Liese, B. S. (1993). *Cognitive therapy for substance abuse.* New York: Guilford Press.

Beitman, B. D., Soth, A. M., & Good, G. E. (2006). Integrating the psychotherapies through their emphases on the future. In G. Stricker & J. Gold (Eds.), *A casebook of psychotherapy integration* (pp. 55–63). Washington, DC: American Psychological Association.

Beutler, L. E. (1983). *Eclectic psychotherapy: A systematic approach.* New York: Pergamon Press.

Beutler, L. E., & Clarkin, J. E. (1990). *Systematic treatment selection: Toward targeted therapeutic interventions.* New York: Brunner/Mazel.

Beutler, L. E., Clarkin, J. E., & Bongar, B. (2000). *Guidelines for the systematic treatment of the depressed patient.* New York: Oxford University Press.

Beutler, L. E., Crago, M., & Arizmendi, T. G. (1986). Research on therapist variables in psychotherapy. In S. L. Garfield & A. E. Bergin (Eds.), *Handbook of psychotherapy and behavior change* (3rd ed., pp.257–310). New York: Wiley.

Beutler, L. E., Engle, D., Mohr, D., Daldrup, R. J., Bergan, J., Meredith, K., et al. (1991). Predictors of differential and self-directed psychotherapeutic procedures. *Journal of Consulting and Clinical Psychology, 59,* 333–340.

Beutler, L. E., & Harwood, T. M. (2000). *Prescriptive psychotherapy: A practical guide to systematic treatment selection.* New York: Oxford University Press.

Beutler, L. E., & Harwood, T. M. (2001). Antiscientific attitudes: What happens when scientists are unscientific? *Journal of Clinical Psychology, 57,* 43–51.

Beutler, L. E., Blatt, S. J., Alamohamed, S., Levy, K. N., & Angtuaco, L. A. (2006). Participant factors in treating dysphoric disorders. In L. G. Castonguay & L. E. Beutler (Eds.), *Principles of therapeutic change that work* (pp. 13–63). New York: Oxford University Press.

Beutler, L. E., Malik, M., Alimohamed, S., Harwood, T. M., Talebi, H., Noble, S., et al. (2004). Therapist variables. In M. J. Lambert (Ed.), *Bergin and Garfield's handbook of psychotherapy and behavior change* (5th ed., pp. 227–306). New York: Wiley.

Beutler, L. E., & Mitchell, R. (1981). Psychotherapy outcome in depressed and impulsive patients as a function of analytic and experiential treatment procedures. *Psychiatry, 44,* 297–306.

Beutler, L. E., Moleiro, C., Malik, M., Harwood, T. M., Romanelli, R., Gallagher-Thompson, D., et al. (2003). A comparison of the Dodo, EST, and ATI factors among comorbid stimulant dependent, depressed patients. *Clinical Psychology and Psychotherapy, 10,* 69–85.

Beutler, L. E., Mohr, D. C., Grawe, K., Engle, D., & MacDonald, R. (1991). Looking for differential effects: Cross-cultural predictors of differential psychotherapy efficacy. *Journal of Psychotherapy Integration, 1,* 121–142.

Beutler, L. E., Sandowicz, M., Fisher, D., & Albanese, A. (1996). Resistance in psychotherapy: What conclusions are supported by research? *In Session: Psychotherapy in Practice, 2,* 77–86.

Beutler, L. E., Williams, R. E., & Wakefield, P. J. (1993). Obstacles to disseminating applied psychological science. *Journal of Applied and Preventive Psychology, 2,* 53–38.

Beutler, L. E., Williams, R. E., Wakefield, P. J., & Entwistle, S. R. (1995). Bridging scientist and practitioner perspectives in clinical psychology. *American Psychologist, 50,* 984–994.

Billings, A. B., & Moos, R. H. (1984). Coping, stress, and social resources among adults with unipolar depression. *Journal of Personality and Social Psychology, 46,* 877–891.

Binder, J. L., & Strupp, H. H. (1997). Negative process: A recurrently discovered and underestimated facet of therapeutic process and outcome in the individual psychotherapy of adults. *Clinical Psychology: Science and Practice, 4,* 121–139.

Blackburn, I. M. (1998). Cognitive therapy. In A. S. Bellack & M. Hersen (Eds.), *Comprehensive clinical psychology* (Vol. 1, pp. 51–84). New York: Pergamon.

Blackburn, I. M., Jones, S., & Lewin, R. J. (1986). A two year naturalistic follow-up of depressed patients treated with cognitive therapy, pharmacotherapy, and combination of both. *Journal of Affective Disorders, 10,* 67–75.

Bowers, W. A. (1990). Treatment of depressed in-patients: Cognitive therapy plus medication, relaxation plus medication, and medication alone. *British Journal of Psychiatry, 156,* 73–78.

Bowlby, J. (1977). The making and breaking of affectional bonds: II. Some principles of psychotherapy. *British Journal of Psychiatry, 130,* 421–431.

Brink, N. E. (2005). Book review of *Cognitive Therapy and Dreams* (2004). R. I. Rosner, Lyddon, W. L. J., & Freeman, A. New York: Springer. *Dreaming, 15,* 58–62.

Brown, G. W. (1997). A psychosocial perspective and the aetiology of depression. In A. Honig & H. M. van Praag (Eds.), *Depression: Neurological, psychopathological, and therapeutic advances* (pp. 343–362). Chichester, UK: Wiley.

Brown, T. A., & Barlow, D. H. (1995). Long-term outcome in cognitive-behavioral treatment of panic disorder: Clinical predictors and alternative strategies for assessment. *Journal of Consulting and Clinical Psychology, 63,* 754–765.

Calvert, S. J., Beutler, L. E., & Crago, M. (1988). Psychotherapy outcome as a function of therapist–patient matching on selected variables. *Journal of Social and Clinical Psychology, 6,* 104–117.

Castonguay, L. G., & Beutler, L. E. (2006a). Common and unique principles of therapeutic change: What do we know and what do we need to know? In L. G. Castonguay & L. E. Beutler (Eds.), *Principles of therapeutic change that work* (pp. 353–369). New York: Oxford University Press.

Castonguay, L. G., & Beutler, L. E. (2006b). Principles of therapeutic change: A task force on participants, relationships, and technique factors. *Journal of Clinical Psychology, 62,* 631–638.

Castonguay, L. G., & Beutler, L. E. (2006c). Therapeutic factors in dysphoric disorders. *Journal of Clinical Psychology, 62,* 639–647.

Choi, Y., Vincelli, F., Riva, G., Wiederhold, B., Lee, J., & Park, K. (2005). Effects of group experiential cognitive therapy for the treatment of panic disorder with agoraphobia. *CyberPsychology and Behavior, 8,* 387–393.

Clark, D. A., & Beck, A. T. (1991). Personality in dysphoria: A psychometric refinement of Beck's Sociotropy–Autonomy Scale. *Journal of Psychopathology and Behavioral Assessment, 13,* 369–388.

Clark, D. A., Steer, R. A., Beck, A. T., & Ross, L. (1995). Psychometric character-istics of revised sociotropy and autonomy scales in college students. *Behaviour Research and Therapy, 33*, 325–334.

Crider, A., Glaros, A. G., & Gevirtz, R. (2005). Efficacy of biofeedback-based treat-ments for temporomandibular disorders. *Applied Psychophysiology and Bio-feedback, 30*, 333–345.

DiGiorgio, K. E., Arnkoff, D. B., Glass, C. R., Lyhus, K. E., & Walter, R. C. (2004). EMDR and theoretical orientation: A qualitative study of how therapists inte-grate eye movement desensitization and reprocessing into their approach to psy-chotherapy. *Journal of Psychotherapy Integration, 14*, 227–252.

Dobson, K. S. (1989). A meta-analysis of the efficacy of cognitive therapy for depres-sion. *Journal of Consulting and Clinical Psychology, 57*(3), 414–419.

Dowd, T. E. (2004). Foreword. In R. I. Rosner, W. L. J. Lyddon, & A. Freeman (Eds.), *Cognitive therapy and dreams*. New York: Springer.

Ellis, A. (2005). Can rational-emotive behavior therapy (REBT) and acceptance and commitment therapy (ACT) resolve their differences and be integrated? *Journal of Rational-Emotive and Cognitive-Behavior Therapy, 23*, 153–168.

Fairburn, C. G., Jones R., Peveler, R. C., Hope, R. A., & O'Connor, M. (1993). Psy-chotherapy and bulimia nervosa: Longer-term effects of interpersonal psycho-therapy, behavior therapy, and cognitive behavior therapy. *Archives of General Psychiatry, 50*, 419–428.

Fava, G. A. (1986). Psychotherapy research: Clinical trials versus clinical reality. *Psy-chotherapy and Psychosomatics, 46*, 6–12.

Finucane, A., & Mercer, S. W. (2006). An exploratory mixed methods study of the acceptability and effectiveness of mindfulness-based cognitive therapy for patients with active depression and anxiety in primary care. *BMC Psychiatry, 6*, 14.

Forsyth, N. L., & Forsyth, D. R. (1982). Internality, control ability, and the effective-ness of attributional interpretation in counseling. *Journal of Counseling Psychol-ogy, 29*, 140–150.

Frank, J. D., & Frank, J. B. (1991). *Persuasion and healing* (3rd ed.). Baltimore: Johns Hopkins University Press.

Freedheim, D. K., Freudenberger, H. J., Kessler, J. W., & Messer, S. B. (1992). *History of psychotherapy: A century of change*. Washington, DC: American Psychologi-cal Association.

Freeman, A., & White, B. (2004). Dreams and the dream image: Using dreams in cog-nitive therapy. In R. I. Rosner, W. L. J. Lyddon, & A. Freeman (Eds.), *Cognitive therapy and dreams* (pp. 69–88). New York: Springer.

Futterman, R., Lorente, M., & Silverman, S. W. (2005). Beyond harm reduction: A new model of substance abuse treatment further integrating psychological tech-niques. *Journal of Psychotherapy Integration, 15*, 3–18.

Gaffan, E. A., Tsaousis, J., & Kemp-Wheeler, S. M. (1995). Researcher allegiance and meta-analysis: The case of cognitive therapy for depression. *Journal of Consult-ing and Clinical Psychology, 63*, 966–980.

Garfield, S. L. (1981). Evaluating the psychotherapies. *Behavior Therapy, 12*, 295–307.

Garratt, G., Ingram, R. E., Rand, K. L., & Sawalani, G. (2007). Cognitive processes in cognitive therapy: Evaluation of the mechanisms of change in the treatment of depression. *Clinical Psychology: Science and Practice, 14*, 224–239.

Gaudiano, B. A., & Herbert, J. D. (2006). Acute treatment of inpatients with psychotic symptoms using acceptance and commitment therapy: Pilot results. *Behaviour Research and Therapy, 44,* 415–437.

Gitlin, M. J. (1995). Effects of depression and antidepressants on sexual functioning. *Bulletin of the Menninger Clinic, 59,* 232–248.

Goldfried, M. R. (1995). *From cognitive-behavior therapy to psychotherapy integration.* New York: Springer.

Goldfried, M. R. (2006). Cognitive-affective relational behavior therapy. In G. Stricker & J. Gold (Eds.), *Casebook of psychotherapy integration* (pp. 153–164). Washington, DC: American Psychological Association.

Goldstein, A. P., & Stein, N. (1976). *Prescriptive psychotherapies.* New York: Pergamon Press.

Haddock, G., & Slade, P. D. (Eds.). (1996). *Cognitive behavioural interventions with psychotic disorders.* New York: Routledge.

Hamamçi, Z. (2006). Integrating psychodrama and cognitive behavioral therapy to treat moderate depression. *The Arts in Psychotherapy, 33,* 199–207.

Harwood, T. M., & Beutler, L. E. (2008). EVTs, EBPs, ESRs, and RIPs: Inspecting the varieties of research based practices. In L. L'Abate (Ed.), *Toward a science of clinical psychology* (pp. 161–176). New York: Nova Science.

Harwood, T. M., Beutler, L. E., Castillo, S., & Karno, M. (2006). Common and specific effects of couples treatment for alcoholism: A test of the generic model of psychotherapy. *Psychology and Psychotherapy: Theory Research and Practice, 79,* 365–384.

Harwood, T. M., & Williams, O. B. (2003). Identifying treatment relevant assessment: Systematic treatment selection. In L. E. Beutler & G. Groth-Marnat (Eds.), *Integrative assessment of adult personality* (pp. 65–81). New York: Guilford Press.

Hawkins, R. S., Tan, S. -Y., & Turk, A. A. (1999). Secular versus Christian inpatient cognitive behavioral therapy programs: Impact on depression and spiritual well-being. *Journal of Psychology and Theology, 27,* 309–331.

Hayes, S. C., & Smith, S. (2005). *Get out of your mind and into your life: The new acceptance and commitment therapy.* New Harbinger.

Hayes, S. C., & Strosahl, K. D. (2004). *A practical guide to acceptance and commitment therapy.* New York: Springer.

Hayes, S. C., Strosahl, K. D., & Wilson, K. G. (2003). *Acceptance and commitment therapy: An experiential approach to behavior change.* New York: Guilford Press.

Heppner, P. P., & Anderson, W. P. (1985). On the perceived non-utility of research in counseling. *Journal of Counseling and Development, 63,* 545–547.

Higgins, S. T., Budney, A. J., & Bickel, W. K. (1994). Applying behavioral concepts and principles to the treatment of cocaine dependence. *Drug and Alcohol Dependence, 34,* 87–97.

Hogg, J. A., & Deffenbacher, J. L. (1988). A comparison of cognitive and interpersonal-process group therapies in the treatment of depression among college students. *Journal of Counseling Psychology, 35*(3), 304–310.

Hollon, S. D. (1996). The efficacy and effectiveness of psychotherapy relative to medications. *American Psychologist, 51,* 1025–1030.

Hollon, S. D., & Beck, A. T. (2004). Cognitive and cognitive behavioral therapies. In M. J. Lambert (Ed.). *Bergin and Garfield's handbook of psychotherapy and behavior change* (5th ed., pp. 447–492). New York: Wiley.

Horvath, A. (1989, June). *There are no main effects, only interactions.* Paper presented at the annual meeting of the Society for Psychotherapy Research, Toronto, Canada.

Hwang, W., Wood, J. J., Lin, K., & Cheung, F. (2006). Cognitive-behavioral therapy with Chinese Americans: Research, theory, and clinical practice. *Cognitive and Behavioral Practice, 13,* 293–303.

Jacobson, N. S., & Hollon, S. D. (1996). Cognitive-behavioral therapy versus pharmacotherapy: Now that the jury's returned its verdict, it's time to present the rest of the evidence. *Journal of Consulting and Clinical Psychology, 64,* 74–80.

Kadden, R. M., Cooney, N. L., & Getter, H. (1989). Matching alcoholics to coping skills or interactional therapy: Posttreatment results. *Journal of Consulting and Clinical Psychology, 56*(1), 48–55.

Keisler, D. J. (1996). *Contemporary interpersonal theory and research: Personality, psychopathology, and psychotherapy.* New York: Wiley.

Kellogg, S. (2004). Dialogical encounters: Contemporary perspectives on "chairwork" in psychotherapy. *Psychotherapy: Theory, Research, Practice and Training, 41,* 310–320.

Kenny, M. A., & Williams, J. M. G. (2007). Treatment-resistant depressed patients show a good response to mindfulness-based cognitive therapy, *Behaviour Research and Therapy, 45,* 617–625.

Kenny, M. C. (2006). An integrative therapeutic approach to the treatment of a depressed American Indian client. *Clinical Case Studies, 5,* 37–52.

Kingdon, D. G., & Turkington, D. (1994). *Cognitive-behavioral therapy of schizophrenia.* New York: Guilford Press.

Knight-Law, A., Sugerman, A., & Pettinati, H. (1988). An application of an MMPI classification system for predicting outcome in a small clinical sample of alcoholics. *American Journal of Drug and Alcohol Abuse, 14*(3), 325–334.

Kovacs, M., Rush, A. J., & Beck, A. T., & Hollon, S. D. (1981). Depressed outpatients with cognitive therapy or pharmacotherapy. *Archives of General Psychiatry, 38,* 33–39.

Kushner, M. G., Donahue, C., Sletten, S., Thuras, P., Abrams, K., Peterson, J., et al. (2006). Cognitive behavioral treatment of co-morbid anxiety disorder in alcoholism treatment patients: Presentation of a prototype program and future directions. *Journal of Mental Health, 15,* 697–707.

LaCroix, M., Clarke, M., Bock, C., & Doxey, N. (1986). Physiological changes after biofeedback and relaxation training for multiple-pain tension-headache patients. *Perceptual and Motor Skills, 63,* 139–153.

Lambert, M. J., Garfield, S. L., & Bergin, A. E. (2004). Overview, trends, and future issues. In M. J. Lambert (Ed.), *Bergin and Garfield's handbook of psychotherapy and behavior change* (5th ed., pp. 805–821). New York: Wiley.

Lambert, M. J., & Ogles, B. (2004). The efficacy and effectiveness of psychotherapy. In M. J. Lambert (Ed.), *Bergin and Garfield's handbook of psychotherapy and behavior change* (5th ed., pp. 139–193). New York: Wiley.

Lambert, M. J., Shapiro, D. A., & Bergin, A. E. (1986). The effectiveness of psychotherapy. In S. L. Garfield & A. E. Bergin (Eds.), *Handbook of psychotherapy and behavior change* (3rd ed., pp. 157–211). New York: Wiley.

Lazarus, A. (1996). The utility and futility of combining treatments in psychotherapy. *Clinical Psychology: Science and Practice, 3,* 59–68.

Lent, R. W., Russell, R. K., & Zamostry, K. P. (1981). Comparison of cue-controlled desensitization, rational restructuring, and a credible placebo in the treatment of speech anxiety. *Journal of Consulting and Clinical Psychology, 49,* 608–610.

Linehan, M. M., & Dimeff, L. (2001). Dialectical behavior therapy in a nutshell. *The California Psychologist, 34,* 10–13.

Liotti, G. (1991). Patterns of attachment and the assessment of interpersonal schemata: Understanding and changing difficult patient–therapist relationships in cognitive psychotherapy. *Journal of Cognitive Psychotherapy, 5,* 105–114.

Mahoney, M. J. (1991). *Human change processes.* New York: Basic Books.

Marlatt, G. A. (Ed.). (1998). *Harm reduction: Pragmatic strategies for managing high- risk behaviors.* New York: Guilford Press.

Marlatt, G. A., Blume, A. W., & Parks, G. A. (2001). Integrating harm reduction therapy and traditional substance abuse treatment. *Journal of Psychoactive Drugs, 33,* 13–21.

Marlatt, G. A., & Gordon, J. R. (Eds.). (1985). *Relapse prevention: Maintenance strategies in the treatment of addictive behaviors.* New York: Guilford Press.

McCullough, J. P. (2000). *Treatment for chronic depression: Cognitive behavioral analysis system of psychotherapy (CBASP).* New York: Guilford Press.

McMinn, M. R., & Campbell, C. D. (2007). *Integrative psychotherapy: Toward a comprehensive Christian approach.* Downers Grove, IL: InterVarsity Press.

Moore, R. G., & Blackburn, I. M. (1996). The stability of sociotropy and autonomy in depressed patients undergoing treatment. *Cognitive Therapy and Research, 20,* 69–80.

Morrow-Bradley, C., & Elliott, R. (1986). Utilization of psychotherapy research by practicing psychotherapists. *American Psychologist, 41*(2), 188–197.

Murphy, G. E., Simons, A. D., Wetzel, R. D., Lustman, P. J. (1984). Cognitive therapy and pharmacotherapy: Singly and together in the treatment of depression. *Archives of General Psychiatry, 38,* 33–39.

Norcross, J. C., & Halgin, R. P. (2005). Training in psychotherapy integration. In J. C. Norcross & M. R. Goldfried (Eds.), *Handbook of psychotherapy integration* (pp. 439–458). New York: Oxford University Press.

Norcross, J. C., Martin, J. R., Omer, H., & Pinsof, W. M. (1996). When and how does psychotherapy integration improve clinical effectiveness?: A roundtable. *Journal of Psychotherapy Integration, 6,* 295–332.

Norcross, J. C., & Goldfried, M. R. (1992). *Handbook of psychotherapy integration.* New York: Basic Books.

Ogles, B. M., Sawyer, J. D., & Lambert, M. J. (1995). Clinical significance of the National Institute of Mental Health Treatment of Depression Collaborative Research Program data. *Journal of Consulting and Clinical Psychology, 63*(2), 001–006.

Orlinsky, D. E., Grawe, K., & Park, B. K. (1994). Process and outcome in psychotherapy: Noch einmal. In A. E. Bergin & S. L. Garfield (Eds.), *Handbook of psychotherapy and behavior change* (4th ed., pp. 270–376). New York: Wiley.

Orlinsky, D. E., & Howard, K. I. (1986). Process and outcome in psychotherapy. In S. L. Garfield & A. E. Bergin (Eds.), *Handbook of psychotherapy and behavior change* (3rd ed., pp 311–384). New York: Wiley.

Parsons, J. T., Rosof, E., Punzalan, J. C., & Di Maria, L. (2005). Integration of motivational interviewing and cognitive behavioral therapy to improve HIV medication adherence and reduce substance use among HIV-positive men and women: Results of a pilot project. *AIDs Patient Care and STDs, 19,* 31–39.

Piaget, J. (1981). *Intelligence and affectivity: Their relationship during child development*. Palo Alto, CA: Annual Reviews. (Original work published 1954)

The Princeton Religious Research Center. (1996). *Religion in America 1996*. Princeton, NJ: Princeton Religious Research Center.

Robins, C. J., & Hayes, A. M. (1993). An appraisal of cognitive therapy. *Journal of Consulting and Clinical Psychology, 61*, 1–10.

Robinson, L. A., Berman, J. S., & Neimeyer, R. A. (1990). Psychotherapy for the treatment of depression: A comprehensive review of controlled outcome research. *Psychological Bulletin, 108*, 30–49.

Rosner, R. I., Lyddon, W. L. J., & Freeman, A. (2004). *Cognitive therapy and dreams*. New York: Springer.

Roth, A., & Fonagy, P. (1996). *What works for whom?* New York: Guilford Press.

Rush, A. J. (1982). Comparison of the effects of cognitive therapy and pharmacotherapy on hopelessness and self-concept. *American Journal of Psychiatry, 139*, 862–866.

Rush, A. J., Beck, A. T., & Kovacs, M., & Hollon, S. T. (1977). Comparative efficacy of cognitive therapy and pharmacotherapy in the treatment of depressed outpatients. *Cognitive Therapy and Research, 1*(1), 17–37.

Rush, A. J., Beck, A. T., Kovacs, M., Weissenburger, J., & Hollon, S. T. (1982). Comparison of the effects of cognitive therapy and pharmacotherapy on hopelessness and self-concept. *American Journal of Psychiatry, 139*, 862–866.

Ryle, A., & McCutcheon, L. (2006). Cognitive analytic therapy. In G. Stricker & J. Gold (Eds.), *Casebook of psychotherapy integration* (pp. 121–136). Washington, DC: American Psychological Association.

Safran, J., Alden, L., & Davison, P. (1980). Client anxiety level as a moderator variable in assertion training. *Cognitive Therapy and Research, 4*(2), 189–200.

Safran, J., & Messer, S. (1997). Psychotherapy integration: A postmodern critique. *American Psychologist, 4*, 140–152.

Safran, J., & Segal, Z. V. (1990). *Interpersonal process in cognitive therapy*. New York: Basic Books.

Safran, J. D., & Muran, J. C. (2000). *Negotiating the therapeutic alliance: A relational treatment guide*. New York: Guilford Press.

Schlicter, K. J., & Horan, J. J. (1981). Effects of stress inoculation on the anger and aggression management skills of institutionalized juvenile delinquents. *Cognitive Therapy and Research, 5*, 359–365.

Scogin, F., Bowman, D., Jamison, C., Beutler, L., & Machado, P. P. (1994). Effects of initial severity of dysfunctional thinking on the outcome of cognitive therapy. *Clinical Psychology and Psychotherapy, 1*(3), 179–184.

Scogin, F., Hamblin, D., & Beutler, L. E. (1987). Bibliotherapy for depressed older adults: A self-help alternative. *Gerontologist, 27*, 383–387.

Seltzer, L. F. (1986). *Paradoxical strategies in psychotherapy: A comprehensive overview and guidebook*. New York: Wiley.

Shaffer, C. S., Shapiro, J., Sark, L. I., & Coghlan, D. J. (1981). Positive changes in depression, anxiety, and assertion following individual and group cognitive behavior therapy intervention. *Cognitive Therapy and Research, 5*, 149–157.

Shapiro, D. A., Barkham, M., Rees, A., & Hardy, G. E. (1994). Effects of treatment duration and severity of depression on the effectiveness of cognitive-behavioral and psychodynamic-interpersonal psychotherapy. *Journal of Consulting and Clinical Psychology, 62*, 522–534.

Sheppard, D., Smith, G. T., & Rosenbaum, G. (1988). Use of MMPI subtpyes in predicting completion of a residential alcoholism treatment program. *Journal of Consulting and Clinical Psychology, 50,* 590–596.

Shoham-Salomon, V., Avner, R., & Neeman, R. (1989). You are changed if you do and changed if you don't: Mechanisms underlying paradoxical interventions. *Journal of Consulting and Clinical Psychology, 57,* 590–598.

Shoham-Saloman, V., & Hannah, M. T. (1991). Client–treatment interactions in the study of differential change process. *Journal of Consulting and Clinical Psychology, 59,* 217–225.

Shoham-Salomon, V., & Rosenthal, R. (1987). Paradoxical interventions: A meta-analysis. *Journal of Consulting and Clinical Psychology, 55,* 22–27.

Simons, A. D., & Thase, M. E. (1992). Biological markers, treatment outcome, and 1–year follow-up in endogenous depression: Electroencephalographic sleep studies and response to cognitive therapy. *Journal of Consulting and Clinical Psychology, 60,* 392–401.

Sloane, R. B., Staples, F. R., Cristol, A. H., Yorkston, N. J., & Whipple, K. (1975). *Psychotherapy versus behavior change.* Cambridge, MA: Harvard University Press.

Smith, M. L., Glass, G. V., & Miller, T. I. (1980). *The benefits of psychotherapy.* Baltimore: Johns Hopkins University Press.

Stiles, W. B., Barkham, M., Twigg, E., Mellor-Clark, & Cooper, M. (2006). Effectiveness of cognitive-behavioural, person-centered and psychodynamic therapies as practiced in UK National Health Service settings. *Psychological Medicine, 10,* 1–12.

Stricker, G. (1994). Reflections on psychotherapy integration. *Clinical Psychology: Science and Practice, 1*(1), 3–12.

Stricker, G., & Gold, J. (1996). Psychotherapy integration: An assimilative, psychodynamic approach. *Clinical Psychology: Science and Practice, 3*(1), 47–58.

Stricker, G., & Gold, J. (2006). *A casebook of psychotherapy integration.* Washington DC: American Psychological Association.

Tasca, G. A., Russell, V., & Busby, K. (1994). Characteristics of patients who choose between two types of group psychotherapy. *International Journal of Group Psychotherapy, 44*(4), 499–508.

Taylor, S. (2006). The interface between cognitive behavior therapy and religion: Comment on Andersson and Asmundson (2006). *Cognitive Behaviour Therapy, 35,* 125–127.

Thase, M. E., & Simons, A. D. (1992). The applied use of psychotherapy in the study of the psychobiology of depression. *Journal of Clinical Psychiatry, 53,* 32–44.

Thorne, F. C. (1962). Self-consistency theory and psychotherapy. *Annals of the New York Academy of Sciences, 96,* 877–888.

Tichelaar, V., Geertzen, Y. I. G., Jan, H. B., Keizer, D., & van Wilgren, P. (2007). Mirror box therapy added to cognitive behavioral therapy in three chronic complex regional pain syndrome type I patients: A pilot study. *International Journal of Rehabilitation Research, 30,* 181–188.

Tref, D. M., & Yuan, H. A. (1983). The use of the MMPI in a chronic back pain rehabilitation program. *Journal of Clinical Psychology, 39*(1), 46–53.

Wachtel, P. L. (1978). On some complexities in the application of conflict theory to psychotherapy. *Journal of Nervous and Mental Disease, 166,* 457–471.

West, A. E., Henry, D. B., & Pavuluri, M. N. (2007). Maintenance model of integrated psychosocial treatment in pediatric bipolar disorder: A pilot feasibility study. *Journal of the American Academy of Child and Adolescent Psychiatry, 46,* 205–212.

Whitfield, H. J. (2006). Towards case-specific applications of mindfulness-based cognitive-behavioral therapies: A mindfulness-based rational emotive behaviour therapy. *Counselling Psychology Quarterly, 19,* 205–207.

Wilson, G. T. (2008). Behavior therapy. In R. J. Corsini & D. Wedding (Eds.), *Current psychotherapies* (8th ed., pp. 223–262). Belmont, CA: Thomson.

Wilson, P. H., Goldin, J. C., & Charbouneau-Powis, M. (1983). Comparative efficacy of behavioural and cognitive treatments of depression. *Cognitive Therapy and Research, 7,* 111–124.

Woody, G. E., McClellan, A. T., Luborsky, L., & O'Brien, C. P. (1984). Sociopathy and psychotherapy outcome. *Archives of General Psychiatry, 42,* 1081–1086.

Young, J. E. (1990). *Cognitive therapy for personality disorders: A schema-focused approach.* Sarasota, FL: Professional Resource Exchange.

PART II

ASSESSMENT CONSIDERATIONS

CHAPTER 5

Cognitive Assessment
Issues and Methods

David M. Dunkley
Kirk R. Blankstein
Zindel V. Segal

There are a thousand thoughts lying within a man
that he does not know till he takes up the pen to write.
—WILLIAM MAKEPEACE THACKERY, *Henry Esmond*

This chapter addresses conceptual and methodological issues relevant to the practice of cognitive assessment. We assume that human cognitive functioning can be described in information-processing terms, and that this perspective can inform clinical assessment practices (e.g., Williams, Watts, MacLeod & Mathews, 1998). Within this model, humans are portrayed as actively seeking, selecting, and utilizing information (both internal and external) in the process of constructing the mind's view of reality (Gardner, 1985). Such activity is an essential feature of the cognitive system and produces varied contents at different levels of operation. While the passage of information through the system is conceived of as both a synthetic and a reciprocal process (Neisser, 1976), most of the attention in the literature is directed at three distinct levels of analysis. Numerous writers (e.g., Segal & Swallow, 1994) have identified cognitive structures (hypothesized inaccessible schemas guiding information processing), processes (means of transforming environmental input and inferring meaning from it), and products or content (conscious thoughts and images) as a framework through which knowledge about the world is organized, described how this framework guides ongoing processing, and defined the most accessible products of this processing.

PROCESS AND METHODS OF COGNITIVE ASSESSMENT

Various classification systems have been presented for the numerous methods of assessing thoughts (Glass & Arnkoff, 1982; Kendall & Hollon, 1981). In their more recent work, Glass and Arnkoff (1997) have organized the methods of cognitive assessment according to each of four dimensions: temporality or timing (retrospective, concurrent, or about future events), degree of structure (endorsement vs. production), response mode (written or oral), and nature of the stimulus (thoughts in general, imagined situation, situation viewed on videotape, role play, or in vivo situation). We propose a fifth dimension, which is the source of thought evaluation (respondent or independent judge; Blankstein & Flett, 1990).

The resulting scheme yields a continuum of assessment procedures ranging from concurrent evaluations to retrospective evaluations. Figure 5.1 illustrates the placement of some common measures on this continuum and provides a brief description of each. Cognitive assessment procedures may also be organized on the basis of structure, wherein the extent to which the assessment imposes its own limits or format on the individual determines its placement on this dimension. While structured self-statement endorsement measures are most commonly used, researchers have developed numerous production strategies to complement the use of questionnaires and inventories. Production measures require participants to generate or recall their thoughts. With this classification in mind, we now introduce the reader to the various methods of assessing the thoughts of participants or clients.

Recordings of spontaneous speech have been employed in a number of studies purportedly assessing respondents' or clients' actual self-talk. These recordings can be taken unobtrusively or following specific instructions. They

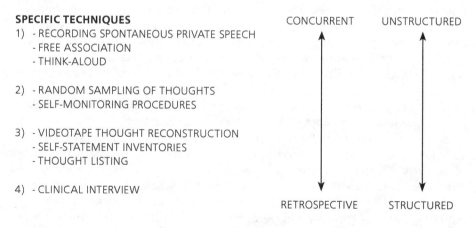

FIGURE 5.1. Continuum of temporal and structural dimensions of cognitive assessment. Adapted from Glass and Arnkoff (1982). Copyright 1982 by Elsevier. Adapted by permission.

represent verbal behavior that can then be transcribed and coded into categories (Kendall & Hollon, 1981). This format is one of the most common
methods for assessing private speech, yet the investigator is limited to subjects'
verbalizations and can never be fully certain that silences are synonymous
with the lack of cognitive processing. Think-aloud procedures require subjects
to provide a continuous monologue of their thoughts during the performance
of a specific task or in a particular situation. Davison and his colleagues (e.g.,
Davison, Robins, & Johnson, 1983; Davison, Vogel, & Coffman, 1997) have
researched a paradigm they refer to as articulated thoughts in simulated situations (ATTS). ATSS provides the researcher or clinician control over stimulus
situations that are usually presented on audiotape (e.g., a social criticism tape
designed to elicit thoughts associated with social anxiety). Participants imagine being in the situation and think aloud after each 10- to 15-second segment
of the 2- to 3-minute stimulus. As is the case with most cognitive production,
this approach requires trained raters or judges to make inferences about the
meaning of respondents' internal dialogues, usually in light of categories of
interest specified by a particular cognitive theory.

At the next level on the continuum, we find methods such as random thought sampling in the natural environment and techniques for self-
monitoring. Hurlburt (1997) reviewed two methods that quantify thinking as
it occurs as people move through their natural environment: "thought sampling" and the "experience sampling method" (ESM). The procedures attempt
to provide an unbiased estimate of cognitive activity as people record their
current thoughts when cued either in person or, more typically, by a portable
mechanical device (beeper) at random or quasi-random intervals. On hearing
the beep participants immediately record their thoughts (and other aspects of
their experience and behavior) by completing quantitative questionnaires and/
or writing narrative descriptions. This procedure enables data to be gathered
over relatively long periods of time in the subjects' own milieu at intervals that
are not contingent on the occurrence of any particular environmental events
(see also Hurlburt & Akhter, 2006).

Self-monitoring procedures ask the individual to record the occurrence
of specific thoughts in a particular stimulus situation or at a particular time.
Their utility lies in the fact that they maximize the probability of gathering
clinically relevant information about important but possibly infrequent situations. For example, Westling and Ost (1993) studied the nature and relation of distressing cognitions and symptoms experienced during panic attacks
prospectively, via self-monitoring. A number of problems are inherent in self-
monitoring procedures, including reactivity, social desirability, and evaluation
apprehension.

A fundamental component of Beck's cognitive theory and therapy per-
tains to how individuals assess and respond to their daily stressful situations.
Daily process designs are a form of self-monitoring that assesses daily stress
and mood symptoms over the course of days or weeks (see Dunkley, Zuroff, &
Blankstein, 2003; Gunthert, Cohen, Butler, & Beck, 2007). Relative to retro-

spective self-report questionnaires that require individuals to summarize their stress and mood over time and across situations, daily process designs reduce retrospective bias and obtain a closer approximation of how individuals actually think on a day-to-day basis as they confront stressors. Statistical analyses of repeated daily assessments within persons can give a more detailed picture of how fluctuations in certain cognitive appraisals (e.g., perceived criticism from others) are associated with changes in mood (see Dunkley et al., 2003; Gunthert et al., 2007).

Videotape thought reconstruction is a relatively infrequently used research strategy that allows a subject to reconstruct his or her train of thought at the time as accurately as possible by viewing a videotape of an actual or role-played problematic situation (Genest & Turk, 1981). These production procedures are classified as more retrospective than techniques discussed earlier, since their aim is to facilitate the subject's "re-living" and reporting of a prior experience, as opposed to reporting on the original experience while it is occurring. In a somewhat related methodology, "thought listing," the subject lists everything about which he or she is (or was) thinking. This production procedure can be more constrained than think-aloud methods, since the assessment typically takes place once the subject is out of the situation. However, although thought listings are frequently collected retrospectively (e.g., recording thoughts immediately following an examination), they can also be obtained in anticipation of a task or situation (e.g., listing thoughts prior to an exam), and even during the task or situation (e.g., listing one's thoughts at different points during the actual exam). Thought listing is an open-response strategy to acquire and categorize the reportable products of people's cognitive processes, such as thoughts, expectations, appraisals, images, and feelings (Cacioppo, von Hippel, & Ernst, 1997). Detailed discussion of the procedures and instructions for administering the thought listing and for coding data can be found in Blankstein, Toner, and Flett (1989).

Endorsement methods, such as self-report inventories or questionnaires, are designed to assess conscious self-verbalizations or thoughts. They contain a predetermined set of thoughts that respondents typically rate with respect to whether or not they experienced the specific positive- or negative-valenced thought in the assessment situation, as well as its frequency of occurrence (Glass & Arnkoff, 1997; Kendall & Hollon, 1981). Self-report measures have also been used to assess respondents' retrospective views of their thoughts, feelings, dysfunctional attitudes, attributions, and related cognitive activity over a long period of time. Although some have expressed skepticism about the value of these questionnaire measures of cognition (e.g., Segal & Dobson, 1992), they are undoubtedly the most commonly used formal cognitive assessment method in clinical practice (Haaga, 1997). A number of endorsement measures have been developed specifically for use with children (e.g., Ronan, Kendall, & Rowe, 1994).

The clinical interview can also be used as a retrospective cognitive assessment tool. For example, the clinician can ask the client to recall an upsetting situation, then recount what he or she was thinking and feeling at the time (Glass & Arnkoff, 1982). Mumma (2004) described an intraindividual empirical approach to the validation of patients' idiosyncratic cognitive schemas (ICSs) in cognitive case formulations (CCFs). This three-stage approach begins with a semi-structured interview to elicit thoughts and beliefs in response to a number of clinically important events and situations. Second, the patient's cognitions are reviewed for relevance and integrated into a CCF. The clinician then evaluates the convergent and discriminant validity of the ICS using construct validation; for example, by predicting daily variability in distress symptoms.

Although our primary focus thus far has been on approaches that assess cognition relatively directly, a variety of other self-report and performance-based approaches have been used by clinical researchers to infer cognitive processes and cognitive structures, such as negative self-schemas (e.g., Segal, Gemar, Truchon, Guirguis, & Horowitz, 1995). Segal and Cloitre (1993) reviewed many of the methodologies available to study the cognitive features of emotional disorders, such as attention, interpretation of ambiguous stimuli, judgments, and memory processes. Some of these experimental measures are discussed further in relation to the cognitive assessment of anxiety and depression. Most of these measures are used primarily in clinical cognitive research, however, and are not likely to be employed in clinical practice.

ADVANTAGES AND LIMITATIONS
OF DIFFERENT SELF-REPORT METHODS

Structured assessments such as endorsement approaches to thought assessment offer the benefits of economy, ease of scoring and administration, a potential for use in clinical practice, standardization across studies, and the accrual of normative data and psychometric information (Schwartz, 1997). The trade-off, however, is against a potentially richer data source and the investigator's ability to uncover information about unpredicted relationships (Davison et al., 1997). Deciding on the degree of structure in an assessment often requires specification of the extent to which the individual's ongoing cognitive activity can be "punctuated" while still providing an accurate picture of its flow. As structure is added, the demand characteristics of the assessment also increase (Glass & Arnkoff, 1982). Furthermore, structured measures typically provide only a few summary scores (Glass & Arnkoff, 1997). Production methods such as the think-aloud procedures have an appeal due to their provision of the unaltered flow of subjects' thoughts (Davison et al., 1997). Constraints on ATSS data are imposed later through strategies to analyze the content, according to experimenter interest, and a virtually unlimited number of different coding schemes can be used on the same dataset. Clearly, the instructions given to subjects to "think aloud" are consequential and can result in the reporting of varying contents.

There is a consensus that a convergent operations approach is optimal in assessment (Webb, Campbell, Schwartz, & Sechrest, 1966). This approach minimizes the drawbacks of any one format and, if dissimilar measures produce similar findings, increases construct validity. However, studies that use multiple cognitive assessment methods often demonstrate little convergent validity, especially between endorsement (e.g., questionnaire) and production (e.g., thought listing) methods (see Chamberlain & Haaga, 1999). These findings raise concerns about whether these measures are assessing different cognitive constructs. Nevertheless, in situations that require diverse information, it may be advantageous to select multiple methods rather than a single method or measure. We turn our focus to questions of threats to psychometrics and the validity of the assessment process.

THREATS TO THE VALIDITY OF COGNITIVE ASSESSMENT

Questions regarding the construct validity of cognitive assessment focus not on the prediction of a criterion or the match between the content of a test and a specific domain, but on the ability of the test itself to measure the cognitive processes of interest (Ghiselli, Campbell, & Zedeck, 1981). This issue particularly applies to questionnaire or self-report formats that supply the subject with a particular content. He or she then provides ratings on dimensions, such as presence or absence, frequency, or degree of belief in the cognitions. The best example of this format is the self-statement inventory, which as we have pointed out, remains one of the most popular formats for assessing self-talk. The question of content validity should not be confused with concerns regarding construct validity, for while we can establish that the self-statements that comprise the inventory are representative of what people in general think in the assessment situation, we are less clear on what actual meaning an endorsement of one of these statements carries for the individual. Furthermore, meaning checks or inquiries are rarely conducted in conjunction with the administration of self-statement inventories (Arnkoff & Glass, 1982), leaving us with the assumption that self-statements have the same personal meanings for all individuals involved. One step toward remediation can be found in the "degree of belief" ratings that some inventories, such as the Automatic Thoughts Questionnaire (Hollon & Kendall, 1980), require in addition to the usual frequency tallies.

Glass and Arnkoff (1982, 1997) provided a cogent critique of the assumption of an isomorphic relationship between cognition and its representation on self-statement inventories. They list four possibilities that reflect different processes underlying item endorsement. One possibility is that subjects who report having a thought "very frequently" may be indicating the impact or the importance of the thought to them, and not necessarily its frequency. This concern is problematic for most self-statement inventories, since scores usually reflect a simple tally of items endorsed. The other possibility is that respondents translate the idiosyncratic or fragmented thoughts the subject experiences in the situation into grammatically correct sentences as they appear on the inventory. Alternatively, endorsement may reflect the view that the thought matches one's view of oneself rather than the actual experience of that specific thought. For example, a woman who sees herself as poorly skilled at solving math problems may endorse an item such as "I'm no good at math, so why even try?" on a questionnaire, because it corresponds to her self-image, rather than whether she necessarily had the thought. A final possibility is that endorsement may reflect the translation of affective experiences into a language-based format. For example, self-statement inventories may provide the opportunity for converting an experience of arousal into a linguistic representation of the event. In this sense, the subject may endorse a thought, such as "I'm really getting worked up about this," without necessarily having experienced it at the time (Glass & Arnkoff, 1982).

Despite concerns about what endorsements actually measure and the meaning of responses, many of these questionnaires (see examples below and the 1997 review by Glass and Arnkoff) have established criterion and predictive validity, and have proved useful to researchers studying cognitive theories. Furthermore, because they are sensitive to treatment effects, they are widely used as outcome measures by clinical researchers (Haaga, 1997). Glass and Arnkoff (1997) suggest that interpretation of frequency scores could be facilitated by rating additional aspects of each thought (intensity, salience, believability, controllability, importance, etc.), and believe that expansion of the dimensions assessed would allow endorsement measures to approach the flexibility of production methods. They further suggest that practicing clinicians can probe their clients as to the subjective meaning of questionnaire-endorsed thoughts.

It is clear that assessors must pay attention to the contextual cues associated with different assessment approaches. Targeted cognitions may not be available within the assessment context unless they are "primed" or activated, usually by induced mood states (Segal & Ingram, 1994). Clark (1997, p. 997) has argued that the accuracy of some cognition questionnaires might be improved if external priming manipulations were added, such as having individuals complete a questionnaire in a situation or context that is known to elicit the relevant cognitions, or through the induction of a mood state that is congruent with the target cognitions.

In summary, although in the past cognitive assessment techniques have been employed with minimal attention to psychometric issues, attention to the psychometric properties of cognitive assessment measures has increased (Clark, 1998). The psychometric status of the widely used endorsement methods is better established than production methods; however, increased emphasis has been placed on psychometric evaluation of thought-listing, think-aloud, and thought-sampling approaches to cognitive assessment. In addition to issues of reliability, content validity, criterion validity, and construct validity, it is important to address the issue of clinical utility. The fact that so few of these measures are used routinely in clinical practice questions their external validity.

COGNITIVE ASSESSMENT OF ANXIETY

In light of recognition that the phenomenology of anxiety is predominantly cognitive, a number of theorists posit a significant role for maladaptive cognitions in the development and maintenance of anxiety disorders (Beck & Emery, 1985; Mathews & MacLeod, 1994). Cognitive assessment is, therefore, especially suited to this domain, yet it cannot be considered a sufficient description until it is integrated with the other response modes (behavioral, physiological) characteristic of anxiety (Nelson, Hayes, Felton, & Jarrett, 1985).

Cognitive Products

Questionnaires that purport to measure some of the general cognitive features of anxiety have been used for some time. The Fear of Negative Evaluation Scale (FNE; Watson & Friend, 1969) is a 30-item, true–false questionnaire designed to measure the degree of apprehension about receiving others' disapproval in social situations, whereas the Social Avoidance and Distress Scale (SAD; Watson & Friend, 1969) uses a similar, 28-item format to measure the experience of distress and discomfort in social situations. Both scales show good internal consistency and test–retest reliability.

Other questionnaires are available to the clinical researcher for the assessment of certain cognitive features related to anxiety. For example, "anxiety sensitivity" is the fear of anxiety-related bodily sensations, based on beliefs that the sensations signal catastrophic somatic, social, or psychological consequences. According to Reiss's expectancy theory (1991) anxiety sensitivity is an individual-difference variable that contributes to general fearfulness and acts as a risk factor in the development of various forms of anxiety disorders, including panic disorder and social anxiety disorder (Taylor, 1999). Anxiety sensitivity was originally conceptualized as a unidimensional construct, as assessed by the 16-item Anxiety Sensitivity Index (ASI; Peterson & Reiss, 1992). ASI scores predict who will respond anxiously to panic-provocation challenges, and who is likely to develop panic attacks and panic disorder (Taylor, 1999). Taylor et al. (2007) developed an 18-item measure, the Anxiety Sensitivity Index–3 (ASI-3), to assess the physical (e.g., "When my stomach is upset, I worry that I might be seriously ill"), cognitive (e.g., "When my thoughts speed up, I worry that I might be going crazy"), and social concerns (e.g., "I worry that other people will notice my anxiety") factors replicated in prior research. In international nonclinical samples of thousands of participants and clinical samples of hundreds of patients, Taylor et al. found support for the factorial validity, and internal consistency of the ASI-3, and evidence of improved psychometric properties relative to the original ASI.

Several other anxious self-statement measures are worth noting. The Anxious Self-Statements Questionnaire (ASSQ; Kendall & Hollon, 1989), a 32-item measure of the frequency of anxious thoughts, has excellent reliability, concurrent validity, and ability to discriminate between known groups, although Glass and Arnkoff (1997) question its discriminant validity with respect to depression. The Cognition Checklist (CCL) developed by Beck, Brown, Steer, Eidelson, and Riskind (1987) assesses the frequency of 12 cognitions related to danger and presumed to be characteristic of anxiety disorders (CCL-Anxiety), and 12 thoughts centered on loss and failure characteristic of depression (CCL-Depression). In a meta-analysis of 13 studies, R. Beck and Perkins (2001) found that the CCL-Anxiety scale did not discriminate between anxious and depressive symptomatology.

To rectify these specificity problems, Woody, Taylor, McLean, and Koch (1998) developed the 77-item University of British Columbia Cognitions Inventory to maximize the specificity of cognitive content and to assess a wide variety of cognitions. Cognitions were sorted by raters into several problem areas based on prototypicality: Panic, Worry, Somatic Preoccupation, Social Fears, and Depression. Woody et al. found better support for the specificity position in their initial study of groups of patients with panic disorder or depressive disorder. The *Negative Affect Self-Statement Questionnaire* (NASSQ) developed by Ronan et al. (1994) also yields anxiety- and depression-specific subscales for children of different ages. The investigator or practitioner interested in employing thought endorsement measures with children should refer to Glass and Arnkoff's (1997) discussion of this issue.

A number of self-report measures have been developed to assess cognitive aspects of specific anxiety disorders, including generalized anxiety disorder, social anxiety disorder, panic disorder and agoraphobia, obsessive–compulsive disorder, and posttraumatic stress disorder (PTSD). In terms of cognitive aspects of generalized anxiety disorder, the Penn State Worry Questionnaire (PSWQ; Meyer, Miller, Metzger, & Borkovec, 1990), a widely used, 16-item measure, assesses an individual's tendency to worry in general. The items reflect a tendency to worry excessively and chronically (e.g., "Once I start worrying I cannot stop"). The PSWQ provides a reliable and valid measure of worry (e.g., Startup & Erickson, 2006). The PSWQ has demonstrated utility across a wide range of diagnostic groups, while exhibiting sufficient specificity to distinguish generalized anxiety disorder from other disorders. The Worry Domains Questionnaire (WDQ; Tallis, Eysenck, & Mathews, 1992) was developed as a measure of five domains of nonpathological worry: (1) Relationships, (2) Lack of Confidence, (3) Aimless Future, (4) Work Incompetence, and (5) Financial. The WDQ has demonstrated adequate internal consistency and validity in nonclinical (e.g., Startup & Erickson, 2006) and clinical (McCarthy-Larzelere et al., 2001) samples. The WDQ is a possible complementary measure to the PSWQ that can guide clinicians in highlighting areas of intervention. In a recent study of 432 university students, Verkuil, Brosschot, and Thayer (2007) found that both the PSWQ and WDQ predicted the frequency and duration of worry assessed daily over 6 days. However, these questionnaires did not account for the larger proportion of variance in daily worry, which suggests that future studies of worry should consider using daily assessments.

The Anxious Thoughts Inventory (AnTI; Wells, 1994), a 22-item content and process measure of proneness to health, social, and meta- (worry about worry) dimensions of worry, has demonstrated adequate internal consistency, validity, and sensitivity to treatment effects (Wells, 2006). "Intolerance of uncertainty" is a cognitive construct that emerging empirical evidence suggests might play an important role in explaining anxiety and worry (e.g., Carleton, Sharpe, & Asmundson, 2007). Intolerance of uncertainty, assessed by the Intolerance of Uncertainty Scale (e.g., Buhr & Dugas, 2002), refers to the tendency of an individual to consider it unacceptable that a negative event may occur, regardless of the likelihood of its occurrence. Although intolerance of uncertainty is related to anxiety sensitivity, research suggests that these two constructs are independently related to fear and anxiety (Carleton et al., 2007).

A differentiated assessment of current (or recent) conscious thoughts is provided by self-statement inventories that sample content specific to particular problem areas, such as social phobia. The Social Interaction Self-Statement Test (SISST: Glass, Merluzzi, Biever, & Larsen, 1982) was designed to assess self-statements after participation in a live heterosexual social interaction. The SISST has 15 positive and 15 negative thoughts, and patients with social phobia have been found to score significantly higher on the Negative subscale and significantly lower on the Positive subscale than other anxiety disorder patients in rating thoughts before, during, and after social interactions (Becker, Namour, Zayfert, & Hegel, 2001). Beazley, Glass, Chambless, and Arnkoff (2001) examined the thoughts of individuals with social phobia across three different social situations—same-sex interactions, heterosexual interactions, and an impromptu speech—and found support for the validity of the SISST Negative subscale across all situations, and of the Positive subscale in the two social interaction situations.

Telch et al. (2004) contended that an SISST weakness is that it does not assess the individual's concerns about observable signs of anxiety, which is considered to be an important component of social phobia. Telch et al. developed the Appraisal of Social Concerns (ASC) scale, a 20-item self-report measure that asks participants to rate the degree to which they feel concerned about social threat. The ASC has three subscales: Negative Evaluation, Observable Symptoms, and Social Helplessness. It has exhibited adequate internal consistency, validity in nonclinical samples (Telch et al., 2004), as well as sensitivity to the effects of treatment in patients with social anxiety disorder (Schultz et al., 2006; Telch et al., 2004).

Self-report inventories of panic disorder and agoraphobia can be grouped into two categories. The first group assesses the degree to which individuals with panic disorder experience dysfunctional cognitions during panic attacks. The Agoraphobic Cognitions Questionnaire (ACQ) was developed by Chambless, Caputo, Bright, and Gallagher (1984). This 14-item measure comprises thoughts concerning negative consequences of experiencing anxiety, and clients are asked to judge the frequency of thoughts when they are in an anxious state. Reliability data show good test–retest stability but low internal consistency. Validity analyses have shown that this scale is sensitive to treatment-induced changes and can discriminate the scores of an agoraphobic and normal control sample.

The 45-item Panic Appraisal Inventory (PAI; Telch, Brouillard, Telch, Agras, & Taylor, 1987) comprises three scales that assess the perceived likelihood of a panic attack in agoraphobic situations (Anticipated Panic), concern about possible catastrophic consequences (Panic Consequences), and confidence in coping with future panic attacks (Coping). Feske and De Beurs (1997) concluded that the PAI shows excellent internal consistency, treatment sensitivity, and good convergent and divergent validity. Although they conclude that the Panic Consequences scale is redundant with, and should not replace, the ACQ, they noted that the Anticipated Panic and Coping scales assess important features not captured by other instruments, and recommend the inclusion of these scales in the assessment of panic disorder.

A second group of measures assesses the degree to which individuals with panic disorder experience fear and anxiety in the context of uncomfortable physiological and psychological sensations. The Body Sensations Questionnaire (BSQ; Chambless et al., 1984), a companion scale to the ASQ, measures the degree to which individuals are frightened or worried by physical sensations associated with autonomic arousal (e.g., heart palpitations). Khawaja and Oei (1998) noted that Chambless and colleagues' (1984) measures do not accurately reflect cognitions with a theme of danger. The modified Catastrophic Cognitions Questionnaire (CCQ-M; Khawaja, Oei, & Baglioni, 1994) is a 21-item measure that reflects danger-related schemas. It comprises three factors that reflect the dimensions of catastrophic cognitions: emotional, physical, and mental catastrophes. Subsequent research may determine that the CCQ-M is a useful tool for the assessment of panic disorder; however, to date, it has not been widely used.

A number of scales have been developed in the areas of obsessions and compulsions. The Padua Inventory—Washington State University Revision (PI-WSUR; Burns, Keortge, Formea, & Sternberger, 1996), a 39-item measure of obsessions and compulsions, was produced to reduce the overlap of the original Padua Inventory with worry. The 28-item Obsessive Compulsive Thoughts Checklist (OCTC; Bouvard, Mollard, Cottraux, & Guerin, 1989) provides a measure of obsessive thoughts over the past week. Freeston and Ladouceur (1993) developed the Cognitive Intrusions Questionnaire to assess intrusive thoughts, images, or impulses (past month) on six proposed themes (Health, Embarrassing Situations, Unacceptable Sexual Behavior, etc.). Glass and Arnkoff (1997) suggested that Purdon and Clark's (1994) Revised Obsessional Intrusions Inventory (ROII) may have greater potential as a measure of the frequency of intrusive obsessive thoughts, images, and impulses. The ROII determines respondents' appraisal and thought control strategies of the most upsetting thought on 10 dimensions. The ROII has good psychometric properties; however, its sensitivity to treatment effects has not been reported.

The Posttraumatic Cognitions Inventory (PTCI; Foa, Ehlers, Clark, Tolin, & Orsillo, 1999), a 33-item self-report measure, was developed to assess trauma-related thoughts and beliefs. The PTCI comprises three factors: Negative Cognitions about Self, Negative Cognitions about the World, and Self-Blame. In an initial study, the three PTCI factors exhibited good internal consistency, test–retest reliability, and validity, and distinguished between traumatized individuals with and without PTSD (Foa et al., 1999). Because sexual assault survivors were overrepresented in Foa et al.'s PTSD sample, J. G. Beck et al. (2004) examined the psychometric properties of the PTCI in individuals who had experienced a serious motorcycle accident. Support was found for the psychometric properties of the two subscales that assessed negative thoughts of the self and the world. However, the Self-Blame subscale did not perform well, perhaps because motorcycle accidents might be less likely to result in self-blame reactions than a sexual assault. Further research should examine how differing forms of trauma might impact the psychometric properties of the PTCI.

The importance of maladaptive metacognitions in anxiety disorders is increasingly being recognized by researchers and clinicians. Beliefs about one's thoughts, or metacognitive beliefs, have been linked to both generalized anxiety disorder and obsessive–compulsive disorder. Cartwright-Hatton and Wells (1997) developed the Meta-Cognitions Questionnaire (MCQ), a 65-item measure that has five metacognitive belief subscales: Positive Worry Beliefs; Negative Beliefs about Thought Uncontrollability and Danger; Lack of Cognitive Confidence; Negative Beliefs about Thoughts in General (themes of superstition, punishment, and responsibility); and Cognitive Self-Consciousness. The MCQ has demonstrated good reliability and construct validity, and discriminates between patients with generalized anxiety disorder or obsessive–compulsive disorder and patients with panic disorder or social phobia (Wells, 2006). Wells and Cartwright-Hatton (2004) have also developed a shortened, 30-item version of the MCQ (MCQ-30), which has exhibited a five-factor structure that is comparable to the original MCQ, and has been found to have acceptable psychometric properties (Wells, 2006).

The *Consequences of Worrying Scale* (Davey, Tallis, & Capuzzo, 1996), developed to assess a range of beliefs that individuals have about the consequences of worrying, may be useful for assessing individuals with generalized anxiety disorder. This 29-item self-report inventory comprises three scales representing negative consequences (Worry Disrupting Effective Performance, Worry Exaggerating the Problem, Worry Causing Emotional Distress) and two scales representing positive consequences (Motivational Influence of Worry, Worry Helping Analytical Thinking). The five consequences of worrying subscales demonstrated adequate internal consistency and validity (Davey et al., 1996).

Two self-report scales have been developed to assess metacognitive content in obsessive–compulsive disorder. The Interpretation of Intrusions Inventory (III), developed by the Obsessive Compulsive Cognitions Working Group (OCCWG; 2003), comprises 31 items that assess interpretations of unwanted, distressing intrusive thoughts, images, or impulses. Participants rate their level of belief within the past 2 weeks of two intrusions that they have experienced recently. In a study of hundreds of outpatients with obsessive–compulsive disorder, nonobsessional anxious patients, community adults, and undergraduate students, the III was demonstrated to be an internally consistent and valid measure of obsessive–compulsive cognitive phenomenology (OCCWG, 2003). The Meta-Cognitive Beliefs Questionnaire (MCBQ; Clark, Purdon, & Wang, 2003) is a 67-item self-report measure developed to assess beliefs about the importance of control and negative consequences related to unwanted, distressing intrusive thoughts (Clark et al., 2003). In a study of large samples of undergraduate students, Clark et al. found support for the construct validity of the MCBQ. Further research of the MCBQ is warranted to examine the generalizability of these findings to clinical samples.

Cognitive Processes

In addition to self-statement inventories, a number of structured measures of thought have been employed in the cognitive assessment of anxiety. Consistent with cognitive models of anxiety, a number of authors have assessed the constructs of perceived danger or the overestimation of personal risk as the salient cognitive processes in anxiety.

Butler and Mathews (1983) asked subjects to fill out separate questionnaires that required interpretations of 20 threatening but ambiguous scenarios. Items were rated in terms of their subjective cost to the subject (e.g., "How bad would it be for you?"), and in terms of their subjective probability of occurrence. Anxious subjects interpreted the ambiguous material as more threatening and rated the subjective cost of the threatening events higher than did a control group of nonanxious subjects. Butler and Mathews interpreted their findings as indicative of an interaction between anxiety and the availability of "danger schemas." Similarly, Williams (1985) described a measure of "perceived danger," defined as a subject's perception of the probability of a negative event occurring given a specific performance.

Other research has examined the relation between anxiety and/or depression, interpretation of ambiguous information, estimates of the probability of both negative and positive futures, and recall of past specific situations or a range of events. For example, MacLeod, Tata, Kentish, Carroll, and Hunter (1997) reported that panic disorder was associated with generating memories of more negative experiences but fewer positive experiences, whereas depression was associated with generating fewer positive experiences but not more negative experiences than controls. This work supports the notion that cognitions differ in anxiety and depression, and that while anxious participants can think negatively about the past, their negative thoughts are more typically focused on the future. These studies also suggest that measures of retrospective and prospective cognitions are useful in clinical cognitive research and are of potential value in clinical practice.

Less structured formats for the cognitive assessment of anxiety have included attempts to sample thinking during *in vivo* (Last, Barlow, & O'Brien, 1985) or simulated (Davison et al., 1983) anxiety-arousing situations. Thought listing has been used in a number of studies whose aim has been to record subjects' thoughts immediately following *in vivo* performance. For example, Last et al. (1985) had agoraphobic participants report what was going through their minds during an exposure session at a shopping mall. Similarly, Hofmann, Moscovitch, Kim, and Taylor (2004) used thought-listing to examine changes in self-perception among socially phobic individuals during cognitive-behavioral therapy (CBT) treatment. Treated subjects reported a greater reduction in negative self-focused thoughts while anticipating socially stressful situations than others assigned to a waiting-list control group. Williams and Rappoport (1983) employed thought sampling in their research comparing cognitive- and exposure-based treatments for agoraphobia. Each subject was provided with a beeper that would activate periodically, thus cueing the individual to record whatever he or she was thinking on a tape recorder. The assessments had high ecological validity, because they were taken during behavioral tests of driving capability.

Think-aloud procedures can be especially informative in anxiety, when the precise contents of the internal dialogue are elusive. Molina, Borkovec, Peasley, and Person (1998) analyzed content of worrisome cognitive activity on stream of consciousness reports obtained from "neutral" and "worry" periods. Participants who met DSM-IV criteria for generalized anxiety disorder used a higher relative frequency of statements suggesting catastrophic interpretations of events, implying a rigid, rule-bound interpretive style and use of somatic anxiety words. Szabo and Lovibond (2002) expanded on this work by investigating whether worry entails problem-solving attempts. Participants monitored and listed their worrisome thoughts in a diary for 7 days. Results showed that approximately 50% of the content of naturally occurring worry reflected a problem-solving process (e.g., solutions are generated and evaluated with respect to their anticipated consequences), whereas approximately 20% reflected concerns with anticipated negative outcomes. These findings illuminated a conceptualization of worry as an ineffective problem-solving process.

Cognitive Structures/Organizations

Despite the fact that current cognitive conceptualizations presume that individuals with anxiety disorders possess maladaptive beliefs that underlie specific negative cognitions related to each disorder, only recently have self-report inventories been developed to assess these dysfunctional attitudes and beliefs in various anxiety disorders. The Social Thoughts and Beliefs Scale (STABS; Turner, Johnson, Beidel, Heiser, & Lydiard, 2003) is a 21-item self-report questionnaire designed to assess various pathological cognitions in individuals with social phobia. Respondents rate the degree to which a particular thought or belief typifies their thinking when anticipating or participating in a social interaction. An initial STABS study found support for the internal consistency and test–retest reliability. The STABS discriminated individuals with social phobia from individuals with other anxiety disorders and those without disorders (Turner et al., 2003). The Panic Beliefs Inventory (PBI; Wenzel, Sharp, Brown, Greenberg, & Beck, 2006), a 35-item self-report inventory, was developed to assess the dysfunctional attitudes and beliefs that increase the probability that panic disorder patients will have catastrophic responses to physical and emotional experiences. Preliminary evidence demonstrated that the PBI is internally consistent, valid, and sensitive to clinical change (Wenzel et al., 2006). The Obsessive Beliefs Questionnaire (OBQ) was developed to assess dysfunctional beliefs (assumptions, attitudes) identified by a large group of international researchers, the OCCWG (2003, 2005), to represent the critical belief domains of obsessive–compulsive disorder. A factor-analytic study (OCCWG, 2005) of 87 belief items found support for three factors: Responsibility/Threat Estimation, Perfectionism/Certainty, and Importance/Control of Thoughts. A 44-item version (OBQ-44) exhibited good internal consistency and validity in clinical and nonclinical samples (OCCWG, 2005).

Whereas the majority of material we have covered in this section describes efforts to measure cognitive aspects of anxiety within an individual's awareness, we have also attempted to assess the "deep" structure representations of anxious individuals; processes that are inferred from behavior (e.g., Rudy, Merluzzi, & Henahan, 1982). For example, Goldfried, Padawer, and Robins (1984), using multidimensional scaling with a sample of socially anxious college males, found that they weighted the dimension of Chance of Being Evaluated the highest with respect to the likelihood of generating anxiety, while giving lower weights to dimensions of Intimacy and Academic Relevance. Nonanxious males weighted Intimacy twice as heavily as Chance of Being Evaluated, which suggests a possible difference in the saliencies that stand out for these two groups when confronted by an opportunity for heterosexual interaction.

Finally, several paradigms have confirmed that people with anxiety disorders show selective processing of threat cues (Mathews & MacLeod, 1994; for a review, see Bar-Haim, Lamy, Pergamin, Bakermans-Kranenburg, & van IJzendoorn, 2007). Mathews and his colleagues (Butler & Mathews, 1983; MacLeod, Mathews, & Tata, 1986; Mathews & MacLeod, 1985) propose that activation of schemas biased toward the processing of information related to personal danger or other threats is characteristic of anxiety states. Mathews and MacLeod, for instance, used the emotional Stroop color-naming task and found that anxious subjects took longer than controls to color-name words with a threatening ("disease," "coffin") as opposed to a neutral ("welcome," "holiday") content. Another measure derived from cognitive science, the dot probe paradigm (MacLeod et al., 1986), assesses the degree of visual capture associated with a particular stimulus. Studies consistently report that anxious subjects are more vigilant for or have more difficulty disengaging from threat-related stimuli than normal controls (Bar-Haim et al., 2007). These results support the existence of cognitive "danger" schemas, which, when activated, bias information processing at a preattentive level. In the context of social anxiety disorder, modified dot probe studies using facial expressions as stimuli have yielded more positive findings in comparison to studies that measure attention to visually presented words. Facial expressions may have more ecological validity in the context of studying social phobia, because real social threat stimuli involve other peoples' reactions, facial expressions, and verbal responses (see Bögels & Mansell, 2004, for a review).

Whether cognitive biases are perceptual or attentional in nature, they play an important role in the maintenance of anxiety, since they affect the interpretations that individuals make at a later point in the information-processing stream. Moreover, the study of attentional biases might have potentially important treatment implications. MacLeod, Rutherford, Campbell, Ebsworthy, and Holker (2002) demonstrated that nonanxious students can be trained successfully to direct their attention away from threatening stimuli. Future research is warranted to see whether these encouraging experimental findings with nonclinical samples generalize to clinical populations.

Remaining Issues

Before leaving this section and moving on to the cognitive assessment of depression, it is important to consider a number of issues that interface with both domains. More work is needed to refine and evaluate measures that exist in these already method-rich areas (Clark, 1997). For example, scoring criteria for thought listing of think-aloud protocols are a good example of an area in which injection of some degree of regularity in the scored dimensions or attributes would aid comparability among investigations. Similarly, the increasing attention to cognitive structures or "deeper" levels of processing would benefit from a focus on resolving some of the definitional issues surrounding the operation of these constructs.

Readers should also bear in mind the close relationship between anxiety and depression symptoms (e.g., Clark & Watson, 1991). Most researchers have set out to differentiate the various syndromes of anxiety and depression using diagnostic systems or symptom inventories. However, Mogg and Bradley's (2005) review suggests that there are noteworthy differences in attentional biases between generalized anxiety disorder and depressive disorder. Consistent evidence indicates that individuals with generalized anxiety disorder exhibit an attentional bias across a wide range of minor, external negative cues (e.g., threatening words, pictures of angry faces) relative to nonanxious individuals. On the other hand, an attentional bias in depression is mainly apparent for negative, self-referent stimuli presented under conditions that permit more extensive processing (see Mogg & Bradley, 2005). Lim and Kim (2005) compared patients with panic disorder and depressive disorder on emotional Stroop tasks using conditions that prevented conscious perception (subliminal exposure), and that allowed clear awareness (supraliminal exposure). Patients with panic disorder showed subliminal selective attention for physical threat and negative words, whereas patients with depressive disorder showed supraliminal selective attention for negative words. Furthermore, investigators have only recently attempted to document the relative contribution of anxiety- and depression-related cognitions in an individual diagnosed with an anxiety and/ or a depressive disorder (see Bar-Haim et al., 2007). Considerably more work is needed to clarify the value of cognition and cognitive processes that differentiate between anxiety and depression.

COGNITIVE ASSESSMENT OF DEPRESSION

The majority of cognitive assessment measures in depression are paper-and-pencil instruments designed to capture either the content of patients' thinking or their underlying attitudes or beliefs. Other significant efforts have addressed the manner in which depressed patients process information, particularly self-referent descriptions or feedback from task performances. Only a few investigators have concerned themselves with thought-listing or think-aloud procedures although the recall of automatic thoughts or self-statements in specific situations is widely employed in the clinical interview format (Beck, Rush, Shaw, & Emery, 1979).

Cognitive Products

The Automatic Thoughts Questionnaire (ATQ; Hollon & Kendall, 1980) measures the frequency with which each of 30 negative automatic thoughts have "popped" into subjects' heads during the past week. In addition, the extent to which subjects tend to believe each of these thoughts is rated on a 5-point scale. The 30 thoughts that comprise the ATQ were derived empirically on the basis of their ability to discriminate between depressed and nondepressed subjects. Sample items include "I don't think I can go on," "No one understands me," and "It's just not worth it." Support for the ATQ's internal consistency and construct validity has been found in a number of studies (e.g., Dobson & Breiter, 1983; Hollon & Kendall, 1980). Hollon and Kendall's factor analysis of the ATQ yielded four factors: (1) personal maladjustment and desire for change, (2) negative self-concepts and expectations, (3) low self-esteem, and (4) helplessness and giving up, which are consistent with Beck's (1967, 1976) theory of depression.

Investigators have emphasized the importance of assessing positive, as well as negative, thinking patterns in depression. Ingram and Wisnicki (1988) developed the Positive Automatic Thoughts Questionnaire (ATQ-P), which assesses the frequency of positive automatic thoughts. The ATQ-P has demonstrated excellent internal consistency and adequate convergent and discriminant validity in relation to other cognitive measures, such as the ATQ (Ingram, Kendall, Siegle, Guarino, & McLaughlin, 1995). Thus, the ATQ-P may supplement the ATQ and provide a more comprehensive picture of automatic thinking patterns in depression.

Flett, Hewitt, Blankstein, and Gray (1998) developed a measure of automatic thoughts similar in format to the ATQ. However, it differs from the ATQ because of its specific focus on automatic thoughts involving perfectionism. The 25-item Perfectionism Cognitions Inventory (PCI) has demonstrated adequate levels of reliability and validity in both nonclinical (Flett et al., 1998) and clinical (Flett, Hewitt, Whelan, & Martin, 2007) samples. Additional research confirmed that the experience of frequent perfectionism thoughts is associated with dysphoria and anxiety, over and above the variance predicted by existing trait measures of perfectionism (Flett et al., 2007) and alternative measures of negative automatic thoughts (Flett et al., 1998).

The Attributional Style Questionnaire (ASQ; Peterson et al., 1982), developed in light of the reformulated learned helplessness model of depression (Abramson, Seligman, & Teasdale, 1978), is the most frequently cited measure of depressive attributions. It presents to subjects 12 hypothetical scenarios that involve themes of achievement or affiliation. Six of the scenarios have positive outcomes, whereas the other six have negative outcomes. Subjects imagine themselves in each situation and rate the extent to which they believe that (1) the outcome was due either to themselves or to other people or circumstances (i.e., internal vs. external factors); (2) the same cause would be operative in the future, under similar circumstances (i.e., stable vs. unstable factors); and (3) the same cause may influence a variety of life situations (i.e., global vs. specific factors).

Internality, Stability, and Globality scores are calculated separately for good and bad outcomes (i.e., six subscales based on six items each) on the ASQ. The internal consistency of these scales is weak, however, so two composite "attributional style" scores are often calculated, one each for good and bad events. This compromise attenuates the ASQ's theoretical relevance. Another major psychometric problem is that, for good events, the ASQ is completely unable to distinguish the three attributional dimensions (Peterson et al., 1982), and it does only marginally better for bad events. Indeed, a factor-analytic study (Bagby, Atkinson, Dickens, & Gavin, 1990) found that the ASQ's factor structure was best represented by a two-factor solution corresponding to the good outcome–bad outcome distinction, which suggests that outcome valence influences attributional style more than individual differences.

In response to these problems (particularly those relating to reliability) an *Extended ASQ* has been developed (EASQ; Metalsky, Halberstadt, & Abramson, 1987). The EASQ is similar in format to the original ASQ, but its 12 scenarios describe only bad events. Indeed, reliability estimates for this scale are more respectable than those reported for the ASQ (Metalsky et al., 1987). As with the ASQ, however, its relevance as a measure of cognition in more severely depressed individuals remains to be tested (Bagby et al., 1990).

An alternative approach to measuring attributions in depression involves examining individuals' attributions for actual negative or distressing life events. Like the ASQ, studies employing this strategy have failed to find support for the orthogonality of the three attributional dimensions (e.g., Gong-

Guy & Hammen, 1980). However, correlations between depression and attributions about actual life events may be somewhat stronger (Brewin & Furnham, 1986) than those involving hypothetical scenarios.

Negative expectancies and hopeless thoughts represent another central theme in the thinking of depressed individuals (Beck, 1976). The Hopelessness Scale (HS; Beck, Weissman, Lester, & Trexler, 1974) is a 20-item self-report scale designed to measure the extent to which individuals harbor a hopeless outlook on the future. Beck et al. reported good internal consistency and validity for the HS. Its scores have been shown to predict eventual suicide in psychiatric outpatients (Brown, Beck, Steer, & Grisham, 2000). The HS may be useful as a screening tool, because high scores may alert clinicians to the risk of self-destructive behavior. Furthermore, all three variance components (trait, state, random error) related to hopelessness scores are related to suicidal behavior (Goldston, Reboussin, & Daniel, 2006). Clinicians need to focus on not only the reduction of acute or short-lived hopelessness to prevent suicide but also reduction of individuals' relatively enduring trait levels of hopelessness.

An emerging and less direct approach to assess hopelessness cognitions involves having subjects rate the probability of positive or negative outcomes in a variety of scenarios (real or hypothetical). Alloy and Ahrens (1987) asked depressed and nondepressed students to rate the likelihood of success or failure in the academic domain, both for themselves and for others. Depressed individuals viewed success as less likely, and failure as more likely outcomes, both for themselves and for others, than did nondepressed participants. This approach may represent a somewhat less transparent strategy than the HS for assessing depressive pessimism, particularly in individuals who exhibit rather mild levels of depression.

Most cognitive accounts emphasize the role of negative or disparaging self-evaluations in depressive phenomenology. The Beck Self-Concept Test (BST; Beck, Steer, Epstein, & Brown, 1990) is a self-report measure designed to evaluate the negative view of self that Beck (1967, 1976) described as a central feature of depression. The BST asks subjects to evaluate themselves relative to their acquaintances on 25 dimensions, representing personality (e.g., good-natured, selfish), abilities (e.g., knowledgeable, successful), aptitudes (intelligent, athletic), virtues (e.g., kind, tidy) and vices (e.g., lazy, greedy). Beck et al. (1990) reported support for the internal consistency, test–retest reliability, and validity of the BST. The BST was not related to a measure of anxiety (the Beck Anxiety Inventory), thus indicating the potential of specificity to depression.

A central theme in Beck's (1967, 1976) formulation of depression is that depressive phenomenology is mediated by faulty, irrational thinking patterns. The Cognitive Bias Questionnaire (CBQ; Hammen & Krantz, 1976; Krantz & Hammen, 1979) comprises six vignettes of problematic situations that involve interpersonal or achievement themes. For each vignette, subjects imagine as vividly as possible what the protagonist might think and feel about the situation, then select from among four response alternatives the one that most closely resembles this response. The response options were constructed to reflect two dichotomous and crossed dimensions: (1) depressive versus non-depressive; and (2) distorted (i.e., irrational) versus nondistorted. An example of a depressive–nondistorted response to the situation "being alone on a Friday night" would be "upsets me and makes me feel lonely." A depressive–distorted (overgeneralization) response would be "upsets me and makes me start to imagine endless days and nights by myself" (Hammen & Krantz, 1976, p. 580). Scores on the CBQ reflect the use frequency of each of the four response categories, although the frequency of depressive–distorted responses are of particular interest. The CBQ has relatively modest internal consistency and reasonable 4- and 8-week test–retest reliabilities. Several studies have differentiated depressed and nondepressed individuals on the basis of CBQ depressive–distorted scores (e.g., Krantz & Hammen, 1979). Mixed findings are reported concerning the discriminant validity of depressive–distorted CBQ scores with anxiety (Krantz & Hammen, 1979).

The Cognitive Response Test (CRT; Watkins & Rush, 1983) is a less structured measure of cognitive distortion in depression than the CBQ. Its 36 items are presented in an open-ended, sentence completion format. Subjects complete each sentence with the first thought that comes to mind. Sample items are "My employer says he will be making some major staff changes. I immediately think: _____" and "When I consider being married, my first thought is: _____." Although this open-ended format has the advantage of obviating the "transparency problems" of fixed-choice tests (Rush, 1984), it is more time-consuming to score. On the basis of rules set out in a standardized test manual, responses are classified as Rational, Irrational, or Nonscorable. Irrational responses are further classified as Irrational–Depressed (i.e., incorporating a negative view of the self, the past, or the future) or irrational-other. Watkins and Rush (1983) reported good inter-reliability across subjects and response types. In terms of discriminant validity, they reported that the irrational-depressed subscale distinguished depressed individuals from a variety of medical, psychiatric, and normal control groups.

Barton, Morley, Bloxham, Kitson, and Platts (2005) argued that the lengthy and highly structured sentence stems of the CRT constrain referential freedom and result in predictable completion patterns. The Sentence Completion Test for Depression (SCD) was developed to encourage diverse responses, and comprises 48 short-sentence stems that tap known areas of depressive thinking (e.g., "I think ... "; "Things in general ... "). The sentence completions are coded according to a manual as negative, positive, or neutral thoughts. Depressed patients have been found to produce more negative thoughts and fewer positive thoughts than controls. Despite its open-ended format, the SCD has demonstrated good construct validity, internal consistency, interrater reliability, sensitivity, and specificity. Moreover, the SCD is novel in that it elicits idiographic information that can be helpful in identifying target problems and dysfunctional beliefs in the CBT case formulation (Barton et al., 2005).

Cognitive Processes

A variety of self-regulatory mechanisms have been implicated in the development and maintenance of depressive phenomenology. Theorists have suggested
that excessive self-focused attention may be related to affective self-regulatory
deficits (Carver & Scheier, 1982). One prominent measure of self-focused
attention is the Self-Focused Sentence Completion task (SFSC; Exner, 1973),
a 30-item scale in which subjects read sentence stems (e.g., "I wish ... " or
"When I look in the mirror ... ") and complete them any way they choose.
In the scoring system detailed by Exner, the SFSC yields 10 scores: total self-
focus (S); self-focus positive, negative and neutral; total external focus (E);
external focus positive, negative and neutral; total ambivalent (A); and total
neutral (N). Exner has reported adequate scoring reliabilities for both experienced and novice raters. A variety of studies have indicated that both mildly
and clinically depressed individuals generate more self-focused responses and
fewer external-focused responses than nondepressives (e.g., Ingram, Lumry,
Cruet, & Sieber, 1987).

Another frequently employed measure of self-focused attention is the Self-
Consciousness Scale (SCS; Fenigstein, Scheier, & Buss, 1975). The SCS comprises three factor-analytically derived subscales: Private Self-Consciousness
(10 items); Public Self-Consciousness (7 items); and Social Anxiety (6 items).
The Private Self-Consciousness subscale (e.g., "I'm always trying to figure
myself out") is considered the dispositional equivalent of the self-focused
attention state. This subscale's reliability and validity have been demonstrated
in several studies (e.g., Fenigstein et al., 1975). It also has been shown to
be associated significantly with depression across a number of studies (for a
review, see Mor & Winquist, 2002).

The Response Styles Questionnaire (RSQ; Nolen-Hoeksema & Morrow,
1991) is designed to measure dispositional responses to depressed mood by
asking respondents what they generally do when they feel depressed. The RSQ
comprises two subscales: a 21-item Rumination Response Scale (RRS), and
an 11-item Distraction Response Scale (DRS). The RRS and DRS have each
demonstrated good internal reliability and are independent of one another
(e.g., Just & Alloy, 1997). The stability of RRS is critical, in that rumination
is proposed to be a reliable individual-difference variable that plays a role in
the onset, maintenance, and recurrence of depression. The RRS test–retest
reliability coefficients have been largest in studies where the level of depression
of participants remained stable (e.g., Nolen-Hoeksema, 2000), and smaller
in studies where depressed mood did change (Kasch, Klein, & Lara, 2001;
see Bagby, Rector, Bacchiochi, & McBride, 2004). This has raised concerns
that RRS scores change significantly as a function of changes in clinical state
(Kasch et al., 2001). However, in a study of patients being treated for major
depression, Bagby et al. (2004) found that RRS scores exhibited equivalent
test–retest reliability for both remitted ($r = .59$) and nonremitted ($r = .62$)
patients, in support for the relative stability of the RRS. The RRS has dem-

onstrated validity for predicting depression (e.g., Nolen-Hoeksema, 2000; Nolen-Hoeksema & Morrow, 1991).

CBT treatment for depression is based, at least in part, on the assumption that changes in cognitive appraisals of daily events are ingredients of a successful therapy. Daily process designs can contribute to a better understanding of the interplay between minor daily events and mood in depressed individuals. For example, Dunkley et al. (2003) found that high-self-critical perfectionists, relative to low-self-critical perfectionists, experienced more negative affect on days when they experienced elevated levels of achievement-related hassles and perceived criticism from others, and low levels of confidence in their ability to cope. In contrast, high-dependent individuals, relative to low-dependent individuals, experienced increases in negative affect on days when they experienced more social hassles. Although Dunkley et al.'s study was of university students, other studies have used daily process designs in clinically depressed samples. For example, in an outpatient sample, Gunthert et al. (2007) found that, for those with high levels of depression, there were greater increases in negative thoughts and affect on days following an interpersonal stressor relative to days following a noninterpersonal stressor. Overall, the daily assessment paradigm holds considerable promise as a means of providing a better understanding of the day-to-day cognitive reactivity of depressed individuals.

Cognitive Structures/Organization

Beck (1967; Beck et al., 1979) proposed that negative self-schemas become activated in depression, which results in the tendency to view oneself unfavorably and to interpret one's past, current, and future experiences in a predominantly negative fashion. Activated negative self-schemas also facilitate the retrieval of schema-congruent information. According to Beck's formulation, negative self-schemas comprise a highly organized network of stored personal information, primarily unfavorable, along with rules for evaluating one's worth or value as a person. The measurement of self-schemas, both at the level of content and of organization, represents an ongoing challenge for depression investigators.

The Dysfunctional Attitude Scale (DAS) is a self-report inventory designed to identify the relatively stable set of attitudes associated with depressive disorders (Weissman, 1979; Weissman & Beck, 1978). As dysfunctional attitudes are thought to reflect prepotent self-schemas, the DAS has been proposed as one measure of cognitive vulnerability to major depressive disorder (Ingram, Miranda, & Segal, 1998). The DAS is available in three forms. The original 100-item inventory (DAS-T) is only occasionally employed in research studies. From the DAS-T, two 40-item parallel forms (DAS-A and DAS-B) have been derived, with the former being the most commonly used.

DAS items are typically stated as contingencies concerning approval from others, prerequisites for happiness, or perfectionistic standards. Items include "It is difficult to be happy unless one is good looking, intelligent, rich and creative," "People will probably think less of me if I make a mistake," and "If someone disagrees with me, it probably indicates he or she does not like me." The DAS has been widely researched on depressed and psychiatric control patients. Both short forms of the DAS have good internal consistency and stability over time (Oliver & Baumgart, 1985; Weissman, 1979). Factor analyses of the DAS-A have consistently yielded two factors: Perfectionism and Need for Approval (e.g., Imber et al., 1990). These factors have good internal consistency and strongly correlate with each other (Zuroff, Blatt, Sanislow, Bondi, & Pilkonis, 1999). DAS-A Perfectionism, but not Need for Approval, has predicted negative outcome in the treatment of depression (Blatt & Zuroff, 2005), which suggests that it might be important to study the DAS-A Perfectionism and Need for Approval scores separately in addressing certain research questions.

One area of controversy concerns the stability of DAS scores in samples of treated depressed patients. Some investigators report a relatively stable pattern of DAS scores, whereas others find a marked change in scores. In a study of adults treated for major depression, Zuroff et al. (1999) found that not only did DAS mean scores change with level of depressed mood but also individuals tended to maintain their relative standing on levels of dysfunctional attitudes despite decreases in depressive symptomatology. Zuroff et al. proposed a state–trait model of dysfunctional attitudes, in which DAS scores are to some degree not only mood state–dependent but also considerably trait-like and consistent over time. This model has been found to capture best subsequent observations of DAS scores (e.g., Otto et al., 2007).

The concurrent validity of the DAS has been tested in several studies, but there are few evaluations of construct validity. The DAS has exhibited moderate correlations with measures of depressive severity and with measures of negative automatic thoughts, or cognitive distortions (e.g., Dobson & Shaw, 1986; Hamilton & Abramson, 1983; Hollon, Kendall, & Lumry, 1986). Although the DAS discriminates groups of depressed and psychiatric control patients, it is not specific to depression. Patients with generalized anxiety disorder, anorexia nervosa, panic disorder, or dysthymia may manifest abnormal DAS scores (Dobson & Shaw, 1986).

The DAS has been employed to evaluate hypothesized attitude change in cognitive therapy or other treatments of depression. Several studies have found that the DAS is sensitive to clinical improvement. For example, Jarrett, Vittengl, Doyle, and Clark (2007) found the magnitude of change in dysfunctional attitudes to be large, clinically significant, and durable over a 2-year follow-up in outpatients with recurrent major depressive disorder after treatment with cognitive therapy. Limited change in DAS-A scores has also been found to predict shorter time to return of depressive symptoms in depressed patients who were at least partially asymptomatic following treatment (Beevers, Keitner, Ryan, & Miller, 2003).

Recently, item response theory methods were used to develop two 9-item short forms of the DAS-A (Beevers, Strong, Meyer, Pilkonis, & Miller,

2007). The short forms were highly correlated with each other and the original 40-item DAS-A (r's ranging from .91 to .93). The short forms exhibited adequate internal consistency, similar change as the DAS-A over the time of treatment, convergent validity, and predicted concurrent depressive severity and change in depression from before treatment to after treatment (Beevers et al., 2007).

Although previous research has demonstrated that DAS-A Perfectionism predicts poor treatment outcome in depression (see Blatt & Zuroff, 2005), interpretation of these findings has only recently been clarified with other information about this variable. Although DAS-A Perfectionism is widely assumed to reflect high personal standards, factor-analytic studies have consistently distinguished between personal standards and self-critical evaluative concerns in higher-order latent dimensions of perfectionism (see Dunkley, Blankstein, Masheb, & Grilo, 2006). Contrary to assumption, results suggest that DAS-A Perfectionism reflects the self-critical dimension, as opposed to the personal standards dimension of perfectionism (Dunkley et al., 2006). Thus, in interpreting previous findings demonstrating the DAS-A Perfectionism scale as a negative predictor of treatment outcome, clinicians should focus more on self-critical evaluative concerns than on personal standards dimensions of perfectionism.

The Role of Priming in Cognitive Assessment of Depression

Several studies (e.g., Miranda, Persons, & Byers, 1990) indicate that individuals prone to depression do obtain higher DAS scores, but only in the presence of a negative mood. Segal and Ingram (1994) reviewed over 40 studies and found positive findings of depressive cognitive processing in 20% of studies that assessed without using a prime, whereas over 80% of studies that employed a prime reported detection of depressotypic cognitions. These findings suggest that transient negative mood states may prime negative self-schemas and increase the accessibility of dysfunctional attitudes.

It appears that the effect of priming cuts across several different levels of cognitive analysis (Ingram, 1990). In the presence of negative mood, dysfunctional cognition for those at risk appears evident in cognitive content (i.e., DAS scores), information encoding and retrieval (adjective recall), and attention (tracking errors in a dichotic listening task; for a review, see Scher, Ingram, & Segal, 2005). This pattern suggests that once a maladaptive cognitive structure/schema is activated by the priming manipulation, it may be the organizing construct linked to each of these more specific cognitive effects. Sad mood, in these studies, may serve as an analogue to potent environmental triggers, and appears to contribute to activating cognitive structures that heretofore have only minimally been involved in online information processing. Moreover, greater cognitive reactivity following sad mood provocation has shown promise in predicting relapse/recurrence in recovered depressed patients (e.g., Segal et al., 2006).

An important question concerns the use of questionnaires as primes. If self-report inventories have the capacity to activate subjects' mental representations, then they would confer distinct advantages in terms of convenience, standardization and time efficiency compared to other methods now in use. One important concern, however, is that prime specificity varies greatly among inventories, yielding uneven levels of construct activation. For example, the ASQ (Peterson & Villanova, 1988), the ATQ (Hollon & Kendall, 1980), and the CBQ (Krantz & Hammen, 1979) demonstrate a number of differences that could affect the degree of activation achieved. There are differences in (1) the type of response requested from subjects, (2) the amount of imaginal input required to respond to the item, and (3) the level of cognition being assessed. For these reasons, use of questionnaires as primes needs to be viewed with caution.

To address the drawbacks associated with using self-report measures, clinical researchers have recently used tasks that permit the study of dysfunctional beliefs that are not influenced by consciously controlled cognitive processes. One such task that has generated interest, the Implicit Association Test (Greenwald, McGhee, & Schwartz, 1998), uses a modified reaction time paradigm to assess implicit associations between the self and negative trait adjectives among individuals vulnerable to depression (Gemar, Segal, Sagrati, & Kennedy, 2001). Formerly depressed participants exhibited a negative evaluative bias for self-relevant information relative to control participants after a negative mood induction (Gemar et al., 2001).

The Self-Referent Encoding Task (SRET; Kuiper & Olinger, 1986) is an adaptation of a laboratory paradigm, originally developed by cognitive psychologists to test Craik and Lockhart's (1972) "levels of processing" model of memory. In the SRET, subjects are serially presented a number of personal adjectives (positive and negative) and asked to decide, in a categorical fashion (i.e., yes or no), whether the adjective is self-descriptive. After all the adjectives have been rated, an incidental recall test is administered.

The SRET yields several schema-related measures. First, consistent with schema-based models of depression, depressed subjects endorse more negative adjectives than do nondepressed controls, who tend to rate more positive adjectives as self-descriptive (e.g., Dozois & Dobson, 2001a; Gotlib, Kasch, et al., 2004; MacDonald & Kuiper, 1984). Second, and certainly less transparent, index of schematic processing relates to the time required for subjects to make their yes or no judgments. Theoretically, schemas should facilitate the processing of schema-congruent information. This notion is supported in SRET studies demonstrating quicker rating times by nondepressed subjects for positive adjectives (Kuiper & MacDonald, 1983), and by depressed subjects for negative adjectives (MacDonald & Kuiper, 1984). However, other studies have failed to replicate these effects (e.g., Dozois & Dobson, 2001a; Gotlib, Kasch, et al., 2004). The third self-schema measure yielded by the SRET relates to incidental recall. Depressed subjects have been shown to recall more negative adjectives following the SRET, whereas nondepressives recall more positive ones (e.g., Dozois & Dobson, 2001a; Gotlib, Kasch, et al., 2004; Kuiper & MacDonald, 1983). The SRET paradigm has been adapted for studies on information processing in children. For example, Timbremont and Braet (2004) found that following a negative mood induction, currently depressed and remitted children rated more negative words as self-descriptive compared to never-depressed children. Never-depressed children recalled more positive self-descriptive words relative to currently depressed and remitted children.

Taken together, results from studies with the SRET provide evidence for the operation of a negative self-schema in depression. However, the SRET's validity as a measure of self-schema content and function has been questioned (for a review, see Segal, 1988). One of the more serious concerns relates to the possibility that observed depression-related differences may reflect mood congruency effects rather than differences in cognitive organization. However, despite its limitations, the SRET is a good illustration of how paradigms from cognitive psychology may be adapted to the cognitive assessment of some of the more inferred features of depression.

The Psychological Distance Scaling Task (Dozois & Dobson, 2001a, 2001b) involves the calculation of interstimulus distances among self-referent adjective stimuli and assesses the structure, or interconnectedness, of cognitive patterns in depression. Dozois and Dobson (2001a) found that depressed individuals demonstrated stronger associations between negative adjective self-descriptors and less interconnectedness for positive self-relevant content. Furthermore, negative cognitive structures remained interconnected in depressed participants whose symptoms had remitted 6 months later, even without a mood or other prime (Dozois & Dobson, 2001b).

Another measure that has been employed to assess cognitive processing in depression is the emotional Stroop color-naming task. Depressed patients generally take longer to name the presentation color of negative words on the emotional Stroop task than positive or neutral words (e.g., Gotlib & McCann, 1984), whereas nondepressed controls show no difference in color-naming speed as a function of the valence of the word. The greater interference shown by depressed patients for negative material is thought to result from extended processing of the semantic content of stimuli, perhaps because this material is more accessible for the subject and is therefore harder to suppress in favor of rapid color naming (Williams et al., 1998).

Although the emotional Stroop paradigm can indicate the extent of semantic processing of valenced material, this particular methodology cannot examine whether material is organized in some fashion. Segal et al. (1995) modified the emotional Stroop paradigm to incorporate a priming design in which the color naming of a target word, relevant to the individual's view of self, was preceded by a prime word thought to be related or unrelated to the subject's self-concept. By previously activating one element in the cognitive system, other interconnected elements of the system might also become activated and influence performance on these related elements. In this way, interconnection among elements of self-representation can be studied. Using this approach, Segal et al. found that depressed patients showed increased interference for negative self-referent material when it was primed by similar negative information than when it was primed by negative information that was not self-descriptive. These results indicate that negative self-attributes are more highly organized in the self-concept of depressed patients than attributes that are negative but not particularly descriptive of the self.

Studies with the dot probe task (e.g., Gotlib, Kasch, et al., 2004; Gotlib, Krasnoperova, Yue, & Joormann, 2004) have consistently found that clinically depressed participants selectively attend to sad faces. Furthermore, Joormann and Gotlib (2007) found support for the stability of these attentional biases, which were evident after individuals recovered from a depressive episode, and even without a priming manipulation. In addition, following a mood induction, never-depressed daughters whose mothers had experienced recurrent episodes of depression were found to attend selectively to negative facial expressions (see Joormann, Talbot, & Gotlib, 2007). As there has been emerging evidence that children of depressed mothers are at increased risk of developing a depressive episode, these findings suggest a potential mechanism related to the intergenerational transmission of risk for depression.

These results are consistent with accounts of depression that emphasize the importance of cognitive organization in the maintenance of the disorder. Because cognitive-behavioral therapy (CBT) is thought to alter the negative nature of such organizations (Beck, 1967), successful treatment of this nature should reduce the strong associations among negative elements in an individual's cognitive system, thus affecting the amount of interference noted on tasks such as the primed Stroop task. Segal and Gemar (1997) found that patients who were less depressed at posttreatment following CBT showed less color-naming interference for self-descriptive negative information. This result supports the view that negative self-information is highly interconnected in the cognitive system of depressed patients, and suggests that possible changes to this organization may result from successful treatment of depression.

Remaining Issues

Research on depression has resulted in a range of measures addressing the content, process, and "deep structure" of cognition. It remains to be seen whether cognitive variables are markers of a vulnerability to depression. The clinician has many ways to assess cognitive changes during a depressive episode. Depending on particular theoretical concerns, measures of cognition may be taken prior to, during, and following treatment. Furthermore, normative data on several cognitive measures have been presented for adults (Dozois, Covin, & Brinker, 2003), as well as children and adolescents (Ingram, Nelson, Steidtmann, & Bistricky, 2007). These data should assist the evaluation of cognition, cognitive change, and treatment effectiveness.

On the other hand, it is not easy to determine which cognitive changes are uniquely influenced by cognitive-behavioral treatment. Any treatment (or "spontaneous remission") that alters the state of depression also results in substantial cognitive change. The extant evidence is mixed regarding whether cognitive changes are specific to cognitive therapy (see Garratt, Ingram, Rand, & Sawalani, 2007). There is some evidence, however, to suggest that cognitive therapy reduces cognitive reactivity to depressed mood more effectively than do pharmacological treatments (Segal, Gemar, & Williams, 1999; Segal et al., 2006). Because cognitive reactivity to depressed mood has been found to be associated with a higher probability of relapse (Segal et al., 1999, 2006), these results suggest that cognitive therapy might be more effective than pharmacotherapy at producing more substantive change in cognitive functioning (see Garratt et al., 2007).

FUTURE DIRECTIONS

The field of cognitive assessment is almost 30 years old, if dated from the seminal work of Kendall and Korgeski (1979). Many advances in both conception and methodology have occurred over the past three decades. Nonetheless, Clark (1997) has outlined a number of challenges that confront researchers and practitioners in the area of cognitive assessment, especially with respect to the assessment of cognitive products. What is evident is a strong trend toward diversification, which is a healthy development within cognitive assessment. Instead of stagnating behind rigid and narrow conceptualizations of what constitutes "acceptable" modes of assessment, cognitive clinical researchers provide a more enriched and vital armamentarium of assessment tools for the study of the relationship among cognition, emotion, and behavior.

We concur with Clark (1997) and also with those who recommend integration within cognitive assessment, and with other approaches. For example, Glass and Arnkoff (1997) lament the fact that so little research has examined relations among measures of cognitive structures, processes, and products. Furthermore, the links among traditional self-report questionnaires, like the DAS, and other approaches borrowed from cognitive psychology, such as the Stroop color–word test (e.g., Segal et al., 1995) need to be more carefully examined to assess further the convergent validity of the various cognitive assessment methods. A reliance on self-report methodologies is insufficient, especially when it is desirable to assess relatively automatic cognitive processes and schemas that are difficult to articulate verbally. Glass and Arnkoff (1997) have nonetheless outlined prescriptions for the improvement and development of self-statement inventories, and there is still much to learn about the products and processes of cognition from the judicious use of production methods, such as the thought-listing and think-aloud approaches. Thought sampling is a useful strategy, especially given its high ecological validity. Reviewers (e.g., Glass & Arnkoff, 1997; Segal & Dobson, 1992) have also pointed to the possible benefit of instrument standardization. Constructs, such as automatic thoughts, schemas, and dysfunctional beliefs and assumptions, are notoriously difficult to measure; standardization would at least ensure that the data from different studies could be integrated in the evaluation of any single construct.

Segal and Dobson (1992) noted the potential value of a typology of cognitions related to stress, particularly in the interpersonal and achievement domains given the ongoing research on the congruency between achievement or interpersonal stress and depression onset and predictors of relapse (Segal, Shaw, Vella, & Katz, 1992). It will also be useful to examine the links among personality constructs that have been posited as vulnerability factors for emotional disorders, especially in relation to matching life events. Further study of cognitive structures, processes, and products that are hypothesized to contribute to the onset, maintenance, and relapse of psychological disorders such as anxiety and depression are needed. For example, Beck (1983) proposed sociotropy and autonomy as two personality styles or modes as vulnerability markers for depression. Sociotropic individuals are excessively invested in interpersonal relationships, whereas autonomous individuals are excessively invested in autonomy and achievement.

Gotlib and Hammen (1992) called for researchers in the depression area to begin to integrate cognitive and interpersonal aspects. Segal and Dobson (1992) recommended expansion of assessment of cognitive representations of social relationships. Gotlib, Kurtzman, and Blehar (1997) proposed that researchers should examine the intersections of biological approaches to the study of depression. A number of investigations have recently demonstrated points of contact between cognitive and neurobiological perspectives with regard to anxiety disorders (e.g., Van den Heuvel et al., 2005) and depressive disorders (e.g., Booij & Van der Does, 2007). If acted on, these proposals will enrich the field of cognitive assessment.

REFERENCES

Abramson, K. Y., Seligman, M. E. P., & Teasdale, J. D. (1978). Learned helplessness in humans: Critique and reformulation. *Journal of Abnormal Psychology, 87,* 102–109.

Alloy, L. B., & Ahrens, A. H. (1987). Depression and pessimism for the future: Biased use of statistically relevant information in predictions for self versus others. *Journal of Personality and Social Psychology, 52,* 366–378.

Arnkoff, D. B., & Glass, C. R. (1982). Clinical cognitive constructs: Examination, evaluation, and elaboration. *Advances in cognitive behavioural research and therapy* (Vol. 1, pp. 1–34). New York: Academic Press.

Bagby, R. M., Atkinson, L., Dickens, S., & Gavin, D. (1990). Dimensional analysis of the Attributional Style Questionnaire: Attributions or outcomes and events. *Canadian Journal of Behavioral Science, 22,* 140–150.

Bagby, R. M., Rector, N. A., Bacchiochi, J. R., & McBride, C. (2004). The stability of the Response Styles Questionnaire Rumination scale in a sample of patients with major depression. *Cognitive Therapy and Research, 28,* 527–538.

Bar-Haim, Y., Lamy, D., Pergamin, L., Bakermans-Kranenburg, M. J., & van IJzendoorn, M. H. (2007). Threat-related attentional bias in anxious and nonanxious individuals: A meta-analytic study. *Psychological Bulletin, 133,* 1–24.

Barton, S., Morley, S., Bloxham, G., Kitson, C., & Platts, S. (2005). Sentence Completion Test for Depression (SCD): An idiographic measure of depressive thinking. *British Journal of Clinical Psychology, 44,* 29–46.

Beazley, M. B., Glass, C. R., Chambless, D. L., & Arnkoff, D. B. (2001). Cognitive self-statements in social phobia: A comparison across three types of social situations. *Cognitive Therapy and Research, 25,* 781–799.

Beck, A. T. (1967). *Depression: Clinical, experimental and therapeutic aspects.* New York: Harper & Row.

Beck, A. T. (1976). *Cognitive therapy and the emotional disorders.* New York: International Universities Press.

Beck, A. T. (1983). Cognitive therapy of depression: New perspectives. In P. J. Clayton & J. E. Barnett (Eds.), *Treatment of depression: Old controversies and new approaches* (pp. 265–290). New York: Raven Press.

Beck, A. T., Brown, G., Steer, R. A., Eidelson, J. L., & Riskind, J. H. (1987). Differentiating anxiety and depression: A test of the cognitive-content specificity hypothesis. *Journal of Abnormal Psychology, 96,* 179–183.

Beck, A. T., & Emery, G. (1985). *Anxiety disorders and phobias.* New York: Basic Books.

Beck, A. T., Rush, A. J., Shaw, B. F., & Emery, G. (1979). *Cognitive therapy of depression.* New York: Guilford Press.

Beck, A. T., Steer, R. A., Epstein, R. A., & Brown, G. (1990). Beck Self-Concept Test. *Psychological Assessment, 2,* 191–197.

Beck, A. T., Weissman, A., Lester, D., & Trexler, L. (1974). The measurement of pessimism: The Hopelessness Scale. *Journal of Consulting and Clinical Psychology, 42,* 861–865.

Beck, J. G., Coffey, S. F., Palyo, S. A., Gudmundsdottir, B., Miller, L. M., & Colder, C. (2004). Psychometric properties of the Posttraumatic Cognitions Inventory (PTCI): A replication with motor vehicle accident survivors. *Psychological Assessment, 16,* 289–298.

Beck, R., & Perkins, S. T. (2001). Cognitive content-specificity for anxiety and depression: A meta-analysis. *Cognitive Therapy and Research, 25,* 651–663.

Becker, C. B., Namour, N., Zayfert, C., & Hegel, M. T. (2001). Specificity of the Social Interaction Self-Statement Test in social phobia. *Cognitive Therapy and Research, 25,* 227–233.

Beevers, C. G., Keitner, G., Ryan, C., & Miller, I. W. (2003). Cognitive predictors of symptom return following depression treatment. *Journal of Abnormal Psychology, 112,* 488–496.

Beevers, C. G., Strong, D. R., Meyer, B., Pilkonis, P. A., & Miller, I. W. (2007). Efficiently assessing negative cognition in depression: An item response theory analysis of the Dysfunctional Attitude Scale. *Psychological Assessment, 19,* 199–209.

Blankstein, K. R., & Flett, G. L. (1990). Cognitive components of test anxiety: A comparison of assessment and scoring methods. *Journal of Social Behavior and Personality, 5,* 187–202.

Blankstein, K. R., Flett, G. L., Boase, P., & Toner, B. B. (1990). Thought listing and endorsement measures of self-referential thinking in test anxiety. *Anxiety Research, 2,* 103–111.

Blankstein, K. R., Toner, B. B., & Flett, G. L. (1989). Test anxiety and the contents of consciousness: Thought listing and endorsement measures. *Journal of Research in Personality, 23,* 269–286.

Blatt, S. J., & Zuroff, D. C. (2005). Empirical evaluation of the assumptions in identifying evidence based treatments in mental health. *Clinical Psychology Review, 25,* 459–486.

Bögels, S. M., & Mansell, W. (2004). Attention processes in the maintenance and treatment of social phobia: Hypervigilance, avoidance and self-focused attention. *Clinical Psychology Review, 24,* 827–856.

Booij, L., & Van der Does, A. J. W. (2007). Cognitive and serotonergic vulnerability to depression: Convergent findings. *Journal of Abnormal Psychology, 116,* 86–94.

Bouvard, M., Mollard, E., Cottraux, J., & Guerin, J. (1989). Etude preliminaire d' une liste de pensees obsedantes: Validation et analyse factorielle [A preliminary study of a list of obsessive thoughts: Validation and factor analysis]. *L'Encéphale, XV,* 351–354.

Brewin, C. R., & Furnham, A. (1986). Attributional versus preattributional variables in self-esteem and depression: A comparison and test of learned helplessness theory. *Journal of Personality and Social Psychology, 50,* 1013–1020.

Brown, G. K., Beck, A. T., Steer, R. A., & Grisham, J. R. (2000). Risk factors for suicide in psychiatric outpatients: A 20–year prospective study. *Journal of Consulting and Clinical Psychology, 68,* 371–377.

Buhr, K., & Dugas, M. J. (2002). The intolerance of uncertainty scale: Psychometric properties of the English version. *Behaviour Research and Therapy, 40,* 931–945.

Burns, G., Keortge, S. G., Formea, G. M., & Sternberger, L. G. (1996). Revision of the Padua Inventory of Obsessive Compulsive Disorder Symptoms: Distinctions between worry, obsessions and compulsions. *Behaviour Research and Therapy, 34,* 163–173.

Butler, G., & Mathews, A. (1983). Cognitive processes in anxiety. *Advances in Behaviour Research and Therapy, 5,* 51–62.

Cacioppo, J. T., von Hippel, W., & Ernst, J. M. (1997). Mapping cognitive structures and processes through verbal content: The thought listing technique. *Journal of Consulting and Clinical Psychology, 65,* 928–940.

Carleton, R. N., Sharpe, D., & Asmundson, G. J. G. (2007). Anxiety sensitivity and intolerance of uncertainty: Requisites of the fundamental fears? *Behaviour Research and Therapy, 45,* 2307–2316.

Cartwright-Hatton, S., & Wells, A. (1997). Beliefs about worry and intrusions: The Meta-Cognitions Questionnaire and its correlates. *Journal of Anxiety Disorders, 11,* 279–296.

Carver, C. G., & Scheier, M. F. (1982). Control therapy: A useful conceptual framework for personality–social, clinical, and health psychology. *Psychological Bulletin, 92,* 111–135.

Chamberlain, J., & Haaga, D. A. F. (1999). Convergent validity of cognitive assessment methods. *Behavior Modification, 23,* 294–315.

Chambless, D. L., Caputo, G. C., Bright, P., & Gallagher, R. (1984). Assessment of fear in agoraphobics: The body sensations questionnaire and the agoraphobic cognition questionnaire. *Journal of Consulting and Clinical Psychology, 52,* 1090–1097.

Clark, D. A. (1997). Twenty years of cognitive assessment: Current status and future directions. *Journal of Consulting and Clinical Psychology, 65,* 996–1000.

Clark, D. A. (1998). The validity of measures of cognition: A review of the literature. *Cognitive Therapy and Research, 12,* 1–20.

Clark, D. A., Purdon, C. L., & Wang, A. (2003). The Meta-Cognitive Beliefs Questionnaire: Development of a measure of obsessional beliefs. *Behaviour Research and Therapy, 41,* 655–669.

Clark, L. A., & Watson, D. (1991). Tripartite model of anxiety and depression: Psychometric evidence and taxonomic implications. *Journal of Abnormal Psychology, 100,* 316–336.

Craik, F. M., & Lockhart, R. S. (1972). Levels of processing: A framework for memory research. *Journal of Verbal Learning and Verbal Behaviour, 11,* 671–684.

Davey, G. C. L., Tallis, F., & Capuzzo, N. (1996). Beliefs about the consequences of worrying. *Cognitive Therapy and Research, 20,* 499–520.

Davison, G. C., Robins, C., & Johnston, M. K. (1983). Articulated thoughts during simulated situations: A paradigm for studying cognition in emotion and behaviour. *Cognitive Therapy and Research, 7,* 17–40.

Davison, G. C., Vogel, R. S., & Coffman, S. G. (1997). Think-aloud approaches to cognitive assessment and the articulated thoughts in simulated situations paradigm. *Journal of Consulting and Clinical Psychology, 65,* 950–958.

Dobson, K. S., & Breiter, H. J. (1983). Cognitive assessment of depression: Reliability and validity of three measures. *Journal of Abnormal Psychology, 92,* 107–109.

Dobson, K. S., & Shaw, B. F. (1986). Cognitive assessment with major depressive disorders. *Cognitive Therapy and Research, 10,* 13–29.

Dozois, D. J. A., Covin, R., & Brinker, J. K. (2003). Normative data on cognitive measures of depression. *Journal of Consulting and Clinical Psychology, 71,* 71–80.

Dozois, D. J. A., & Dobson, K. S. (2001a). Information processing and cognitive organization in unipolar depression: Specificity and comorbidity issues. *Journal of Abnormal Psychology, 110,* 236–246.

Dozois, D. J. A., & Dobson, K. S. (2001b). A longitudinal investigation of information processing and cognitive organization in clinical depression: Stability of schematic interconnectedness. *Journal of Consulting and Clinical Psychology, 69,* 914–925.

Dunkley, D. M., Blankstein, K. R., Masheb, R. M., & Grilo, C. M. (2006). Personal standards and evaluative concerns dimensions of "clinical" perfectionism: A reply to Shafran et al. (2002, 2003) and Hewitt et al. (2003). *Behaviour Research and Therapy, 44,* 63–84.

Dunkley, D. M., Zuroff, D. C., & Blankstein, K. R. (2003). Self-critical perfectionism and daily affect: Dispositional and situational influences on stress and coping. *Journal of Personality and Social Psychology, 84,* 234–252.

Exner, J. E. (1973). The self-focus sentence completion: A study of egocentricity. *Journal of Personality Assessment, 37,* 437–455.

Fenigstein, A., Scheier, M., & Buss, A. (1975). Public and private self-consciousness: Assessment and theory. *Journal of Consulting and Clinical Psychology, 37,* 522–577.

Feske, U., & De Beurs, E. (1997). The Panic Appraisal Inventory: Psychometric properties. *Behaviour Research and Therapy, 35,* 875–882.

Flett, G. L., Hewitt, P. L., Blankstein, K. R., & Gray, L. (1998). Psychological distress and the frequency of perfectionistic thinking. *Journal of Personality and Social Psychology, 75,* 1363–1381.

Flett, G. L., Hewitt, P. L., Whelan, T., & Martin, T. R. (2007). The Perfectionism Cognitions Inventory: Psychometric properties and associations with distress and deficits in cognitive self-management. *Journal of Rational-Emotive and Cognitive-Behavior Therapy, 25,* 255–277.

Foa, E. B., Ehlers, A., Clark, D. M., Tolin, D. F., & Orsillo, S. M. (1999). The Post-traumatic Cognitions Inventory (PTCI): Development and validation. *Psychological Assessment, 11,* 303–314.

Freeston, M. H., & Ladouceur, R. (1993). Appraisal of cognitive intrusions and response style: Replication and extension. *Behaviour Research and Therapy, 31,* 185–191.

Gardner, H. (1985). *The mind's new science: A history of the cognitive revolution.* New York: Basic Books.

Garratt, G., Ingram, R. E., Rand, K. L., & Sawalani, G. (2007). Cognitive processes in cognitive therapy: Evaluation of the mechanisms of change in the treatment of depression. *Clinical Psychological Science and Practice, 14,* 224–239.

Gemar, M. C., Segal, Z. V., Sagrati, S., & Kennedy, S. J. (2001). Mood-induced changes on the Implicit Association Test in recovered depressed patients. *Journal of Abnormal Psychology, 110,* 282–289.

Genest, M., & Turk, D. C. (1981). Think- aloud approaches to cognitive assessment. In T. V. Merluzzi, C. R. Glass, & M. Genest (Eds.), *Cognitive assessment* (pp. 233–269). New York: Guilford Press.

Ghiselli, E. E., Campbell, J. P., & Zedeck, S. (1981). *Measurement theory for the behavioural sciences.* San Francisco: Freeman.

Glass, C. R., & Arnkoff, D. B. (1982). Think cognitively: Selected issues in cognitive assessment and therapy. In P. C. Kendall (Ed.), *Advances in cognitive-behavioral research and therapy* (Vol. 1, pp. 35–71). New York: Academic Press.

Glass, C. R., & Arnkoff, D. B. (1997). Questionnaire methods of cognitive self-statement assessment. *Journal of Consulting and Clinical Psychology, 65,* 911–927.

Glass, C. R., Merluzzi, T. V., Biever, J. L., & Larsen, K. H. (1982). Cognitive assessment of social anxiety: Development and validation of a self-statement questionnaire. *Cognitive Therapy and Research, 6,* 37–55.

Goldfried, M. R., Padawer, W., & Robins, C. (1984). Social anxiety and the semantic structure of heterosocial interactions. *Journal of Abnormal Psychology, 93,* 86–97.

Goldston, D. B., Reboussin, B. A., & Daniel, S. S. (2006). Predictors of suicide attempts: State and trait components. *Journal of Abnormal Psychology, 115,* 842–849.

Gong-Guy, E., & Hammen, C. L. (1980). Causal perceptions of stressful events in depressed and nondepressed oupatients. *Journal of Abnormal Psychology, 89,* 662–669.

Gotlib, I. H., & Hammen, C. L. (1992). *Psychological aspects of depression: Toward a cognitive-interpersonal integration.* Chichester, UK: Wiley.

Gotlib, I. H., Kasch, K. L., Traill, S., Joormann, J., Arnow, B. A., & Johnson, S. L. (2004). Coherence and specificity of information-processing biases in depression and social phobia. *Journal of Abnormal Psychology, 113,* 386–398.

Gotlib, I. H., Krasnoperova, E., Yue, D., & Joormann, J. (2004). Attentional biases for negative interpersonal stimuli in clinical depression. *Journal of Abnormal Psychology, 113,* 127–135.

Gotlib, I. H., Kurtzman, H. S., & Blehar, M. C. (1997). The cognitive psychology of depression: Introduction to the special issue. *Cognition and Emotion, 5,* 497–675.

Gotlib, I . H., & McCann, C. D. (1984). Construct accessibility and depression: An examination of cognitive and affective factors. *Journal of Personality and Social Psychology, 47,* 427–439.

Greenwald, A. G., McGhee, D. E., & Schwartz, J. L. K. (1998). Measuring individual differences in implicit cognition: The Implicit Association Test. *Journal of Personality and Social Psychology, 74,* 1464–1480.

Gunthert, K. C., Cohen, L. H., Butler, A. C., & Beck, J. S. (2007). Depression and next-day spillover of negative mood and depressive cognitions following interpersonal stressors. *Cognitive Therapy and Research, 31,* 521–532.

Haaga, D. A. (1997). Introduction to the special section on measuring cognitive products in research and practice. *Journal of Consulting and Clinical Psychology, 65,* 907–919.

Hamilton, E. W., & Abramson, L. Y. (1983). Cognitive patterns and major depressive disorder: A longitudinal study in a hospital setting. *Journal of Abnormal Psychology, 92,* 173–184.

Hammen, C. L., & Krantz, S. E. (1976). Effects of success and failure on depressive cognitions. *Journal of Abnormal Psychology, 85,* 577–586.

Hofmann, S. G., Moscovitch, D. A., Kim, H., & Taylor, A. (2004). Changes in self-perception during treatment of social phobia. *Journal of Consulting and Clinical Psychology, 72,* 588–596.

Hollon, S. D., & Kendall, P. C. (1980). Cognitive self-statements in depression: Development of an automatic thoughts questionnaire. *Cognitive Therapy and Research, 4,* 383–396.

Hollon, S. D., Kendall, P. C., & Lumry, A. (1986). Specificity of depressotypic cognitions in clinical depression. *Journal of Abnormal Psychology, 95,* 52–59.

Hurlburt, R. T. (1997). Randomly sampling thinking in the natural environment. *Journal of Consulting and Clinical Psychology, 65,* 941–948.

Hurlburt, R. T., & Akhter, S. A. (2006). The descriptive experiences sampling method. *Phenomenology and the Cognitive Sciences, 5,* 271–301.

Imber, S. D., Pilkonis, P. A., Sotsky, S. M., Elkin, I., Watkins, J. T., Collins, J. F., et al. (1990). Mode-specific effects among three treatments for depression. *Journal of Consulting and Clinical Psychology, 58,* 352–359.

Ingram, R. E. (1990). Self-focused attention in clinical disorders: Review and a conceptual model. *Psychological Bulletin, 107,* 156–176.

Ingram, R. E., Lumry, A. B., Cruet, D., & Sieber, W. (1987). Attentional processes in depressive disorders. *Cognitive Therapy and Research, 11,* 351–360.

Ingram, R. E., Miranda, J., & Segal, Z. V. (1998). *Cognitive vulnerability to depression.* New York: Guilford Press.

Ingram, R. E., Kendall, P. C., Siegle, G., Guarino, J., & McLaughlin, S. C. (1995). Psychometric properties of the Positive Automatic Thoughts Questionnaire. *Psychological Assessment, 7,* 495–507.

Ingram, R. E., Nelson, T., Steidtmann, D. K., & Bistricky, S. L. (2007). Comparative data on child and adolescent cognitive measures associated with depression. *Journal of Consulting and Clinical Psychology, 75,* 390–403.

Ingram, R. E., & Wisnicki, K. S. (1988). Assessment of positive automatic cognition. *Journal of Consulting and Clinical Psychology, 56,* 898–902.

Jarrett, R. B., Vittengl, J. R., Doyle, K., & Clark, L. A. (2007). Changes in cognitive content during and following cognitive therapy for recurrent depression: Substantial and enduring, but not predictive of change in depressive symptoms. *Journal of Consulting and Clinical Psychology, 75,* 432–446.

Joormann, J., & Gotlib, I. H. (2007). Selective attention to emotional faces following recovery from depression. *Journal of Abnormal Psychology, 116,* 80–85.

Joormann, J., Talbot, L., & Gotlib, I. H. (2007). Biased processing of emotional information in girls at risk for depression. *Journal of Abnormal Psychology, 116,* 135–143.

Just, N., & Alloy, L. B. (1997). The response theory of depression: Test and an extension for the theory. *Journal of Abnormal Psychology, 106,* 221–229.

Kasch, K. L., Klein, D. N., & Lara, M. E. (2001). A construct validation study of the Response Styles Questionnaire Rumination scale in participants with a recent-onset major depressive episode. *Psychological Assessment, 13,* 375–383.

Kendall, P. C., & Hollon, S. D. (1981). Assessing self-referent speech: Methods in the measurement of self-statements. In P. C. Kendall & S. D. Hollon (Eds.), *Assessment strategies for cognitive-behavioural interventions* (pp. 85–118). New York: Academic Press.

Kendall, P. C., & Hollon, S. D. (1989). Anxious self-talk: Development of the Anxious Self- Statements Questionnaire (ASSQ). *Cognitive Therapy and Research, 13,* 81–93.

Kendall, P. C., & Korgeski, G. P. (1979). Assessment and cognitive-behavioural interventions. *Cognitive Therapy and Research, 3,* 1–21.

Khawaja, N. G., & Oei, T. P. S. (1998). Catastrophic cognitions in panic disorder with and without agoraphobia. *Clinical Psychology Review, 18,* 341–365.

Khawaja, N. G., Oei, T. P. S., & Baglioni, A. (1994). Modification of the Catastrophic Cognitions Questionnaire (CCQ-M) for normals and patients: Exploratory and LISREL analyses. *Journal of Psychopathology and Behavioral Assessment, 16,* 325–342.

Krantz, S., & Hammen, C. L. (1979). Assessment of cognitive bias in depression. *Journal of Abnormal Psychology, 88,* 611–619.

Kuiper, N. A., & MacDonald, M. R. (1983). Schematic processing in depression: The self-consensus bias. *Cognitive Therapy and Research, 7,* 469–484.

Kuiper, N. A., & Olinger, L. J. (1986). Dysfunctional attitudes and a self-worth contingency model of depression. In P. C. Kendall (Ed.), *Advances in cognitive-behavioural research and therapy* (Vol. 5, pp. 115–142). New York: Academic Press.

Last, C. G., Barlow, D. H., & O'Brien, G. (1985). Assessing cognitive aspects of anxiety: Stability over time and agreement between several methods. *Behavior Modification, 9,* 72–93.

Lim, S. L., & Kim, J. H. (2005). Cognitive processing of emotional information in depression, panic, and somatoform disorder. *Journal of Abnormal Psychology, 114,* 50–61.

MacDonald, M. R., & Kuiper, N. A. (1984). Self-schema decision consistency in clinical depressives. *Journal of Social and Clinical Psychology, 2,* 264–272.

MacLeod, C., Mathews, A., & Tata, P. (1986). Attentional bias in emotional disorders. *Journal of Abnormal Psychology, 95,* 15–20.

MacLeod, C., Rutherford, E., Campbell, L., Ebsworthy, G., & Holker, L. (2002). Selective attention and emotional vulnerability: Assessing the causal basis of their association through experimental manipulation of attentional bias. *Journal of Abnormal Psychology, 111,* 107–123.

MacLeod, A. K., Tata, P., Kentish, J., Carroll, F., & Hunter, E. (1997). Anxiety, depression and explanation-based pessimism for future positive and negative events. *Clinical Psychology and Psychotherapy, 4,* 15–24.

Mathews, A., & MacLeod, C. (1985). Selective processing of threat cues to anxiety states. *Behaviour Research and Therapy, 23,* 563–569.

Mathews, A., & MacLeod, C. (1994). Cognitive approaches to emotion and emotional disorders. *Annual Review of Psychology, 45,* 25–50.

McCarthy-Larzelere, M., Diefenbach, G. J., Williamson, D. A., Netemeyer, R. G., Bentz, B. G., & Manguno-Mire, G. M. (2001). Psychometric properties and factor structure of the Worry Domains Questionnaire. *Assessment, 8,* 177–191.

Metalsky, G. I., Halberstadt, L. J., & Abramson, L. Y. (1987). Vulnerability to depressive mood reactions: Toward a more powerful test of the diathesis–stress and causal mediation components of the reformulated theory of depression. *Journal of Personality and Social Psychology, 52,* 386–393.

Meyer, T. J., Miller, M. L., Metzger, R. L., & Borkovec, T. D. (1990). Development and validation of the Penn State Worry Questionnaire. *Behaviour Research and Therapy, 26,* 169–177.

Miranda, J., Persons, J. B., & Byers, C. N. (1990). Endorsement of dysfunctional beliefs depends on current mood state. *Journal of Abnormal Psychology, 99,* 237–241.

Mogg, K., & Bradley, B. P. (2005). Attentional bias in generalized anxiety disorder versus depressive disorder. *Cognitive Therapy and Research, 29,* 29–45.

Molina, S., Borkovec, T. D., Peasley, C., & Person, D. (1998). Content analysis of worrisome streams of consciousness in anxious and dysphoric participants. *Cognitive Therapy and Research, 22,* 109–123.

Mor, N., & Winquist, J. (2002). Self-focused attention and negative affect: A meta-analysis. *Psychological Bulletin, 128,* 638–662.

Mumma, G. (2004). Validation of idiosyncratic cognitive schema in cognitive case formulations: An intraindividual idiographic approach. *Psychological Assessment, 16,* 211–230.

Neisser, S. (1976). *Cognition and reality: Principles and implications of cognitive psychology.* San Francisco: Freeman.

Nelson, R. D., Hayes, S. C., Felton, J. L., & Jarrett, R. B. (1985). A comparison of data produced by different behavioural assessment technique with implications for models of social-skills inadequacy. *Behaviour Research and Therapy, 23,* 1–11.

Nolen-Hoeksema, S. (2000). The role of rumination in depressive disorders and mixed anxiety/depressive symptoms. *Journal of Abnormal Psychology, 109,* 504–511.

Nolen-Hoeksema, S., & Morrow, J. (1991). A prospective study of depression and posttraumatic stress symptoms after a natural disaster: The 1989 Loma Prieta earthquake. *Journal of Personality and Social Psychology, 61,* 115–121.

Obsessive Compulsive Cognitions Working Group. (2003). Psychometric validation of the Obsessive Belief Questionnaire and the Interpretation of Intrusion Inventory: Part I. *Behaviour Research and Therapy, 41,* 863–878.

Obsessive Compulsive Cognitions Working Group. (2005). Psychometric validation of the Obsessive Belief Questionnaire and Interpretation of Intrusion Inventory: Part I. Factor analyses and testing of a brief version. *Behaviour Research and Therapy, 43,* 1527–1542.

Oliver, J. M., & Baumgart, E. P. (1985). The Dysfunctional Attitude Scale: Psychometric properties and relation to depression in an unselected adult population. *Cognitive Therapy and Research, 9,* 161–168.

Otto, M. W., Teachman, B. A., Cohen, L. S., Soares, C. N., Vitonis, A. F., & Harlow, B. L. (2007). Dysfunctional attitudes and episodes of major depression: Predictive validity and temporal stability in never-depressed, depressed, and recovered women. *Journal of Abnormal Psychology, 116,* 475–483.

Peterson, C., Semmel, A., von Baeyer, C., Abramson, L., Metalsky, G., & Seligman, M. (1982). The Attributional Style Questionnaire. *Cognitive Therapy and Research, 6,* 287–299.

Peterson, C., & Villanova, P. (1988). An expanded Attributional Style Questionnaire. *Journal of Abnormal Psychology, 97,* 87–89.

Peterson, R. A., & Reiss, S. (1992). *Anxiety sensitivity index manual* (2nd ed.). Worthington, OH: International Diagnostic Systems.

Purdon, C., & Clark, D. A. (1994). Perceived control and appraisal of obsessional and intrusive thoughts: Replication and extension. *Behavioural and Cognitive Psychotherapy, 22,* 269–285.

Reiss, S. (1991). Expectancy theory of fear, anxiety, and panic. *Clinical Psychology Review, 11,* 141–153.

Ronan, K., Kendall, P. C., & Rowe, M. (1994). Negative affectivity in children: Development and validation of a self-statement questionnaire. *Cognitive Therapy and Research, 18,* 509–528.

Rudy, T. E., Merluzzi, T., & Henahan, P. (1982). Construal of complex assertive situations: A multidimensional analysis. *Journal of Consulting and Clinical Psychology, 50,* 125–137.

Rush, A. J. (1984, March). *Measurement of the cognitive aspects of depression.* Paper presented at the NIMH Workshop on Measurement of Depression, Honolulu, HI.

Scher, C. D., Ingram, R. E., & Segal, Z. V. (2005). Cognitive reactivity and vulnerability: Empirical evaluation of construct activation and cognitive diatheses in unipolar depression. *Clinical Psychology Review, 25,* 487–510.

Schultz, L. T., Heimberg, R. G., Rodebaugh, T. L., Schneier, F. R., Liebowitz, M. R., & Telch, M. J. (2006). The Appraisal of Social Concerns Scale: Psychometric validation with a clinical sample of patients with social anxiety disorder. *Behavior Therapy, 37,* 392–405.

Schwartz, R. M. (1997). Consider the simple screw: Cognitive science, quality improvement, and psychotherapy. *Journal of Consulting and Clinical Psychology, 65,* 970–983.

Segal, Z. (1988). Appraisals of the self-schema construct in cognitive models of depression. *Psychological Bulletin, 103,* 147–162.

Segal, Z. V., & Cloitre, M. (1993). Methodologies for studying cognitive features of emotional disorder. In K. S. Dobson & P. C. Kendall (Eds.), *Psychopathology and cognition* (pp. 19–50). San Diego: Academic Press.

Segal, Z. V., & Dobson, K. S. (1992). Cognitive models of depression: Report from a consensus conference. *Psychological Inquiry, 3,* 219–224.

Segal, Z. V., & Gemar, M. (1997). Changes in cognitive organization for negative self-referent material following cognitive behavior therapy for depression: A primed Stroop study. *Cognition and Emotion, 11,* 501–516.

Segal, Z. V., Gemar, M., Truchan, C., Gurguis, M., & Hurowitz, L. M. (1995). A priming methodology for studying self-representation in major depressive disorder. *Journal of Abnormal Psychology, 104,* 205–213.

Segal, Z. V., Gemar, M., & Williams, S. (1999). Differential cognitive response to a mood challenge following successful cognitive therapy or pharmacotherapy for unipolar depression. *Journal of Abnormal Psychology, 108,* 3–10.

Segal, Z. V., & Ingram, R. E. (1994). Mood priming and construct activation in tests of cognitive vulnerability to unipolar depression. *Clinical Psychology Review, 14,* 663–695.

Segal, Z. V., Kennedy, S., Gemar, M., Hood, K., Pederson, R., & Buis, T. (2006). Cognitive reactivity to sad mood provocation and the prediction of depressive relapse. *Archives of General Psychiatry, 63,* 749–755.

Segal, Z. V., Shaw, B. F., Vella, D. D., & Katz, R. (1992). Cognitive and life stress predictors of relapse in remitted unipolar depressed patients: Test of the congruency hypothesis. *Journal of Abnormal Psychology, 101,* 26–36.

Segal, Z. V., & Swallow, S. R. (1994). Cognitive assessment of unipolar depression: Measuring products, processes and structures. *Behaviour Research and Therapy, 32,* 147–158.

Startup, H. M., & Erickson, T. M. (2006). The Penn State Worry Questionnaire. In G. C. L. Davey & A. Wells (Eds.), *Worry and its psychological disorders: Theory, assessment, and treatment* (pp. 101–119). Hoboken, NJ: Wiley.

Szabo, M., & Lovibond, P. F. (2002). The cognitive content of naturally occurring worry episodes. *Cognitive Therapy and Research, 26,* 167–177.

Tallis, F., Eysenck, M., & Mathews, A. M. (1992). A questionnaire for the measurement of nonpathological worry. *Personality and Individual Differences, 13,* 161–168.

Taylor, S. (1999). *Anxiety sensitivity: Theory, research, and treatment of the fear of anxiety.* Mahwah, NJ: Erlbaum.

Taylor, S., Zvolensky, M. J., Cox, B. J., Deacon, B., Heimberg, R. G., Ledley, D. R., et al. (2007). Robust dimensions of anxiety sensitivity: Development and initial validation of the Anxiety Sensitivity Index–3. *Psychological Assessment, 19,* 176–188.

Telch, M. J., Brouillard, M., Telch, C. F., Agras, W. S., & Taylor, C. B. (1987). Role of cognitive appraisal in panic-related avoidance. *Behaviour Research and Therapy, 27,* 373–383.

Telch, M. J., Lucas, R. A., Smits, J. A. J., Powers, M. B., Heimberg, R., & Hart, T. (2004). Appraisal of social concerns: A cognitive assessment instrument for social phobia. *Depression and Anxiety, 19,* 217–224.

Timbremont, B., & Braet, C. (2004). Cognitive vulnerability in remitted depressed children and adolescents. *Behaviour Research and Therapy, 42,* 423–437.

Turner, S. M., Johnson, M. R., Beidel, D. C., Heiser, N. A., & Lydiard, R. B. (2003). The Social Thoughts and Beliefs Scale: A new inventory for assessing cognitions in social phobia. *Psychological Assessment, 15,* 384–391.

Van den Heuvel, O. A., Veltman, D. J., Groenewegen, H. J., Witter, M. P., Merkelbach, J., Cath, D. C., et al. (2005). Disorder-specific neuroanatomical correlates of attentional bias in obsessive–compulsive disorder, panic disorder, and hypochondriasis. *Archives of General Psychiatry, 62,* 922–933.

Verkuil, B., Brosschot, J. F., & Thayer, J. F. (2007). Capturing worry in daily life: Are trait questionnaires sufficient? *Behaviour Research and Therapy, 45,* 1835–1844.

Watkins, J., & Rush, A. J. (1983). The Cognitive Response Test. *Cognitive Therapy and Research, 7,* 425–436.

Watson, D., & Friend, R. (1969). Measurement of social-evaluative anxiety. *Journal of Consulting and Clinical Psychology, 33,* 448–457.

Webb, E. J., Campbell, D. T., Schwartz, R. D., & Sechrest, L. (1966). *Unobtrusive measures: Non-reactive research in the social sciences.* Chicago: Rand McNally.

Weissman, A. N. (1979). *The Dysfunctional Attitude Scale: A validation study.* Unpublished dissertation, University of Pennsylvania, Philadelphia.

Weissman, A. N., & Beck, A. T. (1978). *Development and validation of the Dysfunctional Attitude Scale: A preliminary investigation.* Paper presented at the 86th annual meeting of the American Educational Research Association, Toronto, Canada.

Wells, A. (1994). A multidimensional measure of worry: Development and preliminary validation of the Anxious Thoughts Inventory. *Anxiety, Stress and Coping, 6,* 289–299.

Wells, A. (2006). The Anxious Thoughts Inventory and related measures of metacognition and worry. In G. C. L. Davey & A. Wells (Eds.), *Worry and its psychological disorders: Theory, assessment, and treatment* (pp. 121–136). Hoboken, NJ: Wiley.

Wells, A., & Cartwright-Hatton, S. (2004). A short form of the Metacognitions Questionnaire: Properties of the MCQ-30. *Behaviour Research and Therapy, 42,* 385–396.

Wenzel, A., Sharp, I., Brown, G., Greenberg, R., & Beck, A. T. (2006). Dysfunctional beliefs in panic disorder: The Panic Belief Inventory. *Behaviour Research and Therapy, 44,* 819–833.

Westling, B. E., & Ost, L.-B. (1993). Relationship between panic attack symptoms and cognitions in panic disorder patients. *Journal of Anxiety Disorders, 7,* 181–194.

Williams, J. M. G., Watts, F., MacLeod, C., & Mathews, A. (1998). *Cognitive psychology and emotional disorders.* Chichester, UK: Wiley.

Williams, S. L. (1985). On the nature and measurement of agoraphobia. In M. Hersen, R. M. Eisler, & P. M. Miller (Eds.), *Progress in behaviour modification* (Vol. 19, pp. 109–144). New York: Academic Press.

Williams, S. L., & Rappoport, A. (1983). Cognitive treatment in the natural environment for agoraphobics. *Behavior Therapy, 14,* 299–313.

Woody, S. R., Taylor, S., McLean, P. D., & Koch, W. (1998). Cognitive specificity in panic and depression: Implications for comorbidity. *Cognitive Therapy and Research, 22,* 427–443.

Zuroff, D. C., Blatt, S. J., Sanislow, C. A., Bondi, C. M., & Pilkonis, P. A. (1999). Vulnerability to depression: Reexamining state dependence and relative stability. *Journal of Abnormal Psychology, 108,* 76–89.

CHAPTER 6

Cognitive-Behavioral
Case Formulation

Jacqueline B. Persons
Joan Davidson

Hazel came to her therapy session feeling depressed and discouraged. She had failed to follow through with her plan to visit her cousin Rose on Sunday. In the previous session her therapist had worked with her on a Thought Record that focused on the upcoming visit and elicited these thoughts about the trip: "I feel too depressed, I have no energy," I can't make the visit when I feel like this," and "I'll do it later when I feel better." The therapist's formulation was that Hazel had a schema of herself as weak, fragile, and helpless, and that this belief was the root of many of her symptoms of depression, especially her passivity and behavioral inactivity. The therapist had worked collaboratively with Hazel to develop this formulation, and had shown Hazel how that view of herself produced the thoughts she had in the situation involving the trip to visit her cousin. Guided by this formulation, Hazel and her therapist had worked to develop some responses to Hazel' s automatic thoughts using the anti-do-nothingism intervention that Dr. Burns describes in *Feeling Good* (Burns, 1999). These were responses like, "I can do this even though I feel lousy," "I'll feel better after I do it," and "I can't wait until I feel better; I need to take action first."

However, this line of intervention failed. Hazel came to the next session feeling more depressed than before (her Beck Depression Inventory [BDI] score was 6 points higher) and reporting that she had not been able to push herself to make the visit. This setback led Hazel's therapist to take another look at her conceptualization of the situation involving the trip. The therapist collected more assessment data to get a clearer picture of what was going on and with some probing, elicited from Hazel some feelings and thoughts about the trip that the therapist previously had not known about. Hazel felt resentful and guilty about the trip, and had the thoughts, "I don't want to visit her, but Rose is ill and really needs me, so I should go" and "If I don't make this trip, I'm a bad cousin." This information suggested that in addition to self-schemas of being weak and helpless, Hazel also held what Young, Klosko, and Weishaar (2003) call the "subjugation" schema, that is, the view that she is unimportant, and that her role in life is to meet others' needs.

Guided by this new formulation hypothesis, Hazel and the therapist agreed to shift their tack. Instead of working to help Hazel overcome her do-nothing thoughts and push ahead to make the trip, the therapist worked to help Hazel identify and overcome her subjugation beliefs and guilt, pay better attention to her needs, and speak up assertively to let her cousin know that she would not be able to visit but would check in by phone. This intervention was successful. Hazel was able to call her cousin and cancel her visit. She came to her next session feeling less depressed and more energized than she had in some time.

This vignette illustrates the role of the cognitive-behavioral (CB) formulation in treatment. The formulation is a hypothesis about the factors that cause and maintain the patient's problems, and it guides assessment and intervention.

This chapter begins with a description of the hypothesis-testing approach to clinical work, of which the case formulation is a part. We discuss the role of the case formulation in treatment and review evidence that the formulation contributes to the effectiveness of treatment. We also describe the elements of the CB case formulation and present a case to illustrate the process of developing a formulation and using it to guide treatment.

We describe our own approach to CB case formulation (see also Persons (2008). Others include functional analysis (Haynes & O'Brien, 2000) and the methods described by Judy Beck (1995) and others (Koerner, 2006; Kuyken, Padesky, & Dudley, 2009; Nezu, Nezu, & Lombardo, 2004; Tarrier, 2006).

CASE FORMULATION AS PART
OF A HYPOTHESIS-TESTING MODE OF CLINICAL WORK

The case formulation is an element of a hypothesis-testing empirical mode of clinical work that is described in Figure 6.1. The therapist begins the process by carrying out an assessment to collect information that is used to develop an initial formulation of the case. The case formulation is a hypothesis about the psychological mechanisms and other factors that cause and maintain a par-

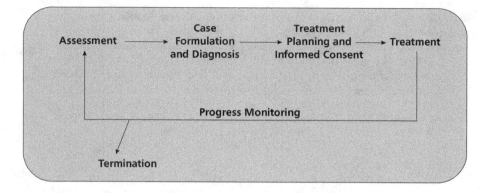

FIGURE 6.1. Case formulation-driven cognitive-behavioral therapy. Shading indicates the therapeutic relationship.

ticular patient's disorders and problems. The formulation is used to develop a treatment plan and to assist in obtaining the patient's informed consent to it. After obtaining informed consent, the therapist moves forward with treatment. At every step in the treatment process, as the backward arrow in Figure 6.1 indicates, the therapist returns repeatedly to the assessment phase; that is, the therapist collects data to monitor the process and progress of the therapy and uses those data to test the hypotheses (formulations) that underpin the intervention plan and to revise them as needed.

Thus, the four elements of case formulation-driven cognitive-behavioral therapy (CBT) are (1) assessment to obtain a diagnosis and case formulation; (2) treatment planning and obtaining the patient's informed consent to the treatment plan; (3) treatment; and (4) continuous monitoring and hypothesis-testing. We discuss each element in turn.

Assessment to Obtain a Diagnosis and Initial Case Formulation

Before treatment begins, the therapist collects assessment data to develop a diagnosis and an initial case formulation. To get this information, the therapist uses interviews, self-report data from the patient, and other sources, including reports from family members and other clinicians.

Many clinicians are reluctant to conduct a diagnostic assessment. They do not want to impede the patient from "telling his or her story"; they fear that the patient will have a negative reaction, or they argue that diagnostic classification and CB theories and therapies are difficult to reconcile conceptually (Follette, 1996). Despite the validity of these concerns, diagnosis yields information that is helpful—if not essential—in treatment. For example, the distinction between unipolar and bipolar mood disorders has important implications for both psychotherapy and pharmacotherapy. Furthermore, the psychopathology, epidemiology, and treatment efficacy literatures are organized by diagnosis, and the effective clinician draws on these literatures. In fact, one of the main methods to develop a case conceptualization and treatment plan is for the therapist to rely on evidence-based formulations and treatment protocols, which usually target disorders. Diagnosis can provide the therapist with some immediate formulation hypotheses. For example, a diagnosis of panic disorder suggests the formulation that panic symptoms result from catastrophic interpretations of benign somatic sensations (Clark, 1986).

A case formulation is important, because interventions flow from it, as Hazel's case at the beginning of this chapter illustrates. The formulation also provides a way to tie all of the patient's symptoms and problems into a coherent whole. As described later in more detail, a complete case formulation describes all of the patient's symptoms, disorders, and problems, and proposes hypotheses about the mechanisms causing the disorders and problems, the precipitants of the disorders and problems, and the origins of the mechanisms.

Whenever possible, the case formulation is based on an empirically supported "nomothetic," or general formulation. The therapist's task is to translate from nomothetic knowledge to idiographic practice, where an "idiographic" formulation and treatment plan describe the causes of symptoms or disorders and the plan for treating them in a particular individual. Hazel, the patient described in the vignette at the beginning of the chapter, met criteria for major depressive disorder; therefore, her therapist based the formulation of her case on Beck's cognitive model of depression (Beck, Rush, Shaw, & Emery, 1979), because it offers an evidence-based formulation and treatment for depression. Hazel's therapist individualized Beck's nomothetic formulation by proposing schema hypotheses that were unique to Hazel's case, and that accounted for her particular symptoms and problems.

Treatment Planning and Obtaining Informed Consent for Treatment

The treatment plan follows from the case formulation. In case formulation–driven CBT, the heart of the treatment plan is not the interventions, but what we call the "mechanism change goals of treatment." These are changes in the psychological mechanisms that the treatment is designed to achieve, and they are based directly on the mechanism hypotheses of the case formulation. So, for example, the formulation that depressive symptoms result from a dearth of positive reinforcement leads to a treatment plan in which the therapist proposes to treat the patient's symptoms by increasing the amount of positive reinforcement the individual receives (Lewinsohn & Gotlib, 1995).

Before beginning treatment, the therapist obtains the patient's informed consent to proceed with the proposed treatment. During the consent process, the therapist develops a diagnosis and formulation of the patient's condition and provides this information to the patient; describes available treatment options; recommends a treatment, describes it, and provides a rationale for the recommendation; and obtains the patient's agreement to proceed with the recommended treatment plan or a compromise treatment plan. Informed consent is particularly important in case formulation–driven CBT, because the therapist often adapts the empirically supported treatment (EST) to meet the unique needs of the patient at hand or even develops an experimental treatment when no EST is available.

Treatment

Therapists who use a case formulation–driven approach to treatment do not rely on a protocol. Instead, they rely on the formulation as a guide to the treatment and select appropriate interventions from the protocol tied to the formulation (e. g., in Hazel's case, from (Beck et al., 1979), from other evidence-based protocols for the patient's disorder and for other disorders, and from the therapist's and patient's experience of what has been helpful in the past. Treatment in case formulation–driven CBT follows a sort of technical eclecticism, where the unifying coherence is provided by the formulation of the case.

Monitoring and Hypothesis Testing

As treatment proceeds, patient and therapist collect data at every therapy session to test the formulation and monitor the process and outcome of therapy. These data allow patient and therapist to answer questions such as the following: Are the symptoms remitting? Are the mechanisms changing as expected? Do the mechanisms (e.g., cognitive distortions) and symptoms (e.g., hopelessness) relate to each other as expected? Does the patient accept and adhere to the interventions and recommendations? Do any problems in the therapeutic relationship interfere with treatment? If the process or outcome of therapy is poor, then the therapist works with the patient to collect more data and to determine what is interfering with progress, and whether a different formulation might lead to a different intervention plan that produces better results.

It is important to monitor progress at every session. Monitoring helps the patient and the therapist determine when the patient has achieved his or her goals and is ready to terminate treatment. When monitoring indicates that treatment is failing, monitoring can identify the failure and alert patient and therapist to the need to initiate a problem-solving process in an attempt to turn the therapy around. Useful monitoring tools appear in Antony, Orsillo, and Roemer (2001), Fischer and Corcoran (2007), and Nezu, Ronan, Meadows, and McClure (2000). Colleagues Kelly Koerner, Cannon Thomas, Janie Hong and Jacqueline Persons have developed some software tools for this purpose; information about them is posted at *www.practiceground.org.*

USING THE FORMULATION IN TREATMENT

Levels of Formulation and Intervention

Formulations are developed at three levels of analysis, and formulations at the various levels guide different aspects of treatment. The three levels are symptom, disorder, and case. These three levels are nested. A "disorder" comprises a set of symptoms, and a "case" comprises one or more disorders and problems. As a result, a case-level formulation generally consists of an extrapolation or extension of one or more disorder- and symptom-level formulations.

The case-level formulation guides the process of treatment planning, especially the process of setting goals and making decisions about which problems to tackle first; it also often frequently guides agenda setting in the therapy session and selection of treatment targets. Most intervention happens at the level of the symptom and is guided by a symptom-level formulation. However, the interventions used to treat a symptom do not just depend on the symptom-level formulation. For example, Hazel's therapist's symptom-level formulation (behavioral passivity) was informed by schema hypotheses drawn from the formulations at the level of the disorder, in this case, the schema hypotheses that are central to Beck's formulation of depression. That is, the original formulation of Hazel's core schema as "I'm helpless" guided the therapist to address Hazel's passivity by targeting these thoughts. The schema hypothesis "I'm unimportant; my role is to care for others" helped the therapist treat Hazel's passivity by targeting her failure to identify and validate her own wishes and to speak up assertively to get them met.

Ways the Formulation Helps in Treatment

The formulation helps treatment in many ways. A key role of the formulation is to guide intervention. As the case of Hazel illustrates, different formulations of a problem lead to different interventions. The formulation can also strengthen the alliance and help the patient adhere to the treatment plan, even if it entails a fair amount of distress and hard work, as CBT often does. The case of Steve, described later in this chapter, illustrates the way the therapist's sharing of the formulation enables Steve to play an active, leadership role in his treatment. A detailed discussion of how the formulation helps the therapist overcome failure, with a case example, is provided in (Persons & Mikami, 2002).

Treatment Utility of the Cognitive-Behavioral Case Formulation

CB therapists adopt a functional view of the case formulation. The key question of interest to the CBT therapist is not "Is the formulation accurate?" or "Does the formulation account for every piece of information I have about the patient?" but "Does the formulation add to the effectiveness of treatment?"

The function of the CB formulation is to guide intervention in a way that improves outcome (Hayes, Nelson, & Jarrett, 1987).

A small literature addresses the question of whether use of a formulation leads to better treatment outcome. A handful of randomized trials that compare the outcomes of case formulation–driven and standardized CBT show that formulation-driven treatment produces outcomes that are equal to (Jacobson et al., 1989; Schulte, Kunzel, Pepping, & Schulte-Bahrenberg, 1992) or a bit better than standardized treatment (Schneider & Byrne, 1987). Uncontrolled trials show that treatment of depressed (Persons, Bostrom, & Bertagnolli, 1999; Persons, Burns, & Perloff, 1988) and depressed anxious patients (Persons, Roberts, Zalecki, & Brechwald, 2006) guided by a CB case formulation and weekly progress monitoring has outcomes similar to those of patients receiving CBT or CBT plus pharmacotherapy in the randomized controlled trials. Another uncontrolled trial (Ghaderi, 2006) showed that patients with bulimia nervosa who received individualized treatment guided by a functional analysis had better outcomes than patients who received standardized treatment on some (abstinence from bulimic episodes, eating concerns, and body shape dissatisfaction) but not other (self-esteem, perceived social support from friends, and depression) outcome measures. Reviews by Nelson-Gray (2003) and Haynes, Leisen, and Blaine (1997) have reported that functional analysis has good treatment utility in individuals with severe behavioral problems, such as self-injurious behavior. Overall, the treatment utility of case formulation, especially for the types of outpatients seen in routine clinical practice, has rarely been studied. Thus, the strongest empirical support for the treatment utility of a CB case formulation currently comes from the method's reliance on evidence-based nomothetic formulations that are used as templates for the idiographic case formulation, and from the idiographic data that the therapist collects to monitor each patient's progress.

THE ELEMENTS OF THE CASE-LEVEL FORMULATION

The case formulation describes all of the patient's disorders and problems, and proposes hypotheses about the mechanisms causing the disorders and problems, the precipitants of the disorders and problems, and the origins of the mechanisms, and ties all the elements together into a coherent whole.

Disorders and Problems

The case formulation accounts for all of the disorders and problems a patient is experiencing. To obtain a comprehensive problem list, the therapist assesses the following domains: psychiatric symptoms, interpersonal, occupational, school, medical, financial, housing, legal, leisure, and difficulties with mental health or medical treatment. A comprehensive list is critical for three reasons.

First, the importance of any symptom, problem, or diagnosis depends on the patient's other problems and diagnoses. For example, a symptom of derealization has different implications for a person with panic disorder than for a person who abuses substances or has a dissociative disorder. To understand the case fully, the therapist must know all of the problems. Second, the therapist who simply focuses on the obvious problems or those on which the patient wishes to focus may miss important problems. Patients frequently wish to ignore problems such as substance abuse, self-harming behaviors, or others that can interfere with the successful treatment of the problems on which the patient *does* want to focus. Third, a comprehensive problem list often reveals common elements or themes that cut across problems. Awareness of these themes can help to generate initial mechanism hypotheses.

The problem list overlaps considerably with Axes I, II, III, and IV of a DSM diagnosis. However, in the Problem List the therapist begins to translate diagnostic information into terms that facilitate conceptualization and intervention from a CB point of view. One way that the Problem List facilitates CB treatment planning is by giving higher priority to problems in functioning than does the DSM, which places those problems down the list on Axis IV. Also, the Problem List details the symptoms of the particular Axis I and II psychiatric disorders the patient is experiencing, and symptoms can often be described in terms of the cognitions and behaviors that are the currency of CBT.

Mechanisms

The heart of the case-level formulation is a description of psychological mechanisms that cause and maintain the patient's problems and symptoms. The formulation might also include biological mechanisms (e.g., low thyroid can contribute to depressive symptoms), but we focus here on primarily psychological mechanisms.

To develop a mechanism hypothesis, the therapist can, as already discussed, rely on a nomothetic disorder formulation that underpins an EST, such as the formulation of obsessive–compulsive disorder that underpins exposure and response prevention (ERP) or the formulation of depression that underpins behavioral activation therapy (BA; Martell, Addis, & Jacobson, 2001). A second strategy is to base the case formulation on a more general psychological theory (e.g., the theory of operant conditioning). The case example presented later in this chapter uses both strategies.

Precipitants

The CB formulation is typically a "diathesis–stress" hypothesis; that is, it describes how vulnerability factors or mechanisms ("diatheses") interact with "stressors" to cause and/or maintain symptoms and problems. Stressors can be external events (e.g., death of a parent) or internal factors (e.g., an endocrine disorder). Thus, many CB formulations are biopsychosocial formulations and include a description of the events that triggered the mechanisms to produce the symptoms and problems.

Origins of the Mechanisms

It is useful to develop a hypothesis about how the patient acquired the mechanisms that cause the problems. An understanding of the likely origins of the problems in the patient's history lends the formulation internal coherence and can also encourage the use of interventions that target symptoms that are tied to early learning events (Padesky, 1994; Young, 1999).

Tying All the Elements Together

The case formulation describes what origins led to the development of what mechanisms, which, activated by specific precipitants, cause the patient's symptoms, disorders, and problems, and links all of these elements together into a coherent whole. It identifies treatment targets and the relationships among them that therapy will attempt to change. The elements of the case formulation for Hazel are identified with CAPITAL LETTERS.

As a result of being the oldest female in a large family, in which her mother was overwhelmed and expected Hazel to play a major caretaking role for her siblings (ORIGINS), Hazel learned the schemas "I'm unimportant," "Others are more important," and "My role in life is to meet the needs of others" (MECHANISMS). These schemas were activated by her husband's illness and his need for a great deal of care from Hazel (PRECIPITANT). As a result of exhausting herself to care for him, Hazel began experiencing symptoms of depression (PROBLEM) and became socially isolated (PROBLEM), which exacerbated her depression. She also experienced worsening of chronic hypertension and diabetes (PROBLEMS), because her excessive attention to her husband's needs prevented her from attending to her own medical needs.

DEVELOPING A FORMULATION FOR "STEVE" AND USING IT TO GUIDE HIS TREATMENT

The case of "Steve," who was treated by the second author (J. D.),[1] illustrates the processes of development and use of a case formulation to guide treatment.

---

[1] "Steve" gave permission for his case to be presented here. Identifying information was changed to protect his privacy.

Assessment to Develop a Diagnosis and Initial Case Formulation

Steve called to request a consultation appointment, stating that although he was managing well now, he had found CBT to be quite helpful to treat his depression in the past and wanted "a tune-up." As the therapist spoke with Steve on the telephone to evaluate whether a consultation was appropriate, she also listened for information pertaining to elements of the case-level formulation (origins, mechanisms, precipitants, problems) and other important aspects of Steve's status and history. Steve told the therapist that he had been in treatment for depression for 16 years and hospitalized twice. His most recent treatment had been about 5 years earlier. He had recently adopted a child (a possible precipitant). Steve was pleasant and engaging, and he sounded like a good candidate for CBT. His request for "booster" sessions sounded quite reasonable. However, Steve's brief account of his psychiatric history raised a red flag. His long-term treatment for depression and two hospitalizations indicated a severe level of past psychopathology that seemed discrepant with how cheerful and lighthearted he sounded on the phone.

The therapist offered to meet with Steve for one or more consultation sessions in which she would assess Steve's problems and symptoms, and offer her recommendations. Steve would evaluate whether the therapist's assessment findings and treatment recommendations made sense to him, and if individual CBT was indicated, Steve and the therapist would evaluate whether they were a good match to work together. Steve gave permission for the therapist to send him a packet of questionnaires to complete and bring to the initial consultation session. The intake packet comprised the revised Symptom Checklist–90 (SCL-90R; Derogatis, 2000), the BDI (Beck et al., 1979), the Burns Anxiety Inventory (Burns, 1997), the Functioning and Satisfaction Inventory (FSI; Davidson, Martinez, & Thomas, 2006), and an Adult Intake Questionnaire (reprinted in Persons, 2008) that asked questions about previous and concurrent treatment, substance use, trauma, family and social history, and legal and other potential problems. The intake packet also included a Treatment and Evaluation Agreement that outlined the limits of confidentiality, the therapist's business policies, and other information needed for informed consent. The therapist asked Steve to review the document and, if he was comfortable with it, to sign it and bring it to the first consultation session, or to raise any concerns and questions at the beginning of the initial meeting.

The primary goals in the initial interview were to work collaboratively with Steve to begin to develop a Problem List, some diagnostic hypotheses and initial formulation hypotheses, and a treatment plan. It was also important to begin to develop a good working alliance. The telephone conversation provided the start of a tentative Problem List (symptoms of depression) and a possible precipitant (recent adoption of a child).

When Steve arrived, the therapist asked his permission to take the first 5 minutes of the session to review the intake packet materials before starting the interview. The initial demographic piece of the Adult Intake Questionnaire revealed that Steve was a gay man in his early 30s who worked as a senior project manager for a high-tech firm and lived with his partner and the child they had recently adopted.

Steve's BDI score was 21, which indicated a moderate level of depression. Symptoms included sadness, discouragement about the future, feeling like a failure, self-criticism, self-blame, lack of enjoyment, loss of interest in people, difficulty making decisions, difficulty getting started doing things, and fatigue. He reported suicidal thoughts but no suicidal intent or plan. Steve scored 12 on the Burns Anxiety Inventory, which indicated mild anxiety. Symptoms included anxious feelings, difficulty concentrating and racing thoughts, as well as tight, tense muscles, and feeling tired, weak, or easily exhausted. He denied worry, however. He endorsed SCL-90R items that were consistent with the other inventories. He gave the highest possible score to only one SCL-90R item: "Feeling that something bad is going to happen to you."

On the FSI (Davidson et al., 2006), Steve reported that he functioned "very well" at work and "somewhat well" in relationships with relatives and friends. He maintained good health care behaviors. Although he was happy with his standard of living, he was "very dissatisfied" with his home/neighborhood/community, and the therapist made a note to collect more information about this. Steve reported that he was functioning "a little poorly" in his relationship with his partner, although he felt very satisfied with the relationship.

The Adult Intake Questionnaire also provided information about Steve's symptoms and problems, and some history. Steve reported that he drank one alcoholic drink per week. He denied using recreational drugs and having current or serious past medical problems. Steve had been married to his high school girlfriend for 1 year before divorcing 15 years earlier. He had come out as a gay man 12 years earlier and for 5 years had lived with his male domestic partner. Steve denied a history of trauma or abuse. He reported that he had had two previous inpatient stays and had taken an antidepressant medication for the previous 5 years, and that it was helpful.

As the therapist moved into the interview, she found that Steve again presented as bright, articulate, and interpersonally skilled, and as warm, genuine, and psychologically minded. Steve described again his wish to get CBT to help him tune up how he managed some stressors. These stressors included the need to move to a new home within a good school district, as their child was reaching school age, and the fact that his partner had been recently diagnosed with cancer that was not immediately life threatening but that did require further testing and treatment. Steve reported that he wanted to be certain he could maintain good coping in the face of these stressors.

As the therapist worked with Steve to develop a Problem List, she was surprised to see that he did not describe symptoms of depression or show facial expressions, body postures, or other evidence of depressed mood. This presentation was inconsistent with his report on the BDI and the SCL-90R, where he had endorsed many symptoms of depression. The therapist noticed the discrepancy but did not yet understand it, and knew that she needed to account for it in her formulation of Steve's case.

Steve was an excellent historian, and it was easy for the therapist to collect a good family history. Steve reported that his upbringing had been greatly influenced by the extreme and intolerant religious group to which his parents belonged. They firmly believed and taught him that if he did not excel in school and church activities, and did not follow the path they had laid out for him (to be a missionary and leader in the church, and to marry and produce children who would continue the tradition), then he was unacceptable to God, his parents, and their religious community. In fact, he would be damned to hell and struck down dead if he participated in any of a number of forbidden activities, including masturbation and homosexual acts. Steve tried to follow the path that his parents planned for him. At first he had some success, excelling in school and Bible studies. However, this lifestyle became increasingly incompatible with his own goals, values, and interests. Steve began to realize that he was gay and wanted a career in business rather than to marry and work for the church. Matters came to a head when Steve was 18. He had realized he was gay and felt unworthy and damned to hell. He fell into an acute depressive episode, attempted suicide by hanging himself (but the support to which he tied the rope broke), and spent 1 month in a psychiatric inpatient unit. Reflecting on his hospitalization, Steve reported, "It felt great to be locked in and away from my family's influence, with no religious counselors." When Steve left the hospital and realized that, contrary to his expectation, he had not been "struck down dead," he began to "rebuild" himself. He divorced, moved to another community, and went to college to study business. He sought therapy to help with this transition and in particular to help him come to terms with the fact that he was a homosexual.

Steve experienced a second episode of depression and suicidality at the age of 28, precipitated by beginning to live with and to establish a committed relationship with another gay man. He was again hospitalized for a month. After his discharge, Steve worked with a CB therapist and found CBT to be "extremely helpful." He especially liked activity scheduling, Thought Records, and keeping Positive Data Logs (PDLs).

As the initial consultation session came to a close, Steve and the therapist agreed to meet again to complete the assessment and treatment planning process. Steve agreed to complete an activity schedule, BDI, and Burns Anxiety Inventory before the second session, and to draft a list of treatment goals.

During the second consultation session, the therapist reviewed the activity schedule and learned that Steve was indeed carrying lots of responsibility and functioning at a high level. She also collected diagnostic information. Based on all the information she gathered, her initial diagnostic hypotheses were that Steve met criteria for major depressive disorder, recurrent, moderate, and dysthymia, but not for a bipolar disorder or an anxiety disorder. The therapist summarized the Problem List she had developed with Steve (depression; concerns about coping with stressors, especially his partner's illness;

and dissatisfaction with his neighborhood and school system). She shared her diagnostic hypotheses and advised Steve that he met criteria for both major depression and dysthymia. Steve concurred and emphasized that his goal was to continue functioning and to avoid another severe depressive episode.

The therapist reviewed Beck's cognitive model of depression with Steve and based her initial formulation hypothesis on it. She chose this model because Steve had used it in his previous therapy, and it was the model with which the therapist was most familiar. She shared her initial schema hypotheses with Steve, namely, that Steve had the self-schema "I am unworthy/bad/unacceptable to God," and a schema of others as rejecting and judgmental. These schemas appeared to have their origins in Steve's fundamentalist religious upbringing, and, when triggered, to produce depressive symptoms. The stressors of his partner's illness, the recent adoption of a child, and the need to move to a new community that would provide a good school for his child were likely precipitants to Steve's current depression.

Treatment Planning and Obtaining Informed Consent to Treatment

Based on the diagnoses and formulation, Steve's previous success in CBT, and his own wishes, the therapist proposed an initial treatment plan of weekly individual CBT sessions. The therapist and Steve agreed that they seemed like a good match to work together. As she proposed the treatment plan, Steve's therapist informed him that she did not have a complete formulation of his problems and symptoms, and that she wanted to spend more time working with him to understand what was causing his symptoms and concerns and to clarify the details of what he needed in the therapy. Steve liked this proposal. The therapist also recommended that Steve continue his antidepressant medication, and he agreed. Steve and the therapist set initial treatment goals, including reduction of depressive symptoms and concern about losing his ability to function. The therapist explained that they would monitor Steve's progress throughout the therapy, and that if progress stalled, then they would revisit the formulation and treatment plan. Steve was agreeable to this as well, and he agreed to complete a BDI and Burns Anxiety Inventory before every session to assess progress.

As the second session ended, Steve asked to set a homework plan to resume keeping a PDL, because it had been so helpful to him in the past. The PDL (Padesky, 1994; Tompkins, Persons, & Davidson, 2000) is a list of concrete and specific instances of data that support the healthy schema the patient is attempting to strengthen. The schema Steve chose to address was "I am worthy." From what the therapist had learned about Steve's family history, precipitants to major depressive episodes, and his previous success using a PDL, this homework plan seemed to make good sense. The therapist had some concern that addressing this schema from the get-go as a homework assignment might be premature, because she did not know Steve very well yet, and schema change interventions were usually used later in treatment, not at the beginning, but given Steve's eagerness to use the PDL and his report about how helpful the intervention had been to him in the past, she agreed to the plan.

Treatment, Progress Monitoring, and Hypothesis Testing

The next three sessions fleshed out Steve's case formulation and focused the treatment more precisely. Something striking happened in the third session. Steve had completed his PDL and brought an impressive list of data that supported the new schema of himself as worthy. Steve's therapist was struck by how impressive his data were. Most patients who use the PDL to strengthen a schema have a lot of difficulty generating material for the log and come in with just a handful of items. But Steve had listed numerous small and large accomplishments, and many instances of positive feedback he had received from work colleagues and supervisors, community leaders, and social service agencies that had helped him foster and adopt a child. He had extensive concrete evidence of his worthiness. When the therapist pointed this out, Steve agreed. He reported that he was acutely aware of a huge "mismatch" between the view of himself as worthy and what he called "a core belief that's always present" that he was not worthy and was in fact a failure and a bad person who was damned to hell. The view of himself as a failure was based on what he had learned at home from his parents and at church. By his parents' standards, Steve reported, he was a failure. He was a gay man who had left the church, and he literally deserved to be struck dead or go to hell.

As he talked about the mismatch of his old belief about himself and the new one, Steve became increasingly distressed and began to sob. The therapist waited for Steve to regain his composure, and when she saw that he was having difficulty doing so, she used grounding techniques described in posttraumatic stress disorder (PTSD) treatment protocols to help Steve calm himself. She asked Steve to look directly at her so he could focus on what she was saying, and she instructed him to take slower breaths, then to look around the room and name items and colors one at a time. After about 10 minutes, Steve regained control. As they talked about what had happened, Steve told the therapist that experiencing such intense sadness and distress was quite frightening to him. He reported that he had not realized how strongly he held the belief that he was unworthy and bad. He was terrified of losing control and feared that he would "fall apart" if he acknowledged the mismatch between the old "unworthy" belief and the new one that he was worthy. Steve's fears were strengthened by his observation that he had become depressed and suicidal, and spent a month in a psychiatric unit each time he confronted the mismatch between these beliefs. In fact, what had just happened in the session was the very thing Steve had feared and avoided. He had avoided confronting the mismatch between his conflicting views of himself for fear that he would lose control. The PDL forced him to confront the mismatch, thus activating emotions that felt overwhelming to him.

The fear of emotional dysregulation explained the discrepancy the therapist had noted between Steve's cheerful demeanor and the numerous symptoms he endorsed on the self-report scales of depression. Steve had minimized his depressive symptoms (and had stayed busy, as the activity schedule indicated) to avoid acknowledging his distress, because he believed that if he felt or showed sadness, he was at risk of falling apart. The therapist discussed this issue with Steve, and they agreed to add the fear of intense emotions to the mechanisms part of the formulation. Thus, Steve's emotional reaction in the third session provided data that led to a revised formulation of his case and helped to clarify his treatment goals. The therapist maintained her initial formulation of key schemas as described earlier, and added to the formulation Steve's fears of confronting the mismatch between the old and new views of himself, and especially of experiencing the intense emotions that this confrontation elicited.

The new formulation proposed that Steve was raised in a home (ORIGINS) in which he was taught the belief, "If I deviate from God's rules, I am unacceptable to God and unworthy" (MECHANISM). He also had a view of *himself* as fragile. In particular, he believed, "If I confront the conflict between my views of myself as unworthy and worthy, I will fall apart and be unable to function." He also believed that *others* were judgmental, critical, rejecting, unforgiving; *the world* was confusing, full of contradictions; and *the future* was uncertain, frightening ("because my mental health is fragile") (MECHANISM). As a result of these beliefs, Steve avoided acknowledging his old beliefs, the contradiction of the old and new beliefs, and any emotional distress, including his symptoms of depression (PROBLEM). Life stressors, including the adoption of child, the search for new home, and his partner's cancer (PROBLEMS and PRECIPITANTS) activated his view of himself as fragile (MECHANISM). As a consequence, he began to feel inadequate and overwhelmed, and had symptoms of depression (PROBLEMS).

Based on this new information, Steve and the therapist agreed to add two additional treatment goals. First, Steve agreed that he wanted to decrease his fear of negative emotions and to overcome his belief that he would fall apart and become unable to function if he experienced negative emotions, especially sadness. Second, he agreed to add the goal of developing balanced schemas that "resolve the mismatch between my view of myself as unworthy/unacceptable and the new view of myself as worthy and acceptable."

Over the course of the next two sessions, Steve and his therapist examined the core schemas of being of unworthy and "disgusting" to God, and the mismatch of the old and new schemas. The therapist continued to use grounding techniques from PTSD protocols to help Steve maintain and regain emotion regulation when, in the course of this work, he became distressed. In this way, Steve learned that he could experience negative emotions in therapy sessions and still regain his composure in the office and function well when he left the office. Overcoming the fear of dysregulation allowed Steve to carry out homework assignments to address his mismatched beliefs about himself. He developed detailed lists of "old values" that he learned from his parents and of his new "core values." He decided to reconcile these two value systems rather than to embrace one and reject the other. Steve reported that this process felt "big," but that he felt hopeful about resolving the conflict between his beliefs.

An event occurred between these early treatment sessions that further informed the formulation and the treatment plan. As part of his work to reconcile his two value systems, Steve attended a nondenominational church service. The sermon included the words, "God loves you in all of your imperfections." These words represented a view of God as accepting, which represented values directly opposed to his parent's values. In just the way the PDL had, this event highlighted the mismatch of his two value systems and triggered Steve's fear of losing control. Steve felt so anxious that he fled the church, fearing that if he stayed, he would become emotionally overwhelmed and fall apart. This reaction was a piece of data supporting the formulation hypothesis that fear and avoidance of emotional dysregulation, and the tension between old and new values, were at the heart of Steve's difficulties.

Moreover, the level of fear he experienced and his escape behavior in church suggested to the therapist that Steve might benefit from an exposure-based treatment of the sort used to treat clinical fears and phobias (e.g., Foa, Hembree, & Rothbaum, 2007). The therapist proposed to Steve that an exposure-based treatment component would allow him systematically to face his fears of dysregulation and of the conflict between his belief systems. The therapist explained the anxiety disorders treatment model of graded exposures to feared situations, using a rating system of subjective units of distress (SUDS) levels to allow Steve to approach gradually and overcome feared situations (Foa et al., 2007). Steve reported that although he had not previously thought about his problems in terms of fears of emotional dysregulation and anxiety, this formulation felt right to him. He liked the systematic exposure-based treatment plan, and he agreed to develop a hierarchy of situations and words that activated emotional dysregulation.

The remainder of the therapy was straightforward. Steve and his therapist developed a short hierarchy of emotionally activating words and situations, and assigned SUDS levels (from 1 to 100, with 100 being the most anxiety provoking) to each item. Examples of hierarchy items included writing (SUDS = 60) and saying (SUDS = 70) the phrase "God loves me in all of my imperfections" and listening to a recording of the sermon that had caused him to flee the church (SUDS = 90). Steve first practiced writing and then verbally repeating the phrase in session, until his SUDS rating dropped below 20. He initiated a plan to repeat the phrase as often as he could throughout the day, including while in the shower, on breaks at work, and during free time at home. Steve was so motivated by how much better he felt after doing this for a week that he ordered a tape of the sermon and began listening to it as soon as it arrived in the mail. His SUDS ratings quickly dropped below 20, which provided data that the case formulation and exposure-based treatment plan were on track. Steve learned that he could fully experience the negative emotions associated with the triggers on his hierarchy without becoming dysregulated, and he no longer needed the grounding techniques the therapist had taught him in the early sessions. Steve and his therapist were able to develop and discuss evidence supporting an integrated schema that allowed him to embrace his new values, while still being loved and accepted by God. He became comfortable with the belief: "I am imperfect and God still loves me. God loves me as I am."

After the eighth session, Steve felt ready to take his son for an extended visit to his parents over the holidays. Steve's willingness to undertake this visit was evidence of the progress he had made in treatment, because it indicated his willingness to engage in interactions with his family members that forced him to face conflicting value systems, negative emotions, and the potential for emotional dysregulation. When he returned from his trip home, Steve was pleased to report that he had been more assertive with his family than he had been in the past and had not avoided situations that were emotionally activating. He had experienced a range of emotions, including negative ones, when he interacted with his family and had felt good about his values, his parenting, and his accomplishments. He reported that it felt "so liberating" not to carry the burden of his old schema around with him. He stated that he felt ready to terminate treatment.

Steve's therapist suggested that they review his progress toward his goals to evaluate whether termination made sense, and Steve agreed to that plan. They had most extensive data on his first goal, that of reducing Steve's depressive symptoms. He had begun treatment with a BDI score of 21. By the third session, when he reviewed the PDL and became dysregulated, his score was 11. Steve reported feeling "shaky" at the end of this session ("crying means I'm not OK"), but also that it felt positive to "capture the core problem." In sessions 4 and 5, as he confronted the mismatch between his schemas and experienced a great deal of emotional distress, his BDI scores increased to 15 and then 16. After working in and out of session to confront the ideas that were most frightening to him, Steve improved markedly. When he returned for his sixth session, his BDI score had dropped to 8, and it was 4 in his 10th and final session. With regard to his goal of reducing concern about his ability to handle stressors, Steve reported feeling confident that he now could handle moving to a new neighborhood and coping with his partner's illness, because he was no longer fearful of "falling apart." He and his partner had begun house hunting, which was something Steve had previously avoided. He had evidence (e.g., from his exposure sessions and his visit to his parents) of his ability to tolerate negative emotional states, and he had made significant progress toward reconciling his old and new value systems.

As they prepared for termination, the therapist and Steve reviewed what he had learned in treatment. Steve was delighted with what he had accomplished in such a brief therapy. Steve pointed out that when he had been severely depressed in the past, he was unable to face the conflict between his beliefs and the accompanying activation of affect. He was pleased that he had initiated this treatment while he was high functioning, and that he and the therapist had successfully identified the obstacle (fear of negative emotions and emotion dysregulation) to developing a positive and integrated self-schema.

The therapist expressed some concern that Steve might be ending treatment prematurely and be vulnerable to relapse. This concern was consistent with the formulation hypothesis that Steve's fears of emotional dysregulation and of acknowledging symptoms or problems might cause him to perceive the need for therapy as an indicator of not being OK, which he previously had equated with catastrophic consequences. Steve was receptive to considering the points the therapist raised but insisted that he had done the necessary work and felt ready to end therapy. Also, Steve had achieved his treatment goals, and the data from the weekly BDI scores indicated that his depressive symptoms had remitted. Steve and the therapist agreed that he would contact her to arrange for additional sessions if they were needed in the future.

Follow-Up

One and a half years after the end of therapy, the therapist contacted Steve to obtain some follow-up data for this chapter. Steve reported that he had been well in the interim and was flourishing. He reported a BDI score of 0 and a Burns Anxiety Inventory score of 1. He endorsed only a few symptoms on the SCL-90R and no longer endorsed the item "Feeling that something bad is going to happen to you." On the FSI, he reported that he was functioning "very well" to "extremely well" and was satisfied in most areas of life. The only domain in which he felt only "a little satisfied" was his home/neighborhood/community. He and his partner were considering another move, because Steve had been promoted and his new job entailed a very long commute from their current home. His partner's cancer was in remission. The therapist felt some concern that Steve's scores were too low—that is, that Steve had not entirely overcome his fear of negative emotions but was simply avoiding them. Nevertheless, the scores and Steve's report about how well he had been doing provided evidence that treatment had had lasting results, as did a beautiful letter Steve wrote that described how much he had gotten from the therapy. He reflected back on the beginning of treatment and described himself as having been "in the middle of a crisis of confidence." He reported that in therapy he had resolved the "deep inner conflict between value systems." He wrote: "I was able to sink the juggernaut of my old beliefs and reconcile my new values with a much friendlier, humane God with the grace to accept me as I am. In some ways I had to learn to tolerate doubt, be honest and authentic, take care of myself, and trust myself to do my best in the process (and it's OK because I can never be 'perfect' anyhow)."

Overview of the Case

The case of Steve illustrates several points. First, although Beck's model provided a foundation for the case formulation and the treatment, the therapist also relied on other models to guide her formulation and treatment. After she learned that Steve was afraid of the mismatch of his beliefs about himself and the negative emotions that resulted, the therapist relied on the learning theory–based formulation underpinning exposure-based treatment of anxiety disorders to guide treatment of those fears. She and Steve developed a hierarchy of the thoughts and emotions he feared and systematically carried out exposures to them.

Second, the conceptualization and interventions Steve's therapist used are also consistent with several other CB models. Steve's formulation and treatment are consistent with the exposure-based cognitive therapy (EBCT) developed by Adele Hayes and her colleagues (2007), which applies principles of exposure and schema-focused therapies to the treatment of depression. In fact, the spike in Steve's BDI scores early in treatment is quite consistent with the Hayes et al. model of the change process in their therapy.

Steve's conceptualization and treatment also fit nicely with the conceptualization and treatment of PTSD developed by Ehlers and Clark (2000). PTSD often includes fears of negative emotions that arise when patients confront conflicting belief systems (e.g., the old belief that "the world is safe," and a new one that "the world can be dangerous") that are not integrated into a coherent biographical narrative. Ehlers and Clark encourage the person with PTSD to approach the feared emotions to learn that they are not dangerous and to work to integrate apparently conflicting ideas into a coherent narrative. Steve's treatment could also be viewed as including elements of acceptance and commitment therapy (Hayes, Strosahl, & Wilson, 1999), especially the emphasis on overcoming experiential avoidance.

The observation that the conceptualization and interventions Steve's therapist used were consistent with several models and therapies highlights the point that multiple CB models are available to guide conceptualization and treatment. Steve's therapist used more than one model to guide his treatment. We suspect that the use of multiple models to guide treatment for one patient is common in clinical practice, although, to our knowledge, this practice has not been subjected to formal study.

Although the availability of multiple models is a boon in many ways, it can also make the therapist's job more difficult. The therapist can get lost in the forest of options. A case formulation provides a clear path through the woods. The strategy of developing a clear formulation, then using it to select interventions from multiple sources, can provide overall clarity and coherence to the treatment.

Third, Steve's case was an unusually successful one. We speculate that contributing factors included the moderate severity of Steve's symptoms and his strengths, especially the degree of leadership he took in his therapy. For example, Steve himself proposed repeated exposure to the sermon that was so frightening to him, and he took steps to order a copy that he could listen to repeatedly. Steve was an unusually full collaborator in his treatment. We suspect that many patients could play a more active role in their treatment if therapists worked harder to permit and encourage such activity. As Miller and Rollnick (2002) point out, patients truly are the expert on their problems and can contribute hugely to their own treatment. We encourage therapists to engage their patients fully in the formulation and treatment processes.

FINAL DISCUSSION

This chapter describes and illustrates a framework for providing individualized CBT, of which the case formulation is a key element. The framework is depicted in Figure 6.1. The formulation (or formulations, because the therapist develops and uses multiple formulations at multiple levels over the course of treatment) serves as a hypothesis that the therapist uses to guide intervention and tests by collecting data to evaluate the process and progress of therapy. McCrady and Epstein (2003) have discussed the need for such a framework in the substance abuse field, and the American Psychological Association (2005) has described the need for such a framework in psychotherapy more generally. These frameworks, including the one described here, are not new therapies. They simply provide a heuristic for adapting evidence-based treatments to the case at hand in a thoughtful and systematic way. Nevertheless, these frameworks require evaluation in controlled studies to determine their utility in clinical practice.

REFERENCES

American Psychological Association. (2005). *Report of the 2005 Presidential Task Force on Evidence-Based Practice.* Washington, DC: American Psychological Association.

Antony, M. M., Orsillo, S. M., & Roemer, L. (Eds.). (2001). *Practitioner's guide to empirically based measures of anxiety.* New York: Kluwer Academic/Plenum Press.

Beck, A. T., Rush, J. A., Shaw, B. F., & Emery, G. (1979). *Cognitive therapy of depression.* New York: Guilford Press.

Beck, J. S. (1995). *Cognitive therapy: Basics and beyond.* New York: Guilford Press.

Burns, D. D. (1997). *Therapist toolkit.* Available at *www.feelinggood.com.*

Burns, D. D. (1999). *Feeling good: The new mood therapy.* New York: Morrow.

Clark, D. M. (1986). A cognitive approach to panic. *Behaviour Research and Therapy, 24,* 461–470.

Davidson, J., Martinez, K. A., & Thomas, C. (2006, November). *Validation of a new measure of functioning and satisfaction for use in outpatient clinical practice.*

Paper presented at the meeting of the Association for Behavioral and Cognitive Therapies, Chicago, IL.

Derogatis, L. R. (2000). *SCL-90-R.* Washington, DC: American Psychological Association.

Ehlers, A., & Clark, D. M. (2000). A cognitive model of posttraumatic stress disorder. *Behaviour Research and Therapy, 38,* 319–345.

Fischer, J., & Corcoran, K. (2007). *Measures for clinical practice and research: A sourcebook: Vol. 2. Adults.* Oxford, UK: Oxford University Press.

Foa, E. B., Hembree, E., & Rothbaum, B. (2007). *Prolonged exposure therapy for PTSD: Emotional processing of traumatic experiences: Therapist Guide: Treatments that work.* New York: Oxford University Press.

Follette, W. C. (1996). Introduction to the special section on the development of theoretically coherent alternatives to the DSM system. *Journal of Consulting and Clinical Psychology, 64,* 1117–1119.

Ghaderi, A. (2006). Does individualization matter?: A randomized trial of standardized (focused) versus individualized (broad) cognitive behavior therapy for bulimia nervosa. *Behaviour Research and Therapy, 44,* 273–288.

Hayes, A. M., Feldman, G. C., Beevers, C. G., Laurenceau, J.-P., Cardaciotto, L., & Lewis-Smith, J. (2007). Discontinuities and cognitive changes in an expsoure-based cognitive therapy for depression. *Journal of Consulting and Clinical Psychology, 75*(3), 409–421.

Hayes, S. C., Nelson, R., & Jarrett, R. (1987). The treatment utility of assessment: A functional approach to evaluating assessment quality. *American Psychologist, 42,* 963–974.

Hayes, S. C., Strosahl, K. D., & Wilson, K. G. (1999). *Acceptance and commitment therapy: An experiential approach to behavior change.* New York: Guilford Press.

Haynes, S. N., Leisen, M. B., & Blaine, D. D. (1997). Design of individualized behavioral treatment programs using functional analytic clinical case models. *Psychological Assessment, 9,* 334–348.

Haynes, S. N., & O'Brien, W. H. (2000). *Principles and practice of behavioral assessment.* New York: Kluwer Academic/Plenum Press.

Jacobson, N. S., Schmaling, K. B., Holtzworth-Munroe, A., Katt, J. L., Wood, L. F., & Follette, V. M. (1989). Research-structured vs. clinically flexible versions of social learning-based marital therapy. *Behaviour Research and Therapy, 27,* 173–180.

Koerner, K. (2006). Case formulation in dialectical behavior therapy for borderline personality disorder. In T. D. Eells (Ed.), *Handbook of psychotherapy case formulation* (2nd ed., pp. 317–348). New York: Guilford Press.

Kuyken, W., Padesky, C. A., & Dudley, R. (2009). *Collaborative case conceptualization: Working effectively with clients in cognitive-behavioral therapy.* New York: Guilford Press.

Lewinsohn, P. M., & Gotlib, I. H. (1995). Behavioral theory and treatment of depression. In E. E. Beckham & W. R. Leber (Eds.), *Handbook of depression* (2nd ed., pp. 352–375). New York: Guilford Press.

Martell, C. R., Addis, M. E., & Jacobson, N. S. (2001). *Depression in context: Strategies for guided action.* New York: Norton.

McCrady, B. S., & Epstein, E. E. (2003, November). *Treating alcohol and drug problems: Individualized treatment planning and intervention.* Paper presented at the meeting of the Association for Advancement of Behavior Therapy, Boston, MA.

Miller, W. R., & Rollnick, S. (2002). *Motivational interviewing: Preparing people for change* (2nd ed.). New York: Guilford Press.

Nelson-Gray, R. O. (2003). Treatment utility of psychological assessment. *Psychological Assessment, 15,* 521–531.

Nezu, A. M., Nezu, C. M., & Lombardo, E. (2004). *Cognitive-behavioral case formulation and treatment design: A problem-solving approach.* New York: Springer.

Nezu, A. M., Ronan, G. F., Meadows, E. A., & McClure, K. S. (Eds.). (2000). *Practioner's guide to empirically based measures of depression.* New York: Kluwer Academic.

Padesky, C. A. (1994). Schema change processes in cognitive therapy. *Clinical Psychology and Psychotherapy, 1,* 267–278.

Persons, J. B. (2008). *The case formulation approach to cognitive-behavior therapy.* New York: Guilford Press.

Persons, J. B., Bostrom, A., & Bertagnolli, A. (1999). Results of randomized controlled trials of cognitive therapy for depression generalize to private practice. *Cognitive Therapy and Research, 23,* 535–548.

Persons, J. B., Burns, D. D., & Perloff, J. M. (1988). Predictors of dropout and outcome in cognitive therapy for depression in a private practice setting. *Cognitive Therapy and Research, 12,* 557–575.

Persons, J. B., & Mikami, A. Y. (2002). Strategies for handling treatment failure successfully. *Psychotherapy: Theory, Research, Practice and Training, 39,* 139–151.

Persons, J. B., Roberts, N. A., Zalecki, C. A., & Brechwald, W. A. G. (2006). Naturalistic outcome of case formulation-driven cognitive-behavior therapy for anxious depressed outpatients. *Behaviour Research and Therapy, 44,* 1041–1051.

Schneider, B. H., & Byrne, B. M. (1987). Individualizing social skills training for behavior-disordered children. *Journal of Consulting and Clinical Psychology, 55,* 444–445.

Schulte, D., Kunzel, R., Pepping, G., & Schulte-Bahrenberg, T. (1992). Tailor-made versus standardized therapy of phobic patients. *Advances in Behaviour Research and Therapy, 14,* 67–92.

Tarrier, N. (Ed.). (2006). *Case formulation in cognitive behaviour therapy: The treatment of challenging and complex cases.* New York: Routledge.

Tompkins, M. A., Persons, J. B., & Davidson, J. (2000). Cognitive-behavior therapy for depression: Schema change methods [Videotape]. Washington, DC: American Psychological Association.

Young, J. E. (1999). *Cognitive therapy for personality disorders: A schema-focused approach.* Sarasota, FL: Professional Resource Exchange.

Young, J. E., Klosko, J. S., & Weishaar, M. E. (2003). *Schema therapy: A practitioner's guide.* New York: Guilford Press.

PART III

THE THERAPIES

CHAPTER 7

Problem-Solving Therapy

Thomas J. D'Zurilla
Arthur M. Nezu

Problem-solving therapy (PST) is a positive approach to clinical intervention that focuses on training in constructive problem-solving attitudes and skills. The aims of PST are both to reduce psychopathology and to enhance psychological and behavioral functioning to prevent relapses and the development of new clinical problems, as well as to maximize quality of life. PST was originally introduced by D'Zurilla and Goldfried (1971) during the early 1970s as part of the growing trend in the field of behavior modification toward a greater emphasis on cognitive mediation in an attempt to facilitate self-control and maximize the generalization and maintenance of behavior changes (Kendall & Hollon, 1979). In subsequent years, D'Zurilla, Nezu, and their associates have continued to refine and revise the theory and practice of PST and to evaluate its efficacy for a variety of different psychological, behavioral, and health disorders (D'Zurilla, 1986; D'Zurilla & Nezu, 1999, 2007; C. M. Nezu, D'Zurilla, & Nezu, 2005; Nezu, Nezu, & D'Zurilla, 2007; Nezu, Nezu, Friedman, Faddis, & Houts, 1998; Nezu, Nezu, & Perri, 1989).

A large number of outcome studies evaluating the efficacy of PST have been reported in the clinical, counseling, and health psychology literature. In populations that range from children to adolescents, adults, and older adults, PST has been employed as a stand-alone treatment method and as part of a treatment package, a maintenance strategy, and a prevention program. These interventions have been applied within a variety of clinical and nonclinical settings, including individual, group, marital, and family therapy, primary care settings, workshops, seminars, and academic courses. Clinical participants have presented with a wide range of adjustment problems and disorders, including schizophrenia, depression, stress and anxiety disorders, suicidal ideation and behavior, substance abuse, weight problems, offending behavior, relationship problems, mental retardation, cancer, and other medical problems. This chapter focuses on PST for adolescents and adults (for a discussion of PST programs for children, see Frauenknecht & Black, 2004). The chapter is divided into two major sections. In the first section, we discuss the theory underlying PST and the empirical evidence supporting it. In the second, we describe the clinical practice of PST and discuss evidence supporting the efficacy of PST for a variety of psychological, behavioral, and health disorders.

THEORETICAL AND EMPIRICAL FOUNDATIONS

The goals of PST are to reduce and/or prevent psychopathology and enhance positive well-being by helping individuals cope more effectively with stressful problems in living. Depending on the nature of the problematic situation, effective coping may involve improving the situation (e.g., achieving a performance goal, removing an aversive condition, resolving a conflict) and/or reducing the emotional distress generated by the situation (e.g., acceptance, tolerance, making something good come from the problem, reducing physical tension). The theory on which PST is based involves two interrelated conceptual models: (1) the social problem-solving model and (2) the relational/problem-solving model of stress and well-being.

The Social Problem-Solving Model

"Social problem solving" refers to problem solving as it occurs in the natural social environment (D'Zurilla & Nezu, 1982). Social problem solving is at the same time a learning process, a general coping strategy, and a self-control method. Because problem solution results in a change in performance capability in specific situations, social problem solving qualifies as a learning process (Gagné, 1966), but as it also increases the probability of adaptive coping outcomes across a wide range of problematic situations, it is a general, versatile coping strategy. Finally, because social problem solving is a *self-directed* learning process and coping strategy, it is also a self-control method with important implications for the maintenance and generalization of treatment effects (D'Zurilla & Goldfried, 1971; Mahoney, 1974; Nezu, 1987). The social problem-solving model described below was originally introduced by D'Zurilla and Goldfried (1971), and later expanded and refined by D'Zurilla, Nezu, and Maydeu-Olivares (2002; D'Zurilla & Nezu, 1982, 1990, 1999, 2007; Maydeu-Olivares & D'Zurilla, 1995, 1996).

Definitions of Major Concepts

The three major concepts in social problem-solving theory are (1) social problem solving, (2) the problem, and (3) the solution. In this context, "social problem solving" is defined as the self-directed cognitive-behavioral process by which an individual, couple, or group attempts to identify or discover effective solutions for specific problems encountered in everyday living. Social problem solving is thus conceived as a conscious, rational, effortful, and purposeful activity aimed at improving a problematic situation, reducing or modifying the negative emotions generated by the situation, or both of these outcomes. Hence, it is best viewed as the metaprocess of understanding, appraising, and adapting to stressful life events, rather than simply a singular coping strategy or activity. As defined here, social problem solving deals with all types of real-life problems, including impersonal problems (e.g., insufficient finances, property damage), personal/intrapersonal problems (cognitive, emotional, behavioral, health), as well as interpersonal problems (e.g., interpersonal disputes, marital conflicts).

A "problem" (or problematic situation) is defined as an imbalance or discrepancy between adaptive demands and the availability of effective coping responses. Specifically, a problem is any life situation or task (present or anticipated) that demands an effective response to achieve a goal or resolve a conflict, when no effective response is immediately apparent or available to the person. The demands of a problematic situation may originate in the environment (e.g., job demands, behavioral expectations of significant others) or within the person (e.g., a personal goal, need, or commitment). The obstacles might include novelty, ambiguity, unpredictability, conflicting demands, performance skills deficits, or lack of resources. A specific problem might be a single, time-limited event (e.g., forgetting an important appointment, an acute illness); a series of similar or related events (e.g., repeated demands at work, repeated substance use by an adolescent daughter); or a chronic, ongoing situation (e.g., continuous pain or loneliness).

A "solution" is a situation-specific coping response or pattern of responses that is the outcome of the problem-solving process when it is applied to a specific problematic situation. An "effective" solution is one that achieves the problem-solving goal (e.g., changing the situation for the better, reducing negative emotions, increasing positive emotions), while it also maximizes other positive consequences and minimizes negative consequences. These consequences include long-term, as well as short-term, personal and social outcomes.

Problem solving should be distinguished from solution implementation. These two processes are conceptually different and require different sets of skills. "Problem solving" refers to the process of discovering solutions to specific problems, whereas "solution implementation" refers to the process of carrying out those solutions in the actual problematic situations. Problem-solving skills are assumed to be general, whereas solution implementation skills vary across situations and depend on the type of problem and solution. Problem-solving skills and solution implementation skills are not always correlated; some individuals might possess poor problem-solving skills but good solution implementation skills, or vice versa. Because both sets of skills are required for effective functioning or social competence, it is often necessary in PST to combine training in problem-solving skills with training in other social and behavioral performance skills to maximize positive outcomes (D'Zurilla & Nezu, 2007).

Major Problem-Solving Dimensions

The original social problem-solving model (D'Zurilla & Goldfried, 1971; D'Zurilla & Nezu, 1982, 1990) hypothesized that problem-solving ability comprises two major, partially independent processes: (1) problem orientation and (2) problem-solving skills (later referred to as "problem-solving proper" [e.g., D'Zurilla & Nezu, 1999] and more recently as "problem-solving style" [e.g., D'Zurilla & Nezu, 2007; D'Zurilla et al., 2002]). "Problem orientation" is a metacognitive process that primarily serves a motivational function in social problem solving. It involves the operation of a set of relatively stable cognitive-emotional schemas that reflect a person's general awareness and appraisals of problems in living, as well as his or her own problem-solving ability (e.g., threat vs. challenge appraisals, self-efficacy beliefs, outcome expectancies). "Problem-solving skills," on the other hand, are the activities by which a person attempts to understand problems in everyday living and to discover effective "solutions," or ways of coping with them. In this model, four major problem-solving skills are identified: (1) problem definition and formulation, (2) generation of alternative solutions, (3) decision making, and (4) solution implementation and verification (D'Zurilla & Goldfried, 1971). The latter component comprises self-monitoring and solution evaluation skills during and following solution implementation; it does *not* include solution implementation skills.

Based on this theoretical model, D'Zurilla and Nezu (1990) developed the Social Problem-Solving Inventory (SPSI), which comprises two major scales: the Problem Orientation Scale (POS) and the Problem-Solving Skills Scale (PSSS). The items in each scale reflect both constructive and dysfunctional problem-solving characteristics (cognitive, emotional, and behavioral). The assumption that problem orientation and problem-solving skills are different, albeit related, components of social problem-solving ability was supported by data indicating that the POS items were more highly correlated with the total POS score than with the total PSSS score, whereas the reverse was true for the PSSS items (D'Zurilla & Nezu, 1990).

Based on an integration of the original social problem-solving model and subsequent factor analyses of the SPSI, D'Zurilla et al. (2002; Maydeu-Olivares & D'Zurilla, 1995, 1996) developed a revised, five-dimensional social problem-solving model that comprises two different, albeit related, problem orientation dimensions and three different problem-solving styles. The two problem orientation dimensions are positive problem orientation and negative problem orientation, whereas the three problem-solving styles are rational problem solving, impulsivity/carelessness style, and avoidance style. Positive problem orientation and rational problem solving are constructive dimensions that increase the likelihood of positive problem-solving outcomes, whereas negative problem orientation, impulsivity/carelessness style, and avoidance style are dysfunctional dimensions that disrupt or inhibit effective problem solving, resulting in negative personal and social outcomes.

"Positive problem orientation" is a constructive problem-solving cognitive set that involves the general disposition to (1) appraise a problem as a "challenge" (i.e., opportunity for benefit or gain); (2) believe that problems are solvable (positive outcome expectancies, or "optimism"); (3) believe in one's personal ability to solve problems successfully ("problem-solving self-efficacy"); (4) believe that successful problem solving takes time, effort, and persistence; and (5) commit oneself to solving problems with dispatch rather than avoiding them. "Negative problem orientation" is a dysfunctional or inhibitive cognitive-emotional set that involves a tendency to (1) view a problem as a significant threat to psychological, social, behavioral, or health well-being; (2) doubt one's personal ability to solve problems successfully; and (3) become emotionally upset when confronted with problems in living (i.e., low frustration and uncertainty tolerance).

"Rational problem solving" is a constructive problem-solving style that involves the rational, deliberate, and systematic application of four major problem-solving skills: (1) problem definition and formulation, (2) generation of alternative solutions, (3) decision making, and (4) solution implementation and verification. The rational problem solver gathers facts and information about a problem carefully and systematically, identifies demands and obstacles, sets realistic problem-solving goals, generates a variety of possible solutions, anticipates the consequences of the different solutions, judges and compares the alternatives, chooses the "best" solution, implements that solution, and carefully monitors and evaluates the outcome. This dimension does not include the solution implementation skills that are also necessary for effective problem-solving performance in specific problematic situations.

"Impulsivity/carelessness style" is a dysfunctional problem-solving pattern characterized by active attempts to apply problem-solving strategies and techniques, but these attempts are narrow, impulsive, careless, hurried, and incomplete. A person with this problem-solving style typically considers only a few solution alternatives, often impulsively going with the first idea that comes to mind. In addition, he or she scans alternative solutions and consequences quickly, carelessly, and unsystematically, and monitors solution outcomes carelessly and inadequately.

"Avoidance style" is another dysfunctional problem-solving pattern characterized by procrastination, passivity or inaction, and dependency. The avoidant problem solver prefers to avoid problems rather than confront them immediately, puts off problem solving for as long as possible, waits for problems to resolve themselves, and attempts to shift the responsibility for solving his or her problems to other people.

The five problem-solving dimensions are measured by the Social Problem-Solving Inventory—Revised (SPSI-R; D'Zurilla et al., 2002). Effective social problem-solving ability is indicated on this instrument by high scores on posi-

tive problem orientation and rational problem solving and low scores on negative problem orientation, impulsivity/carelessness style, and avoidance style,
whereas ineffective social problem-solving ability is indicated by low scores
on positive problem orientation and rational problem solving, and high scores
on negative problem orientation, impulsivity/carelessness style, and avoidance style. The five-dimension model of the SPSI-R has been cross-validated
in samples of young adults (D'Zurilla et al., 2002) and adolescents (Sadowski, Moore, & Kelley, 1994). Translated versions of the SPSI-R have been
cross-validated in samples of Spanish (Maydeu-Olivares, Rodríquez-Fornells,
Gómez-Benito, & D'Zurilla, 2000), German (Graf, 2003), and Chinese adults
(Siu & Shek, 2005).

A RELATIONAL/PROBLEM-SOLVING MODEL
OF STRESS AND WELL-BEING

A major assumption underlying the use of PST is that symptoms of psychopathology can often be understood and effectively prevented or treated if they
are viewed as ineffective, maladaptive, and self-defeating coping behaviors
that in turn have negative psychological and social consequences, such as
anxiety, depression, low self-esteem, and impaired interpersonal functioning
(D'Zurilla & Goldfried, 1971). Hence the theory of PST is also based on a
relational/problem-solving model of stress and well-being in which the concept of social problem solving is given a central role as a general and versatile coping strategy. This strategy increases adaptive functioning and positive
well-being, which, in turn, reduce and prevent the negative impact of stress on
well-being and adjustment (D'Zurilla, 1990; D'Zurilla & Nezu, 1999, 2007;
Nezu, 1987; Nezu & D'Zurilla, 1989).

The relational/problem-solving model integrates Richard Lazarus's relational model of stress (Lazarus, 1999; Lazarus & Folkman, 1984) with the
social problem-solving model presented earlier. In Lazarus's model, "stress" is
defined as a person–environment relationship in which demands are appraised
by the person to tax or exceed coping resources and threaten his or her well-
being (Lazarus & Folkman, 1984). This relational definition of stress is similar to the definition of a "problem" in social problem-solving theory. Hence, a
problem is also a "stressor," if it is at all difficult and significant for well-being.
In the relational/problem-solving model, stress is viewed as a function of the
reciprocal relations among three major variables: (1) stressful life events, (2)
emotional stress/well-being, and (3) problem-solving coping.

"Stressful life events" are life experiences that present a person with
demands for personal, social, or biological readjustment (Bloom, 1985). In
this model, two major types of stressful life events are major negative events
and daily problems. A "major negative event" is a broad life experience, such
as a major negative life change, that often requires sweeping readjustments
in a person's life (e.g., divorce, death of a loved one, job loss, major illness or
injury). In contrast, a "daily problem" is a more narrow and specific stress-

ful life event (see definition of "problem"). Although major negative events and daily problems may develop independently in a person's life, they are often causally related (Nezu & D'Zurilla, 1989). For example, a major negative event, such as a divorce, usually creates many new stressful problems for a person (e.g., difficulty paying bills, dealing with children's needs, meeting new people). Conversely, an accumulation of unresolved daily problems (e.g., marital conflicts, job problems, excessive alcohol use) may eventually cause or contribute to a divorce.

In this model, the concept of "emotional stress" refers to the immediate emotional responses of a person to stressful life events, as modified, modulated, or transformed by cognitive appraisal and coping processes (Lazarus, 1999). Depending on the nature of stressful life events (e.g., aversiveness, controllability), cognitive appraisals, and coping behavior, emotional stress responses may be negative (e.g., anxiety, anger, depression) or positive (e.g., hope, relief, exhilaration, joy). Negative emotions are likely to predominate when the person (1) appraises a stressful event as threatening or harmful to well-being, (2) doubts his or her ability to cope effectively, and (3) performs coping responses that are ineffective, maladaptive, or self-defeating. On the other hand, positive emotions may compete with negative emotions and sometimes dominate when the person (1) appraises a stressful event as a significant "challenge" or opportunity for benefit, (2) believes that he or she is capable of coping with the problem effectively, and (3) performs coping responses that are effective, adaptive, and self-enhancing.

Emotional stress is a key part of a broader construct of "well-being" that also encompasses cognitive, behavioral, social, and physical functioning (Lazarus & Folkman, 1984). Hence, the relational/problem-solving model assumes that stressful life events, cognitive appraisals, and coping processes have a significant impact on general well-being, and on the person's adjustment status (e.g., development of a clinical disorder vs. positive mental and physical health).

The most important concept in the relational/problem-solving model is "problem-solving coping," a process that integrates all cognitive appraisal and coping activities within a general social problem-solving framework. A person who applies the problem-solving coping strategy effectively (1) perceives a stressful life event as a challenge or "problem to be solved," (2) believes that he or she is capable of solving the problem successfully, (3) carefully defines the problem and sets a realistic goal, (4) generates a variety of alternative "solutions" or coping options, (5) chooses the "best" or most effective solution, (6) implements the solution effectively, and (7) carefully observes and evaluates the outcome. Unlike Lazarus's relational model of stress (Lazarus & Folkman, 1984), which views problem solving as a form of "problem-focused coping" that is limited to mastery goals (i.e., changing or controlling the stressful situation), problem solving is conceived here as a broader, more versatile coping strategy that may have problem-focused goals (i.e., changing the situation for the better), emotion-focused goals (i.e., reducing or modifying one's emotions), or both types of goals, depending on the nature of the particular problematic situation and how it is defined and appraised. When the situation is appraised as changeable or controllable, then problem-focused goals are emphasized, although the person might also set an emotion-focused goal, if emotional distress is high. On the other hand, if the situation is appraised as largely unchangeable, then emotion-focused goals are emphasized (e.g., acceptance, making something good come from the problem). Regardless of what goals are set, the ultimate expected outcome of problem solving is to enhance adaptive coping and positive well-being, and to reduce the negative impact of stress on well-being and adjustment.

The hypothesized relationships among the major variables in the relational/problem-solving model of stress and well-being are summarized in Figure 7.1, which shows that major negative events and daily problems are the two types of stressful life events in the model, and that they are assumed to influence each other. For example, a major negative event, such as a job loss, is likely to result in many new daily problems for an individual (e.g., difficulty paying bills, job search). Conversely, an accumulation of unresolved daily problems on the job (e.g., failure to meet performance goals, conflicts with coworkers, tardiness) may eventually result in loss of the job (i.e., getting fired or quitting). Both types of stressful life events are also assumed to have a direct negative impact on well-being, as well as an indirect negative effect via problem solving. The relationship between stressful life events and well-being is well established (Bloom, 1985). Moreover, a number of studies have suggested that an accumulation of unresolved daily problems may have

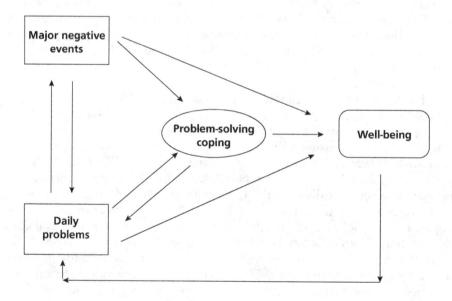

FIGURE 7.1. Hypothesized relationships among the major concepts of the relational/problem-solving model of stress and well-being. From D'Zurilla and Nezu (2007). Copyright by Springer Publishing Company, LLC. Reprinted by permission.

a greater negative impact on well-being than the number of major negative events (e.g., Burks & Martin, 1985; DeLongis, Coyne, Dakof, Folkman, & Lazarus, 1982; Nezu, 1986a; Weinberger, Hiner, & Tierney, 1987). These findings suggest that it is important in PST to identify the daily problems that might be created by major negative events and to focus on solving these daily problems, as well as coping with the major negative event itself.

The model assumes that problem solving influences the relationship between stressful life events and well-being by functioning as a mediator or a moderator. The model recognizes two different mediational hypotheses. The first hypothesis is based on the ABC model, where stressful life events (A) are assumed to set the occasion for problem-solving behavior (B), which, in turn results in personal and social consequences (C) that affect well-being. If problem solving is ineffective, negative well-being ensues (e.g., anxiety, depression), but effective problem solving has positive consequences for well-being (e.g., fewer negative emotions, more positive emotions). The second mediational hypothesis assumes that problem solving is an intervening variable in a causal chain, in which stressful life events have a negative impact on problem-solving ability and performance, which in turn have a negative effect on well-being. In contrast with the preceding ABC hypothesis, the arrows from stressful life events to problem solving are interpreted as negative causal relationships rather than prompting effects.

In the moderator hypothesis, the major assumption is that stressful life events interact with problem-solving ability to influence well-being. Specifically, the negative relationship between stress and well-being is stronger when problem-solving ability is low rather than high. In other words, poor problem-solving ability increases the negative impact of stressful life events on well-being, whereas good problem-solving ability functions as a "buffer" to reduce the negative impact of stress on well-being. In this hypothesis, the assumption of a causal relationship between stressful life events and problem-solving ability is not necessary. In this respect, the moderator hypothesis is consistent with the first mediational hypothesis described earlier.

As Figure 7.1 shows, the model also hypothesizes that a *reciprocal* relationship exists between daily problems and problem solving. Specifically, in addition to the assumption that stressful events may have a negative impact on problem solving, the model also assumes that problem solving is likely to influence the frequency of daily problems. Ineffective problem solving is expected to result in an increase in daily problems, whereas effective problem solving is expected is to reduce the frequency of daily problems. Finally, the relationship between stressful events and well-being is viewed as reciprocal. Specifically, in addition to the direct and indirect impact of stressful events on well-being, the model assumes that well-being is likely to have an impact on future stressful events. Negative adjustment outcomes (e.g., anxiety, depression, impaired social and behavioral functioning) are likely to result in an increase in daily problems and major negative events, whereas positive adjustment outcomes (e.g., hope, self-esteem, happiness, competence) are likely to reduce the frequency of these stressful events.

The relational/problem-solving model of stress and well-being provides a theoretical rationale for PST, as well as a useful framework for assessment prior to PST. During assessment, the therapist identifies major negative life events, current daily problems, emotional stress responses, problem orientation deficits and distortions, problem-solving style deficits, and solution implementation skills deficits. Based on this assessment, PST is applied to (1) increase positive problem orientation, (2) reduce negative problem orientation, (3) improve rational problem-solving skills, (4) reduce or prevent impulsive/careless problem solving, and (5) minimize the tendency to avoid problem solving. Other cognitive-behavioral methods (e.g., social skills training, exposure methods) may be used to teach effective solution implementation skills and/or to reduce anxiety that might inhibit effective solution implementation. Achieving these goals increases adaptive situational coping and positive psychological, social, and physical well-being, and reduces or prevents the negative effects of stress on well-being and adjustment.

EMPIRICAL SUPPORT FOR THE THEORY OF PROBLEM-SOLVING THERAPY

Support for the theory of PST comes from research on the hypothesized relationships that involve the problem-solving variable, as well as research on the process of PST. While most of the studies have focused on the relationship between social problem-solving ability and well-being or adjustment, some studies have examined the role of problem solving as a mediator or a moderator of the relationship between stressful life events and well-being or adjustment. In addition, a few studies on the process of PST have examined the relationship between improvements in adjustment following PST and increases in social problem-solving ability.

According to the theory of PST, social problem solving is a general and versatile coping strategy that enhances adaptive functioning and positive well-being, and reduces the negative effects of stress on well-being across a wide range of stressful situations. Based on this assumption, it can be hypothesized that social problem-solving ability is related to a wide range of positive and negative adjustment outcomes. Reviews of the vast research literature during the past three decades provide substantial support for this basic hypothesis (see Chang, D'Zurilla, & Sanna, 2004; D'Zurilla & Nezu, 2007; Nezu, 2004). Problem-solving ability has been found to be positively related to adaptive situational coping strategies, behavioral competence (e.g., social skills, academic performance, job performance), and positive psychological functioning (e.g., positive affectivity, self-esteem, a sense of mastery and control, life satisfaction). In addition, problem-solving deficits have been found to be associated with general psychological distress, depression, suicidal ideation, anxiety, substance abuse and addictions, offending behavior (e.g., aggression, criminal behavior), severe psychopathology (e.g., schizophrenia), health-related distress, and health-compromising behaviors. These results have been found using different measures of social problem-solving ability in a wide range of participants, including both clinical and nonclinical samples and medial patients. Participants have also varied widely in age, nationality, ethnic/racial status, and severity of symptomatology.

A number of studies have provided support for the hypotheses that social problem-solving ability is a mediator and a moderator of the relationship between stressful life events and well-being or adjustment. Specifically, problem-solving ability has been found to moderate the relationship between major negative events and depression (Nezu, Nezu, Saraydarian, Kalmar, & Ronan, 1986; Nezu, Perri, Nezu, & Mahoney, 1987; Nezu, Nezu, Faddis, DelliCarpini, & Houts, 1995) and anxiety (Nezu, 1986b; Nezu et al., 1995). Problem-solving ability has also been found to moderate the relationship between personal and/or interpersonal problems and daily hassles, and anxiety (Londahl, Tverskoy, & D'Zurilla, 2005), aggression (Tverskoy, Londahl, & D'Zurilla, 2007), internalizing symptoms, and externalizing symptoms (Bell & D'Zurilla, in press). Problem-solving ability also mediates the relationship between daily stressful events and emotional well-being (Folkman & Lazarus, 1988), depression (Kant, D'Zurilla, & Maydeu-Olivares, 1997; Nezu & Ronan, 1985; Nezu, Perri, & Nezu, 1987), anxiety (Kant et al., 1997), and internalizing and externalizing symptoms (Bell & D'Zurilla, in press).

Support for the theory of PST has been provided by several outcomes studies that have examined the *process* of PST. In support of the hypothesis that PST reduces maladjustment and psychopathology by increases in social problem-solving ability, several studies have found significant relationships between increases on measures of problem-solving ability following PST and reductions on measures of negative psychological conditions, including psychological stress (D'Zurilla & Maschka, 1988), clinical depression (Nezu, 1987; Nezu & Perri, 1989), and cancer-related anxiety and depression (Nezu, Nezu, Felgoise, McClure, & Houts, 2003a).

Overall, these results are consistent with the assumptions of the social problem-solving model and the relational/problem-solving model of stress and well-being. Therefore, we can conclude that there is strong empirical support for the theory on which PST is based (for a comprehensive review, see also Chang et al., 2004; D'Zurilla & Nezu, 2007; Nezu, 2004).

CLINICAL APPLICATIONS

Practice of Problem-Solving Therapy: General Guidelines and Clinical Considerations

A comprehensive generic manual for conducting PST in an optimal manner is presented in D'Zurilla and Nezu (2007). A companion, "self-help" manual designed for patients, research participants, or laypersons is also available (Nezu et al., 2007). In this section, we offer a general outline of our generic manual as well as some clinical considerations and recommendations that facilitate the effective implementation of PST.

Because PST is effective for a wide range of individuals with diverse psychological, behavioral, and health problems, it is unlikely that any single, standardized manual would be equally appropriate for all participants. Depending on the particular therapy goals, the relevant problematic situations related to these goals, and the problem-solving strengths and weaknesses of particular participants, the emphasis that is required for different aspects or components of problem-solving ability and performance vary. Hence, our generic manual is organized into a set of 14 training modules that focus on different aspects, or components, of social problem-solving ability, or performance, rather than a standard sequence of components with a standard time period for each component. Each module has a different problem-solving objective (e.g., fostering problem-solving self-efficacy beliefs, controlling disruptive emotions, increasing the ability to generate alternative solutions, improving decision-making ability).

Clinicians and researchers can use these modules to design their own PST programs tailored to meet the needs of specific patients or specific research projects. In a clinical setting, the choice of which modules to implement would be based on the treatment goals, the relevant problematic situations, and a comprehensive and individualized assessment of the participants' problem-solving strengths and weaknesses. In a research setting, the choice of modules would be based on specific research questions (e.g., whether to evaluate the entire PST package or specific components of PST).

The modules in our generic manual describe general behavior change principles or "strategies" (e.g., modeling, behavior rehearsal, cognitive restructuring), as well as a variety of specific training exercises, or "tactics," for achieving the problem-solving objectives of each module. However, the specific training activities that are most appropriate or effective are likely to vary across programs, and depend on the goals of the program, the particular mode of implementation (e.g., face-to-face individual therapy, group therapy, telephone counseling), and specific characteristics of the participants (e.g., age, educational level, type of disorder, degree of deficiency in problem-solving abilities and skills). As such, we focus on general behavior change principles and do not equate PST with any "prescribed" set of training exercises or any particular mode of implementation. Hence, when designing a specific PST program for a particular patient or research project, we recommend that clinicians and researchers use their own brainstorming capabilities to identify or design the most appropriate or effective means for achieving the problem-solving objectives of each module, both in terms of different training exercises and different modes of implementation.

PST Training Modules

Table 7.1 provides a list of the 14 modules that comprise our generic PST manual. These modules are geared collectively to achieve the following overall problem-solving treatment goals: (1) Enhance one's positive problem orienta-

TABLE 7.1. **Problem-Solving Training Modules**

Topic	Key training objectives and activities
1. Initial Structuring	• Establish a positive therapeutic relationship. • Present overall rationale and structure of PST and how it can be of specific help to a given client. • Encourage optimism.
2. Assessment	• Formally (e.g., administer SPSI-R) or informally (e.g., interview) assess problem-solving strengths and weaknesses. • Assess areas of a client's life that are stressful.
3. Obstacles to Effective Problem Solving	• Discuss cognitive limits of conscious mind (i.e., difficulties in "multitasking," especially when under stress) • Discuss ways to foster multitasking: (a) "externalization" (e.g., make lists of ideas); (b) "visualization" (e.g., covertly rehearse implementing a solution plan); and (c) "simplification" (e.g., break down complex problem into more manageable subproblems).
4. Problem Orientation: Fostering Self-Efficacy	• Introduce concept and importance of maintaining a positive problem orientation. • Foster client's self-efficacy, for example, use visualization exercise to help client "experience" having successfully solved a problem (i.e., facilitate sense of being able to "see the light at the end of the tunnel").
5. Problem Orientation: Recognizing Problems	• Enhance client's ability to recognize problems when they occur. • Use feelings, ineffective behavior, and certain thoughts as cues that a problem exists. • Use problem checklist to help "normalize" the experience of problems.
6. Problem Orientation: Viewing Problem as Challenges	• Foster the patient's ability to identify and subsequently alter negative thinking, dysfunctional attitudes, and restricted ways of thinking. • Engage in a "reversed advocate role-play" exercise, where the client argues a contrasting point of view from a given maladaptive belief that he or she holds.
7. Problem Orientation: Use and Control of Emotions	• Foster the client's understanding of the role of emotions in problem solving. • Teach patients to (a) "use" emotions to inform the problem-solving process (e.g., as a cue that a problem exists, to facilitate motivation); and (b) manage disruptive emotions (e.g., via cognitive reframing techniques, relaxation exercises).
8. Problem Orientation: STOP & THINK!	• Teach the STOP & THINK technique to inhibit tendencies to be impulsive or avoidant (i.e., to visualize a red STOP sign or traffic light as a cue to "stop" and then to "think" in a problem-solving mode).

(cont.)

TABLE 7.1. *(cont.)*

Topic	Key training objectives and activities
9. Problem Definition and Formulation	• Foster the client's ability to understand better the nature of the problem (e.g., the reasons why it is a problem for that given individual) and to set realistic problem-solving goals and objectives.
10. Generation of Alternatives	• Facilitate the patient's creative ability to produce a wide range and variety of potential solution ideas for a given problem using various brainstorming techniques (e.g., "the more the better").
11. Decision Making	• Enhance the client's ability to make effective decisions by being able to (a) better identify possible consequences to a given action, and (b) conduct a cost–benefit analysis regarding the value and likelihood of various outcomes of a given action.
12. Solution Implementation and Verification	• Foster the individual's ability to (a) carry out a solution plan effectively, (b) monitor its outcome, (c) evaluate its effectiveness, and (d) engage in self- reinforcement in the process of problem solving, as well as the possible success of the actual outcome.
13. Guided Practice	• Maximize proficiency in the application of problem-solving attitudes and skills, and facilitate the transfer and generalization of these attitudes and skills to a variety of current and future stressful problems in the natural environment.
14. Rapid Problem Solving	• Teach the client a set of problem-solving questions/guidelines that help him or her to apply the overall model in just a few minutes.

tion; (2) decrease one's negative orientation; (3) foster one's ability to apply rational problem-solving skills; (4) reduce one's tendency to avoid problem solving; and (5) minimize one's tendency to be impulsive and careless. To be considered a sufficient test of PST, we suggest that a stand-alone intervention, at a minimum, contain training in the goals represented in modules 1 through 13.

Depending on the population, training can proceed in one of three ways after an initial introductory session: (1) Each subsequent session is devoted to a specific problem-solving dimension (e.g., training in problem orientation is provided in session 2, problem definition and formulation (PDF) training in session 3, generation of alternatives (GOA) training in session 4, and so forth; (see Nezu & Perri, 1989, Nezu et al., 2003a, for examples of outcome investigations that used this approach); (2) training in problem orientation is conducted in the next one (or two) sessions, followed by a session devoted to all four rational problem-solving skills, followed by multiple sessions devoted to guided practice; and (3) training in problem orientation is highlighted across several sessions in the beginning, if research findings identify a given population that requires such training (see Nezu, 2004).

Use of Adjunctive Training Strategies

Similar to many other directive forms of psychotherapy or counseling, in particular those under a cognitive-behavioral umbrella, the success of PST to a large degree depends on the effectiveness of its implementation. The PST therapist needs to be competent in various adjunctive treatment strategies that foster competent PST implementation, including the following:

- Didactic instruction (e.g., teaching specific problem-solving principles)
- Coaching (e.g., verbal prompting of possible alternative solutions to a problem)
- Modeling (e.g., demonstrating specific ways to apply various problem-solving principles)
- Shaping (e.g., training in progressively more difficult steps)
- Rehearsal (e.g., practicing applying various problem-solving exercises to real-life problems)
- Feedback (e.g., providing corrective evaluations)
- Positive reinforcement (e.g., praising a client's efforts)

Beyond these skill sets, the following list of PST "Dos and Don'ts" are offered as important clinical considerations based on our experience in both clinical and research settings regarding the competent implementation of PST (see also Nezu et al., 1998):

- DO attempt to build a positive therapeutic relationship.
- DO be enthusiastic and optimistic.
- DO encourage active participation.
- DO make PST highly relevant to a particular client or group.
- DO include homework assignments.
- DO follow-up on homework.
- DO focus on solution implementation.
- DO use both "problem-focused" goals (i.e., goals involving changing the problematic nature of a stressful situation), and "emotion-focused" goals (i.e., objectives focused on minimizing one's emotional distress related to the problem).
- DO use handouts as adjuncts to training.
- DO conduct an assessment of an individual's problem-solving strengths and weaknesses.
- DON'T present PST in a mechanistic manner.
- DON'T focus only on superficial problems.

Patient Manual

As noted earlier, we have recently developed a self-help problem-solving training guidebook for the patient, research participant, or any layperson interested in the enhancement of his or her ability to cope effectively with stress (Nezu et al., 2007). This self-help manual reflects the recommendations for the clinician or researcher just presented. Because PST helps individuals to adapt more successfully to their environments, this approach uses the acronym ADAPT, as described below, to remind individuals to engage in the five problem-solving steps of our model:

A = *Attitude*. Before attempting to solve the problem, individuals should adopt a positive, optimistic *attitude* (i.e., problem orientation) toward the problem and their problem-solving ability.

D = *Define*. This step recommends that individuals, after adopting a positive attitude, *define* the problem by obtaining relevant facts, identifying obstacles that inhibit goal achievement, and specifying a realistic goal.

A = *Alternatives*. Based on a well-defined problem, persons are directed to generate a variety of different alternatives to overcome any identified obstacles and achieve the problem-solving goal.

P = *Predict*. After generating a list of alternatives, people are directed to predict both the positive and negative consequences of each alternative, and to choose the one(s) that has the highest probability to achieve the problem-solving goal, while minimizing costs and maximizing benefits.

T = *Try out*. When individuals have chosen a solution, they are then asked to try out the solution in real-life and monitor its effects. If they are satisfied with the results, the problem is solved and they should engage in self-reinforcement. If they are not satisfied, they are then directed to go back to the "A" step and search for a more effective solution.

EFFICACY OF PROBLEM-SOLVING THERAPY: OVERVIEW OF OUTCOME STUDIES

In this last section, we provide an overview of the outcome literature regarding the efficacy of PST. To prevent redundancy, however, we focus only on a representative sample of those investigations published since 2000, because studies prior to that date have already been reviewed in previous versions of this volume (D'Zurilla & Nezu, 1999). The described studies include the following categories: schizophrenia, depression, generalized anxiety disorder, caregivers, obesity, headaches, cancer, diabetes, and offenders. Although no related studies have been published since 2000, PST was previously found to be effective for the following problems and patient groups: suicide, social phobia, distressed couples, parent–child problems, primary care patients, persons with mental retardation, back pain, substance abuse, head-injured patients, and arthritis (see D'Zurilla & Nezu, 2007, for a review).

Patients with Schizophrenia

Liberman, Eckman, and Marder (2001) randomly assigned 75 adult outpatients diagnosed with schizophrenia either to 4 months of weekly PST group sessions or an equal amount of supportive group therapy. Results indicated that although both sets of patients improved at posttreatment regarding their ability to identify problems, PST participants demonstrated significant improvements in other assessed problem-solving dimensions, such as generating alternatives, decision making, role-play skills, and overall role-play performance.

Glynn et al. (2002) compared a clinic-based skills training approach with a similar program supplemented by manual-based generalization sessions in the community. PST training was one of three major skills sets included in both treatment conditions; the other two involved medication management and effective living skills. Results indicated that generalization training in the community led to significant posttreatment improvements in instrumental role functioning, social relations, and overall adjustment. Moreover, these rates of improvement in social functioning were coupled with low rates of psychiatric exacerbation.

Depression

Based on a model of depression that underscores the important role that problem-solving deficits play in its etiopathogenesis (Nezu et al., 1989), early treatment studies found PST to be particularly effective in reducing depressive symptomatology (e.g., Nezu, 1986c). Researchers continue to find PST to be an evidenced-based intervention for major depressive disorder. In fact, the authors of one recent meta-analysis focusing specifically on PST for depression concluded that although additional research is needed, "there is no doubt that PST can be an effective treatment for depression" (Cuijpers, van Straten, & Warmerdam, 2007, p. 9). Another recent meta-analysis led to the same conclusion for both post-treatment and follow-up results (Bell & D'Zurilla, 2009). In addition, although PST was not found to be more effective than alternative psychosocial therapies or psychiatric medication, it was more effective than supportive therapy/attention control groups. Significant moderators of treatment effectiveness included whether the PST program included problem orientation training, whether all four problem-solving skills were included, and whether all five components were included (i.e., problem orientation and the four problem-solving skills). Another moderator that approached significance ($p = .06$) was whether the SPSI-R (D'Zurilla et al., 2002) was administered before treatment to assess strengths and weaknesses in social problem-solving abilities.

As an example, Alexapoulos, Raue, and Areán (2003) compared PST with supportive therapy (ST) in a group of depressed older adult individuals who also exhibited impairment in executive functioning. Results indicated that PST was more effective than ST in engendering remission of depression, fewer posttreatment depressive symptoms, and less overall neurocognitive disability. In another trial, Mynors-Wallis, Gath, Day, and Baker (2000) compared the following four treatment conditions regarding depressed primary care patients: (1) PST as provided by research general practitioners; (2) PST as given by research practice nurses; (3) antidepressant medication (either fluvoxamine or paroxetine) provided by research general practitioners; and (4) a combined PST and medication package. Results indicated that patients in all four conditions improved over the course of 12 weeks. The combined treatment was found to be no more effective than either PST or medication treatment alone. In addition, there was no difference in outcome based on whether physicians or nurses delivered PST.

PST has been studied as a treatment for dysthymia and minor depression in primary care. The Treatment Effectiveness Project (Barrett et al., 1999) was the first large-scale evaluation in the United States of PST for primary care patients (PST-PC). PST-PC is described as a collaborative treatment approach in which a patient's symptoms are first identified and linked to various problems in living. Such problems are then defined and clarified, and attempts are made next to solve them in a structured manner (Hegel, Barrett, & Oxman, 2000). Williams et al. (2000) provide the results of an evaluation comparing PST-PC to either paroxetine or placebo with specific regard to a group of 415 older primary care adults. Patients receiving the active medication were found to show greater symptom resolution than did placebo patients. Whereas no differences at posttreatment were found between PST-PC and placebo patients, PST-PC patients' symptoms improved more rapidly than those of placebo patients during the latter treatment weeks. With regard to patients diagnosed with minor depression, both the paroxetine and PST-PC conditions led to improved overall mental health functioning compared with the placebo condition, but only with regard to those individuals in the lowest tertile of baseline functioning. Moreover, it appeared that the PST-PC effects were more subject to site differences than those of the drug treatment.

Generalized Anxiety Disorder

Ladouceur, Dugas, Freeston, Gagnon, and Thibodeau (2000) compared a generalized anxiety disorder (GAD) intervention that targeted intolerance of uncertainty, erroneous beliefs about worry, poor problem orientation, and cognitive avoidance with a delayed treatment control. Training in problem orientation was included in a larger treatment package and had patients remain focused on the problem and not pay undue attention to related minor details. Worries about situations not amenable to problem solving were treated with cognitive exposure to decrease the threatening nature of the worry itself. Results indicated that the overall treatment package led to both statistically and clinically significant changes at posttreatment, and that these gains were maintained at 6- and 12-month follow-ups.

Dugas et al. (2003) treated GAD by targeting intolerance of uncertainty via the reevaluation of positive beliefs about worry, cognitive exposure, and PST. Treatment comprised 14 weekly, 2-hour group sessions and was compared with a waiting-list control. The cognitive-behavioral intervention demonstrated significantly greater improvement on all dependent measures (i.e., self-report and clinician ratings of GAD symptoms, intolerance of uncertainty, anxiety, depression, and social adjustment) compared with the control. Moreover, treated participants made further gains over the course of a 2-year follow-up period. In an examination of the efficacy of each of the two major treatment components of their GAD intervention, Provencher, Dugas, and Ladouceur (2004) conducted a case replication series of 18 primary GAD patients who received 12 sessions of their cognitive-behavioral treatment. The therapy was individualized according to the main worries of a given patient, PST was provided for worries about current problems, and cognitive exposure was applied to worries about hypothetical situations. Results indicated that both intervention strategies led to significant improvements on all outcome measures, which were maintained at a 6-month follow-up.

Caregivers

Due to the often significant distress and levels of burden experienced by family caregivers of persons with medical problems, PST has also been evaluated as a potentially important intervention for such individuals (C. M. Nezu, Palmatier, & Nezu, 2004). For example, Gallagher-Thompson et al. (2000) compared PST with a program geared to increase pleasant events and to a waiting-list control, with regard to reductions in depression and feelings of burden in family caregivers of physically or cognitively impaired older adults. Results indicated that both treatments engendered significant improvement compared with the waiting-list control.

Grant, Elliott, Weaver, Bartolucci, and Giger (2002) also compared PST, a sham intervention, and a control with regard to 74 caregivers of individuals who suffered a stroke. Results indicated that, compared with the sham and control conditions, family caregivers receiving PST training evidenced better problem-solving skills, greater caregiver preparedness, less depression, and significant improvements in measures of vitality, social functioning, mental health, and role limitations related to emotional problems.

Wade, Wolfe, Brown, and Pestian (2005) conducted an open trial of a Web-based family problem-solving intervention geared to improve parent and child adaptation in families of children who suffered moderate to severe traumatic brain injury. Families were provided with computers, Web cameras, and high-speed Internet access. Therapists conducted weekly videoconferences with the families who completed self-guided Web exercises about problem solving, communication, and antecedent behavior management strategies. Results revealed significant improvements in injury-related burden, parental psychiatric symptoms, depression, and parenting stress. Although no significant improvement was found for children's self-reported depression, there was a significant decrease in antisocial behaviors in the injured children.

Obesity

In addition to evaluations as a stand-alone treatment, PST has been used as an adjunct to foster the effectiveness of other intervention strategies (Nezu & Nezu, 2006). For example, Perri et al. (2001) hypothesized that PST would foster adherence to a behavioral weight loss intervention by helping individuals to overcome barriers to adherence such as scheduling difficulties, completing homework assignments, or the interference of psychological distress. After completion of 20 weekly group sessions of standard behavioral treatment therapy (BT) for obesity, 80 women were randomly assigned to one of three conditions: (1) no further contact (BT only); (2) relapse prevention training (RP); and (3) PST. At the end of 17 months, no differences in overall weight loss were observed between RP and BT-only, or between RP and PST. However, PST participants had significantly greater long-term weight reductions than BT-only participants, and a significantly larger percentage of PST participants achieved "clinically significant" losses of 10% or more body weight that did BT-only members (approximately 35 vs. 6%).

Recurrent Headaches

PST was combined with applied relaxation to treat recurrent headaches in a delivery mode that included the Internet and e-mail (Ström, Pettersson, & Andersson, 2000). Headache sufferers ($N = 102$) were randomly assigned to either the treatment condition or to a waiting-list control. The intervention was delivered over the course of 6 weeks, with a new segment sent to participants on a weekly basis to encourage consistent participation. Pre- and post-treatment analyses indicated that the PST plus relaxation intervention led to a statistically significant reduction in headaches and that among 50% of these, the reduction was clinically significant. One of the more important outcomes of this study was the notion that a low-cost method of treatment delivery could be clinically effective.

Cancer

Given the high prevalence of psychological distress experienced by cancer patients and their families, researchers have looked at the potential efficacy of various psychosocial interventions to address this public health concern (Nezu, Nezu, Felgoise, & Zwick, 2003b). For example, Mishel et al. (2002) paired training in problem solving with a cognitive reframing strategy to help males diagnosed with localized prostate carcinoma to manage their levels of uncertainty and symptom control. Participants were randomly assigned to one of three experimental conditions: combined psychosocial treatment provided to the patient, treatment provided to the patient and a selected family member, and a treatment-as-usual control. Participants who received either form of the intervention improved significantly by the 4-month assessment period, which is a critical period of time when cancer treatment side effects are most prevalent. As such, it is particularly noteworthy that the combined PST and cognitive reframing treatment led to significant improvement in control of incontinence 4-months postbaseline.

Allen et al. (2002) assessed the efficacy of PST as a stand-alone intervention compared to a no-treatment control in a sample of 164 women diagnosed with breast cancer, and for whom a first course of chemotherapy had been recently initiated. PST comprised two in-person and four telephone sessions with an oncology nurse who provided PST to the women over a 12-week period. At a 4-month evaluation, participants in general tended to have significantly fewer unmet needs and better mental health compared to baseline. Differences between the two conditions emerged at the 8-month assessment, which pointed to the efficacy of PST training. In general, PST led to improved mood and more effective coping with problems associated with daily living tasks. Furthermore, the intervention helped the majority of women to resolve a range of problems related to cancer and its treatment, including physical side effects, marital and sexual difficulties, and psychological problems. However, an unexpected finding emerged, because women who had baseline scores characteristic of "poor problem solving" were less likely to resolve cancer-related problems, relative to the control participants.

Nezu et al. (2003a) evaluated the efficacy of PST for 132 adult cancer patients. In this clinical trial, adult cancer patients who were experiencing significant distress (e.g., depression) were randomly assigned to one of three conditions: (1) individual PST; (2) PST provided simultaneously to the cancer patient and to his or her designated significant other (e.g., spouse, family member); and (3) a treatment-as-usual control. Results at posttreatment supported the efficacy of PST with respect to decreases in emotional distress and improvement in overall quality of life across several self-report ratings, clinician ratings, and ratings by the significant other. Specifically, patients in both treatment conditions were found to evidence significant improvement compared to individuals in the control condition. At posttreatment, no differences were found between these two conditions. However, at a 6-month follow-up assessment, patients who received PST along with a significant other continued to improve significantly beyond those individuals receiving PST by themselves, highlighting the advantage of the formal inclusion of a collaborative person in treatment.

Sahler et al. (2002) randomly assigned 92 mothers of newly diagnosed pediatric cancer patients to one of two conditions: PST and standard psychosocial care. The results indicated that mothers in the PST condition has significantly enhanced problem-solving skills and significantly decreased negative affectivity at posttreatment compared to the control group. Moreover, analyses revealed that changes in self-reports of problem-solving behaviors accounted for 40% of the difference in mood scores between the two conditions, and that the intervention had the greatest impact on improving constructive problem solving, whereas improvement in mood was most influenced by decreases in dysfunctional problem solving.

In an extension of this work, Sahler et al. (2005) assessed the efficacy of an 8-week PST compared to a usual care control in a sample of 430 English- and Spanish-speaking mothers of pediatric cancer patients. Results from this investigation replicated the 2007 study, indicating that mothers who received the PST protocol had significantly enhanced problem-solving skills and decreased negative affectivity. Whereas treatment effects appeared to be greatest at posttreatment, several differences were maintained at the 3-month follow-up.

Diabetes

Problem solving is often identified as a key ingredient of chronic illness self-management (Bodenheimer, Lorig, Holman, & Grumbach, 2002) and is a component of many successful diabetes management programs (Glasgow, Toobert, Barrera, & Stryker, 2004). Glasgow et al. conducted a series of mediational analyses to determine whether problem solving was related to improved outcomes regarding a multiple-lifestyle behavior change program (called the Mediterranean Lifestyle Program; MLP) developed for postmenopausal women with type 2 diabetes and at risk for coronary heart disease. The MLP program (Toobert, Glasgow, Barrera, & Bagdade, 2002) addressed changes in diet, physical activity, stress management, and social support. Patients were randomly assigned to a usual care control condition ($N = 116$) and to the MLP program ($N = 163$). Mediational analyses indicated that (1) problem solving improved significantly more in the MLP group than in controls, and (2) this increase was a partial mediator of positive outcome (e.g., changes in self-efficacy, decreases in caloric intake).

Offenders

PST has for the past several decades been a component of several different programs geared to decrease recidivism rates among a variety of offender populations, both in Europe and in the United States (McMurran & McGuire, 2005). This work is based in part on empirical literature that has identified links between social problem solving and aggression (Keltikangas-Järvinen, 2005), personality disorders (Dreer, Jackson, & Elliott, 2005; McMurran, Egan, & Duggan, 2005), and sex offending (C. M. Nezu, Nezu, Dudek, Peacock, & Stoll, 2005).

Think First, a treatment program that relies heavily on PST as a major intervention component, includes problem-solving training, self-management training, social interaction training, and values education. The overall goals of Think First are to help individuals acquire, develop, and apply a series of social problem-solving and allied skills that will enable them to manage difficulties in their lives and avoid future reoffending (McGuire, 2005). Due to the inherent difficulties in conducting such research with this population (e.g., a community's intolerance of having offenders in "no-treatment control" conditions), there are no randomized controlled trials of the Think First program as implemented in either community (i.e., probation) or institutional (i.e., prison) settings. However, McGuire and Hatcher (2001) provide pre- and posttreatment data from an open trial of 225 offenders who completed the program in probation settings. Significant improvements were identified regarding problems, criminal attitudes, impulsivity, self-esteem, and empathy. Furthermore, although other, similar short-term and follow-up evaluation studies are generally positive and encouraging, the program's efficacy has yet to be demonstrated within the context of a methodologically well-controlled study.

We are currently in the process of analyzing the results of a randomized controlled trial of PST for paroled sex offenders (C. M. Nezu, Nezu, Heilbrun, Clair, & DiFrancisco, 2009). Subjects were initially allocated to one of two conditions: 20 sessions of group PST versus a waiting-list control. At posttreatment, offenders who previously received PST were further assigned to either a no-further-contact control or a maintenance protocol (practicing application of PST with a "buddy"). Rearrest/reoffense data are being collected for both 1-year and 5-year follow-up assessments. This study will provide information regarding the potential efficacy of PST as an intervention for this population, as well as its relevance as a maintenance strategy.

Summary

Similar to previous reviews, this overview of outcome investigations strongly suggests that PST is both an efficacious and flexible intervention for a variety of patient populations and problems. In fact, in addition to the positive conclusions from the meta-analyses specific to PST investigations focused on depression cited earlier (Bell & D'Zurilla, 2009; Cuijpers et al., 2007), another recent meta-analysis conducted across 32 studies, with a total of 2,895 participants with a variety of mental and physical health problems, provides strong quantitative evidence of its efficacy (Malouff, Thorsteinsson, & Schutte, 2007). Specifically, although not found to be significantly more effective than other psychosocial treatments ($d = 0.22$), PST was significantly more effective than either no treatment ($d = 1.37$) or attention placebo ($d = 0.54$). Significant moderators of these results included whether the PST protocol included training in problem orientation (see Nezu, 2004; Nezu & Perri, 1989), whether homework was assigned, or whether a developer of PST (i.e., A. M. Nezu) helped to conduct the investigation.

SUMMARY AND CONCLUSIONS

PST is a positive approach to clinical intervention that focuses on training in adaptive problem-solving attitudes and skills. The theory of PST is based on a relational/problem-solving model of stress and well-being, in which the concept of "social problem solving" (i.e., real-life problem solving) is assumed to play an important role as a general and versatile coping strategy. According to this model, PST reduces and prevents psychopathology by increasing a person's ability to cope effectively with a wide range of stressful problems in living. Within this approach, effective coping includes (1) changing stressful situations for the better (problem-focused coping) and (2) adapting to adverse conditions that cannot be changed or controlled (emotion-focused coping).

The generic PST manual (D'Zurilla & Nezu, 2007) comprises a set of training modules that focus on different aspects or components of social problem-solving ability and performance. These modules describe general behavior change principles or strategies, as well as a variety of specific training exercises or tactics. Using these modules, clinicians and researchers can design their own unique PST programs tailored for specific patients or research projects. A companion, "self-help" manual designed for patients, research participants, or laypersons is also available (Nezu, Nezu, & D'Zurilla, 2007).

Over the past three decades, a large body of accumulated research evidence has provides substantial support for the theory of PST, as well as the efficacy of this approach for a wide range of psychological, behavioral, and health disorders. Based on this research evidence, it can be concluded that PST is a potentially useful and effective intervention for any disorder in which stress and coping deficits play an important role as maintaining conditions.

REFERENCES

Alexopoulus, G. S., Raue, P., Areán, P. (2003). Problem-solving therapy versus supportive therapy in geriatric major depression with executive dysfunction. *American Journal of Geriatric Psychiatry, 11*, 46–52.

Allen, S. M., Shah, A. C., Nezu, A. M., Nezu, C. M., Ciambrone, D., Hogan, J., et al. (2002). A problem-solving approach to stress reduction among younger women with breast carcinoma: A randomized controlled trial. *Cancer, 94*, 3089–3100.

Barrett, J. E., Williams, J. W., Oxman, T. E., Katon, W., Frank, E., Hegel, M. T., et al. (1999). The Treatment Effectiveness project: A comparison of the effectiveness of paroxetine, problem-solving therapy, and placebo in the treatment of minor depression and dysthymia in primary care patients: Background and research plan. *General Hospital Psychiatry, 21*, 260–273.

Bell, A. C., & D'Zurilla, T. J. (in press). The influence of social problem solving on the relationship between daily stress and adjustment. *Cognitive Therapy and Research*.

Bell, A. C., & D'Zurilla, T. J. (2009). Problem-solving therapy for depression: A meta-analysis. *Clinical Psychology Review, 29*, 348–353.

Bloom, B. L. (1985). *Stressful life event theory and research: Implications for primary prevention* [D.H.H.S. Publication No. (AMD) 85-1385]. Rockville, MD: National Institute of Mental Health.

Bodenheimer, T. S., Lorig, K., Holman, H., & Grumbach, K. (2002). Patient self-management of chronic disease in primary care. *Journal of the American Medical Association, 288*, 2469–2475.

Burks, N., & Martin, B. (1985). Everyday problems and life change events: Ongoing vs. acute sources of stress. *Journal of Human Stress, 11*, 27–35.

Chang, E. C., D'Zurilla, T. J., & Sanna, L. J. (Eds.). (2004). *Social problem solving: Theory, research, and training.* Washington, DC: American Psychological Association.

Cuijpers, P., van Straten, A., & Warmerdam, L. (2007). Problem solving therapies for depression: A meta-analysis. *European Psychiatry, 22*, 9–15.

DeLongis, A., Coyne, J., Dakof, G., Folkman, S., & Lazarus, R. S. (1982). Relationship of daily hassles, uplifts, and major life events to health status. *Health Psychology, 1*, 119–136.

Dreer, L. E., Jackson, W. T., & Elliott, T. R. (2005). Social problem solving, personality disorder, and substance abuse. In M. McMarran & J. McGuire (Eds.), *Social problem solving and offending: Evidence, evaluation, and evolution* (pp. 67–90). Chichester, UK: Wiley.

Dugas, M. J., Ladouceur, R., Léger, E., Freeston, M. H., Langlois, F., Provencher, M. D., et al. (2003). Group cognitive-behavioral therapy for generalized anxiety disorder: Treatment outcome and long-term follow-up. *Journal of Consulting and Clinical Psychology, 71*, 821–825.

D'Zurilla, T. J. (1986). *Problem-solving therapy: A social competence approach to clinical intervention.* New York: Springer.

D'Zurilla, T. J. (1990). Problem-solving training for effective stress management and prevention. *Journal of Cognitive Psychotherapy: An International Quarterly, 4*, 327–355.

D'Zurilla, T. J., & Goldfried, M. R. (1971). Problem solving and behavior modification. *Journal of Abnormal Psychology, 78*, 107–126.

D'Zurilla, T. J., & Maschka, G. (1988, November). *Outcome of a problem-solving approach to stress management: I. Comparison with social support.* Paper presented at the Association for Advancement of Behavior Therapy Convention, New York, NY.

D'Zurilla, T. J., & Nezu, A. (1982). Social problem solving in adults. In P. C. Kendall (Ed.), *Advances in cognitive-behavioral research and therapy* (Vol. 1, pp. 202–274). New York: Academic Press.

D'Zurilla, T. J., & Nezu, A. M. (1990). Development and preliminary evaluation of the Social Problem-Solving Inventory (SPSI). *Psychological Assessment: A Journal of Consulting and Clinical Psychology, 2*, 156–163.

D'Zurilla, T. J., & Nezu, A. M. (1999). *Problem-solving therapy: A social competence approach to clinical intervention* (2nd ed.). New York: Springer.

D'Zurilla, T. J., & Nezu, A. M. (2007). *Problem-solving therapy: A positive approach to clinical intervention* (3rd ed.). New York: Springer.

D'Zurilla, T. J., Nezu, A. M., & Maydeu-Olivares, A. (2002). *Social Problem-Solving Inventory—Revised: Technical manual.* North Tonawanda, NY: Multi-Health Systems.

Folkman, S., & Lazarus, R. S. (1988). Coping as a mediator of emotion. *Journal of Personality and Social Psychology, 54*, 466–475.

Frauenknecht, M., & Black, D.R. (2004). Problem-solving training for children and adolescents. In E. C. Chang, T. J. D'Zurilla, & L. J. Sanna (Eds.), *Social problem solving: Theory, research, and training* (pp. 153–170). Washington, DC: American Psychological Association.

Gagné, R.M. (1966). Human problem solving: Internal and external events. In B.

Kleinmutz (Ed.), *Problem solving: Research, method, and theory*. New York: Wiley.

Gallagher-Thompson, D., Lovett, S., Rose, J., McKibbin, C., Coon, D., Futterman, A., et al. (2000). Impact of psychoeducational interventions on distressed caregivers. *Journal of Clinical Geropsychology, 6*, 91–110.

Glasgow, R. E., Toobert, D. J., Barrera, M., & Stryker, L. A. (2004). Assessment of problem-solving: A key to successful diabetes self-management. *Journal of Behavioral Medicine, 27*, 477–490.

Glynn, S. M., Marder, S. R., Liberman, R. P., Blair, K., Wirshing, W. C., Wirshing, D. A., et al. (2002). Supplementing clinic-based skills training with manual-based community support sessions: Effects on social adjustment of patients with schizophrenia. *American Journal of Psychiatry, 159*, 829–837.

Graf, A. (2003). A psychometric test of a German version of the SPSI-R. *Zeitschrift für Differentielle und Diagnostische Psychologie, 24*, 277–291.

Grant, J. S., Elliott, T., Weaver, M., Bartolucci, A., & Giger, J. N. (2002). Telephone intervention with family caregivers of stroke survivors after rehabilitation. *Stroke, 33*, 2060–2065.

Hegel, M. T., Barrett, J. E., & Oxman, T. E. (2000). Training therapists in problem-solving treatment of depressive disorders in primary care: Lessons learned from the "Treatment Effectiveness Project." *Families, Systems, and Health, 18*, 423–435.

Kant, G. L., D'Zurilla, T. J., & Maydeu-Olivares, A. (1997). Social problem solving as a mediator of stress-related depression and anxiety in middle-aged and elderly community residents. *Cognitive Therapy and Research, 21*, 73–96.

Keltikangas-Järvinen, L. (2005). Social problem solving and the development of aggression. In M. McMurran & J. McGuire (Eds.), *Social problem solving and offending: Evidence, evaluation and evolution* (pp. 31–50). Chichester, UK: Wiley.

Kendall, P. C., & Hollon, S. D. (Eds.). (1979). *Cognitive-behavioral interventions: Theory, research, and procedures*. New York: Academic Press.

Ladouceur, R., Dugas, M. J., Freeston, M. H., Gagnon, F., & Thibodeau, N. (2000). Efficacy of a cognitive-behavioral treatment for generalized anxiety disorder: Evaluation in a controlled clinical trial. *Journal of Consulting and Clinical Psychology, 68*, 957–964.

Lazarus, R. S. (1999). *Stress and emotion: A new synthesis*. New York: Springer.

Lazarus, R. S., & Folkman, S. (1984). *Stress, appraisal, and coping*. New York: Springer.

Liberman, R. P., Eckman, T., & Marder, S. R. (2001). Training in social problem solving among persons with schizophrenia. *Psychiatric Services, 52*, 31–33.

Londahl, E.A., Tverskoy, A., & D'Zurilla, T.J. (2005). The relations of internalizing symptoms to conflict and interpersonal problem solving in close relationships. *Cognitive Therapy and Research, 29*, 445–462.

Mahoney, M. J. (1974). *Cognition and behavior modification*. Cambridge, MA: Ballinger.

Malouff, J. M., Thorsteinsson, E. B., & Schutte, N. S. (2007). The efficacy of problem solving therapy in reducing mental and physical health problems: A meta-analysis. *Clinical Psychology Review, 27*, 46–57.

Maydeu-Olivares, A., & D'Zurilla, T.J. (1995). A factor analysis of the Social

Problem-Solving Inventory using polychoric correlations. *European Journal of Psychological Assessment, 11,* 98–107.

Maydeu-Olivares, A., & D'Zurilla, T. J. (1996). A factor-analytic study of the Social Problem-Solving Inventory: An integration of theory and data. *Cognitive Therapy and Research, 20,* 115–133.

Maydeu-Olivares, A., Rodríguez-Fornells, A., Gómez-Benito, J., & D'Zurilla, T. J. (2000). Psychometric properties of the Spanish adaptation of the Social Problem-Solving Inventory—Revised (SPSI-R). *Personality and Individual Differences, 29,* 699–708.

McGuire, J. (2005). The Think First programme. In M. McMurran & J. McGuire (Eds.), *Social problem solving and offending: Evidence, evaluation and evolution* (pp. 183–206). Chichester, UK: Wiley.

McGuire, J., & Hatcher, R. (2001). Offense-focused problem solving: Preliminary evaluation of a cognitive skills program. *Criminal Justice and Behavior, 28,* 564–587.

McMurran, M., Egan, V., & Duggan, C. (2005). Stop & Think!: Social problem-solving therapy with personality-disordered offenders. In M. McMurran & J. McGuire (Eds.), *Social problem solving and offending: Evidence, evaluation and evolution* (pp. 207–220). Chichester, UK: Wiley.

McMurran, M., & McGuire, J. (Eds.). (2005). *Social problem solving and offending: Evidence, evaluation and evolution.* Chichester, UK: Wiley.

Mishel, M. H., Belyea, M., Gemino, B. B., Stewart, J. L., Bailey, D. E., Robertson, C., et al. (2002). Helping patients with localized prostate carcinoma manage uncertainty and treatment side effects: Nurse delivered psychoeducational intervention over the telephone. *Cancer, 94,* 1854–1866.

Mynors-Wallis, L. M., Gath, D. H., Day, A., & Baker, F. (2000). Randomised controlled trial of problem solving treatment, antidepressant medication, and combined treatment for major depression in primary care. *British Medical Journal, 2,* 26–30.

Nezu, A. M. (1986a). Effects of stress from current problems: Comparisons to major life events. *Journal of Clinical Psychology, 42,* 847–852.

Nezu, A. M. (1986b). Negative life stress and anxiety: Problem solving as a moderator variable. *Psychological Reports, 58,* 279–283.

Nezu, A. M. (1986c). Efficacy of a social problem-solving therapy approach for unipolar depression. *Journal of Consulting and Clinical Psychology, 54,* 196–202.

Nezu, A. M. (1987). A problem-solving formulation of depression: A literature review and proposal of a pluralistic model. *Clinical Psychology Review, 7,* 121–144.

Nezu, A. M. (2004). Problem solving and behavior therapy revisited. *Behavior Therapy, 35,* 1–33.

Nezu, A. M., & D'Zurilla, T. J. (1989). Social problem solving and negative affective conditions. In P. C. Kendall & D. Watson (Eds.), *Anxiety and depression: Distinctive and overlapping features* (pp. 285–315). New York: Academic Press.

Nezu, A. M., & Nezu, C. M. (2006). Problem solving to promote treatment adherence. In W. T. O'Donohue & E. Livens (Eds.), *Promoting treatment adherence: A practical handbook for health care providers* (pp. 135–148). New York: Sage.

Nezu, A. M., Nezu, C. M., & D'Zurilla, T. J. (2007). *Solving life's problems: A 5-step guide to enhanced well-being.* New York: Springer.

Nezu, A. M., Nezu, C. M., Faddis, S., DelliCarpini, L. A., & Houts, P. S. (1995,

November). *Social problem solving as a moderator of cancer-related stress.* Paper presented to the Association for Advancement of Behavior Therapy, Washington, DC.

Nezu, A. M., Nezu, C. M., Felgoise, S. H., McClure, K. S., & Houts, P. S. (2003a). Project Genesis: Assessing the efficacy of problem-solving therapy for distressed adult cancer patients. *Journal of Consulting and Clinical Psychology, 71,* 1036–1048.

Nezu, A. M., Nezu, C. M., Felgoise, S. H., & Zwick, M. L. (2003b). Psychosocial oncology. In I. B. Weiner (Editor-in-Chief) & A. M. Nezu, C. M. Nezu, & P. A. Geller (Eds.), *Handbook of psychology: Vol. 9. Health psychology* (pp. 267–292). New York: Wiley.

Nezu, A. M., Nezu, C. M., Friedman, S. H., Faddis, S., & Houts, P. S. (1998). *Helping cancer patients cope: A problem-solving approach.* Washington, DC: American Psychological Association.

Nezu, A. M., Nezu, C. M., & Perri, M. G. (1989). *Problem-solving therapy for depression: Therapy, research, and clinical guidelines.* New York: Wiley.

Nezu, A. M., Nezu, C. M., Saraydarian, L., Kalmar, K., & Ronan, G. F. (1986). Social problem solving as a moderator variable between negative life stress and depressive symptoms. *Cognitive Therapy and Research, 10,* 489–498.

Nezu, A. M., & Perri, M. G. (1989). Social problem solving therapy for unipolar depression: An initial dismantling investigation. *Journal of Consulting and Clinical Psychology, 57,* 408–413.

Nezu, A. M., Perri, M. G., & Nezu, C. M. (1987, August). *Validation of a problem-solving/stress model of depression.* Paper presented at the American Psychological Association Convention, New York, NY.

Nezu, A. M., Perri, M. G., Nezu, C. M., & Mahoney, D. J. (1987, November). *Social problem solving as a moderator of stressful events among clinically depressed individuals.* Paper presented at the Association for Advancement of Behavior Therapy Convention, Boston, MA.

Nezu, A. M., & Ronan, G. F. (1985). Life stress, current problems, problem solving, and depressive symptomatology: An integrative model. *Journal of Consulting and Clinical Psychology, 53,* 693–697.

Nezu, C. M., D'Zurilla, T. J., & Nezu, A. M. (2005). Problem-solving therapy: Theory, practice, and application to sex offenders. In M. McMurran & J. McGuire (Eds.), *Social problem solving and offenders: Evidence, evaluation and evolution* (pp. 103–123). Chichester, UK: Wiley.

Nezu, C. M., Nezu, A. M., Dudek, J. A., Peacock, M., & Stoll, J. (2005). Social problem-solving correlates of sexual deviancy and aggression among adult child molesters. *Journal of Sexual Aggression, 11,* 27–36.

Nezu, C. M., Nezu, A. M., Heilbrun, K., Clair, M., & DiFrancisco, M. (2009). *Problem-solving therapy for sexual offenders: A randomized clinical trial.* Manuscript submitted for publication.

Nezu, C. M., Palmatier, A., & Nezu, A. M. (2004). Social problem-solving training for caregivers. In E. C. Chang, T. J. D'Zurilla, & L. J. Sanna (Eds.), *Social problem solving: Theory, research, and training* (pp. 223– 238). Washington, DC: American Psychological Association.

Perri, M. G., Nezu, A. M., McKelvey, W. F., Schein, R. L., Renjilian, D. A., & Viegener, B. J. (2001). Relapse prevention training and problem-solving therapy in the long-term management of obesity. *Journal of Consulting and Clinical Psychology, 69,* 722–726.

Provencher, M. D., Dugas, M. J., & Ladouceur, R. (2004). Efficacy of problem-solving training and cognitive exposure in the treatment of generalized anxiety disorder: A case replication series. *Cognitive and Behavioral Practice, 11,* 404–414.

Sadowski, C., Moore, L. A., & Kelley, M. L. (1994). Psychometric properties of the Social Problem-Solving Inventory (SPSI) with normal and emotionally disturbed adolescents. *Journal of Abnormal Child Psychology, 22,* 487–500.

Sahler, O. J. Z., Fairclough, D. L., Phipps, S., Mulhern, R. K., Dolgin, M. J., Noll, R. B., et al. (2005). Using problem-solving skills training to reduce negative affectivity in mothers of children with newly diagnosed cancer: Report of a multisite randomized trial. *Journal of Consulting and Clinical Psychology, 73,* 272–283.

Sahler, O. J. Z., Varni, J. W., Fairclough, D. L., Butler, R. W., Noll, R. B., Dolgin, M. J., et al. (2002). Problem-solving skills training for mothers of children with newly diagnosed cancer: A randomized trial. *Developmental and Behavioral Pediatrics, 23,* 77–86.

Siu, A.M.H., & Shek, D.T.L. (2005). The Chinese version of the Social Problem-Solving Inventory: Some initial results on reliability and validity. *Journal of Clinical Psychology, 61,* 347–360.

Ström, L., Pettersson, R., & Andersson, G. (2000). A controlled trial of self-help treatment of recurrent headache conducted via the internet. *Journal of Consulting and Clinical Psychology, 68,* 722–727.

Toobert, D. J., Glasgow, R. E., Barrera, M., & Bagdade, J. (2002). Enhancing support for health behavior change among women at risk for structure heart disease: The Mediterranean Lifestyle Trial. *Health Education and Research, 17,* 547–585.

Tverskoy, A., Londahl, E. A., & D'Zurilla, T. J. (2007). *The role of social problem solving in the relationship between conflict and aggression in close relationships.* Unpublished manuscript. Department of Psychology, Stony Brook University, NY.

Wade, S. L., Wolfe, C., Brown, T. M., & Pestian, J. P. (2005). Putting the pieces together: Preliminary efficacy of a Web-based family intervention for children with traumatic brain injury. *Journal of Pediatric Psychology, 30,* 437–442.

Weinberger, M., Hiner, S. L., & Tierney, W. M. (1987). In support of hassles as a measure of stress in predicting health outcomes. *Journal of Behavioral Medicine, 10,* 19–31.

Williams, J. W., Barrett, J., Oxman, T., Frank, E., Katon, W., Sullivan, M., et al. (2000). Treatment of dysthymia and minor depression in primary care: A randomized controlled trial in older adults. *Journal of the American Medical Association, 284,* 1519–1526.

CHAPTER 8

Rational Emotive Behavior Therapy

Windy Dryden
Daniel David
Albert Ellis

Rational emotive behavior therapy (REBT) was founded in 1955 by Albert Ellis (1997). As such, it has the longest history of any of the cognitive-behavioral therapies (CBTs) covered in this handbook. Like many originators of new therapeutic systems of that time, Ellis had become increasingly disenchanted with the traditional psychoanalytic therapies as effective and efficient helping systems. Although this disillusionment was in part responsible for the creation of REBT, other influences can be detected in this regard. Ellis had had a long-standing interest in philosophy and was particularly influenced by the writings of Stoic philosophers, such as Epictetus and Marcus Aurelius. The oft-quoted phrase of Epictetus, "People are disturbed not by things but by their view of things," crystallized Ellis's view that philosophical factors are more important than psychoanalytic and psychodynamic factors in accounting for psychological disturbance. An up-to-date version of this famous saying, "People disturb themselves by the rigid and extreme beliefs that they hold about things," shows the central role given to rigid and extreme beliefs by REBT theory in understanding the roots of psychopathology.

In addition to the influence of the Stoics, the impact of other philosophers can be discovered in Ellis's ideas. For example, Ellis (1981a) was influenced by Immanuel Kant's writings on both the power and the limitations of cognition and ideation, particularly those found in *The Critique of Pure Reason*. Ellis has argued that REBT is founded upon the logico-empirical methods of science, and in this respect he, along with George Kelly (1955), pointed to the writings of Popper (1959, 1963) and Reichenbach (1953) as having a distinct impact on his efforts to make these philosophical ideas core features of the therapeutic system of REBT.

REBT is closely identified with the tenets of ethical humanism (Russell, 1930, 1965). Furthermore, REBT has distinct existential roots; Ellis has said in this respect that he was particularly influenced by the ideas of Paul Tillich (1953). Like other existentialists (e.g., Heidegger, 1949), REBT theorists agree that humans are "at the centre of their universe (but not of the universe) and have the power of choice (but not of unlimited choice) with regard to their emotional realm" (Dryden & Ellis, 1986, p. 130). Ellis (1984a) has claimed that REBT is doubly humanistic in its outlook, in that it

a) helps people maximize their individuality, freedom, self-interest, and self-control, and
b) helps them live in an involved, committed, and selectively loving manner. It thereby strives to facilitate individual and social interest. (p. 23)

Although Ellis himself espoused atheistic values, a number of rational emotive behavioral theorists and practitioners do subscribe to religious faiths (e.g., Hauck, 1972; Powell, 1976). REBT is not against religion per se; rather, it opposes "fanatic religiosity"—a dogmatic and rigid belief in faith, which is deemed to lie at the heart of psychological disturbance (Ellis, 1983a). Indeed, REBT shares with the philosophy of Christianity the view that we would do better to condemn the sin but forgive (or, more accurately, accept) the sinner.

Finally, Ellis's ideas were influenced by the work of the general semanticists, who argued that our psychological processes are to a great extent determined by our overgeneralizations and by the careless language we employ. Like Korzybski (1933), Ellis held that modification of the errors in our thinking and our language have a marked effect on our emotions and actions.

Although Ellis claimed that the creation of REBT owes more to the work of philosophers than to (pre-1959) psychologists, he was in fact influenced by the writings of a number of psychologists. Ellis was originally trained in psychoanalytic methods by a training analyst of the Karen Horney school; the influence of Horney's (1950) ideas on the "tyranny of the shoulds" is certainly apparent in the conceptual framework of REBT. However, whereas Horney saw that this mode of thought had a profound impact on the development and maintenance of neurotic problems, she did not, as Ellis later did, emphasize the dogmatic and absolutistic nature of these cognitions. Furthermore, although Horney saw that these "shoulds" had a tyrannical effect on psychological disturbance, she did not take a vigorous and active stance in helping people to challenge and change them, as is favored by REBT therapists.

Ellis (1973) stated that REBT owes a unique debt to the ideas of Alfred Adler (1927), who held that a person's behavior springs from his or her ideas. Adler's concept of the important role played by feelings of inferiority in psychological disturbance predates Ellis's view that ego anxiety based on the concept of self-rating constitutes a fundamental human disturbance. REBT also emphasizes the role of social interest in determining psychological health, as did Adler (1964). Other Adlerian influences on REBT are the importance that humans attribute to goals, purposes, values, and meanings; the emphasis on active–directive teaching; the employment of a cognitive-persuasive form of therapy; and the teaching method of holding live demonstrations of therapy sessions before an audience. However, REBT differs from Adlerian therapy in that it emphasizes the biological roots (Ellis, 1976), but places less stress on the role of early childhood experience and birth-order factors in accounting for such disturbance. Furthermore, Adler did not discriminate among the various types of cognitions and did not mention the absolutistic "musts" that are a central feature of the REBT perspective on psychological disturbance. Finally, whereas Adler did not use behavioral techniques, REBT espouses many specific therapeutic techniques and methods, and is both cognitive and behavioral (Dryden, 1984a; Ellis, 1998).

When Ellis first gave presentations on what he then called "rational psychotherapy" in the mid-1950s, he stressed the cognitive–philosophical aspects of the therapy to emphasize its differences with the psychoanalytic therapies. This stance led critics to accuse rational psychotherapy of neglecting its clients' emotions, which was not the case. Consequently, in 1961, Ellis changed the name of his approach to rational emotive therapy (RET), which was used until 1993, when he again changed the name of the approach to rational emotive behavior therapy (REBT) in reply to critics who argued that RET neglected clients' behaviors (Ellis, 1993a). However, REBT has always advocated the use of active behavioral methods, and Ellis acknowledged the influence of some of the earliest pioneers of behavioral therapy on his ideas and therapeutic practice. Also, from its inception, REBT has actively and systematically employed homework assignments to encourage clients to practice newly acquired therapeutic insights in their own life situation. Ellis saw the importance of such assignments in his early work as a sex and marriage counselor, in overcoming his own early anxieties about approaching women and speaking in public, and in the pioneering work of Herzberg (1945), who advocated the use of such assignments.

Students of the history of the development of psychotherapy will be interested to note that at the same time Ellis was creating REBT, a number of other therapists each independently developed therapeutic systems that had some cognitive-behavioral emphasis (Eric Berne, George Kelly, Abraham Low, E. Lakin Phillips, and Julian Rotter). Of these, only REBT is today recognized as a major form of CBT and as such is represented in this handbook.

BASIC THEORY

REBT has a perspective on (1) the nature of human beings, psychological health, and disturbance; (2) the acquisition of psychological disturbance; and (3) how such disturbance is perpetuated. Following discussion of these issues, we examine REBT's theory of therapeutic change and conclude this section by comparing the REBT theoretical model with those posited by other CBTs.

The Image of the Person

REBT theory conceives of the person as a complex, biosocial organism with a strong tendency to establish and pursue a variety of goals and purposes. Although people differ enormously in what brings them happiness, the fact that they construct and pursue valued goals shows that they strive to bring a sense of meaning to their lives. Humans are thus seen as hedonistic, in that their major goals appear to be to stay alive and actively pursue happiness. In this respect, they are further seen as having the related tasks of satisfying both their self-interests and their social interests.

The concept of rationality is central to an understanding of the person, where "rational" means that which is true, logical, and/or aids people to achieve their basic long-term goals and purposes. REBT theory holds that while people would do better to satisfy some of their short-range goals, they should adopt a philosophy of long-range hedonism if they are to achieve their basic goals and purposes. Consequently, "irrational" is that which is false, illogical, and/or hinders or obstructs people from achieving their basic long-range goals and purposes. Rationality is thus not defined in any absolute sense in REBT theory, since that which aids or hinders this goal achievement is dependent on the individual in his or her own particular situation.

While REBT theory stresses the role played by cognitive factors in human functioning, cognition, emotion, and behavior are not viewed as separate psychological processes but rather as highly interdependent and interactive processes. Thus, the statement "Cognition leads to emotion" tends to accentuate a false picture of psychological separatism. In the famous "ABCs" of REBT, A has traditionally stood for an "activating" event (i.e., the aspect of the situation that activates the person's beliefs); B for the beliefs the person holds about this aspect; and C for the emotional, behavioral, and cognitive consequences that stem from B (Ellis, 1985a, 1994). Yet the adherence to a particular set of beliefs tends to influence the inferences humans make and the environments they seek out. While beliefs do affect our emotion and behavior, the way we feel and act has a profound reciprocal effect on our beliefs. Our emotional and behavioral reactions can help to create environments and skew our perceptions of these environments, which in turn constrain our emotional and behavioral repertoires (as in the self-fulfilling prophecy effect). Thus, REBT theory sees the person as having overlapping intrapsychic processes, in constant interaction with his or her social and material environment. Having said that, we emphasize that the relation between A and C is almost always mediated by B, be it conscious and/or unconscious information processing/computation; hence, C is postcognitive. Obviously, an emotion (C) can act as an A, being apparently precognitive (i.e., the emotion appears before the belief).

This is a mere misinterpretation, because an emotion at A must have been generated at a previous point in time, and the computational (i.e., conscious or unconscious information processing) component involved in its generation makes it postcognitive.

Ellis (1976, 1979a) stressed that humans have two major biological tendencies. First, they have a strong tendency to think irrationally. According to rational emotive behavioral theory, humans show great ease in converting their strong preferences into devout absolutistic demands (psychological inflexibility; rigid/absolutistic thinking). Although Ellis (1984a) acknowledged that social influences affect this process, he also noted that "even if everybody had had the most rational upbringing, virtually all humans would often irrationally transform their individual and social preferences into absolutistic demands on (a) themselves, (b) other people, and (c) the universe around them" (p. 20). Ellis (1976, 1979a) argued that the following evidence supports his hypothesis of the biological basis of human irrationality, which in many ways is linked to modern evolutionary psychology (Buss, 2001; Cosmides & Tooby, 2006):

1. Virtually all humans, including bright and competent people, show evidence of major human irrationalities.
2. Virtually all the disturbance-creating irrationalities have been found in just about all social and cultural groups that have been studied historically and anthropologically.
3. Many irrational behaviors, such as procrastination and lack of self-discipline, go counter to the teachings of parents, peers, and the mass media.
4. Even bright and competent people often adopt other irrationalities after giving up former ones.
5. People who vigorously oppose various kinds of irrational behaviors often fall prey to these very irrationalities: Atheists and agnostics exhibit zealous and absolutistic philosophies, and highly religious individuals act immorally.
6. Insight into irrational thoughts and behaviors helps only partially to change them.
7. Humans often return to irrational behavioral patterns even though they have worked hard to overcome them.
8. People often find it easier to learn self-defeating rather than self-enhancing behaviors. Thus, people very easily overeat but have great trouble following a sensible diet.
9. Psychotherapists, who should presumably be good role models of rationality, often act irrationally in their personal and professional lives.
10. People frequently delude themselves into believing that bad experiences (e.g., divorce, stress, and other misfortunes) will not happen to them.

However, lest these hypotheses create the impression that REBT has a gloomy image of humans, REBT theory stresses the existence of a second basic biological tendency, which is that humans have both the ability to think about their thinking and the ability to exercise their power to choose to work toward changing their irrational thinking. Thus, people are by no means slaves to their tendency toward irrational thinking; they can strive to transcend its effects through active choice and continual effort to change this thinking through cognitive, emotive, and behavioral methods. The overall REBT image of the person is quite an optimistic one.

REBT views humans by nature as fallible and probably not perfectible. Humans "naturally" make errors, and often defeat and obstruct themselves in pursuit of their long range goals. Therapeutically, they are thus encouraged to accept their fallibility, and to challenge their self-created demands for perfection and the self-depreciation that accompany such demands. REBT emphasizes that the person is also a complex organism, one that is constantly in flux. As such, REBT theory considers that humans have great potential to utilize the many opportunities they encounter to effect changes in the ways they think, feel, and act.

REBT is a constructivistic approach to psychotherapy, holding that although people's preferences are influenced by their upbringing and their culture, when their desires are not met they disturb themselves by constructing irrational beliefs in such situations. However, REBT disagrees with constructivistic approaches, which argue that all constructions are equally viable, because REBT theory holds that some rational constructions are more consistent with reality, more logical, and more functional than others. A major goal of REBT is to encourage clients to make rational in preference to irrational constructions. Figure 8.1 shows where REBT stands on 10 personality dimensions put forward by Corsini (1977). A unidirectional arrow (← or →) indicates the pole that is stressed in the theoretical underpinnings of REBT. The sign indicates that the theory encompasses both poles of the dimension equally.

THE NATURE OF PSYCHOLOGICAL DISTURBANCE AND HEALTH

Psychological Disturbance

REBT theory posits that the tendency of humans to create and hold rigid evaluative beliefs (i.e., psychological inflexibility) about actual and inferred events lies at the heart of disturbance. These beliefs (i.e., appraisals) are couched in the form of dogmatic "musts," "shoulds," "have to's," and "oughts." Ellis (1983a) argued that these absolutistic cognitions are at the core of a philosophy of dogmatic religiosity that he claimed is the central feature of human emotional and behavioral disturbance. Absolute "musts" do not invariably lead to psychological disturbance, however, because it is possible for a person

Focus on explicit, observable behavior that can be counted and numbered.	OBJECTIVE	→	SUBJECTIVE	Concern with the inner personal life of the individual—his or her ineffable self.
Person seen as composed of parts, organs, units, elements put together to make the whole.	ELEMENTARISTIC	→	HOLISTIC	The person is seen as having a certain unity, and the parts as aspects of the total entity. The individual is seen as indivisible.
Apersonal theories are impersonal, statistically based, and consider generalities rather than individuals. They are based on group norms.	APERSONAL	→	PERSONAL	Personal theories deal with the single individual. They are ideographic.
Focus on the measurement of units of behavior.	QUANTITATIVE	→	QUALITATIVE	Behavior is seen as too complex to be measured exactly.
The individual is seen as a unit reactor, not a learner, filled with instincts and based on generalizations preestablished by heredity.	STATIC	→	DYNAMIC	The individual is seen as a learner, with interactions between behavior and consciousness and between consciousness, and unconsciousness.
The person is predominantly biologically based.	ENDOGENISTIC	←	EXOGENISTIC	The person is predominantly influenced by social and environmental factors.
The individual is seen as not responsible for his or her behavior as being the pawn of society, heredity, or both.	DETERMINISTIC	→	INDETERMINISTIC	The person is seen as basically under his or her own direction. Control is within the person, and prediction is never completely possible.

(cont.)

FIGURE 8.1. Rational-emotive therapy described on 10 personality dimensions. Adapted from Corsini (1977). Copyright 1977 by Wadsworth, a part of Cengage Learning. Adapted by permission.

	PAST	PRESENT/ FUTURE	FUTURE	
The individual is seen in terms of what he or she has inherited or learned in the past.	PAST	PRESENT/ FUTURE	FUTURE	The individual is seen as explained by his or her anticipations of future goals.
The person is seen as operating on an emotional basis, and with the intellect at the service of the emotions.	AFFECTIVE	↔	COGNITIVE	The person is seen as essentially rational, with the emotions subserving the intellect.
The individual is seen as rational and affected by factors within his or her awareness span.	CONSCIOUS	↔	UNCONSCIOUS	The person is seen as having considerable investment below the level of awareness.

FIGURE 8.1. *(cont.)*

to believe devoutly that he or she must succeed at all important projects, have confidence that he or she will be successful in these respects, and actually succeed in them and thereby not experience psychological disturbance. However, the person remains vulnerable to disturbance, because there is always the possibility that he or she may fail in the future. Thus, while REBT theory argues that an absolutistic, rigid philosophy frequently leads to disturbance, it does not claim that this is invariably so. In this way, even with respect to its view of the nature of human disturbance, REBT adopts an antiabsolutistic position.

REBT theory posits that if humans adhere to a philosophy of demands, or "musturbation," then they will also tend to create a number of extreme conclusions that are deemed to be derivatives of these "musts." These derivatives are viewed as irrational because they too are false, illogical, extreme, and tend to sabotage a person's basic goals and purposes. "Awfulizing" occurs when an event is rated as being more than 100% bad and/or as the worst thing that could happen—a truly exaggerated and magical conclusion that stems from the belief "This must not be as bad as it is." "Low frustration tolerance" (LFT) means believing that one cannot bear it if an event that must not happen actually occurs or threatens to occur, and that if it does, one cannot experience virtually any happiness at all. "Depreciation" is the tendency for humans to rate themselves and others as subhuman or undeserving if they do something that they "must" not do, or fail to do something that they "must" do. Depreciation can also be applied to others whom the person rates as being "rotten" for failing to give what he or she must have, and/or to life conditions. Some theorists use the term "global evaluation" here to indicate the problematic aspects of both global and positive evaluations.

Although Ellis (1984a) argued that awfulizing, LFT, and depreciation are secondary irrational processes, in that they stem from the philosophy of "musts," these processes can sometimes be primary. Indeed, Wessler (1984) argued that they are more likely to be primary, and that "musts" are often derived from them. However, recent empirical research (DiLorenzo, David, & Montgomery, 2007) supports the idea that whereas demandingness is a primary irrational appraisal process, awfulizing, LFT, and depreciation are secondary irrational appraisal processes. Nevertheless, demandingness may still follow the other irrational processes as part of the reappraisal (i.e., metacognition) processes that follow the initial appraisal (see David, 2003; Lazarus, 1991). Therefore, the philosophy of "musts" on the one hand, and those of awfulizing, LFT, and depreciation on the other are in all probability interdependent processes that often seem to be different sides of the same cognitive coin.

In summary, REBT theory discerns two major categories of human psychological disturbance in ego disturbance and discomfort disturbance (Ellis, 1979b, 1980a). In "ego disturbance" the person depreciates him- or herself as a result of making rigid demands on self, others, and the world. In "discomfort disturbance," the person makes demands, but these demands reflect the belief that comfort and comfortable life conditions must exist.

Ellis (1984a, 1985a) noted that humans make numerous kinds of illogical assumptions when they are disturbed. In this respect, REBT agrees with the early writings of cognitive therapists (e.g., Beck, Rush, Shaw, & Emery, 1979; Burns, 1980) that such cognitive distortions are a feature of psychological disturbance. However, REBT theory holds that such distortions almost always stem from the "musts" (see Table 8.1). Abelson and Rosenberg (1958) introduced the terms "hot" and "cold" cognitions to mark the distinction between appraising (hot) and knowing (cold). The term "cold cognitions" refers to the way people develop representations (i.e., accurate and/or distorted description of inferences) of relevant circumstances (i.e., activating events), whereas the term "hot cognitions" refers to the way people appraise/evaluate cold cognitions (David, 2003). Thus, during a specific activating event, there seem to be four different situations in which cold and hot cognitions regarding the activating event are related (based on David, 2003): (1) distorted representation/non-negatively appraised; (2) nondistorted representation/non-negatively appraised; (3) distorted representation/negatively appraised; and (4) nondistorted representation/negatively appraised. Although past research suggested that cold cognitions (e.g., inferences in the form of attributions) are strongly related to emotions (e.g., Schachter & Singer, 1962; Weiner, 1985), it is now generally accepted that as long as cold cognitions remain unevaluated, they are insufficient to produce emotions (David, 2003; Lazarus, 1991); therefore, emotional suffering is related only in situations 3 and 4, described earlier. Although REBT clinicians at times discover all the illogicalities just listed, and a number of others that are less frequently found in clients, they particularly focus on the unconditional "shoulds," "oughts," and "musts" constituting

TABLE 8.1. Common Cognitive Distortions

1. *All-or-none thinking:* "If I fail at any important task, as I must not, I'm a *total* failure and *completely* unlovable!"
2. *Jumping to conclusions and negative nonsequiturs:* "Since they have seen me dismally fail, as I *absolutely should* not have done, they will view me as an incompetent worm."
3. *Fortune-telling:* "Because they are laughing at me for failing, they know that I *absolutely should* have succeeded, and they will despise me forever. "
4. *Focusing on the negative:* "Because I *can't stand* things going wrong, as they *must* not, I can't see any good that is happening in my life."
5. *Disqualifying the positive:* "When they compliment me on the good things I have done, they are only being kind to me and forgetting the foolish things that I *absolutely should* not have done."
6. *Allness and neverness:* "Because conditions of living *ought* to be good and actually are so bad and so intolerable, they'll always be this way and I'll never have any happiness."
7. *Minimization:* "My accomplishments are the result of luck and are unimportant. But my mistakes, which I *absolutely should* never have made, are as bad as could be and are totally unforgivable."
8. *Emotional reasoning:* "Because I have performed so poorly, as I *absolutely should* not have done, I feel like a total nincompoop, and my strong feeling proves that I *am* no damned good."
9. *Labeling and overgeneralization:* Because I must not fail at important work and have done so, I am a complete loser and failure!"
10. *Personalizing:* "Since I am acting far worse than I *absolutely should* act and they are laughing, I am sure they are only laughing at me, and that is *awful*!"
11. *Phonyism:* "When I don't do as well as I *ought* to do and they still praise and accept me, I am a real phony and will soon fall on my face and show them how despicable I am!"
12. *Perfectionism:* "I realize that I did fairly well, but I *absolutely should* have done perfectly well on a task like this, and am therefore really an incompetent! "

Note. REBT theory holds that these tend to be derived from rigid beliefs.

the philosophical core of irrational beliefs that lead to emotional disturbance. REBT clinicians help clients to relinquish these core beliefs, and to refrain from creating new irrational derivatives from them. They usually encourage their clients, however, to have strong and persistent desires, wishes, and preferences, and to avoid feelings of detachment, withdrawal, and lack of involvement (Ellis, 1984b, 1984c, 1994, 1996a). More importantly, REBT holds that unrealistic and illogical distortions do not in themselves create emotional disturbance. People may unrealistically think that because they frequently fail, they always have done so and always will. In both of these instances, however, they could rationally conclude, "Too bad! Even though I often fail, there is no reason why I must succeed. I would prefer to, but I don't have to do well. So I'll be as happy as I can be even with my constant failures." They would then rarely be emotionally disturbed.

To reiterate, REBT considers the essence of emotional disturbance to consist of people's absolutistic "musts" and demands about their failure, their rejections, their poor treatment by others, and life's frustrations and losses. REBT therefore differs from other CBTs in that it particularly encourages therapists to look for clients' dogmatic, unconditional "musts"; to differentiate them from client's preferences; and to teach clients how to relinquish the former and retain the latter (Dryden, 2008).

Psychological Health

If rigid beliefs are at the core of much psychological disturbance, then REBT theory argues that a philosophy of relativism or "desiring" is a central feature of psychologically healthy humans. This philosophy—psychological flexibility—acknowledges that humans have a large variety of desires, wishes, wants, and preferences, but that if they refuse to transform these nondogmatic values into grandiose and dogmatic demands, they will not become psychologically disturbed. They will, however, experience healthy negative emotions, such as sadness, regret, disappointment, and healthy anger when their desires are unfulfilled. Many people new to REBT think that preferences are the hallmark of rational beliefs. However, it is the nondogmatic nature of preferences that is critical. For example, one might transform a preference, such as "I want to do well ..., " but disturb oneself by implicitly transforming this into a rigid belief "therefore, I have to do so." However, when one holds a nondogmatic preference, one both asserts the preference and negates the demand (i.e., "I want to do well, and I will do my best to do so, but I accept that this might not happen, and I don't necessarily have to do well").

REBT theory posits that if humans adhere to a philosophy of "nondogmatic preferences," then they can create three major nonextreme belief conclusions. "Antiawfulizing" occurs if a person does not get what he or she wants and acknowledges the lack of fulfillment of these desires, but also acknowledges that this deprivation is bad but not "awful." In general, when persons adhere to the nondogmatic desiring philosophy, the stronger their desire, the greater their rating of badness when they do not get what they want. "High frustration tolerance" (HFT) means that the person (1) acknowledges that an undesirable event has happened (or may happen); (2) believes that the event should empirically occur if it does; (3) considers that the event can be and is worth tolerating; (4) attempts to change the undesired event or accepts the "grim" reality if it cannot be modified; and (5) actively pursues other goals even though the situation cannot be altered. Acceptance occurs when the person accepts him- or herself and others as fallible human beings. In addition, life conditions are accepted as they exist. People who have the philosophy of acceptance fully acknowledge that the world is complex and events are often outside of personal control. Acceptance does not imply resignation, however. A philosophy of acceptance means that a person acknowledges that whatever does exists should exist, but does not have to exist forever. These conclusions are rational in that they are not only nonextreme, but they are also consistent with reality, sensible, and tend to help people reach their goals or formulate new goals, if their old ones cannot be realized.

REBT distinguishes between healthy and unhealthy negative emotions. The same distinction could be applied to positive emotions; however, we do not discuss this issue here (for details see Tiba & Szentagotai, 2005). Healthy negative emotions are associated with rational beliefs and unhealthy negative emotions, with irrational beliefs. For example, concern is an emotion associated with the belief "I hope that this threat does not happen to me, but I am not immune from it and nor do I have to be. If it does happen, it would be unfortunate, but not terrible." In contrast, anxiety occurs when a person believes, "This threat must not happen to me and it would be awful if it does." Healthy anger (also called "annoyance") occurs when another person disregards an individual's rule of living. Such a person tends to believe, "I wish the other person had not done that and I don't like what he or she did, but it does not follow that he or she must not break my own rule of conduct." In unhealthy anger, however, the person believes that the other must not break this rule and damns the other for doing so (Ellis, 1977c). Rational emotive behavior therapists do not target healthy negative emotions (sadness as opposed to depression; remorse vs. guilt; disappointment vs. shame) for change during therapy, because they are deemed to be consequences of rational thinking.

If ego disturbance and discomfort disturbance based on demands (psychological inflexibility) are the cornerstones of the REBT view of human psychological problems, then self-acceptance and a high level of discomfort tolerance, based on desiring and accepting (psychological flexibility), are the cornerstones of psychological health and are implicit in a philosophy of nondevout desire. Ellis (1979a) has outlined nine other criteria of positive mental health: (1) enlightened self-interest; (2) social interest; (3) self-direction; (4) acceptance of ambiguity and uncertainty; (5) scientific thinking; (6) commitment and being vitally absorbed in important projects; (7) flexibility; (8) calculated risk taking; and (9) acceptance of reality.

The Acquisition and Perpetuation of Psychological Disturbance

REBT does not advance a very elaborate view concerning the acquisition of psychological disturbance, in part because humans have a distinct biological tendency to think and act irrationally, but also because theories of acquisition do not necessarily suggest therapeutic interventions. Although Ellis acknowledged that environmental variables contribute to psychological disturbance, he argued that these do not account for the presence of such disturbances since people tend to generate their own biologically-based demands (Ellis, 1979a). Thus, Ellis (1984c) said, "Parents and culture usually teach children which superstitions, taboos and prejudices to abide by, but they do not originate their basic tendency to superstitiousness, ritualism and bigotry" (p. 209).

Rational emotive behavioral theory also posits that humans vary in their disturbability. Some people emerge relatively unscathed psychologically from being raised by uncaring or overprotective parents, whereas others emerge emotionally damaged from more "healthy" child-rearing approaches (Werner & Smith, 1982). Thus, Ellis (1984c) claimed that "individuals with serious aberrations are more innately predisposed to have rigid and crooked thinking than those with lesser aberrations, and consequently they are likely to make lesser advances" (p. 223). In summary, the REBT theory of acquisition views humans as not disturbed simply by our experiences; rather, we bring our ability to disturb ourselves to our experiences.

REBT theory maintains that people tend to perpetuate their psychological problems by their own "naive" theories concerning the nature and attributions of these problems. They lack what Ellis (1979a) called "REBT Insight Number 1": that psychological disturbance is primarily determined by the rigid and extreme beliefs that people hold about negative life events. Rather, they often consider that these situations directly cause their disturbances. Since people make incorrect hypotheses about the major determinants of their problems, they consequently attempt to change activating situations rather than their own beliefs. Second, people may have Insight Number 1 but lack "REBT Insight Number 2," which is that by reindoctrinating themselves with their rigid and extreme beliefs, people remain disturbed. While they may see that their problems are determined by their beliefs, they may distract themselves and thus perpetuate their problems by searching for the historical antecedents of these beliefs instead of directing themselves to change the current beliefs. Third, people may have the first two insights but still sustain their disturbance because they lack "REBT Insight Number 3," which is that only if people diligently work and practice in the present and future to think, feel, and act against their irrational beliefs are they likely to change them and make themselves less disturbed. People who have all three insights clearly see that their rational choice is to continue to challenge their beliefs cognitively, emotively, and behaviorally to break the perpetuation of the disturbance cycle. Merely acknowledging that a belief is irrational is usually insufficient to effect change (Ellis, 1972b).

Ellis (1979a) argued that the major reason people perpetuate their psychological problems is because they adhere to a philosophy of LFT. Such people believe that they must be comfortable; thus, they do not make changes because such work involves discomfort. They are short-range hedonists in that they are motivated to avoid short-term discomfort, even though accepting and working against their temporary uncomfortable feelings would probably help them to reach their long-range goals. Such people rate cognitive and behavioral therapeutic tasks as "too painful," and as even more painful than the psychological disturbance for which they have achieved some measure of tolerance. They prefer to remain with their "comfortable" discomfort rather than face the change-related discomfort that they believe they must not experience. Maultsby (1975) has argued that people often back away from change because they are afraid they will not feel right about it. He actively shows clients that these feelings of "unnaturalness" are natural concomitants of relearning. Another prevalent form of LFT is anxiety about anxiety (i.e., secondary emotion/meta-emotion or secondary disturbance/meta-disturbance). In this case, individuals believe that they must not be anxious; thus, they do not expose themselves to anxiety-provoking situations because they are anxious that they might become anxious if they did so—an experience they would rate as "awful." As such, they perpetuate their problems and overly restrict their lives to avoid experiencing anxiety.

A major way in which people perpetuate their psychological problems is by acting in ways that are consistent with their irrational beliefs. For example, when a person is anxious about making new friends because he believes that he must not be rejected, this irrational belief influences him to act in a variety of dysfunctional ways. If he actually acts in these ways, he strengthens his irrational beliefs, which makes it harder for him to overcome his fear of rejection. Thus, when helping this person to dispute his irrational beliefs, it is important to encourage him to act in ways that are consistent with his newly developed rational beliefs. If he challenges his irrational beliefs cognitively but continues to act in dysfunctional ways, he will easily go back to his irrational beliefs.

REBT theory endorses the Freudian view of human defensiveness to explain how people perpetuate their psychological problems (Freud, 1937). Thus, people employ various defense mechanisms (e.g., rationalization, avoidance) that are designed to help them deny the existence of these problems or to minimize their severity. The REBT view is that these defenses are used to ward off self-damnation tendencies and that, under such circumstances, if these people honestly took responsibility for their problems, they would severely denigrate themselves for having them. In addition, they employ defense mechanisms to ward off discomfort anxiety, because if such people admitted their problems, they would rate them as "too hard to bear" or "too difficult to overcome."

Ellis (1979a) noted that people sometimes experience a form of perceived payoff for their psychological problems, other than the avoidance of discomfort. Such payoffs serve to perpetuate the problems. Thus, a woman who claims to want to overcome her procrastination may avoid tackling the problem because she is afraid that if she became successful she might then be criticized by others as being "too masculine," a situation that she may believe is intolerable. Her procrastination is thus seen as protection from this "unbearable" state of affairs (Dryden, 1984b). Finally, the well-documented "self-fulfilling prophecy" phenomenon helps to explain why people perpetuate their psychological problems (Jones, 1977; Wachtel, 1977). Here people act according to their beliefs and consequent predictions, often eliciting from themselves or others responses that they then interpret in a manner that confirms their initial hypotheses. Thus, a socially anxious man may believe that other people would not want to get to know "how worthless an individual I am." He then attends a social function and acts as if he is worthless, by avoiding others. When such social behavior does not invite approaches from others, he then interprets the event: "I was right; other people don't want to know me. I really am no good."

In conclusion, REBT theory holds that people naturally tend to perpetuate their problems and to have a strong innate tendency to cling to self-defeating, habitual patterns and thereby resist basic change. Helping clients change poses a challenge for REBT practitioners.

Theory of Therapeutic Change

REBT holds that humans have the capacity to choose to work toward changing irrational thinking and its self-defeating effects, and that the most elegant and long-lasting changes that humans can effect are ones that involve the philosophical restructuring of irrational beliefs. Change at this level can be specific or general. Specific philosophical change means that rigid demands ("musts," absolute "shoulds") about given situations are changed to nondogmatic preferences. General philosophical change involves the adoption of a nondogmatic preferential attitude toward life events in general. Ellis distinguished between superelegant and semielegant philosophical change at the general level. Discussing these changes, Ellis said:

> By superelegant I mean that practically under all conditions for the rest of their life they would not upset themselves about anything. Very few will ever do this because it is against the human condition and people fall back to musturbating and thereby disturbing themselves. Some will effect a semielegant solution, meaning that in most instances they will call up a new rational-emotive philosophy that will enable them to feel sad or annoyed but not anxious, depressed, or angry when poor conditions occur. (cited in Weinrach, 1980, p. 156)

To effect a philosophical change at either the specific or general level, people need to do the following:

1. Realize that, to a large degree, humans create their own psychological disturbances. Whereas environmental conditions can contribute to their problems, they are in general of secondary consideration in the change process.
2. Recognize that they do have the ability to change these disturbances significantly.
3. Understand that emotional and behavioral disturbances stem largely from rigid and extreme irrational beliefs.
4. Detect their irrational beliefs and discriminate between irrational and rational alternatives.
5. Dispute these irrational beliefs using the logico-empirical methods of science.
6. Work toward internalization of their new rational beliefs with cognitive, emotive, and behavioral methods of change, and ensure that their behavior is consistent with their rational beliefs.
7. Continue this process of challenging irrational beliefs and using multimodal methods of change for the rest of their lives.

When people effect a philosophical or belief change, they often are able to correct their distorted inferences of reality (overgeneralizations, faulty attributions, etc.; Dryden, Ferguson, & Clark, 1989; Wessler & Wessler, 1980). However, they often need to challenge these distorted inferences more directly, as REBT has emphasized (Ellis, 1973; Ellis & Harper, 1961a, 1961b; see also Beck et al., 1979). People may also effect inferentially based changes, without making a profound philosophical change, to get better and stay better. Thus, they may regard their inferences as hunches about reality rather than facts, may generate alternative hypotheses, and may seek evidence and/or carry out experiments that test out each hypothesis. They may then accept the hypothesis that represents the "best bet" of those available. Consider a man who thinks that his coworkers view him as a fool. To test this hypothesis he may first specify their negative reactions to him. These constitute the data from which he quickly draws the conclusion "They think I'm a fool." He might realize that what he has interpreted to be negative responses to him may not be negative, or, if they seem to be negative, he might carry out an experiment to test the meaning he attributes to their responses. For example, he could test his hunch by directly asking them for their view of him. As a result, this person may conclude that his coworkers find some of his actions foolish rather than consider him to be a complete fool. His mood may lift because his inference of the situation has changed, but he may still hold to his negative belief: "People must not think I am a fool. If they did, I would indeed be a fool." Thus, he has made an inferential change but not a philosophical one, which would be more of the form: "Even if I act foolishly, that makes me a person with foolish behavior, not a foolish person. And even if they deem me a total idiot, that is simply their view, with which I can choose to disagree." Rational emotive behavior therapists hypothesize that people are more likely to make a profound philosophical change if they first assume that their inferences are true, then challenge their irrational beliefs, rather than first correct their inferential distortions, then challenge their underlying irrational beliefs.

People can also make direct changes of the situation. Thus, in the earlier example, the man could leave his job or distract himself from the reactions of his colleagues by taking on extra work and devoting himself to that effort. Or he might carry out relaxation exercises whenever he comes in contact with his coworkers, distracting himself once again from their perceived reactions. Additionally, the man may have a word with his supervisor, who may then instruct the other workers to change their behavior toward the man. Such strategies may lead to relief from distress, to feeling better, but they do not modify the irrational belief so that the man gets better and stays better.

A person can change his or her behavior to effect inferential and/or philosophical change. For example, the man whose coworkers view him as a fool might change his own behavior toward them, thus eliciting a different set of responses from them that would lead him to reinterpret his previous inference. However, if he could determine that they indeed consider him to be a fool, then the man could actively seek them out and show himself that he could stand the situation, and that just because they think him a fool doesn't make him one, thus effecting philosophical change and learning to accept himself regardless of their views.

While rational emotive behavior therapists prefer to help their clients make profound philosophical changes to get better and stay better, they do not dogmatically insist that their clients make such changes. If a client is not able at any given time to change his or her irrational beliefs, then the rational emotive behavior therapist would endeavor to help the client either to change A directly (by avoiding the troublesome situation, or by behaving differently) or to change his or her distorted inferences about the situation to feel better.

Differences with Other Cognitive-Behavioral Therapies

Ellis (1980b) distinguished between specialized REBT and general REBT. He argued that general REBT is synonymous with broad-based CBT, but that specialized REBT differs from CBT in a number of important respects:

1. REBT has a distinct philosophical emphasis as a central feature, which other forms of CBT omit. It stresses that humans appraise themselves, others, and the world in terms of (1) rational, preferential, flexible, and tolerant philosophies (i.e., psychological flexibility) and (2) irrational, musturbatory, rigid, intolerant, and absolutistic philosophies (i.e., psychological inflexibility).

2. REBT has an intrinsic existential–humanistic outlook, unlike most other CBT approaches. It sees people "as holistic, goal-directed individuals who have importance in the world just because they are human and alive; it unconditionally accepts them with their limitations, and it particularly focuses upon their experiences and values, including their self-actualizing potentialities" (Ellis, 1980b, p. 327). It also has an ethical humanism, because it encourages people to emphasize human interest before the interests of deities, material objects, and lower animals.

3. REBT favors striving for pervasive and long-lasting (philosophically based) rather than symptomatic change.

4. REBT attempts to eliminate self-ratings, but encourages unconditional self-acceptance. It views self-esteem as a self-defeating concept, based on conditional self-evaluations (Dryden, 1998).

5. REBT sees psychological disturbance as a partial outcome of taking life too seriously. It advocates the appropriate use of humorous therapeutic methods (Ellis, 1977a, 1977b, 1981b).

6. REBT stresses the use of antimusturbatory techniques that go to the philosophical core of emotional disturbance, and the disputation of irrational beliefs at this core, rather than merely antiempirical inferences that are more peripheral. REBT teaches clients how to become their own scientists and use forceful logico-empirical disputation of irrational beliefs rather than only stressing the employment of rationally oriented, coping self-statements whenever possible.

7. REBT employs, but only mildly encourages, the use of cognitive methods that serve to distract people (e.g., relaxation methods) from their disturbed philosophies. Specialized REBT holds that such techniques may help clients better in the short term but do not encourage them to identify or change the devout philosophies that underpin their psychological problems in the long term. REBT also employs problem-solving and skills training methods, along with, but not instead of, teaching people to work at understanding and changing their irrational beliefs.

8. While other CBTs recognize specific instances of discomfort anxieties (e.g., "fear of fear" [Mackay, 1984] and affect intolerance [Linehan, 1993]), REBT gives a more central role to the concept of discomfort disturbance than do other CBTs. "Discomfort disturbance" is defined as disturbance that appears when people think (1) that their life or comfort is seriously threatened and/or lost, (2) that they must not feel uncomfortable and have to feel at ease, and/or (3) that it is awful and/or terrible when they do not get what they supposedly must get (Ellis, 1994).

9. Because humans frequently make themselves disturbed about their original disturbances (i.e., meta-disturbances), rational emotive behavior therapists actively look for secondary and tertiary symptoms of disturbance and encourage clients to work on overcoming these before addressing the primary disturbance.

10. REBT has clear-cut theories of disturbance and its treatment, but it is eclectic or multimodal in its techniques. It favors some techniques (e.g., active disputing) over others (e.g., cognitive distraction) and strives for profound or elegant philosophical change where feasible.

11. REBT discriminates between healthy and unhealthy negative emotions. Negative emotions are constructive affective responses to thwarted desires, when based on a nondogmatic and flexible philosophy of desire, and when they do not needlessly interfere with people's goals and purposes. Unconstructive emotions are based on rigid demands about thwarted desires. REBT considers these latter feelings as symptoms of disturbance, because they often sabotage people's attempts to pursue their goals and purposes constructively.

12. Whereas other CBTs tend not to make this distinction, REBT advocates that therapists give unconditional acceptance to clients rather than warmth or approval. REBT holds that therapist warmth and approval have their distinct dangers, in that they may unwittingly strengthen clients' need for love and approval. Rational emotive behavior therapists encourage clients to accept themselves unconditionally.

13. REBT stresses the importance of vigor and force in counteracting irrational philosophies and behaviors (Dryden, 1984a; Ellis, 1994, 1996b). REBT stresses that because humans are biologically predisposed to originate and perpetuate their disturbances, they often experience difficulty in changing the ideological roots of these problems. It therefore urges both therapists and clients to use considerable force and vigor in interrupting clients' irrationali-

ties. By "force" and "vigor" we mainly mean an active–directive, empathic, and persistent style of cognitive restructuring, not an intrusive one.

14. REBT is more selective than most other CBTs in the use of behavioral change methods. Thus, it sometimes favors the use of penalization to encourage resistant clients to change, such as burning a hundred dollar bill when they fail to stop smoking or fail to come to work on time. Furthermore, REBT has reservations about the use of social reinforcement in therapy. It considers that humans are too reinforceable, and that they may do the right thing for the wrong reason. REBT therapists help clients become maximally nonconformist, nondependent, and individualistic, and thus use social reinforcement techniques sparingly. Finally, REBT favors the use of *in vivo* desensitization and flooding methods rather than gradual desensitization techniques, since it argues that the former procedures best help clients to raise their level of frustration tolerance (Ellis, 1962, 1983c).

15. Although REBT therapists prefer to use specialized REBT whenever feasible, they do not dogmatically insist that it be employed. When they pragmatically employ general REBT, their therapeutic practice may be indistinguishable from that of other cognitive-behavioral therapists (Ellis, 1996b).

A fuller discussion of the distinctive features of REBT can be found in Dryden (2008).

ASSESSMENT CONSIDERATIONS

In this section we discuss additional considerations regarding assessment for REBT. REBT assessment strategies are based on both a "disorder/nosological model" and a "functional model" (e.g., based on listing the problems). Both REBT assessment models are guided by the concept of "evidence-based assessment." Each area of assessment is briefly discussed below.

The Rational Emotive Behavior Therapy Disorder/Nosological Model

The use of the disorder model in REBT is similar to that used in other models of psychotherapy. There are typically four steps to this process, as follows:

Step 1. Evaluate the clinical disorder/condition: This step is guided by DSM criteria and is often based on the SCID (Structured Clinical Interview for DSM-IV), which gives us a categorical measure of symptoms, and on various psychological tests to provide a continuous measure of the symptoms.

Step 2. Evaluate the causal mechanisms (i.e., psychological factors) involved in the clinical disorder/condition according to evidence-based theories or the consensus of the professional community, if necessary. The instruments we use in this step include clinical interviews and psychological tests and/or tasks with rigorous psychometric properties. Factors that can be evaluated include cognitive vulnerability factors related to (1) general cognitions, such as descriptions and inferences (e.g., automatic thoughts, intermediary and core beliefs/schemas), (2) irrational beliefs, and (3) cognitive resilience factors, such as rational beliefs that are important in health promotion and the prevention of relapse and recurrence.

Depending on the theory that relates the clinical condition with the causal mechanisms, other patient-related psychological factors of interest may include coping mechanisms and personality, behavioral, psychophysiological, and/or affective factors. Also, beyond the patient-related factors, we evaluate two other factors: (1) outcome and mechanism of change during the psychotherapeutic process and (2) therapist competence (e.g., the REBT Competency Scale).

Step 3. Establish a list of problems: The same clinical condition does not necessarily affect two different people identically in real life. Thus, the development of a list of real-life problems is fundamental.

Step 4. Conceptualize each problem according to the cognitive and/or behavioral ABC model (Ellis, 1994): This step involves identifying each component of the ABC model (i.e., activating events; specific beliefs; emotional, behavioral, and cognitive consequences), in relation to a specific problem on the list.

These steps lead to (1) a description of the clinical condition; (2) a picture of the main causal mechanisms of the clinical condition that should be targeted during treatment, and of the resilience mechanisms; (3) an understanding of the clinical condition in real life, based on the list of problems; and (4) a clear idea of the needed treatment to be implemented and its likely efficacy/effectiveness.

The Rational Emotive Behavior Therapy Functional Model

REBT is used in cases that have a formal DSM diagnosis, as well as in nonclinical cases, and in health promotion. In such cases, the assessment process is somewhat different than described earlier. In such cases, assessment would normally include the following steps:

- Step 1: Establish a list of problems: Develop a comprehensive list of real-life problems that affect the client and/or specific goals to be attained (e.g., in health promotion).
- Step 2: Conceptualize each problem according to the ABC model, and start the intervention based on this conceptualization.

In addition to the main requirement of being an evidence-based assessment, REBT assessment is based on two main classes of cognitive processes (for details, see David, 2003; David, Szentagotai, Kallay, & Macavei, 2005; David, Montgomery, Macavei, & Bovbjerg, 2005; David & Szentagotai, 2006). Some are explicit (i.e., conscious information processing) and others are implicit (i.e., unconscious information processing). Explicit cognitive processes can function consciously or automatically and may be assessed by interview and self-report measures. Implicit cognitive processes require the use of implicit tests and tasks (see Reber, 1993; Schacter & Tulving, 1994), such as priming procedures (sentence completion tests, drawing completion tests, automatic thoughts in simulated situations tasks, etc.). Because children also have difficulties verbalizing their cognitions, the testing procedure can be conceptualized as a game in such cases.

CLINICAL APPLICATIONS

In this section we first discuss the major clinical applications of REBT. We use individual therapy to consider (1) the therapeutic bonds that rational emotive behavior therapists endeavor to establish with their clients, (2) the clinical process of REBT from inception to termination, and (3) the major therapeutic techniques employed in REBT. Second, we discuss the application of REBT to a case of anxiety and a case of depression. Finally, we consider other clinical applications of REBT.

Individual Therapy

Therapeutic Bonds

Whereas other psychotherapy systems regard the therapeutic relationship as the major vehicle of change, REBT considers the establishment of effective therapeutic bonds to be an important ingredient but not a necessary vehicle for therapeutic change. However, when specific problems appear in the therapeutic bond, they can be approached in the ABC framework, as an *in vivo* opportunity for client and therapist to use REBT. Ellis (1979c) argued that effective REBT is best done in a highly active–directive manner, although he also acknowledged that it can be practiced successfully in more passive therapeutic style (Ellis, 1984a). Since the major goals of REBT therapists are to teach clients to think more rationally and ultimately to help them use its methods for themselves, they see themselves as educators and strive to establish the most appropriate learning climate for each client.

REBT therapists strive to accept their clients unconditionally as fallible human beings. Even if clients' actions are self-defeating, no matter how badly clients behave inside or outside therapy, REBT therapists show clients that they accept them. Although REBT therapists accept their clients, most do not interact with clients in a very warm fashion for two main reasons. First, undue therapist warmth may lead to the entrenchment of clients' needs for love and approval, which can perpetuate the beliefs at the core of much human disturbance. Clients of warm therapists may appear to improve and certainly to feel better, because they come to believe that they must be worthy since their therapists like them. However, their self-acceptance remains dependent on outside approval, and they may never challenge this philosophy of conditional self-acceptance with their warm, loving therapists (who themselves may have dire needs for their clients' approval). Second, undue therapist warmth may reinforce clients' philosophies of LFT (Ellis, 1982). Even so, there may be occasions (e.g., severely depressed clients) when therapist warmth is appropriate for a restricted period of time.

Most REBT therapists interact in an open manner with their clients and do not hesitate to give personal information about themselves if clients ask for it, except when they judge that clients may use such information against themselves. They disclose to their clients when they have experienced similar problems and share how they solved these problems using REBT. They thus serve as good role models and inspire their clients with the hope that it is possible to overcome emotional and behavioral problems.

REBT therapists agree with Carl Rogers (1957) that is in important for therapists to be empathic with clients. However, they offer their clients not only affective empathy but also philosophical empathy, showing their clients that they understand the underlying philosophies upon which their emotions are based.

REBT therapists often favor an informal style of interaction with clients. They employ humor when appropriate, because emotional disturbance can be viewed as a result of taking things too seriously. Thus, humorous style may loosen clients up and encourage them to stand back and laugh at their dysfunctional thinking and behavior, but not at themselves. This latter point is in keeping with the REBT perspective of the self as comprising myriad different, ever-changing aspects rather than one rateable whole. Consequently, therapists direct their own humor at aspects of clients' dysfunction, not at the client as a person. Indeed, REBT therapists often direct their humor against some of their own irrationalities and by so doing show that they do not take themselves too seriously (Ellis, 1983b).

Although REBT therapists tend to favor an informal, humorous, active–directive style of therapeutic participation, they are flexible in this respect and are mindful of which therapeutic style might be most effective for a given client (Eschenroeder, 1979). Varying one's therapeutic style in REBT, however, does not mean a departure from the theoretical principles on which the content of therapy is based (Beutler, 1983; Dryden & Ellis, 1986). The issue of appropriate therapeutic styles in REBT warrants more formal research.

Therapeutic Process

Some clients approach an REBT therapist because they know about REBT, whereas others may know nothing about this therapeutic method. In any event, it is often beneficial to explore clients' expectations for therapy at the outset of the process. Duckro, Beal, and George (1979) have argued that it is important to distinguish between preferences and anticipations when expectations are assessed. Clients' preferences for therapy concern the kind of experience they want, whereas anticipations concern the service they think they will receive. Clients who have realistic anticipations, as well as a preference for the REBT therapeutic process in general require far less induction into REBT than clients who have unrealistic anticipations of the process and/or prefer a different therapeutic experience.

Induction procedures generally involve demonstrations that REBT is an active–directive structured therapy oriented to clients' present and future problems, and requires clients to play an active role in the change process (Dryden, 1999). Induction can take a number of different forms. First, therapists may use pretherapy role induction procedures in which a typical course of REBT is outlined and productive client behaviors are demonstrated (Macaskill & Macaskill, 1983). Second, therapists may give a short lecture at the outset of therapy about the nature and process of REBT. Third, therapists may employ induction-related explanations in the initial therapy sessions, use client material to illustrate how problems may be tackled in REBT, and outline the respective roles of client and therapist.

Some REBT therapists spend little time gathering background information about their clients. Others may try to get this information if they are working with clients who want to understand how their developmental process and past experience have led to an irrational thinking style. In some cases this insight may be important in cognitive restructuring. If the therapist decides that such information is not necessary for a particular patient, he or she may ask the client for a description of current major problem(s). As the client describes his or her problem(s), the therapist intervenes fairly early to break these down into their ABC components. If a client begins by describing A (the inferred event), then the therapist asks for C (most usually the client's emotional and/or behavioral reactions). However, if a client begins by outlining C, then the therapist will ask for a brief description of A. When A is assessed, the rational emotive behavior therapist prefers to assess fully the client's inferences in search of the most relevant inference about which the client disturbs herself (in this case) at C. The following illustrates this process using "Windy's Magic Question" (Dryden, 2001).

WD: So what were you anxious about in the situation where you had to make a presentation?

CLIENT: I am not sure. I was anxious about a few things.

WD: Such as?

CLIENT: The people thinking I did not know what I was talking about, me shaking, my boss giving me a bad evaluation.

WD: OK, so if I gave you one thing that would completely take all or most of your anxiety away, what would that be?

CLIENT: Knowing that my boss would not give me a bad evaluation.

WD: So if you knew that, how would you feel about shaking and people there thinking that you did not know what you were talking about? you would not feel anxious?

CLIENT: Well, I wouldn't like it, but I would not feel anxious.

Because C is assessed mainly by verbal report, clients sometimes experience difficulty in accurate report of their emotional and behavioral problems. REBT therapists may use a variety of emotive (e.g., Gestalt two-chair dialogue, psychodrama), imagery-based, and other techniques (e.g., keeping an emotion/behavior diary) to facilitate this part of the assessment process (Dryden, 1999). If the assessment has revealed unhealthy negative emotions and/or dysfunctional behaviors at C, the therapist helps the client identify irrational beliefs at B. It is important to help clients to see the link between their irrational beliefs and their unhealthy affective and behavioral consequences at C. Some rational emotive behavior therapists like to give a short lecture at this point on the role of the "musts" in emotional disturbance and how they can be distinguished from preferences. Ellis, for example, often gave the following account:

ELLIS: Imagine that it's not essential, but you prefer to have at least $11.00 in your pocket at all times. You discover you only have $10.00. How will you feel?

CLIENT: Frustrated.

ELLIS: Right. Or you'd feel concerned or sad, but you wouldn't kill yourself. Right?

CLIENT: Right.

ELLIS: OK. Now this time imagine that you absolutely have to have a minimum of $11.00 in your pocket at all times. You must have it; it is a necessity. You must, you must, you must have a minimum of $11.00 and again you look and you find you only have $10.00. How will you feel?

CLIENT: Very anxious.

ELLIS: Right, or depressed. Now remember it's the same $11.00 but a different belief. OK, now this time you still have that same belief. You have to have a minimum of $11.00 at all times, you must. It's absolutely essential. But this time you look in your pocket and find that you've got $12.00. How will you feel?

CLIENT: Relieved, content.

ELLIS: Right. But with that same belief you have to have a minimum of $11.00 at all times something will soon occur to you that you would feel very anxious about. What do you think that would be?

CLIENT: What if I lose $2.00?

ELLIS: Right. What if you lose $2.00, what if you spend $2.00, what if you get robbed? That's right. Now the moral of this model applies to all humans, rich or poor, black or white, male or female, young or old, in the past or in the future, and it is that people make themselves disturbed if they don't get what they think they must, but they are also panicked when they do because of the must. For even if they have what they think they must, they could always lose it.

CLIENT: So I have no chance to be happy when I don't have what I think I must and little chance of remaining unanxious when I do have it?

ELLIS: Right! Your *must*urbation will get you nowhere except depressed or panicked!

An important goal of the assessment stage of REBT is to help clients distinguish between their original problems (e.g., depression, anxiety, withdrawal, addiction) and their problems about their primary problems (e.g., depression about depression, anxiety about anxiety, shame about withdrawal, or guilt about addiction). REBT therapists assess meta-problems before they assess clients' original problems, because these often require prior therapeutic attention. For example, clients find it difficult to focus on their original problem of anxiety when they are severely blaming themselves for being anxious.

Meta-problems are assessed in the same manner as original problems. When particular problems have been assessed according to the "ABC" model, and clients recognize the link between their irrational beliefs and their dysfunctional emotional and behavioral consequences, then therapists can proceed to the disputing stage. The initial purpose of disputing is to help clients gain intellectual insight into the fact that no evidence can support their rigid beliefs or the extreme derivatives of these demands. There exists only evidence that if they stay with their nondogmatic preferences, and if these are not fulfilled, then they will get unfortunate or "bad" results, whereas if they are fulfilled, then they will get desirable or "good" results. Intellectual insight in REBT reflects an acknowledgment that an irrational belief frequently leads to emotional disturbance and dysfunctional behavior, and that a rational belief abets emotional health (Ellis, 2002). REBT uses intellectual insight as a springboard for the working-through phase, in which clients are encouraged to use a large variety of techniques to help them achieve emotional insight. "Emotional insight" in REBT is defined as a very strong and frequently held belief that an irrational idea is dysfunctional and that a rational idea is helpful (Ellis, 1963). When a person has achieved emotional insight, he or she thinks, feels, and behaves according to the rational belief.

It is mainly in the working-through phase of REBT that therapists frequently encounter obstacles to client progress. Three major forms of such obstacles are deemed to occur in REBT: (1) relationship obstacles, (2) client obstacles, and (3) therapist obstacles. Relationship obstacles basically take two forms. First, therapist and client may be poorly matched and fail to develop a productive working relationship. Early referral to a more suitable therapist is indicated in such situations. Second, therapist and client may get on too well, with the result that (1) they collude to avoid uncomfortable issues, and (2) the therapist fails to encourage the client to push him- or herself to change irrational beliefs in the life situation. In this case, therapy can become an enjoyable experience for both, but the therapist would do better to remind him- or herself and the client that the major purpose of their relationship is to help the client overcome psychological problems and pursue goals outside of the therapeutic situation. Therapists need to raise their own and their clients levels of frustration tolerance to work toward this end.

Therapist obstacles to client progress also take two basic forms. First, therapists may have skills deficits and conduct REBT in an ineffective manner. In this case, supervision and further training are needed. Second, therapists may bring their own needs for approval, success, and comfort to therapy, and interfere with client progress. In this situation, therapists would do better to use REBT on themselves or seek personal therapy (Ellis, 1983b, 1985b).

Ellis (1983d) found that clients' own extreme level of disturbance may be a significant obstacle to progress. He confirmed that the clients who benefit most from therapy are precisely those who need it least (i.e., those who are less disturbed at the outset), and he (Ellis, 1983e, 1983f, 1984d, 1985b) outlined many therapeutic strategies for use with resistant clients. First, therapists need to maintain an unusually accepting attitude toward resistant clients. Second, they should preferably strive consistently to encourage such clients to change. Third, they should persist in showing clients the negative consequences that undoubtedly follow their refusal to work on their problems. Fourth, a good deal of therapeutic flexibility, innovation, and experimentation is called for in work with resistant clients (Dryden & Ellis, 1986).

Termination in REBT preferably takes place when clients have made some significant progress and are proficient in REBT's self-change techniques. Terminating clients should preferably be able to (1) acknowledge that they will experience unhealthy negative emotions and dysfunctional actions; (2) detect the irrational beliefs that underpin these experiences; (3) discriminate between their irrational beliefs and their rational alternatives; (4) challenge irrational beliefs; and (5) counteract them by using a variety of behavioral self-change methods. It is often helpful for therapists to arrange for their clients to attend follow-up sessions and monitor client progress to deal with any remaining obstacles to sustained improvement.

Major Therapeutic Techniques

The major therapeutic techniques employed in REBT are described here, with an emphasis on the technical aspects of specialized REBT, in which the goal is to effect profound philosophical change. In general REBT, therapists employ a variety of additional techniques that are adequately covered elsewhere in this handbook, and freely employ techniques derived from other schools of therapy. However, REBT "is based on a clear-cut theory of emotional health and disturbance: The many techniques it employs are used in the light of that theory" (Ellis, 1984c, p. 234). Because REBT therapists adhere to the theory's emphasis on long-range hedonism, they rarely employ a technique that has beneficial short-range but deleterious long-range effects. It should also be noted that we list techniques under *cognitive, emotive,* and *behavioral* headings to emphasize the major modality of these techniques. However, consistent with the REBT view that cognition, emotion, and behavior are really interdependent processes, we note that almost all of the following techniques include cognitive, emotive, and behavioral elements.

Cognitive Techniques

The most commonly employed technique in REBT is "disputation" (i.e., cognitive restructuring) of irrational beliefs. Phadke (1982) described the disputing process in three steps. First, therapists help clients to detect the irrational beliefs that underpin their self-defeating emotions and behaviors. Second, they debate/discuss (1) the truth or falsehood and/or (2) the usefulness or lack of usefulness of these irrational beliefs. During this process they help their clients with the third step, which is to discriminate between irrational and rational beliefs. Debating is usually conducted according to the Socratic method of asking questions, such as "Where is the evidence that you must do this?"; "How does it follow that because you want this you must get it?"; and "Is it useful for you to think this way? How does thinking like this help you?" Skillful REBT therapists use a variety of different restructuring/debating styles with their clients (see DiGiuseppe, 1991).

A number of written homework forms are available to assist clients to dispute their irrational beliefs between sessions (see Figure 8.2). Clients can also listen to audiotapes of therapy sessions and dispute their own irrational beliefs on tape. Here they initiate and sustain a dialogue between the rational and irrational parts of themselves. Clients who find the disputing process too difficult are encouraged to develop rational self-statements that they can write on small cards and repeat to themselves at various times between therapy sessions. An example of such a statement might be "I want my boyfriend's love, but I don't need it."

Three cognitive methods that therapists often suggest to help clients reinforce a new rational philosophy are (1) bibliotherapy, in which clients read self-help books and materials (e.g., Ellis & Becker, 1982; Ellis & Harper, 1997; Young, 1974); (2) listening to CDs of REBT lectures on various themes (e.g., Ellis, 1971b, 1972a); and (3) using REBT with others, such as friends and relatives, so that the clients gain practice using rational arguments.

A number of semantic methods are employed in REBT. Defining techniques are sometimes employed that help clients to use less self-defeating language. Thus, instead of "I can't," clients are urged to say "I haven't yet." Referenting techniques are also employed (Danysh, 1974), in which clients

SITUATION = "A" =	
"iB" (irrational belief) =	"rB" (rational belief) =
"C" (emotional consequence) =	"C" (emotional goal) =
(behavioral consequence) =	(behavioral goal) =
(thinking consequence) =	(thinking goal) =
"D" (Disputing) =	
Reexamine "A"	

1) Write down a brief, objective description of the "situation" you were in.

2) Identify your "C"—your major disturbed emotion, your dysfunctional behavior, your distorted subsequent thinking.

3) Identify your "A"—what you were most disturbed about in the situation (steps 2 and 3 are interchangeable).

4) Set emotional, behavioral, and thinking goals.

5) Identify your irrational beliefs ("iBs"; i.e., demand + awfulizing belief), LFT belief, or deprecation belief.

6) Identify the alternative rational beliefs ("rBs") that will enable you to achieve your goals (i.e., nondogmatic preference + antiawfulzing belief), HFT belief, or acceptance belief.

7) Develop persuasive arguments to convince yourself that your irrational beliefs are irrational and your rational beliefs are rational—"D." These arguments will help you to achieve your emotional, behavioral, and thinking goals.

8) Reexamine "A" and consider how realistic it was. Given all the facts, would there have been a more realistic way of looking at "A"? If so, write it down.

FIGURE 8.2. ABCD blank form with instructions. Copyright 2003 by Windy Dryden. Reprinted by permission.

list both the negative and positive referents of a particular concept, such as smoking. This method can be employed to counteract clients' tendencies to focus on the positive aspects of a harmful habit and neglect its negative aspects.

REBT therapists also employ a number of imagery techniques. Rational emotive imagery (Ellis, 1993b; Maultsby & Ellis, 1974) encourages clients to change their unhealthy negative emotions to healthy ones (C), while maintaining a vivid image of the negative event at A. Time projection imagery methods are also employed in REBT (Lazarus, 1984). Thus, a client may say that if a particular event occurred, would be "awful." Rather than directly challenge this irrational belief at this stage, the therapist may help the client to picture what life might be like at regular intervals after the "awful" event has occurred. In this way clients are indirectly helped to change their irrational beliefs, because they come to see that life goes on after the "awful" event, that they will usually recover from it, and that they can continue to pursue their original goals or develop new ones. Such realizations encourage clients to reevaluate their irrational beliefs. Finally, some rational emotive behavior therapists use a hypnosis paradigm (e.g., Golden, 1983).

Emotive Techniques

REBT has often been falsely criticized for neglecting the emotive aspects of psychotherapy. However, this is far from the truth. REBT therapists use cognitive and behavioral techniques to target irrational beliefs to eliminate distress; the change in cognitions is therefore not a goal per se, but a means to impact on distress and unhealthy negative feelings. Moreover, therapists frequently employ a number of emotive techniques that challenge clients' irrational beliefs but not the client as a person. First, a number of humorous methods encourage clients to think rationally by not taking themselves too seriously (Ellis, 1977a, 1977b). Second, REBT therapists model a rational philosophy through self-disclosure. They honestly admit that they have had similar problems and show that they overcame them by using REBT. Thus, Dryden frequently tells clients that he used to feel ashamed of his stammer, then relates how he accepted himself with his speech impediment and forced himself to tolerate the discomfort of speaking in public whenever the opportunity arose. Third, REBT therapists frequently use a number of stories, mottos, parables, witticisms, poems, and aphorisms as adjuncts to cognitive disputing techniques (Wessler & Wessler, 1980). Fourth, Ellis (1977a, 1977b, 1981b) has written a number of humorous songs to present rational philosophies in an amusing and memorable format. The following is a rational humorous song written by Dryden to the tune of "God Save the Queen":

> God save my precious spleen
> Send me a life serene
> God save my spleen!

Protect me from things odious
Give me a life melodious
And if things get too onerous
I'll whine, bawl, and scream!

Ellis (1979d) advocated the use of force and energy in the practice of psychotherapy, whenever it is applicable (depending on the client and his or her clinical situation), and emphasized the employment of such interventions that fully involve clients' emotions. REBT therapists suggest that clients can move from intellectual to emotional insight by vigorously disputing their irrational beliefs (Ellis, 1993c). Vigor is often employed by clients in "rational role reversal," in which they forcefully and dramatically adopt the role of their rational self, and dispute self-defeating beliefs as articulated by their irrational self. Force and energy also play a significant part in REBT's now-famous shame-attacking exercises (Ellis, 1969, 1995; Ellis & Becker, 1982). Here clients deliberately seek to act "shamefully" in public in order to accept themselves and to tolerate the ensuing discomfort. Minor infractions of social rules often serve as suitable shame-attacking exercises, such as calling out the time in a crowded department store, wearing bizarre clothes designed to attract public attention, or going into a hardware store and asking if they sell tobacco. In risk-taking exercises clients deliberately force themselves to take calculated risks in areas where they wish to make changes. While disputing relevant irrational beliefs, Ellis has discussed how he overcame his anxiety about approaching women by deliberately forcing himself to speak to 100 women in the Bronx Botanical Gardens. Dryden pushed himself to speak on national and local radio as part of a campaign to overcome his public speaking anxiety. Both Ellis and Dryden took these risks, showing themselves that nothing "awful" would result from such experiences.

Behavioral Techniques

REBT has advocated the use of behavioral techniques since 1955, because cognitive change is very often facilitated by behavioral change (Emmelkamp, Kuipers, & Eggeraat, 1978). Since REBT therapists are concerned about helping clients raise their level of frustration tolerance, they encourage them to carry out homework assignments based on *in vivo* desensitization and flooding paradigms rather than those based on the gradual desensitization paradigm (Ellis, 1979e; Ellis & Abrahms, 1978; Ellis & Becker, 1982; Ellis & Grieger, 1977). They pragmatically negotiate a compromise, however, and encourage reluctant clients to undertake tasks that are sufficiently challenging for them but not overwhelming given their present status (Dryden, 1985).

Other behavioral methods employed in REBT include (1) "stay in there" activities (Grieger & Boyd, 1980) that encourage clients to remain in uncomfortable situations for a long period of time to learn how to tolerate discomfort; (2) antiprocrastination exercises, in which clients are encouraged to push themselves to start tasks sooner rather than later, and learn to tolerate the discomfort of breaking the "mañana habit"; (3) the use of rewards and penalties to encourage clients to undertake uncomfortable assignments in the pursuit of their long-range goals (Ellis, 1979c; 1985b), and (4) Kelly's "fixed role therapy," in which clients are encouraged to act as if they already think rationally, to enable them to experience the fact that change is possible.

Other behavioral methods are employed in both specialized and general REBT (e.g., various forms of skills training methods). These are used in specialized REBT to encourage philosophical change, whereas in general REBT, they are employed to teach clients skills that are absent from clients' repertoires. When skills training is used in specialized REBT, it is employed along with the disputation of irrational beliefs and after the client has achieved some measure of philosophical change. REBT argues that the most effective way for clients to bring about change is by the repeated use of cognitive, emotive, and behavioral techniques that are consistent with the rational beliefs that they seek to develop. These techniques are particularly important as clients face the adversities about which they previously disturbed themselves.

Techniques That Are Avoided in REBT

It is clear that REBT is a multimodal form of therapy that advocates the employment of techniques in the cognitive, emotive, and behavioral modalities. However, because the choice of therapeutic techniques is inspired by REBT theory, a number of therapeutic techniques are avoided or used sparingly in the practice of REBT (Ellis, 2002). REBT therapists do not absolutely avoid using the following methods, however, as some techniques may be useful for pragmatic purposes (Ellis, 2002):

1. Techniques that help people become more dependent (e.g., undue therapist warmth as a strong reinforcement, the creation and analysis of a transference neurosis).
2. Techniques that encourage people to become more gullible and suggestible (e.g., Pollyannish positive thinking).
3. Techniques that are long-winded and inefficient (e.g., psychoanalytic methods in general and free association in particular, encouraging lengthy descriptions of activating experiences).
4. Methods that help people feel better in the short term rather than get better in the long term (e.g., experiential techniques that fully expressing one's feelings in a dramatic or cathartic manner, some Gestalt methods and primal techniques).
5. Techniques that distract clients from working on their irrational philosophies (e.g., relaxation methods, yoga, and other cognitive distraction methods). These methods may be employed, however, along with cognitive disputing designed to yield some philosophic change.

6. Methods that unwittingly reinforce clients' philosophy of LFT (e.g., gradual desensitization).
7. Techniques that include an antiscientific philosophy (e.g., faith healing and mysticism).
8. Techniques that attempt to change activating events (A) before or without showing clients how to change their irrational beliefs (B) (e.g., some strategic family systems techniques).
9. Techniques that have dubious validity (e.g., neurolinguistic programming).

CASE EXAMPLES

Freda: A Case of Anxiety

Freda was a 40-year-old divorced woman with grown-up children, both of whom lived with her. She was involved in a car accident 18 months previously as a passenger. While not seriously hurt, she had experienced anxiety when driving ever since that time. Freda's anxiety was experienced on two levels. First, she became anxious whenever a large truck approached her from the rear. Second, she became enormously anxious about her anxiety and felt intense panic. She consulted me (W. D.), and I first worked on the larger metaproblem. Her irrational belief was "I must not be anxious and it is horrible when I am." I disputed this belief and helped her to see that anxiety is uncomfortable but not dangerous (Low, 1952). We tackled her original anxiety problem next, with the use of "inference chaining" (Moore, 1983) to reveal that she was terrified about (1) dying "before her time" and (2) what would happen to her two sons in the event of her death. First, I helped her see that no law of the universe declared that she must not die in a car crash and that she must live longer than she would live. Second, I asked her what was the worst fate she could imagine for her sons. She was particularly anxious about her elder son, who seemed somewhat vulnerable. She was also anxious that he might not be able to cope on his own and might become a vagrant, which she evaluated as "terrible." I disputed this irrational belief as well and helped Freda to see that it would be very bad or tragic, but hardly terrible, if he did become a vagrant, since there was no law of the universe that said that he must not become a vagrant. I pointed out further that if he did become a vagrant, he might still obtain some happiness. First, I encouraged her to drive even though she was anxious, and to tolerate this experience as "bad" but not "awful." After this experience brought about some improvement, I urged her to seek out large trucks and tolerate the discomfort of being "hemmed in." Additionally, I helped her to see that her irrational beliefs at B led to her overestimating the likelihood of (1) her dying and (2) her son becoming a vagrant in the event of her death, both of which were cognitive consequences (3) of her irrational beliefs.

The theme of being hemmed in emerged in other ways. She was being romantically pursued by a man in whom she felt no interest. She felt trapped because he was not discouraged by her polite requests for him to leave her alone. I asked her what would stop her from being firm and backing this assertion up with a refusal to talk to him. She thought that this approach would discourage him but said that she would feel guilty if he were hurt by such a direct approach. I helped her to see that her guilt stemmed from the belief "I would be a bad person for causing him pain." First I disputed this belief and showed her that even if she did directly cause the man pain, she could accept herself as a fallible human being for acting badly. I then helped her see that she would be responsible for depriving him rather than cruelly hurting him, since if he felt hurt or denigrated by her rejection, he would create these feelings by irrationally depreciating himself. In the next session, she claimed success at asserting herself with the man and reported further alleviation of her driving anxiety. She spontaneously reported that feeling less trapped in her personal relationships helped her feel less hemmed in while driving.

In subsequent sessions, Freda discussed further problems concerning lack of assertion, guilt, and embarrassment. I helped her to see that there were links among these problems, and she became increasingly proficient at the detection and disputation of her irrational beliefs. I explained the concept of shame-attacking exercises to her, and she reported in the next session undertaking one. For years she had been anxious about bringing men home to meet her two sons. On this occasion she met a much younger man at a dance and took him home that night. She did so to dispute her shame-inducing belief: "My sons would look down on me as a cradle-snatcher and that would prove that I am a shit." She felt that this action was very beneficial, because her sons did make several negative comments, but she had told them that she was going to live her life her way, and that although she would like their approval, if they chose to regard her as "a desperate old woman," then that was unfortunate but hardly the end of the world.

At the end of 12 weekly sessions, Freda had made significant progress in disputing her dire needs for approval and comfort. More importantly, she had internalized the method of disputing and saw the benefits of actively working to counteract her irrational philosophies. A 6-month follow-up revealed that Freda had maintained her progress. She was able to drive quite comfortably, and although she was not anxious, she still did not like having big trucks behind her. She felt much freer about saying what she thought to others and acting more in her own interests, even if others might view her in a negative light. She reported that her sons had changed their attitude toward her: "They seem to respect the 'new me' more than the old one."

Bob: A Case of Depression

Bob was a severely depressed 50-year-old man. His depression emerged after he lost his job and as a result experienced sex problems. Bob was referred to me

(W. D.) after his general practitioner discovered that he was feeling suicidal. In our first session I learned that he was feeling hopeless about his future, because he considered that he was "finished as a man." I persistently showed him that he could accept himself as a man who had temporarily lost employment and erectile sufficiency, rather than damn himself as being less of a man for these two losses. His mood lifted appreciably by the end of the session, but I told him that he could telephone me between sessions if he became suicidal again.

In our second session I discovered he was also ashamed about being depressed and about seeking psychotherapeutic help. Again I helped him to dispute his irrational belief, "I must be able to solve my problems on my own," and also encouraged him to counteract his shame by telling his best friend about his problems.

He reported feeling much better at the start of our third session. Bob did not feel ashamed about telling his friend about his problems, and he had received a sympathetic response from his friend, who in turn confided that he had had similar problems the previous year. This response had a profound effect on Bob, as it helped him to see that he could gain happiness by changing some of his priorities. He began to see that friendship was as important as achievement, and that it was possible for him to redefine what it meant to be a man.

In our fourth session I disputed his anxiety-creating belief about his sexual performance, and his irrational belief that "I must get it up to be a man." It was apparent that Bob clearly understood the difference between rational and irrational beliefs. He went home and enjoyed several sexual experiences with his wife when he resolved to act on the belief that "an erection and orgasm would be nice, but sex can be enjoyed without them." Additionally, Bob decided to do some voluntary work in a local hospital, and he enjoyed it even though he predicted he would gain no satisfaction from doing so.

Bob demonstrated interest in the area of gender identity and read several books on the pressures of being a male in today's society. He began to take a more active role with domestic chores and by the seventh session no longer regarded it as "women's work." In the eighth session Bob relapsed and reported feeling depressed again. It transpired that he was condemning himself for being "an erstwhile male chauvinist." I showed him again that he was a fallible human, and that he could accept himself as such even if he had adhered to a male chauvinistic philosophy in the past, and even if he still retained some of this philosophy today. We had a full discussion of the concept of unconditional self-acceptance, and Bob resolved to act on this philosophy.

In our final two sessions we discussed several career-related issues. Bob decided as a result of this discussion to attend a university and study for a degree in social work. At our final session, he considered how he had changed some fundamental attitudes:

"Looking back, I can realize that I had believed in the concept of the two-dimensional man. I was OK as long as I was in a good job and my cock functioned well. Now I can see that there is much more to being a man than that. I feel you have helped me widen my horizons and I now view myself as being considerably more complex than before. I have an increased enjoyment of friendship, and sex with my wife is incredibly more enriching."

A 6-month follow-up revealed that Bob was enjoying his university course and was free from depression. At his first therapy session, his Beck Depression Inventory score of 42 was in the severe range. At his 10th and final session of regular therapy, his score had gone down to 3, and at the 6-month follow-up it was 1.

THE EMPIRICAL STATUS
OF RATIONAL EMOTIVE BEHAVIOR THERAPY

REBT should be evaluated at two levels: (1) the empirical status of its theory; and (2) the empirical status of its clinical strategies.

Rational Emotive Behavioral Theory

The following summarizes what we know and do not know about the empirical status of REBT theory (based on David, Schnur, & Belloi, 2002; David, Szentagotai, et al., 2005; David, Montgomery, et al., 2005):

What We Know

1. The ABC model as a general framework has received significant empirical support (e.g., Lazarus, 1991), is the fundamental framework of all cognitive-behavioral psychotherapies (e.g., see Dobson, 2000), and is widely accepted in the clinical field.

2. Irrational beliefs, such as particular types of cognitive appraisal (hot cognitions), are considered important causal mechanisms involved in various clinical conditions. For example, awfulizing is involved in both anxiety and pain, whereas running oneself down is a fundamental component of depressed mood (e.g., David et al., 2002; David, Szentagotai, et al., 2005; Solomon, Bruce, Gotlib, & Wind, 2003). The aspect links rational emotive behavioral theory to the major modern motivational and emotion theories.

3. Demandingness (i.e., psychological inflexibility/absolutistic thinking) is a primary irrational cognitive process/mechanism, and LFT, awfulizing, and global evaluation/self-depreciation are secondary irrational appraisal mechanisms (e.g., see DiLorenzo et al., 2007). However, demandingness, as part of the reappraisal process (see David, 2003; Lazarus, 1991) might follow the secondary irrational appraisal mechanism.

4. Irrational beliefs are cognitive vulnerability factors, which means that they only generate a clinical condition in conjunction with some more or less explicit stressful activating events.

5. Irrational beliefs generate distorted descriptions and inferences. For example, Szentagotai and Freeman (2007) found that the depressed mood of patients with major depression is determined by automatic thoughts, which are influenced by irrational beliefs. The way we represent activating events in our mind (i.e., by descriptions and inferences) depends on the interaction between the activating events and our rational and irrational beliefs. Descriptions and inferences ("cold cognitions") may in turn generate various operant behaviors, then both cold cognitions and operant behaviors may be further appraised in a rational–irrational manner, producing feelings and physiological responses (see David, 2003; Szentagotai & Freeman, 2007).

6. There is a specific pattern of irrational beliefs for various clinical feelings: demandingness and LFT for anger, demandingness and global evaluation/depreciation for depressive mood, and demandingness and awfulizing for anxiety, and so forth (e.g., see David et al., 2002).

What We Do Not Know

1. Rational beliefs have often been conceptualized as a low level of irrational beliefs rather than as an independent construct; in other words, they have been conceptualized as poles of a unidimensional construct. Research has shown, however, that rational and irrational beliefs are independent (e.g., Bernard, 1998). Unfortunately, few assessment measures have an independent scale for rational beliefs. Thus, we do not know clearly the role of irrational beliefs in health promotion and the prevention of clinical conditions.

2. We do not know whether rational beliefs generate functional descriptions and inferences during specific activating events.

3. We know very little about the biological implementation of rational and irrational beliefs. For example, an interesting empirical question is whether rational beliefs are mainly related to various prefrontal areas, whereas irrational beliefs are related to both prefrontal cortex and the amygdala; considering that irrational beliefs are highly emotionally laden and difficult to change, and are supposed to have a strong ancient biological and even evolutionary basis, this is a viable hypothesis, with implication for both theory and practice of REBT. For example, do rational beliefs replace irrational beliefs or just control them and their output? Depending on the answer to this question, various new clinical strategies for cognitive restructuring might emerge.

4. We do not know in detail the qualitative and quantitative differences between healthy/functional and unhealthy/dysfunctional feelings (e.g., depressed mood vs. sadness; anxiety vs. concern; anger vs. annoyance; guilt vs. remorse), and how rational and irrational beliefs are related to these differences. Research (e.g., David et al., 2005b) tends to suggest a binary or qualitative model of distress, but the data are not yet compelling.

Myths and Misconceptions
Regarding Rational Emotive Behavioral Theory

The following analysis is based on the work of David, Szentagotai, et al. (2005). REBT theory has often been described by its critics as a "monolithic," inflexible therapy, incapable of addressing specific disorders and of providing a differentiated understanding of the specific pattern of cognitive processes underlying various forms of psychopathology (Beck et al., 1979; Padesky & Beck, 2003). There is a significant empirical basis for these specific cognitive models of various cognitive-behavioral psychotherapies; their implications for various disorders (e.g., anxiety, depression, personality) have been well documented (e.g., Beck & Emery, 1985; Riskind, 1999). Ellis (1994) differentiates between elegant (specialized) and inelegant (general) REBT. Whereas inelegant REBT has assimilated these specific models, elegant REBT, while acknowledging them (see Ellis, 1994), describes the core of psychopathology as comprising a few basic irrational beliefs. Symptoms and specific cognitions (e.g., specific descriptions and inferences in the form of automatic thoughts) described by various specific disorder models are considered the products of these core irrational beliefs.

According to REBT, challenging core irrational beliefs is accompanied by a change in both symptoms and in cognitions described by specific models (DiGiuseppe, 1996; Dryden et al., 1989a; Dryden, Ferguson, & Hylton, 1989b; Dryden, Ferguson, & McTeague, 1989c). This "reductionistic approach" is identical to the neurosciences approach, in which a whole range of psychopathology is reduced to several neurotransmitters and their interactions. However, even if we accept the "reductionistic" label, in a sense similar to that used in neurosciences, the difficulties of REBT in explaining different emotional reactions may still be a myth. Indeed, as we mentioned earlier, David et al. (2002) have described how different core irrational beliefs interact with one another to generate various emotional problems (e.g., demandingness and awfulizing in anxiety; demandingness and LFT in anger; demandingness and self-depreciation in depressed mood etc.).

Some proponents of cognitive therapy (e.g., Padesky & Beck, 2003) launched another criticism of REBT, arguing that it is more a philosophical theory and therapy than a scientific one. This is an epistemological misconstruction of REBT. Any psychotherapeutic system can be described at a paradigmatic level (i.e., philosophical assumptions), a theoretical level (empirically testable hypotheses), and in reference to its models and intervention procedures. In all psychotherapeutic systems, assumptions are neither verifiable nor falsifiable; they are often assumed simply because the influential founder of the paradigm proposed them. REBT as a system might be incompatible with the way the mainstream works and has therefore not been able to penetrate it fully, mainly because REBT typically exposes its philosophical assumptions (e.g., see in this chapter the discussion about the nature of human beings). For example, cognitive therapy has its own untestable assumptions beyond the well-validated models and theories, but they are often not exposed. It has been quite a while now that REBT has modified its original approach by exposing its theory and models for testing, not just its philosophical assumptions. Meta-analyses of the studies focused on these REBT theory and intervention models (e.g., Engels, Garnefsky, & Diekstra, 1993) suggest that REBT is very probably efficacious and an evidence-based form of CBT.

REBT theory has been unfairly criticized. For example, MacInnes (2004) states that limited evidence supports it. Although more research is needed to test REBT theory, the criteria and the method used by MacInnes (2004) are not correct in our view. For example, he confuses the random selection of participants with the randomized distribution of participants in various experimental conditions. A randomized distribution of participants in various groups is fundamental for testing REBT theory, while a randomized selection of participants from the general population would be useful to generalize it. Most REBT studies presented by MacInnes as flawed for not using randomization have, in fact, used a randomized distribution of participants in various groups to test the theory rigorously. Considering that most scientific studies do not involve representative samples of the population, why should this be a fundamental problem only in the case of REBT? Similar to other scientific areas, REBT compensates for this shortcoming by arguing for generalization by means of repeating studies.

The Empirical Status of Rational Emotive Behavior Therapy Clinical Strategies

The following synthesis is based on the work of David, Szentagotai, et al. (2005). Before 1970, rigorous empirical research regarding REBT efficacy (i.e., how REBT works in randomized controlled trials) and effectiveness (i.e., how REBT works in real-life clinical settings) was infrequently conducted. After 1970, a series of outcome studies was published, setting the basis for several qualitative reviews of REBT (e.g., DiGiuseppe, Miller, & Trexler, 1977; Ellis, 1973; Haaga & Davidson, 1989a, 1989b; Zettle & Hayes, 1980; David, Szentagotai, et al., 2005). Although generally supportive, these qualitative reviews have revealed some methodological problems that should be corrected in future research to strengthen the conclusion about the efficacy and/or effectiveness of REBT.

Outcome research has become the basis for a quantitative approach to examine the efficacy and/or effectiveness of REBT, and to address criticisms advanced in previous qualitative REBT reviews (Engels et al., 1993; Lyons & Woods, 1991). Quantitative reviews include both general studies, which focus on cognitive-behavioral psychotherapy, and specific studies of the efficacy and/or effectiveness of REBT. REBT has generally done well in quantitative reviews of psychotherapy. For example, it yielded the second highest average effect size among 10 major forms of psychotherapy in an early meta-analysis (Smith & Glass, 1977). Two rigorous meta-analyses have addressed specifically the efficacy and/or effectiveness of REBT (i.e., Engels et al., 1993; Lyons & Woods, 1991). The following conclusions about REBT's efficacy and/or effectiveness are based on these two quantitative meta-analyses (see also David, Szentagotai, et al., 2005):

- REBT research has been focused on both efficacy and effectiveness studies.
- REBT is effective for a large range of clinical psychiatric problems and clinical outcomes. REBT has a much greater effect on "low reactivity" outcomes, which do not have an evident relationship with the REBT treatment (e.g., physiological measures, grade-point average), than on "high reactivity" measures, which have a direct and evident relationship with the treatment (e.g., irrational beliefs). This suggests that REBT's effects are not due to participants' compliance or task demand characteristics.
- REBT is equally effective for clinical and nonclinical populations with a wide age range (9–70 years), and for males and females.
- Group and individual REBT are equally effective.
- Therapists who have a higher level of training achieve better clinical results in REBT interventions.
- Higher numbers of REBT sessions are associated with better clinical outcomes.
- Higher-quality outcome studies have shown greater REBT efficacy and/or effectiveness.

First, although favorable, the treatment efficacy literature needs to pay more attention to generic methodological criteria (see Haaga & Davidson, 1993), such as (1) formal clinical assessment of psychopathology, (2) adherence to/adequacy of clinical protocols, (3) measures of the clinical significance of change (e.g., effect sizes; normative comparisons), (4) collection of follow-up data, and (5) subject attrition. Second, patients in many of the clinical trials tend to be the YAVIS type (young, attractive, verbal, intelligent, sensitive), and some of their problems are subclinical; hence, generalization of these results to clinical practice should keep this limitation in mind. Third, REBT has evolved; therefore, it is possible that earlier studies contaminate the conclusion regarding the relative efficacy of REBT and other therapies. However, the newer generation of REBT randomized clinical trials, which adhere to broad methodological criteria, has also yielded a positive view on the efficacy of REBT. Overall, these studies have found that REBT is an effective treatment compared to various control conditions, with an efficacy comparable to most behavioral treatments for obsessive–compulsive disorder (Emmelkamp &

Beens, 1991; Emmelkamp, Visser, & Hoekstra, 1988), social phobia (Mersch, Emmelkamp, & Lips, 1991; Mersch, Emmelkamp, Böegels, & van der Sleen, 1989), and social anxiety (DiGiuseppe et al., 1990). Both REBT and self-instructional training seem less effective than *in vivo* exposure in agoraphobia (Emmelkamp, Brilman, Kuiper, & Mersch, 1988).

REBT in conjunction with pharmacotherapy has been found more effective than medication alone for major depression (e.g., Macaskill & Macaskill, 1996). In the case of patients with dysthymia, REBT has been shown to be as efficient as pharmacotherapy, but its combination with pharmacotherapy is much more promising (Wang et al., 1999). Also, REBT seems to be an effective adjunct to pharmacotherapy for inpatients with schizophrenia (e.g., Shelley, Battaglia, Lucely, Ellis, & Opler, 2001). A recent randomized clinical trial of patients with major depressive disorder ($N = 170$ patients) by David, Szentagotai, Lupu, and Cosman (2008) shows that REBT is as efficient as cognitive therapy and pharmacotherapy (i.e., fluoxetine) at the end of treatment and at 6-month follow-up (and more efficient than medication at 6-month follow-up on one of the two measures of depression).

These results encourage future clinical research regarding the efficacy (internal validity) and effectiveness (external validity) of REBT for various clinical conditions. It is important to point out that some of the REBT outcome research has been conducted on nonclinical samples displaying subclinical problems and/or in real-life clinical settings (effectiveness studies). REBT proposes not only a useful theory for clinical groups but also an educational system with implications for nonclinical and subclinical populations that have an interest in self-help and personal development. Overall, we believe that it is safe and correct to say that REBT is very probably an effective form of psychotherapy for clinical and nonclinical problems, and definitely an evidence-oriented therapy. Interestingly, its effectiveness is better validated than its efficacy. Although some REBT proponents suggest that it should be more efficient than other forms of cognitive-behavioral psychotherapy, because it focuses on fundamental evaluative core beliefs (e.g., demandigness/psychological inflexibility), this assumption has not yet received clear empirical support (DiGiuseppe et al., 1990; Warren, McLellarn, & Ponzoha, 1988). The efficacy and effectiveness of REBT should receive more empirical attention to allow a clear answer.

Finally, although irrational beliefs are important causal cognitive factors in psychopathology, it is not yet clear whether the efficacy/effectiveness of REBT can be attributed to challenging irrational beliefs, because this aspect of REBT theory has been insufficiently studied. Component designs that isolate specific beliefs or examine the association between changes in beliefs and changes in other outcome measures would provide important evidence for the basic premises of the REBT theory. Efficacy studies based on well-controlled randomized clinical trials (see, e.g., David et al., 2008), and effectiveness studies examining REBT in real clinical settings are necessary. Finally, a new quantitative meta-analysis to assess recent empirical studies of REBT efficacy and effectiveness is needed.

DIRECTIONS FOR FUTURE DEVELOPMENT

Five main future developments exist for REBT, each of which we examine briefly.

Rational Emotive Behavior Therapy within an Integrated Approach to Psychotherapy

The scientific field does not discuss "medicines" but "Medicine." Paradoxically, in psychotherapy we talk about "psychotherapies" and "schools of psychotherapy" in a scientific context. Our view is that in the future we will talk about "psychotherapy," and what today are called "schools of psychotherapy" will become clinical strategies within an evidence-based field of psychotherapy. REBT will follow the same path. Its main contributions to integrated, evidence-based psychotherapy will be both theoretical and practical.

At a theoretical level, REBT has revealed the role of the irrational cognitive processes of demandingness, awfulizing, and LFT as causal mechanisms in clinical disorders, and corresponding importance of the rational cognitive processes of acceptance-based desiring, nonawfulizing, and HFT as health-promoting mechanisms.

At the practical level, the clinical strategies introduced by REBT include (1) the use of humor and irony in cognitive restructuring, (2) the role of forceful disputation (when applicable) in cognitive restructuring, and (3) the focus on meta-emotions and meta-cognitions (called by Ellis the secondary emotions and secondary beliefs, respectively). These REBT strategies are highly complex and require a very well-trained therapist to implement them after a careful clinical assessment that considers the type of client, the type of problems, the level of the therapeutic alliance, and the level of understanding of the clinical conceptualization on which this strategy is based.

Having said this, we would like to correct an important misconception regarding REBT in the clinical field. Although these are practical innovations introduced by REBT, REBT practice is not based only on these strategies. The main contribution of REBT to the clinical field is related to the ABC model as an etiopathogenetic and sanogenetic theory. Based on this model, practical strategies used to change irrational beliefs and to promote rational beliefs depend on the client and his or her problem. Thus, the use of metaphors and of a less-directive style may be recommended in some cases, whereas in others a more direct approach to cognitive restructuring is indicated. Cognitive restructuring strategies used in REBT typically fall into the following categories: (1) pragmatic; (2) empirical; (3) logical; (4) metaphorical; (5) pastoral; and (6) other (e.g., often borrowed from various therapies, such as Gestalt therapy), depending on the type of client and his or her clinical problem.

Rational Emotive Behavior Therapy in the Era of Virtual Reality

Virtual reality (VR) technology allows a user to interact with a real or imagined computer-simulated environment. A simulated environment can be individualized to help in assessing rational and irrational beliefs and/or to test and restructure irrational beliefs. VR can also be used as a safe exposure procedure. For example, rather than using rational emotive imagery, the client can be projected into a virtual environment and be fully controlled by the therapist, but based on the client's previous descriptions. This process allows an intense and controlled exposure procedure and immersion of the client into the activating event, with a positive impact on cognitive restructuring.

Rational Emotive Behavior Therapy and Evolutionary Psychology

If Ellis (1994) was right about a biological tendency toward irrationality, the understanding of rational and irrational beliefs from the viewpoint of modern evolutionary psychology is fundamental (see Buss, 2001). Is irrationality an evolutionary design, be it a general or a more local adaptation? The implications are serious for both theory and the way therapy is conducted to change irrationality.

Rational Emotive Behavior Therapy in Health Promotion and Self-Help

The REBT perspective has a strong appeal among the cognitive-behavioral approaches. If psychopathology stems from only a few identifiable and modifiable irrational beliefs, an intervention that changes these irrational beliefs may significantly reduce a large spectrum of psychopathology and suffering. Moreover, such an intervention could be designed to address health promotion by targeting cognitive vulnerability and the enhancement of rational beliefs as protective factors. REBT is also popular in the form of pamphlets, books, audio and video recordings, and programmed material. It has already reached and affected literally millions of people via mass media presentations, including many who are not seriously disturbed but have used its principles to enhance and actualize their lives. Because REBT involves a psychoeducational process that involves teaching people how to look for and uproot their irrationalities, because it shows them how to keep doing REBT-based self-help homework as a major part of the therapeutic process, and because it can be stated in simple, self-help terms and made available to large numbers of people, we believe that the future of REBT may well lie in its mass applications and its educational procedures rather than its use for individual and group psychotherapy.

REBT has many applications and has been useful in a number of fields, such as politics, business, education, coaching, parenting, communication, sports, religion, and assertiveness training. Many other applications of REBT in these and other aspects of human life can be expected. Thus, the REBT model is not only efficient and promising in the treatment of mental disorders but also cost-effective and time-efficient in health promotion and in improving normal human functioning. REBT has been less rigorously investigated as a health promotion intervention, and this research should be a focus of future research.

Rational Emotive Behavior Therapy in the Context of Cognitive and Behavioral Sciences

Most cognitive-behavioral psychotherapies use behavioral techniques based on a classic cognitive conceptualization. REBT, however, has expanded the ABC model to assimilate a behavioral conceptualization (see David, 2003). Thus, the B refers to both explicit (conscious) and implicit (unconscious) information processing that generates behavioral consequences (C) maintained by their own effects (e.g., reinforcements). In other words, the modern ABC model has assimilated the cognitive unconscious (i.e., unconscious information processing, such as implicit memory, implicit learning, implicit perception) at the B level, and the behavioral component (e.g., reinforcement) at the C level. For example, although a drinking behavior may initially be generated by an irrational belief (B) (e.g., "I must drink to cope with my depression") during depressed mood (A), by practice, the A–C connection may become procedural (e.g., if A, then C) and automatic (coded in the procedural/implicit memory system), and once generated, the behavior is maintained by its consequences (e.g., negative reinforcement—avoiding depressed mood). Similarly, a state of anxiety can initially be generated by an irrational belief (B), such as "I must succeed; otherwise it is awful." By practice however, anxiety (C) may fall under the control and be mediated by another type of belief, often implicit, known as "response expectancy" (see Montgomery, David, DiLorenzo, & Schnur, 2007), which is defined as expectancy for a nonvolitional response, and it can be conscious (explicit memory) or unconscious (implicit memory) (Kirsch, 1999).

Thus, certain types of information are represented in our memory in a format (e.g., nonverbal associations) and neural substrate (e.g., amygdala) that make them not consciously accessible (David, 2003; Kihlstrom, 1999; Schacter & Tulving, 1994). Other types of information are represented in a format (e.g., propositional networks) and neural substrate (e.g., prefrontal cortex) that make them consciously accessible; by practice, they may end up functioning implicitly, but if and when necessary, they can be retrieved in an explicit format (see the case of automatic thoughts). Thus, contrary to Mahoney (1993) and others, we argue that the "unconscious revolution in cognitive-behavioral therapy" has not yet taken place (but see Dowd &

Courchaine, 1996), and that, in fact, it has to start by being based on a clear understanding of the cognitive unconscious and by incorporating it into the ABC model. For example, (based on David, 2003) unconscious information processes may be countered by activating conscious processes; thus, their effects can be controlled by conscious strategies. Also, an emotion generated by unconscious information processing may not be a clinical problem per se, but it may become an A, and may then be consciously appraised, generating a secondary emotional problem. These are all empirical questions that future research should explore to understand how unconscious and conscious beliefs interact with each other to generate various C's. This expanded ABC model is the modern ground on which REBT is now developing, making REBT a suitable platform for psychotherapy integration.

REFERENCES

Abelson, R., & Rosenberg, M. (1958). Symbolic psycho-logic: A model of attitudinal cognition. *Behavioral Science, 3,* 1–13.

Adler, A. (1927). *Understanding human nature.* New York: Garden City.

Adler, A. (1964). *Social interest: A challenge to mankind.* New York: Capricorn.

Beck, A. T., & Emery, G. (1985). *Anxiety disorders and phobias: A cognitive perspective.* New York: Basic Books.

Beck, A. T., Rush, A. J., Shaw, B. F., & Emery, G. (1979). *Cognitive therapy of depression.* New York: Guilford Press.

Bernard, M. E. (1998). Validations of General Attitude and Beliefs Scale. *Journal of Rational-Emotive and Cognitive-Behavior Therapy, 16,* 183–196.

Beutler, L. E. (1983). *Eclectic psychotherapy: A systematic approach.* New York: Pergamon.

Burns, D. D. (1980). *Feeling good: The new mood therapy.* New York: Morrow.

Bus, D. M. (2001). Human nature and culture: An evolutionary, psychological perspective. *Journal of Personality, 69,* 955–978.

Corsini, R. J. (Ed.). (1977). *Current personality theories.* Chicago: Wadsworth.

Cosmides, L., & Tooby, J. (2006). *Evolutionary psychology: A primer.* Available at *www.psych.ucsb.edu/research/cep/primer.html.*

Danysh, J. (1974). *Stop without quitting.* San Francisco: International Society for General Semantics.

David, D. (2003). Rational emotive behavior therapy (REBT): The view of a cognitive psychologist. In W. Dryden (Ed.), *Rational emotive behavior therapy: Theoretical developments* (pp. 130–159). London: Brunner/Routledge.

David, D., Montgomery, G., Macavei, B., & Bovbjerg, D. (2005). An empirical investigation of Albert Ellis's binary model of distress. *Journal of Clinical Psychology, 61,* 499–516.

David, D., Schnur, J., & Belloiu, A. (2002). Another search for the "hot" cognition: Appraisal irrational beliefs, attribution, and their relation to emotion. *Journal of Rational-Emotive and Cognitive-Behavior Therapy, 20,* 93–131.

David, D., & Szentagotai, A. (2006). Cognitions in cognitive-behavioral therapies; toward an integrative model. *Clinical Psychology Review, 26,* 284–298.

David, D., Szentagotai, A., Kallay, E., & Macavei, B. (2005). A synopsis of rational-emotive behavior therapy (REBT): Fundamental and applied research. *Journal of Rational-Emotive and Cognitive-Behavior Therapy, 23,* 175–221.

David, D., Szentagotai, A., Lupu, V., & Cosman, D. (2008). Rational emotive therapy, cognitive therapy, and medication in the treatment of major depressive disorder: A randomized clinical trial, posttreatment outcomes, and six-month follow-up. *Journal of Clinical Psychology, 6,* 728–746.

DiGiuseppe, R. (1991). Comprehensive cognitive disputing in RET. In M. E. Bernard (Ed.), *Using rational-emotive therapy effectively* (pp. 173–195). New York: Plenum Press.

DiGiuseppe, R. (1996). The nature of irrational and rational beliefs: Progress in rational emotive behavior theory. *Journal of Rational-Emotive and Cognitive-Behavior Therapy, 4,* 5–28.

DiGiuseppe, R., Simon, K. S., McGowan, L., & Gardner, F. (1990). A comparative outcome study of four cognitive therapies in the treatment of social anxiety. *Journal of Rational-Emotive and Cognitive-Behavior Therapy, 8,* 129–146.

DiGiuseppe, R., Miller, N. J., & Trexler, L. D. (1977). A review of rational-emotive psychotherapy studies. *Counseling Psychologist, 7,* 64–72.

DiLorenzo, T. A., David, D., & Montgomery, G. (2007). The interrelations between irrational cognitive processes and distress in stressful academic settings. *Personality and Individual Differences, 42,* 765–776.

Dobson, K. S. (Ed.). (2000). *Handbook of cognitive-behavioral therapies* (2nd ed.). New York: Guilford Press.

Dowd, T. E., & Courchaine, E. K. (1996). Implicit learning, tacit knowledge, and implications for stasis and change in cognitive psychotherapy. *Journal of Cognitive Psychotherapy, 10,* 163–180.

Dryden, W. (1984a). *Rational-emotive therapy: Fundamentals and innovations.* London: Croom-Helm.

Dryden, W. (1984b). Rational-emotive therapy. In W. Dryden (Ed.), *Individual therapy in Britain* (pp. 235–263). London: Harper & Row.

Dryden, W. (1985). Challenging but not overwhelming: A compromise in negotiating homework assignments. *British Journal of Cognitive Psychotherapy, 3*(1), 77–80.

Dryden, W. (1998). *Developing self-acceptance.* Chichester, UK: Wiley.

Dryden, W. (1999). *Rational emotive behaviour therapy: A personal view.* Bicester, UK: Winslow Press.

Dryden. W. (2001). Reason to change: A rational emotive behaviour therapy (REBT) workbook. Hove, East Sussex, UK: Bruner/Routledge.

Dryden, W. (2008). *The distinctive features of rational emotive behavior therapy.* London: Routledge.

Dryden, W., & Ellis, A. (1986). Rational-emotive therapy. In W. Dryden & W. L. Golden (Eds.), *Cognitive-behavioural approaches to psychotherapy* (pp. 129–168). London: Harper & Row.

Dryden, W., Ferguson, J., & Clark, T. (1989a). Beliefs and inferences: A test of rational-emotive hypothesis 1: Performing in an academic seminar. *Journal of Rational-Emotive and Cognitive-Behavior Therapy, 7,* 119–129.

Dryden, W., Ferguson, J., & Hylton, B. (1989b). Beliefs and inference A of rational-emotive hypothesis 3: On expectations about enjoying a party. *British Journal of Guidance and Counselling, 17,* 68–75.

Dryden, W., Ferguson, J., & McTeague, S. (1989c). Beliefs and inferences: A test of rational-emotive hypothesis 2: On the prospect of seeing a spider. *Psychological Reports, 64,* 115–123.

Duckro, P., Beal, D., & George, C. (1979). Research on the effects of disconfirmed role expectations in psychotherapy: A critical review. *Psychological Bulletin, 86,* 260–275.

Ellis, A. (1962). *Reason and emotion in psychotherapy.* Secaucus, NJ: Lyle Stuart.

Ellis, A. (1963). Toward a more precise definition of "emotional" and "intellectual" insight. *Psychological Reports, 13,* 125–126.

Ellis, A. (1969). A weekend of rational encounter. *Rational Living, 4*(2), 1–8.

Ellis, A. (1971a). *Growth through reason.* North Hollywood, CA: Wilshire Books.

Ellis, A. (1971b). *How to stubbornly refuse to be ashamed of anything* [Cassette recording]. New York: Institute for Rational-Emotive Therapy.

Ellis, A. (Speaker). (1972a). *Solving emotional problems* [Cassette recording]. New York: Institute for Rational-Emotive Therapy.

Ellis, A. (1972b). Helping people get better: Rather than merely feel better. *Rational Living, 7,* 2–9.

Ellis, A. (1973). *Humanistic psychotherapy: The rational-emotive approach.* New York: McGraw-Hill.

Ellis, A. (1976). The biological basis of human irrationality. *Journal of Individual Psychology, 32,* 145–168.

Ellis, A. (1977a). Fun as psychotherapy. *Rational Living, 12*(1), 2–6.

Ellis, A. (Speaker). (1977b). *A garland of rational humorous songs* [Cassette recording]. New York: Institute for Rational-Emotive Therapy.

Ellis, A. (1977c). *Anger—how to live with and without it.* Secaucus, NJ: Citadel Press.

Ellis, A. (1979a). The theory of rational-emotive therapy. In A. Ellis & J. M. Whiteley (Eds.), *Theoretical and empirical foundations of rational-emotive therapy* (pp. 33–60). Monterey, CA: Brooks/Cole.

Ellis, A. (1979b). Discomfort anxiety: A new cognitive behavioral construct: Part 1. *Rational Living, 14*(2), 3–8.

Ellis, A. (1979c). The practice of rational-emotive therapy. In A. Ellis & J. M. Whiteley (Eds.), *Theoretical and empirical foundations of rational-emotive therapy* (pp. 61–100). Monterey, CA: Brooks/Cole.

Ellis, A. (1979d). The issue of force and energy in behavioral change. *Journal of Contemporary Psychotherapy, 10,* 83–97.

Ellis, A. (1979e). A note on the treatment of agoraphobics with cognitive modification versus prolonged exposure *in vivo. Behaviour Research and Therapy, 17,* 162–164.

Ellis, A. (1980a). Discomfort anxiety: A new cognitive behavioral construct: Part 2. *Rational Living, 15*(1), 25–30.

Ellis, A. (1980b). Rational-emotive therapy and cognitive behavior therapy: Similarities and differences. *Cognitive Therapy and Research, 4,* 325–340.

Ellis, A. (1981a). The place of Immanuel Kant in cognitive psychotherapy. *Rational Living, 16,* 13–16.

Ellis, A. (1981b). The use of rational humorous songs in psychotherapy. *Voices, 16*(4), 29–36.

Ellis, A. (1982). Intimacy in rational-emotive therapy. In M. Fisher & G. Striker (Eds.), *Intimacy* (pp. 203–217). New York: Plenum Press.

Ellis, A. (1983a). *The case against religiosity.* New York: Institute for Rational-Emotive Therapy.

Ellis, A. (1983b). How to deal with your most difficult client: You. *Journal of Rational-Emotive Therapy, 1*(1), 3–8. Also published 1984 in *Psychotherapy in Private Practice, 2,* 25–36.

Ellis, A. (1983c). The philosophic implications and dangers of some popular behavior therapy techniques. In M. Rosenbaum, C. M. Franks, & Y. Jaffe (Eds.), *Perspectives in behavior therapy in the eighties* (pp. 138–155). New York: Springer.

Ellis, A. (1983d). Failures in rational-emotive therapy. In E. B. Foa & P. M. G. Emmelkamp (Eds.), *Failures in behavior therapy* (pp. 159–171). New York: Wiley.

Ellis, A. (1983e). Rational-emotive therapy (RET) approaches to overcoming resistance: I. Common forms of resistance. *British Journal of Cognitive Psychotherapy, 1,* 28–38.

Ellis, A. (1983f). Rational-emotive therapy (RET) approaches to overcoming resistance: II. How RET disputes clients' irrational resistance-creating beliefs. *British Journal of Cognitive Psychotherapy, 1*(2), 1–16.

Ellis, A. (1984a). The essence of RET. *Journal of Rational-Emotive Therapy, 2*(1), 19–25.

Ellis, A. (1984b, August). *Rational-emotive therapy and transpersonal psychology.* Paper presented at the 92nd Annual Convention of the American Psychological Association, Toronto, Canada.

Ellis, A. (1984c). Rational-emotive therapy. In R. J. Corsini (Ed.), *Current psychotherapies* (3rd ed., pp. 196–238). Itasca, IL: Peacock.

Ellis, A. (1984d). Rational-emotive therapy (RET) approaches to overcoming resistance: III. Using emotive and behavioural techniques of overcoming resistance. *British Journal of Cognitive Psychotherapy, 2*(1), 11–26.

Ellis, A. (1985a). Expanding the ABCs of rational-emotive therapy. In M. J. Mahoney & A. Freeman (Eds.), *Cognition and psychotherapy* (pp. 313–323). New York: Plenum Press.

Ellis, A. (1985b). Rational-emotive therapy (RET) approaches to overcoming resistance: IV. Handling special kinds of clients. *British Journal of Cognitive Psychotherapy, 3,* 26–42.

Ellis, A. (1993a). Changing rational-emotive therapy (RET) to rational emotive behavior therapy (REBT). *Behavior Therapist, 16,* 257–258.

Ellis, A. (1993b). Rational-emotive imagery: RET version. In M. E. Bernard & J. L. Wolfe (Eds.), *The RET source book for practitioners* (pp. II, 8–II, 10). New York: Institute for Rational-Emotive Therapy.

Ellis, A. (1993c). Vigorous RET disputing. In M. E. Bernard & J. L. Wolfe, (Eds.), *The RET resource book for practitioners* (pp. 2–7). New York: Institute for Rational-Emotive Therapy.

Ellis, A. (1994). *Reason and emotion in psychotherapy* (Rev. and updated). Secaucus, NJ: Birch Lane.

Ellis, A. (1995). Rational emotive behavior therapy. In R. Corsini & D. Wedding (Eds.), *Current psychotherapies* (5th ed., pp. 162–196). Itasca, IL: Peacock.

Ellis, A. (1996a). *Better, deeper, and more enduring brief therapy.* New York: Brunner/Mazel.

Ellis, A. (1996b). Responses to criticisms of rational emotive behavior therapy (REBT) by Ray DiGiuseppe, Frank Bond, Windy Dryden, Steve Weinrach, and Richard Wessler. *Journal of Rational-Emotive and Cognitive-Behavior Therapy, 14,* 97–121.

Ellis, A. (1997). The evolution of Albert Ellis and rational emotive behavior therapy. In J. K. Zeig (Ed.), *The evolution of psychotherapy: The third conference* (pp. 69–82). New York: Brunner/Mazel.

Ellis, A. (1998). *How to control your anxiety before it controls you.* Secaucus, NJ: Carol.

Ellis, A. (2002). *Overcoming resistance: A rational emotive behavior therapy integrated approach* (2nd ed.). New York: Springer.

Ellis, A., & Abrahms, E. (1978). *Brief psychotherapy in medical and health practice.* New York: Springer.

Ellis, A., & Becker, I. (1982). *A guide to personal happiness.* North Hollywood, CA: Wilshire Books.

Ellis, A., & Grieger, R. (Eds.). (1977). *Handbook of rational-emotive therapy.* New York: Springer.

Ellis, A., & Harper, R. A. (1961a). *A guide to rational living.* Englewood Cliffs, NJ: Prentice-Hall.

Ellis, A., & Harper, R. A. (1961b). *A guide to successful marriage.* North Hollywood, CA: Wilshire Books.

Ellis, A., & Harper, R. A. (1997). *A guide to rational living* (3rd rev. ed.). North Hollywood, CA: Melvin Powers.

Emmelkamp, P. M., & Beens, H. (1991). Cognitive therapy with obsessive–compulsive disorder: A comparative evaluation. *Behaviour Research and Therapy, 29,* 293–300.

Emmelkamp, P. M., Brilman, E., Kuiper, H., & Mersch, P. P. (1988). The treatment of agoraphobia: A comparison of self-instructional training, rational emotive therapy, and exposure *in vivo. Behavior Modification, 10,* 37–53.

Emmelkamp, P. M. G., Kuipers, A. C. M., & Eggeraat, J. B. (1978). Cognitive modification versus prolonged exposure *in vivo*: A comparison with agoraphobics as subjects. *Behaviour Research and Therapy, 16,* 33–41.

Emmelkamp, P. M., Visser, S., & Hoekstra, R. (1988). Cognitive therapy vs. exposure *in vivo* on the treatment of obsessive–compulsives. *Cognitive Therapy and Research, 12,* 103–114.

Engels, G. I., Garnefsky, N., & Diekstra, F. W. (1993). Efficacy of rational-emotive therapy: A quantitative analysis. *Journal of Consulting and Clinical Psychology, 6,* 1083–1090.

Eschenroeder, C. (1979). Different therapeutic styles in rational-emotive therapy. *Rational Living,* 14(1), 3–7.

Freud, A. (1937). *The ego and the mechanisms of defense.* London: Hogarth.

Golden, W. L. (1983). Rational-emotive hypnotherapy: Principles and practice. *British Journal of Cognitive Psychotherapy,* 1(1), 47–56.

Grieger, R., & Boyd, J. (1980). *Rational-emotive therapy: A skills-based approach.* New York: Van Nostrand Reinhold.

Haaga, D. A. F., & Davidson, G. C. (1989a). Slow progress in rational-emotive therapy outcome research: Etiology and treatment. *Cognitive Therapy and Research, 13,* 493–508.

Haaga, D. A. F., & Davidson, G. C. (1989b). Outcome studies of rational-emotive therapy. In M. E. Bernard & R. DiGiuseppe (Eds.), *Inside rational-emotive therapy: A critical appraisal of the theory and therapy of Albert Ellis* (pp. 155–197). New York: Academic Press.

Haaga, D. A. F., & Davidson, G. C. (1993). An appraisal of rational-emotive therapy. *Journal of Consulting and Clinical Psychology, 61,* 215–220.

Hauck, P. A. (1972). *Reason in pastoral counseling.* Philadelphia: Westminster.

Heidegger, M. (1949). *Existence and being.* Chicago: Henry Regnery.

Herzberg, A. (1945). *Active psychotherapy.* New York: Grune & Stratton.

Horney, K. (1950). *Neurosis and human growth.* New York: Norton.

Jones, R. A. (1977). *Self-fulfilling prophecies: Social, psychological and physiological effects of expectancies.* Hillsdale, NJ: Erlbaum.

Kelly, G. (1955). *The psychology of personal constructs.* New York: Norton.

Kihlstrom, J. F. (1999). The psychological unconscious. In P. A. Lawrence & O. P. John (Eds.), *Handbook of personality: Theory and research* (2nd ed., pp. 424–442). New York: Guilford Press.

Kirsch, I. (1999). *How expectancies shape experience.* Washington, DC: American Psychological Association.

Korzybski, A. (1933). *Science and sanity.* San Francisco: International Society of General Semantics.

Lazarus, A. A. (1984). *In the mind's eye: The power of imagery for personal enrichment.* New York: Guilford Press.

Lazarus, R. S. (1991). *Emotion and adaptation.* New York: Oxford University Press.

Linehan, M. M. (1993). *Cognitive-behavioral treatment of borderline personality disorder.* New York: Guilford Press.

Low, A. A. (1952). *Mental health through will-training.* West Hanover, MA: Christopher.

Lyons, L. C., & Woods, P. J. (1991). The efficacy of rational-emotive therapy: A quantitative review of the outcome research. *Clinical Psychology Review, 11,* 357–369.

Macaskill, N. D., & Macaskill, A. (1983). Preparing patients for psychotherapy. *British Journal of Clinical and Social Psychiatry, 2,* 80–84.

Macaskill, N. D., & Macaskill, A. (1996). Rational-emotive therapy plus pharmacotherapy versus pharmacotherapy alone in the treatment of high cognitive dysfunction depression. *Cognitive Therapy and Research, 20,* 575–592.

MacInnes, D. (2004). The theories underpinning rational emotive behaviour therapy: Where's the supportive evidence? *International Journal of Nursing Studies, 41,* 685–695.

Mackay, D. (1984). Behavioural psychotherapy. In W. Dryden (Ed.), *Individual therapy in Britain* (pp. 264–294). London: Harper & Row.

Mahoney, M. J. (1993). Introduction to special section: Theoretical developments in the cognitive psychotherapies. *Journal of Consulting and Clinical Psychology, 61,* 187–194.

Maultsby, M. C., Jr. (1975). *Help yourself to happiness: Through rational self-counseling.* New York: Institute for Rational-Emotive Therapy.

Maultsby, M. C., Jr., & Ellis, A. (1974). *Technique for using rational-emotive imagery.* New York: Institute for Rational-Emotive Therapy.

Mersch, P. P., Emmelkamp, P. M., Bögels, S. M., & van der Sleen, J. (1989). Social phobia: Individual response patterns and the effects of behavioural and cognitive interventions. *Behaviour Research Therapy, 27,* 421–434.

Mersch, P. P., Emmelkamp, P. M., & Lips, C. (1991). Social phobia: Individual response patterns and the long-term effects of behavioural and cognitive interventions: A follow-up study. *Behaviour Research and Therapy, 29,* 357–362.

Montgomery, G., David, D., DiLOrenzo, T., & Schnur, J. (2007). Response expectancies and irrational beliefs predict exam-related distress. *Journal of Rational-Emotive and Cognitive-Behavior Therapy, 25,* 17–34.

Moore, R. H. (1983). Inference as "A" in RET. *British Journal of Cognitive Psychotherapy, 1*(2), 17–23.

Padesky, C. A., & Beck. A. T. (2003). Science and philosophy: comparison of cognitive therapy and rational emotive behavior therapy. *Journal of Cognitive Psychotherapy 17,* 211–224.

Phadke, K. M. (1982). Some innovations in RET theory and practice. *Rational Living, 17*(2), 25–30.

Popper, K. R. (1959). *The logic of scientific discovery.* New York: Harper & Brothers.

Popper, K. R. (1963). *Conjectures and refutations.* New York: Harper & Brothers.

Powell, J. (1976). *Fully human, fully alive.* Niles, IL: Argus.

Reber, A. (1993). *Implicit learning and tacit knowledge: An essay on the cognitive unconscious.* New York: Oxford University Press.

Reichenbach, H. (1953). *The rise of scientific philosophy.* Berkeley: University of California Press.

Riskind, J. H. (1999). Introduction to Special Issue on Cognitive Styles and Psychopathology. *Journal of Cognitive Psychotherapy: An International Quarterly, 13,* 3–4.

Rogers, C. R. (1957). The necessary and sufficient conditions of therapeutic personality change. *Journal of Consulting Psychology, 21,* 95–103.

Russell, B. (1930). *The conquest of happiness.* New York: New American Library.

Russell, B. (1965). *The basic writings of Bertrand Russell.* New York: Simon & Schuster.

Schachter, S., & Singer, J. E. (1962). Cognitive, social and physiological determinants of emotional state. *Psychological Review, 69,* 379–399.

Schacter, D. L., & Tulving, E. (1994). *Memory systems.* Cambridge, MA: MIT Press.

Shelley, A. M., Battaglia, J., Lucely, J., Ellis, A., & Opler, A. (2001). Symptom-specific group therapy for inpatients with schizophrenia. *Einstein Quarterly Journal of Biology and Medicine, 18,* 21–28.

Smith, M. L., & Glass, G. V. (1977). Meta-analysis of psychotherapy outcome studies. *American Psychologist, 32,* 752–760.

Solomon, A., Bruce, A., Gotlib, I. H., & Wind, B. (2003). Individualized measurement of irrational beliefs in remitted depressives. *Journal of Clinical Psychology, 59,* 439–455.

Szentagotai, A., & Freeman, A. (2007). An analysis of the relationship between irrational beliefs and automatic thoughts in predicting distress. *Journal of Cognitive and Behavioral Psychotherapies, 7,* 1–11.

Tiba, A., & Szentagotai, A. (2005). Positive emotions and irrational beliefs: Dysfunctional positive emotions in healthy individuals. *Journal of Cognitive and Behavioral Psychotherapies, 5,* 53–72.

Tillich, P. (1953). *The courage to be.* New Haven: Yale University Press.

Wachtel, P. L. (1977). *Psychoanalysis and behavior therapy: Toward an integration.* New York: Basic Books.

Wang, C., Jia, F., Fang, R., et al. (1999). Comparative study of rational-emotive therapy for 95 patients with dysthymic disorder. *Chinese Mental Health Journal, 13*, 172–183.

Warren, R., McLellarn, R. W., Ponzoha, C. (1988). Rational-emotive therapy versus general cognitive-behavior therapy in the treatment of low self-esteem and related emotional disturbances. *Cognitive Therapy and Research, 12*, 21–37.

Weiner, B. (1985). *An attributional theory of motivation and emotion.* New York: Springer-Verlag.

Weinrach, S. G. (1980). Unconventional therapist: Albert Ellis. *Personnel and Guidance Journal, 59*(2), 152–160.

Werner, E. E., & Smith, R. S. (1982). *Vulnerable but invincible: A study of resilient children.* New York: McGraw-Hill.

Wessler, R. A., & Wessler, R. L. (1980). *The principles and practice of rational-emotive therapy.* San Francisco: Jossey-Bass.

Wessler, R. L. (1984). Alternative conceptions of rational-emotive therapy: Toward a philosophically neutral psychotherapy. In M. A. Reda & M. J. Mahoney (Eds.), *Cognitive psychotherapies: Recent developments in theory, research, and practice* (pp. 65–79). Cambridge, MA: Ballinger.

Young, H. S. (1974). *A rational counseling primer.* New York: Institute for Rational-Emotive Therapy.

Zettle, R. D., & Hayes, S. C. (1980). Conceptual and empirical status of rational-emotive therapy. *Progress in Behaviour Modification, 9*, 125–166.

CHAPTER 9

Cognitive Therapy

Robert J. DeRubeis
Christian A. Webb
Tony Z. Tang
Aaron T. Beck

Since its introduction by Aaron T. Beck in the 1960s, cognitive therapy (CT) has grown steadily in its influence, as best reflected in its now nearly ubiquitous representation in not training programs in clinical psychology but also social work, nursing, psychiatry, and other professions where education in evidence-based treatments of mental illness is valued. Not coincidentally, the number of research investigations regarding either the benefits of CT or related issues of mechanism or theory has also undergone steady growth. As a consequence, in a variety of disorders, CT is now seen as a viable, if not superior, alternative to hitherto dominant treatments, such as medications for depression.

Although the initial impetus for CT came from Beck's early interviews with depressed patients (Beck, 1963), the content of the treatment has evolved. While operating initially from a classically Freudian perspective, Beck found that Freud's (1917/1957) formulations of the depressive syndrome (melancholia) missed the mark in several respects. Following several systematic studies (Beck, 1961; Beck & Hurvich, 1959; Beck & Ward, 1961), Beck eschewed an anger-turned-inward model and saw that, clinically, a more satisfying formulation focused on the *content* of the depressed person's negative thinking. His early descriptions emphasized the common negative biases and distortions that he found among depressed patients. These descriptions led to hypotheses about the content and processes of cognition that are relatively distinctive to depression. Importantly, he argued that these cognitive aspects are more central to depression and more amenable to verification than the dynamic (motivational) processes posited in work to that time. Early studies were generally supportive of this view (see Hollon & Beck, 1979, for a review).

In this chapter we outline the cognitive theory of psychopathology and describe treatment procedures that follow from the theory. We then consider evidence for the efficacy of the treatment approach, as well as evidence concerning the critical elements of CT. We conclude with future directions for research on CT.

BASIC THEORY

A cognitive theory of depression assumes that the depressed person exhibits distorted information processing, which results in a consistently negative view of him- or herself, the future, and the world. These cognitive contents and processes are presumed to underlie the behavioral, affective, and motivational symptoms of depression. To understand the nature of an emotional episode or disturbance, the cognitive model of emotional disorders focuses on the cognitive content of one's reaction to the upsetting event or stream of thought. The heuristic and therapeutic value of the cognitive model lies in its emphasis on the relatively easily accessed (preconscious or conscious) mental events that patients can be trained to report. It does not depend on "unconscious" motivations, the nature of which in psychoanalytic therapies it is the therapist's responsibility to ascertain.

During the treatment of depression, the beliefs reported by the patient are examined as they pertain to his or her views of him- or herself, the future, and the world. This trio of domains has been labeled the "cognitive triad" (Beck, Rush, Shaw, & Emery, 1979), and is used to help therapist and patient identify areas of concern that are involved in emotional distress. The assumption is that sadness, loss of motivation, suicidal wishes, and so on, are related to concerns in one (or more) of these three domains. Similar relations between overt symptoms and beliefs are assumed to operate in other disorders as well. For example, cognitive aspects of the anxious state, which typically are concerned with future disaster or discomfort, are the focus in anxious patients.

Treatment Mechanisms

CT focuses on beliefs of various kinds: the patient's expectations, evaluations (or ascriptions), and attributions of causality or responsibility (Hollon & Kriss, 1984). Once the patient attends to the content of his or her cognitive reaction, he or she is encouraged to view it as a hypothesis rather than as a fact; that is, as a possible but not necessarily true proposition. Framing a belief as a hypothesis has been called "distancing" to refer to the way one can dissociate oneself from a belief to allow a more objective examination of it (see Hollon, 1999). Through careful scrutiny and consideration of the belief, the patient can gradually arrive at a different view. By virtue of change in the belief, change in the emotional reaction follows; that is, with the attenuation of the cognitive basis for an emotionally upsetting reaction to an event or problem, the emotional reaction will subside.

Several effects are expected from repeated attempts to identify and question the content of the patient's reactions to events. First, concern over troubling events in the recent past diminishes, since the patient no longer holds the initially troubling aspects of the beliefs. This reduced concern limits the negative affect that would normally occur during ruminations about, or recollections of, these events. The result is a less negative "basal" level of emotion or mood.

Second, puzzling emotional reactions become understandable. The sense of control, hopefulness, and comfort that follows the adoption of the cognitive model is said to be common to many forms of psychotherapy (Frank, 1973). Through the adoption of a set of organizing principles or a coherent worldview, the patient comes to see a "light at the end of the tunnel." The simple, commonsense model the patient learns in CT is particularly useful in achieving this effect.

Third, after experience with the successful implementation of CT methods, the patient begins to use them when confronted with day-to-day difficulties. Used appropriately, the methods ameliorate many concerns that would otherwise lead to emotional distress. Since CT is largely a skills-based therapy, the patient eventually comes to employ the approach on his or her own, tackling more and more problems. In the most successful cases, patients continue to employ the cognitive model and its methods in the face of difficult circumstances long after formal therapy is terminated.

Since people are often careless when they make inferences about interpersonal and self-relevant matters (Nisbett & Ross, 1980), the thinking skills taught in cognitive therapy are applicable even after the acute problem remits. Indeed, many of these skills are probably used by people who never experience mental health problems. In addition, the risk of relapse is quite high in most disorders for which CT is used. The patient who can apply the skills learned during therapy is assumed to be at a lower risk for subsequent relapse. As reviewed below, several studies have pointed to a prophylactic effect of CT.

Cognitive Errors

Another perspective on the patient's thinking is discussed as the patient is taught that several "types" of thinking errors to which we are all subject occur more frequently during affective episodes. These are the "cognitive errors" discussed by Beck et al. (1979; see Table 9.1). The labels given to these errors serve a heuristic function, as they remind the patient of different ways in which his or her thinking may be in error. The motivated patient will memorize and identify instances of them in his or her own thinking. When the error is identified, the patient can either discount the inference that involved the error or use more general analytic techniques to question the validity of the inference.

TABLE 9.1. Definitions of 11 Common Cognitive Errors

All-or-nothing thinking: Placing experiences in one of two opposite categories; for example, flawless or defective, immaculate or filthy, saint or sinner.

Overgeneralizing: Drawing sweeping inferences (e.g., "I can't control my temper") from a single instance.

Discounting the positives: Deciding that if a good thing has happened, then it couldn't have been very important.

Jumping to conclusions: Focusing on one aspect of a situation in deciding how to understand it (e.g., "The reason I haven't received a phone call from the job I applied to is that they have decided not to offer it to me").

Mind reading: Believing one knows what another person is thinking, with very little evidence.

Fortune telling: Believing one knows what the future holds, while ignoring other possibilities.

Magnifying/minimizing: Evaluating the importance of a negative event, or the lack of importance of a positive event, in a distorted manner.

Emotional reasoning: Believing that something must be true, because it feels like it is true.

Making "should" statements: Telling oneself that one should do—or should have done—something, when it is more accurate to say that one would like to do—or wishes one had done—the preferred thing.

Labeling: Using a label (bad mother, idiot) to describe a behavior, then imputing all the meanings the label carries.

Inappropriate blaming: Using hindsight to determine what one "should have done," even if one could not have known the best thing to do at the time; ignoring mitigating factors; or ignoring the roles played by others in determining a negative outcome.

Schema Work

CT also aims to work on another, "deeper" level. Through the analysis of many instances of negative emotional experiences, patient and therapist come to see that the patient has certain patterns of thinking, or "schemas" (Beck, 1964, 1972; J. Beck, 1995; Hollon & Kriss, 1984; Persons, 1989). Schemas are the underlying cognitive structures that organize the patient's experience and therefore form the basis for the individual instances of bias or distortion. These schemas are thought to represent the core of the cognitive disturbance, and as such are sometimes referred to as "core beliefs." Schemas can often be stated in the form of "if–then" propositions, and are similar in breadth to irrational beliefs described by Albert Ellis (e.g., "If I am not competent in every way, then I'm a failure"; see Ellis & Harper, 1975). Though not as readily accessible as the individual occurrences of thought (so-called "automatic thoughts"), these schemas become apparent to patient and therapist as they identify the consistencies or themes that run through the automatic thoughts.

When these themes are identified, their utility (balance of the pros and cons of holding them) or validity (their fit with available evidence) can be examined. If these inquiries help to change the patient's schemas, then he or she can begin to recognize situations in which these "core beliefs" are implicit in his or her reactions to potentially disturbing events; the patient can then consider an alternative inference. In addition, the strength with which the patient holds these core beliefs and their corollaries will diminish over time. Presumably, new schemas replace the old. So, for example, the patient may replace the aforementioned schema with something like "If I've given a task the effort it's due, then I can be satisfied with it."

The Nature of the Therapeutic Interaction

Much of what distinguishes CT from other cognitive-behavioral therapies lies in the role assumed by the therapist and the role that he or she recommends to the patient. In the relationship, which is meant to be collaborative, the therapist and patient assume an equal share of the responsibility for solving the patient's problems. The patient is assumed to be the expert on his or her own experience and on the meanings he or she attaches to events; that is, cognitive therapists do not assume that they know why the patient reacted a certain way in a certain situation; they ask for the patient's recollection of ongoing thoughts and images. Furthermore, cognitive therapists do not assume to know why a certain thought was upsetting; they ask the patient.

The reliance on the patient's report of the meaning of his or her thoughts distinguishes CT from Ellis's rational emotive therapy (RET; Ellis, 1984) on the one hand, and from a Meichenbaum-type cognitive-behavior modification (CBM; Meichenbaum, 1972) on the other. In our experience, therapists who have not trained in CT often mistakenly attribute to CT features of one of these two traditions, so it is important to distinguish CT from them. RET employs a deductive approach in which the therapist more readily infers the nature of a patient's thinking errors on the basis of experience with other patients and knowledge of rational emotive theory. In it can be found rules for determining the underlying or basic beliefs implied by the reactions that patients report for upsetting events. Ellis recommends that the therapist be "a step ahead" of the patient, supplying him or her with the meanings of his or her reported thoughts (see, e.g., Ellis, 1984, p. 221). In a learning theory–derived system such as Meichenbaum's CBM, thoughts are treated more as behaviors, so that one thought can replace another, or can be differentially reinforced; there is less emphasis on the *meaning* of the thoughts involved. Though a cognitive therapist may on occasion encourage the patient to view an automatic thought as a habit, and therapy may aim to eliminate the habit or replace it with a new or less distressing alternative, these strategies are not employed before the patient has thoroughly explored the meanings or implications of the thought and decided that the meaning of the habitual thought is not true.

The assumption in CT is that the meaning systems are idiosyncratic. For this reason the patient must take an active role in his or her treatment. He or she is taught to be prepared to question his or her thoughts during a distressing event or shortly thereafter. By contrast, in Meichenbaum's self-instructional training (SIT; Meichenbaum, 1972), the therapist helps the patient to make specific coping statements to him- or herself when confronted with difficulties. A simple way to refer to this difference between CT and SIT is that the therapist teaches the patient to question his or her inferences in CT, whereas in SIT the therapist teaches the patient to change them. The focus on questioning in CT leads advocates to believe that it is a more general approach that can be readily applied by the patient to new situations or to new reactions in familiar situations. Insofar as this distinction captures a major difference between CT and SIT, it also implies that in CT more responsibility is placed on the shoulders of the patient.

When new data are to be gathered, or when experiments that address an idiosyncratic belief of the patient are attempted, the cognitive therapist involves the patient in planning the data collection or the experiment. His or her goal is to help the patient devise tests whose results would be convincing to the *patient*, rather than to a logician, to another patient, or to the therapist. Thus, the patient is actively involved in his or her treatment and, again, is the expert on his or her own case. The cognitive therapist, of course, is the expert on the cognitive model and, especially at the beginning of therapy, is responsible for teaching the patient the principles that underlie the therapy. He or she is also the expert on the analytical methods used to test the beliefs reported by the patient.

As in any interpersonal relationship, problems between therapist and patient may arise. In CT, concerns of the patient that become apparent in relation to the therapy or the therapist are actively discussed. The therapist seeks feedback and responds to it in ways that are consistent with the model. Thus, the therapist helps the patient attend to his or her thoughts about the therapy itself, and together they examine them.

CLINICAL APPLICATIONS

Behavioral Methods

CT has always included procedures or adaptations of procedures that originated in other active–directive schools of therapy. Many of the adaptations are of behavioral methods which, in CT, are used to promote cognitive change. This section highlights the prominent behavioral methods used in CT. Although these methods are used to increase activity or to provide experiences of pleasure or mastery, the focus is on change in beliefs. The cognitive therapist often explains the assignment of behavioral tasks in this way, indicating that the patient's attempts to engage in the assigned task will serve either to test a hypothesis that the patient holds or to provide a setting that provokes the formation of new hypotheses that can be tested subsequently. Jacobson et al. (1996) reported that a 12-week course of treatment with only behavioral methods achieved outcomes similar to those produced by a 12-week course of treatment that included CT procedures in addition to purely behavioral ones. Thus, whereas these methods have traditionally been considered auxiliary in CT, their therapeutic impact should not be underestimated.

Self-Monitoring

Most patients who begin a course of CT are asked to maintain a careful, hour-by-hour record of their activities and associated moods, or other pertinent phenomena, for at least 1 week at the beginning of treatment. One useful variant is to have the patient record his or her mood on a 0- to 100-point scale, where 0 is the worst he or she has ever felt, and 100 is the best. As suggested in Beck et al. (1979), the patient can also record the degree of mastery or pleasure associated with each recorded activity. This record acquaints the therapist with the way the patient spends his or her time. In the process, the patient is often surprised by some aspect of the record, such as how much time he or she spends watching television. It can also serve as a baseline against which later records can be compared.

A variety of hypotheses can be tested using self-monitoring, such as "It doesn't do any good for me to get out of bed," "I'm always miserable; it never lets up," and "My schedule is too full for me to accomplish what I must." Examination of a completed record is a far better basis for judging such hypotheses than is the patient's memory of recent events, since his or her memory will often be selective. Another common use of the self-monitoring record is to obtain a record of particularly bad or particularly good events that can be discussed in the next session. The therapist can then ask the patient to recall the thoughts that occurred at the time in question. Finally, if there are consistencies in the record, such that certain kinds of events are associated with good or bad moods, or with mastery or pleasure, then these activities can be identified and sought out or avoided, through the scheduling or structuring of activities.

Scheduling Activities

The purpose of scheduling activities in CT is twofold: (1) to increase the probability that the patient will engage in activities that he or she has been avoiding unwisely, and (2) to remove decision making as an obstacle in the initiation of an activity. Since the decision has been made in the therapist's office, or in advance by the patient him- or herself, the patient need only carry out what he or she has agreed (or decided) to do.

When the patient does not carry out the agreed-upon activities, it becomes an important topic for resolution in the succeeding therapy session. Nonadherence may result from overambitiousness or lack of clarity on the part of the therapist, in which case the therapist will assume responsibility and adjust accordingly. Since it is often the case that such "failures" are similar in character to what has been troubling the patient generally, in that they also are caused by unrealistic negative beliefs, a thorough analysis of the cognitive obstacles is indicated. For example, a cognitive therapist will work through the pessimistic thoughts that led the patient to give up, pointing out that anyone who believed the proposition (e.g., "I am not capable of writing this letter") at the time would not take the next step. In this example, the validity of the proposition would be examined, and a behavioral test would ensue.

Scheduled activities are often of three types: (1) those that are associated with mastery, pleasure, or good mood during self-monitoring; (2) those that the patient recalls as having been rewarding in the past but that he or she has avoided during the current episode; and (3) new activities agreed upon by the patient and therapist that offer the prospect of generating useful information or providing reward. When scheduling activities, the cognitive therapist tries to help the patient anticipate the environmental or cognitive obstacles that are likely to interfere with the scheduled activities. These obstacles can then be discussed in the session, or the schedule can be shaped or modified in such a way as to eliminate the obstacles or minimize their effects.

A test of a hypothesis discussed in the session may be embedded in the schedule. For example, television watching can be scheduled for some evenings, reading for others, and visiting with friends for still others. The patient can then monitor his or her mood, or the degree of mastery and pleasure he or she experiences in each activity, to test the belief about the utility of these activities. An added benefit of such a suggestion is that the patient is often more willing to carry out an activity if it is couched in terms of an experiment, perhaps because he or she is not at the same time making a commitment to the activity beyond the time of the experiment.

Other Behavioral Strategies

Since tasks that have been avoided by the patient are often exactly those that have been difficult to do, modifying the structure of these tasks is often appropriate. Large tasks (e.g., finding a job, giving a speech) are explicitly broken down into their smaller units (circling want-ads, outlining the main points of the speech, etc.) to make them more concrete and less overwhelming. This intervention has been termed "chunking." "Graded tasks" can also be constructed, such that easier tasks or simpler aspects of larger tasks are set out as the first to be attempted. This process is also called "success therapy," because it is assumed that success on the earlier, easier tasks provides an impetus to move on to the more difficult ones. Though chunking and graded task assignments may seem simplistic, it is often surprising to both patient and therapist how these simple alterations in the structure of a task change the patient's view of the task and, subsequently, the likelihood of its being accomplished.

This overview of common behavioral aspects of CT shows how behavioral assignments can be incorporated into CT, and how the focus on the cognitive aspects of these assignments can produce therapeutic effects. Variations on these simple procedures, suited to the goals of a particular case, are often desirable and can provide a solid foundation for the cognitive change that is the focus of the therapy.

Cognitive Methods

Whereas behavioral procedures are primarily used to alter actions of the patient, many CT procedures aim expressly at change in cognition, since cognitive theory considers that change in affect and behavior comes chiefly as a result of cognitive changes. An overview of the basic concepts employed in procedures that are explicitly aimed at cognitive change is presented below.

Daily Record of Dysfunctional Thoughts

Much of the work in CT centers around the use of a device called the Daily Record of Dysfunctional Thoughts (DRDT; see Beck et al., 1979). The DRDT is presented here to illustrate several of the principles and options embedded in the CT approach. The four most important columns in the DRDT (see Figure 9.1) correspond to the three points in the cognitive model of emotion (situation, belief, emotional consequence), plus the alternative or counterresponses to the beliefs (i.e., the more "rational" or functional beliefs). Patients are typically taught first to use the DRDT by noting those times when they experience an unpleasant or puzzling affective state. Thus, the cognitive therapist must be certain that the patient (1) understands what he or she means by "feelings," "emotions," or "moods"; (2) can identify different feelings; and (3) offers a judgment of the intensity of these states. The therapist also asks the patient to note the situation and stream of thoughts during which the feelings occurred. Most patients readily attend to the situation and the emotional state of their experience at times of emotional disturbance (e.g., "I was hurt because he didn't answer me"). Many patients also view situations as the direct cause of their emotional responses, considering in addition that "something" is wrong with them that leads to their experiencing maladaptive or upsetting emotional reactions. The job of the cognitive therapist is thus to teach the patient to attend to his or her thoughts and images at these times. At least initially, automatic thoughts are often determined retrospectively in response to the queries of the therapist.

Once the patient is able to report situations, thoughts, and emotional reactions, preferably at the time of the event and on paper, intervention can begin. Though termed "rational response" on the DRDT, it is not necessary to assume that patients' beliefs are always irrational, or even incorrect. To say that the work involves "coming up with rational responses" to automatic thoughts is only a rough approximation of the intent of CT. More precisely, it involves the examination of inferences made when the patient is emotionally distressed, and that may be considered necessary for the experience of the distress. Thus, whether the responses to the initial thoughts are called "rational," "adaptive," "alternative," or some other term, the intervention focuses

Directions: When you notice your mood getting worse, ask yourself, "What's going through my mind right now?" and as soon as possible, jot down the thought or mental image in the Automatic Thoughts column. Then consider how accurate or realistic those thoughts are.

Date	Situation	Emotions	Automatic Thoughts	Alternative responses	Outcome
	Where were you—and what was going on—when you got upset?	What emotions (sad, anxious, angry, etc.) did you feel at the time? Rate the intensity of each (0–100%).	What thoughts and/or images went through your mind? Rate your belief in each (0–100%).	Use the questions at the bottom to compose responses to the automatic thoughts. Rate your belief in each (0–100%). Also, consult list of possible distortions.	Rerate your belief in your automatic thoughts (0–100%) and in the intensity of your emotions (0–100%).

(1) What is the **evidence** that the automatic thought is true? What is the evidence that it is not true?

(2) Are there **alternative explanations** for that event, or **alternative ways** to view the situation?

(3) What are the **implications** if the thought is true? What's the most upsetting thing about it? What's the most realistic view? What can I do about it?

Possible distortions: All-or-nothing thinking; overgeneralizing; discounting the positives; jumping to conclusions; mind reading; fortune telling; magnifying/minimizing; emotional reasoning; making "should" statements; labeling; inappropriate blaming.

FIGURE 9.1. Daily Record of Dysfunctional Thoughts. Adapted from Beck, Rush, Shaw, and Emery (1979). Copyright 1979 by Aaron T. Beck, A. John Rush, Brian F. Shaw, and Gary Emery. Adapted with permission from The Guilford Press.

on helping the patient learn to question and examine his or her inferences (Dobson & Dobson, 2009).

Many secondary features of the DRDT are worth mentioning. Patients can record the degree of belief in the "automatic thought," both before and after it is examined, which allows for a check on the effect of the questioning. When a high degree of belief in the automatic thought remains, it indicates that however elegant or thorough the questioning may have seemed, it did not resolve the initial concern. The patient has missed either a key meaning or has made a thorough and accurate characterization of the situation. In the latter case, the therapist may then help the patient examine the significance or meaning of his or her thoughts. Similarly, the degree of the affective response can be recorded both before and after an analysis of the thoughts. Little or no change in affect tells the cognitive therapist that an important element was missed in the analysis, and that further exploration is needed. Finally, there is a space where the degree of belief in the rational response can be recorded. If the response is trite (e.g., "Things will get better soon") or in any way not convincing to the patient, it can be picked up here.

The DRDT can be worked on in the session, but as therapy progresses, it is best used independently by the patient, with the therapist simply checking it over during the session. Though patients eventually do the work of the DRDT without paper and pen, it is quite useful for them to save their completed records, since many of the concerns and responses worked through during therapy are relevant later in the therapy and after therapy has ended. When CT has a prophylactic effect, it is assumed that it is in part because the patient has retained the ability to attend to and question his or her thinking, as was the case during therapy.

Patients are taught to apply three kinds of questions to the beliefs they record:

1. "What is the evidence for and against the belief?"
2. "What are alternative interpretations of the event or situation?"
3. "What are the real implications, if the belief is correct?"

Each of the questions is stated here in a general form and can, of course, be modified to suit the patient's situation or style.

Cognitive Errors

An alternative and often complementary approach to the three questions involves the therapist teaching the patient to learn to recognize when his or her thinking falls into one of the categories of cognitive errors (see Table 9.1). These labels remind the patient that he or she, as is true of all people, is prone to exaggeration or other biased thinking. At these times, the patient can discount the improbable or illogical inference, reframe it in a less extreme form, or analyze the inference using the three questions. For example, a patient in the teaching profession may conclude that he or she has given a poor lecture, since three of the 40 students in the class were inattentive from time to time during the lecture. The patient may then notice that he or she has "personalized," particularly if another reason that can be readily given for the inattentiveness does not involve the quality of the lecture (e.g., it was 80 degrees in the lecture hall, the students are apathetic). Alternatively, the patient may decide that he or she has "overgeneralized," if on reflection he or she recalls that most of the students seemed quite interested during the lecture, and that several students came to him or her after class with thoughtful questions.

Socratic Questioning and Guided Discovery

Perhaps the most distinctive stylistic feature of CT, as well as the most difficult for therapists in training to master, is the judicious and persistent use of the Socratic method of questioning. The term "guided discovery" also refers to the process, through the use of leading yet open questions, of helping patients to arrive at new perspectives that challenge their faulty beliefs. The art of Socratic questioning is to walk the line between leading the patient where the therapist would like him or her to go and allowing the patient to "free associate." The most common error made by inexperienced cognitive therapists is to be in such a hurry, or to be so certain of a conclusion the patient should come to, that he or she either lectures the patient or asks leading questions. As a matter of fact, Socrates' use of questions in the Socratic dialogues (Cooper, 1997; see especially *Euthyphro* and *Crito*) is often quite like the latter, in that Socrates tended to know exactly where he was going with his line of questions. Therefore, good "Socratic" questions of the CT sort are much more open-ended and theory-free than those of the originator (see Overholser [1993a, 1993b] for a discussion of Socratic questioning in therapy). A good practice exercise is for the therapist to listen to a voice recording of a session, to stop the tape each time he or she has uttered a declarative statement or asked a closed-ended question, then to generate a Socratic question that makes the same point but in a potentially more fruitful manner. Socratic questioning is especially productive in therapy, because the patient is maximally engaged to think about the problem under discussion, as well as its solution. Moreover, good Socratic questioning prevents a common problem in nonoptimal CT: The therapist can become quite convinced that the patient's thoughts are in error, but the patient is left with idiosyncratic doubts and concerns that were not addressed in the discussion between patient and therapist.

The Downward Arrow

The thought reported initially by a patient is often in a form that yields little, if analyzed for its validity. For instance, a patient may think, in response to a perceived snub by someone at a party, "She doesn't think I'm exciting enough." Though any therapist can imagine a number of reasons why this thought may be upsetting to the patient, presumably the patient extracts from this inference some implications or meanings that are particularly important to him or her. Thus, rather than first asking questions about how reasonable the inference is (e.g., "Did she give any other indications of her interest or disinterest?"; "Could there be other reasons why she acted that way?"), the therapist might do well to ask a question such as "And what would it mean (regarding you or your future) if it were true that she sees you as not exciting enough for her?" Though essentially a variant of the third of the three questions listed earlier, this approach toward a reported belief has been termed the "downward-arrow" technique. "Downward arrow" refers to a series of questions that can be asked of almost any inference, where each answer begs another question. These questions are of the form "What if it is true that ... ?" or "What about that bothers you?" Each question probes for the personal meaning of the inference to the patient, until an inference is brought out that will profit from the work of CT. In the previous example, the downward arrow might yield the following: "I'm an uninteresting person," "I'll never attract that sort of person," or another meaning that the original inference implies for the patient. It is important for the therapist to realize that the meanings are idiosyncratic and can therefore be difficult to predict, even after he or she has come to know the patient well. Furthermore, although a therapist may ask the first two of the three questions immediately, there are times when it is more productive to employ the downward-arrow technique first.

These efforts are not mutually exclusive, however. In many instances it is worthwhile both to proceed "downward" to discover the meanings of the inference, and to use the first two of the three questions at more than one level during the inquiry. So, in the preceding example, the therapist could encourage the patient to question both the belief that the fellow partygoer finds the patient uninteresting and the idea that even if that belief were true, it follows that the patient is uninteresting or doomed to loneliness.

Identifying Schemas

After several sessions, the therapist and patient likely will notice a consistency to the beliefs that are involved in emotional disturbance for the patient. This consistency will not be found at the "surface" level, but at the level of personal meaning. For example, the therapist and patient may note that many of the patient's entries in the DRDT include beliefs of the form: "If I am not the best X, then it is not worth pursuing, and I am worthless as an X." These beliefs can be examined in ways that are an extension of the application of the three questions and the identification of cognitive errors. In her book *Cognitive Therapy: Basics and Beyond,* Judith Beck (1995) describes a tool called the Cognitive Conceptualization Diagram, which is well-suited to approach this inquiry systematically.

TREATMENT PROCEDURES FOR DEPRESSION

Beginning of Treatment

The cognitive therapist has several complementary goals at the beginning of treatment. They can be categorized as (1) assessment, (2) socializing the patient into the cognitive model, and (3) dealing with the patient's pessimism (about treatment and in general). Assessment efforts can include administration and scoring of the self-report Beck Depression Inventory–II (BDI-II; Beck, Steer, & Brown, 1996), which can then be used as a session-to-session measure of depression level. Though its validity as a depression severity measure has been well demonstrated (Beck, Steer, & Brown, 1996), it is as a within-patient change measure that the BDI-II is of greatest use during the course of therapy.

Patient and therapist need to develop a common understanding of the model that will be used during treatment. To this end, patients are asked to read the booklet *Coping with Depression* (Beck & Greenberg, 1974), or a similar description of the cognitive model of depression and its treatment. Therapist and patient can discuss the patient's reaction to the booklet and framed a recent experience in the cognitive model. Though this early "socialization" of the patient into the cognitive model of treatment often involves didactic explanation, it has the added benefit of giving the patient an account of his or her difficulties that leaves room for understanding and improvement. Thus, the patient's hopelessness, a common feature of depression, is dealt with thoroughly and directly.

At the beginning of treatment, additional interventions often address the patient's pessimism or hopelessness. These interventions can take the form of working through a task that the patient has not been able to tackle, or one that the patient does not believe he or she has the resources to complete. The therapist elicits and records the patient's expectations for his or her performance on the task, then guides the patient through the anticipated obstacles. When the patient is able to accomplish more than he or she expected, the success is used as a foundation upon which further attempts can be built.

The Middle Phase

Although work on cognitive coping skills begins in the early phase of treatment, the middle phase is used to solidify these skills. Between sessions the patient identifies the situations and thoughts that bring about negative affect. Ideally, he or she keeps a written record on the DRDT and is beginning to question his or her thinking either during or soon after a puzzling or maladaptive emotional episode. The therapist helps the patient "fine-tune" his or her responses to initial thoughts, often by using the downward arrow technique described earlier; that is, the therapist reviews the DRDT with the patient to discover where he or she could attempt alternative analyses of his or her automatic thoughts.

It is also during the middle phase that schemas or underlying assumptions are identified. The developmental histories of these schemas are also discussed to help the patient make sense of his or her patterns. Without such an inquiry, the patient is apt to view his or her idiosyncratic way of interpreting events in the world as coming "out of the blue." Unexplained negative affect can also leave the patient feeling helpless and, worse yet, believing that he or she is fundamentally flawed in some way. In this respect CT is similar to the "depth" approaches to psychotherapy, in that it aims to foster an understanding of the influence of early experience upon subsequent attitudes and concerns. These aspects of CT have been especially well-described by J. Beck (1995) and Persons (1989).

The Final Phase

During the final phase of therapy, gains are reviewed and therapy is focused on the prevention of relapse. Therapist and patient anticipate difficult situations or problems that may arise in the future and tax the patient's coping skills. This is a crucial phase of therapy, since it is common for patients to be unclear about the importance of the skills they have learned. Many patients attribute their recovery to changes in their environment, even if these changes have come about through their own effort. Because the patient by this time is feeling better, it is vital that his or her skills be tested and demonstrated to increase the likelihood that he or she will employ them when difficult situations arise, as they inevitably will.

It is also during this phase that the patient's beliefs about his or her ability to leave therapy must be addressed. The patient may believe that he or she can cope with problems as long as he or she remains in therapy, but that it will be impossible to handle them on his or her own. If a collaborative working relationship has already developed, then the therapist will need to place even more responsibility for the treatment on the shoulders of the patient over time, so that he or she becomes more a consultant than an active therapist. This gradual shift can serve as the context for a test of the patient's ability to work problems out on his or her own.

Finally, therapist and patient may agree to schedule "booster sessions" to follow up the work that has been done. Jarrett et al. (1998) describe evidence that such sessions, scheduled at monthly intervals during the period following response to CT for depression, reduce the rate of relapse and recurrence. Clinicians and patients report that even less frequent (e.g., three times per year) booster sessions can be beneficial for maintaining the patient's focus on gains made during the more intensive weekly (or twice weekly) sessions of the acute treatment phase. This lower frequency of booster sessions, employed in the 1-year continuation phase of a study by DeRubeis and colleagues (2005), was associated with a very low relapse rate, as described below.

TREATMENT PROCEDURES
FOR PANIC DISORDERS AND AGORAPHOBIA

CTs have been developed for many disorders, such as generalized anxiety disorder, obsessive–compulsive disorder, and hypochondriasis. These other approaches all follow a form similar to that described earlier for depression (see Clark, 1999; Salkovskis, 1996). Each population requires somewhat different treatment emphases, however, based on the phenomenology that defines the disorder. The phenomenology and treatment of panic disorder have been especially well developed (see Beck, Emery, & Greenberg, 1985; Clark, 1996).

The symptomatology in the development of a panic attack follows an almost stereotyped sequence. First, the patient experiences an unpleasant or puzzling sensation that he or she cannot discount as nonpathological. If the patient has had previous panic attacks, then he or she may "recognize" this symptom as a prelude to such a reaction and, indeed, may anticipate an incipient panic attack. In any event, the progression continues if the patient ascribes pathological significance to the particular sensation or symptom and is unable to dismiss it as not dangerous. The patient's meaning or interpretation will "make sense" to the therapist, in that it will bear a relation to the sensation(s). Thus, a pain in the chest might be interpreted as a heart attack, and tightness or shortness of breath as a sign that one will stop breathing. Lightheadedness is often viewed as a signal of impending loss of consciousness, numbness or tingling in the extremities as having a stroke, and mental confusion as a sign that one is going crazy, and so on.

Often, precipitating factors of which the patient is unaware can readily explain the onset of these experiences. Thus, an individual may feel faint if he or she has risen suddenly from a chair, gone for a long time without eating, or been looking down from a high place. He or she may become generally aroused by hearing unpleasant (or even pleasant) news. Any of these sensations may be interpreted by the individual as a sign of an impending disaster. A large proportion of patients who are subject to panic attacks also seem to experience hyperventilation. A person who is upset or who experiences shortness of breath, for example, may start to breathe rapidly and as a result of "blowing off" carbon dioxide may experience symptoms of "alkalosis" (numbness and tingling in the extremities, generalized discomfort).

A patient who has had a certain amount of "cognitive strain" may have a sudden lapse of memory or difficulty in reasoning that he or she then attributes to a serious mental disorder. A father experiencing a burst of emotion during a quarrel with his children may interpret the accompanying bodily feelings as a sign that he is out of control and about to assault them. As the panic attack develops, the individual focuses on the symptoms. He or she is now aware of a pounding heartbeat, faintness, dizziness, or shortness of breath. The individual then anticipates catastrophic consequences of the symptoms and may fear that if they continue any longer, then he or she will die. Some patients report vivid visual images, such as falling down, being surrounded by people, or being placed in an ambulance and taken to the hospital. Occasionally a patient, particularly one with a high level of depression, may have an image of him- or herself lying dead in a coffin, and feeling extremely lonely and isolated from other people.

One of the most striking aspects of the panic attack is the patient's loss of ability during the attack to view his or her sensations objectively and to apply an appropriate label to them. Even though the patient may have agreed a few moments prior to the attack that the symptoms do not represent any serious threat to life or mental stability, he or she may lose the ability to apply this information once the attack has started. It is not clear whether there is an inhibition of the higher evaluative functions, or whether instead the individual's attention is so focused on the symptoms and their (mistaken) meanings that he or she does not have the cognitive capacity left to evaluate his or her interpretations. In any event, the loss of capacity to apply reason and medical knowledge to the interpretation of the symptoms seems to be a necessary component of the disorder. A patient may have all the features of intense anxiety, but he or she will not have a panic attack, if he or she retains the ability to regard his or her symptoms objectively.

The next stage in the development of the panic disorder takes the form of a vicious cycle. As the individual begins to interpret his or her symptoms (e.g., rapid heart rate, shortness of breath) as pathological, his or her sense of danger increases, which in turn intensifies the symptoms. With the increased focus on the symptoms and their imagined consequences, the patient becomes even less able to apply reason to his or her symptoms, and they continue to escalate. A special feature of this progression is the patient's recognition that his or her usual attempts to ward off fear, such as walking around or trying to divert his or her own attention, do not seem to quell the disturbance. The symptoms appear to be uncontrollable, and he or she begins to believe that they will continue to escalate until a disaster occurs. The patient may engage in "safety behaviors" (e.g., sitting down to avert a heart attack) that then become a problem that needs to be addressed in therapy. In contrast to panic attacks associated with phobias of specific environmental situations (e.g., acrophobia, claustrophobia), the spontaneous "attack" represents a "phobia" (fear) of a set of internal conditions.

General Treatment Approach

The cognitive treatment of panic disorder has evolved since it was first introduced, following the growing recognition of the insidious role played by "safety behaviors" in the maintenance of anxiety disorders (Salkovskis, 1996), including panic disorder (Salkovskis, Clark, Hackmann, Wells, & Gelder, 1999). In the first edition of this book, we recommended that patients be taught to use relaxation procedures, controlled breathing, and distraction as means of diminishing or blunting incipient panic attacks, because these methods seemed indicated at that time (Beck et al., 1985; Clark, Salkovskis,

& Chalkley, 1985). It is now clear that these procedures, while helpful in some cases, can prevent the full benefit of the treatment in other cases. This seeming paradox occurs because patients with panic disorder can come to believe that they *must* engage in these practices, lest the feared consequence ensue. Although the original recommendation of these methods stemmed from the observation that patients can use them to learn that panic attacks are controllable and, thus, essentially harmless, many patients develop the maladaptive inference that the panic-blunting procedures are essential for their well-being. For example, a patient who has learned controlled breathing may become convinced that if, in the beginning of a panic attack, he or she does not gain control of his or her breathing, he or she will faint. This belief is then reinforced (via negative reinforcement) each time the patient engages in the controlled breathing, because, indeed, he or she does not faint. Cognitive therapists actively discourage patients' engagement in safety behaviors. Moreover, the therapist and patient identify and endeavor to cease any safety behaviors the patient already employs during panic attacks. These behaviors can include calling a friend for support, going to the emergency room, leaning against a wall (to prevent falling), or monitoring one's heart rate. Because patients can be highly creative in their use of safety-enhancing thoughts or behaviors, they must be thoroughly educated about the concept of safety behaviors. Some of these behaviors are so automatic that patients are unable to report about them retrospectively, so they need to be on the lookout for them.

The Oxford-Based Cognitive Therapy Package (Clark, 1996) includes four cognitive and two behavioral methods. The cognitive methods are as follows:

1. The therapist and patient together map out the sequence of a recent panic attack, using the "vicious cycle" model.

2. Within this sequence, the patient's beliefs (e.g., "The fact that my heart is pounding means I am having a heart attack") are identified and challenged. One way to test the patient's beliefs is to show the patient that the symptoms reduce during an attack if he or she gains control of breathing or uses a distraction procedure. Most patients will see that heart attacks and other life-threatening events (e.g., stroke) cannot be controlled by distraction or measured breathing, so this can serve as a disconfirmation of their belief. However, as noted earlier, this procedure is used only to test beliefs, not as a means of preventing future panic attacks, lest the method of control become a safety behavior.

3. More realistic beliefs are identified and considered (e.g., "I am anxious; therefore, my heart is pounding more than usual").

4. The images experienced by the patient (e.g., of being placed in an emergency vehicle and taken to a hospital) are altered, so that the next time the patient begins to have such an image, he or she can correct it to a beneficial image, such as the image of a gradual resolution of the anxiety attack.

The behavioral methods in the Oxford-Based Cognitive Therapy Package are as follows:

1. Procedures are engaged to induce the feared sensations. Patients are taught to hyperventilate, to focus attention on their body, or to read pairs of words or phrases in which one member of the pair represents a feared sensation (e.g., heart pounding), and the other a feared catastrophe (e.g., heart attack). These procedures help patients to see that the symptoms can be brought about readily by measures that do not cause the feared catastrophe. Patients therefore learn that these sensations are not reliable signals of impending danger.

2. Patients are encouraged to expose themselves to and remain in the feared situations they have either avoided or fled. For some patients, exposure is primarily to situations that involve physical exertion, such as exercise or sexual activity. For others, anxiety-arousing situations, such as crowded shopping malls, might be targeted. For still others, a theme that ties together the feared situations will not be identified. In those cases, exposure is to those specific situations in which panic attacks have occurred in the past.

ADDITIONAL CONSIDERATIONS

Empirical Status of the Approach

Efficacy of Cognitive Therapy for Depression: Acute Treatment

Over the last three decades, the efficacy of CT and medications as treatments for major depressive disorder have been compared in several randomized clinical trials (Blackburn, Bishop, Glen, Whalley, & Christie, 1981; DeRubeis et al., 2005; Dimidjian et al., 2006; Elkin et al., 1989; Jarrett et al., 1999; Hollon et al., 1992; Murphy, Simons, Wetzel, & Lustman, 1984; Rush, Beck, Kovacs, & Hollon, 1977). The earliest of these trials (Blackburn et al., 1981; Rush et al., 1977) suggested that CT may be more effective than tricyclic antidepressants. However, implementation of the pharmacological conditions in these early trials is generally considered to have been suboptimal (Hollon, Shelton, & Loosen, 1991; Meterissian & Bradwejn, 1989). Subsequent studies in which the pharmacological conditions were better implemented found CT and medication to be about equally efficacious (Hollon et al., 1992; Murphy et al., 1984).

Dobson (1989) published a meta-analysis of outcome research on CT for depression, in which he concluded that the results from efficacy studies "document a greater degree of change for cognitive therapy compared with a waiting list or no-treatment control, pharmacotherapy, behavior therapy, and other psychotherapies" (p. 414). His conclusions were consistent with what many experts in the field had by that time come to believe: that cognitive therapy for depression was the best example of an empirically validated psychological treatment for a serious mental disorder. This emerging consensus began to break down, however, with the publication of a series of articles from the Treatment of Depression Collaborative Research Program (TDCRP; Elkin et al., 1989), a three-site, randomized controlled trial that included a placebo control group and allowed direct comparisons between each of the treatment conditions and a bona fide control condition. Although the main finding was no significant difference in outcome between the CT and antidepressant medication conditions, secondary analyses indicated that medication was more effective than CT, which in turn was not significantly superior to pill-placebo among patients with more severe levels of depressive symptoms (Elkin et al., 1995).

The TDCRP findings generated a great deal of controversy (see the *Journal of Consulting and Clinical Psychology* special issue, which includes papers by Elkin, Gibbons, Shea, & Shaw, 1996; Jacobson & Hollon, 1996a, 1996b; Klein, 1996). Discrepancies in outcomes across the three sites led some to question the quality of the CT delivered in the TDCRP (Jacobson & Hollon, 1996a). Specifically, among the more severely depressed patients, medication and CT were equally effective at the site that was more experienced with CT, whereas medication was superior to CT at the other two sites (see Jacobson & Hollon, 1996b). In addition, findings from a mega-analysis that pooled data from the TDCRP and three other, similar trials (Hollon et al., 1992; Murphy et al., 1984; Rush et al., 1977) indicated that CT was as effective as medications in the treatment of severely depressed patients (DeRubeis, Gelfand, Tang, & Simons, 1999). In fact, although statistically significant differences did not emerge between the two treatment modalities, overall effect size comparisons tended to favor CT.

In the same year as the publication of the DeRubeis et al. (1999) mega-analysis, Jarrett et al. (1999) published the results from another large-scale, placebo-controlled, randomized comparison of medications and CT in major depressive disorder. This study included only patients diagnosed with atypical depression and used a monoamine oxidase inhibitor as the antidepressant. CT and medication were equally effective in the treatment of atypical depression, and both were superior to pill-placebo. Nonetheless, analyses of data from the TDCRP's more severely depressed subsample continued to dominate the perception of the efficacy of CT for depression. For example, the American Psychiatric Association's treatment guidelines recommended, as they still do (2000), that medications rather than CT be initially offered to those with moderate to severe levels of depression, presumably on the basis of findings from the TDCRP alone.

None of these studies included a large sample of patients with moderate to severe levels of depression. Thus, in an effort to clarify conflicting results regarding the relative efficacy of CT and antidepressant medications in the treatment of more severely depressed patients, DeRubeis et al. (2005) conducted a large, two-site, placebo-controlled comparison of CT and antidepressant medication, in which they restricted the study to only those patients with moderate to severe depression. Results from the study, which was conducted at the University of Pennsylvania and at Vanderbilt University, indicated that CT was as effective as medication in the alleviation of depressive symptoms, and that both treatments were superior to pill-placebo. Interestingly, a significant site x treatment interaction emerged in the study. Specifically, the medication condition was superior to CT at Vanderbilt, whereas the average response was (nonsignificantly) better in CT relative to medications at the University of Pennsylvania. This site difference in the relative efficacy of the two treatments was attributed in part to differences in the levels of experience of the cognitive therapists at the two sites. Reminiscent of the pattern observed in the TDCRP, better outcomes in CT tended to be obtained at the site with the more experienced therapists.

In contrast to most previous studies, but consistent with the TDCRP findings, were results from a placebo-controlled comparison of antidepressant medication, CT, and behavioral activation therapy at the University of Washington (Dimidjian et al., 2006). Although Dimidjian et al. did not find significant differences between CT and the other active treatments overall, or in the less severe subsample, they did report that CT was less effective than either medication or behavioral activation in the moderate to severe subsample. The authors attributed this effect to a subset of CT patients who exhibited "extreme nonresponse" (ENR), defined by posttreatment BDI-II (Beck et al., 1996) scores greater than 30. Specifically, at the end of treatment, 22% of patients assigned to CT exhibited ENR, whereas this was true of only 5% of medication patients, and none of the behavioral activation patients.

Efficacy of Cognitive Therapy: Relapse Prevention

Given the high risk for relapse and recurrence in persons who have experienced previous depressive episodes, reducing these risks is an important treatment goal. Most of the studies described earlier have included, in addition to tests of the acute effects of CT, examinations of its relapse prevention effects. In most studies this has taken the form of a comparison of symptom severity or relapse rates evidenced during follow-up by patients who have responded to cognitive therapy relative to those who have responded to antidepressant medication. In both groups, treatment would have terminated at the end of the acute (3- to 4-month) period, and follow-ups have typically been for 1–2 years.

A 1-year naturalistic follow-up of the Rush et al. (1977) study revealed that the CT group scored significantly lower on depression severity measures than the antidepressant medication group at the 12-month (but not the 6-month) follow-up point (Kovacs, Rush, Beck, & Hollon, 1981). Similarly, in a 2-year naturalistic follow-up of the Blackburn et al. (1981) study, Blackburn, Eunson, and Bishop (1986) found that patients who had responded to CT were less likely to experience a relapse/recurrence than those who had responded to medications. Simons, Murphy, Levine, and Wetzel (1986) reported that patients who received CT during the acute treatment phase of the Murphy et al. (1984) study were less likely than drug-treated patients to have relapsed in the year following acute treatment. Evans et al. (1992) reported the 2-year follow-up of the Hollon et al. (1992) study, and found that patients who had responded to CT during the acute phase had a significantly lower relapse rate than did patients who had responded to medication. Findings from the follow-up of the TDCRP were inconsistent with those of the other major studies. Although the CT group fared somewhat better than the medication group, the differences were not large, and they were not statistically significant (Shea et al., 1992).

In the subsequent phase of the DeRubeis et al. (2005) study of patients with moderate to severe depression, treatment responders were followed for a 12-month period (Hollon et al., 2005). The group of patients who had responded to CT evidenced a significantly lower relapse rate during the follow-up period relative to the group that had responded to medication and were withdrawn onto pill-placebo. The relapse rate of those who had previously received CT was also not significantly different, and indeed numerically lower, than that of a continued medication group during the 1-year follow-up period.

A similar pattern of findings was observed during the 2-year follow-up phase of the Dimidjian et al. (2006) study (Dobson et al., 2008). In the first year of the follow-up phase, patients who had previously received CT were significantly less likely to relapse than those who had previously been treated with medications and were subsequently withdrawn onto pill-placebo. At the 2-year follow-up, recurrence rates were also significantly lower for the CT group relative to the medication withdrawal group. Interestingly, behavioral activation therapy appeared to provide similar prophylactic benefits as CT. The group that had received behavioral activation therapy did not differ significantly from the CT group in terms of risk of experiencing a relapse or recurrence during the follow-up phase (although CT generally evidenced a small but nonsignificant advantage over behavioral activation therapy in most comparisons). Moreover, results suggested that acute treatment with either CT or behavioral activation therapy prevented symptom return as effectively as did continuing patients on medication.

Evidence for the prophylactic benefits of CT also comes from studies of the effects of brief CT following successful pharmacotherapy. In several studies a relatively brief course of CT (about 10 sessions) following a successful course of pharmacotherapy has been found to reduce the risk of symptom return (Blackburn & Moore, 1997; Bockting et al., 2005, 2006; Fava, Grandi, Zielezny, Canestrari, & Morphy, 1994; Fava, Grandi, Zielezny, & Canestrari, 1996; Fava, Rafanelli, Grandi, Canestrari, & Morphy, 1998a; Fava, Rafanelli, Grandi, Conti, & Belluardo, 1998b; Fava, Ruini, Rafanelli, Finos, Conti, & Grandi, 2004; Paykel et al., 1999, 2005). In addition, mindfulness-based cognitive therapy (MBCT), an 8-week treatment that combines aspects of CT with mindfulness meditation principles, has shown promise as a means of reducing the risk of relapse (Teasdale et al., 2000; Ma & Teasdale, 2004).

Cognitive Therapy for Other Forms of Psychopathology

Encouraged by the demonstrated successes of CT in the treatment of depression, researchers and clinicians have adapted CT core principles to the treatments of other forms of psychopathology. Beck (2005) provided an overview of the development of these adaptations and outcome evidence in support of their efficacy. Deacon and Abramowitz's (2004) meta-analytic review focused more narrowly on outcome research on the anxiety disorders.

We have already described the Oxford-Based Cognitive Therapy Package. Evidence concerning its efficacy has been reviewed by Clark (1996; see also a meta-analytic review by Gould, Otto, & Pollack, 1995), who showed that across five separate studies, between 74 and 94% of patients assigned to CT became panic-free and maintained this status through the respective follow-up periods, which ranged from 6 to 15 months in length. Moreover, results from these outcome studies indicate that CT not only outperformed waiting-list control conditions but also that it was superior in efficacy to applied relaxation, pharmacotherapy, and exposure therapy.

Chambless and Gillis (1993) reviewed nine clinical trials that evaluated the efficacy of CT for generalized anxiety disorder (GAD; Beck et al., 1985). They found that the evidence mostly supported CT's efficacy in treating GAD (see also DeRubeis & Crits-Christoph, 1998). This conclusion has been bolstered by two additional published studies (Barlow, Rapee, & Brown, 1992; Durham et al., 1994) since the Chambless and Gillis review (1993), as well as the Deacon and Abramowitz (2004) review.

For obsessive–compulsive disorder (OCD), Van Oppen et al. (1995) found that CT (based on Beck et al., 1985; Salkovskis, 1985) was equivalent to exposure and response prevention, an OCD treatment with established efficacy. Research has also found CT to be effective for bulimia nervosa (see Compas, Haaga, Keefe, & Leitenberg, 1998, for a review). Taken together, these results demonstrate that the principles of CT and treatments based on them can be applied successfully to a variety of disorders.

Research on the Process of Cognitive Therapy

Numerous measures have been designed to assess cognitive constructs in depression. Most measures have been developed from an interest in theoretical questions regarding depression. In this section we focus on therapist and patient measures used specifically to address questions about the effects of CT. The measures and applications described below stem from an interest in the following questions: Does it matter what the therapist does in CT (e.g., the extent to which therapists adhere to CT techniques, the quality or appropriateness of the delivery of these techniques)? Do patients change in ways that are predicted by CT theory? Are these changes specific to CT, or do similar changes occur in other effective treatments? These questions guide the type of thorough analysis that should be performed on any successful form of treatment (see Hollon & Kriss, 1984, for a model of change in therapy that incorporates these questions), and several measures have been developed to address some of these questions.

Therapist Behavior

The Cognitive Therapy Scale (CTS; Young & Beck, 1980) and the Collaborative Study Psychotherapy Rating Scale (CSPRS; Hollon, Evans, Auerbach, et al., 1985) are measures of therapist behavior that have been employed in research on CT for depression. The CTS was developed as a measure of a therapist's "competence" in CT. Specifically, it was designed not only to take into account whether therapists adhere to the methods of cognitive therapy but also to assess the quality with which these methods were implemented. The CTS has been used primarily as a means to determine whether therapists in outcome trials are "competent" to deliver CT. Scores on each of the 11 items of the CTS can range from 0 to 6. The CTS has demonstrated good reliability when used by raters trained together in the use of the instrument and who consult with one another periodically in an effort to prevent rater drift. For example, Hollon, Emerson, and Mandell (1982) obtained a very respectable interrater reliability coefficient of .86. However, ratings made by experts on tapes from the Jacobson et al. (1996) outcome study evidenced unusually low reliability, in the range of .10, possibly because those experts neither trained together in the use of the CTS nor checked with one another during the course of the rating study (Jacobson & Gortner, 2000).

The relation between therapist competence and changes in depressive symptoms in CT has been examined (Kingdon, Tyrer, Seivewright, Ferguson, & Murphy, 1996; Kuyken & Tsivrikos, 2009; Shaw et al., 1999; Trepka, Rees, Shapiro, Hardy, & Barkham, 2004), and whereas significant positive associations have been obtained between treatment outcomes and both experts' and patients' ratings of therapist competence (Kuyken & Tsivrikos, 2009), other results are varied. For example, using the TDCRP data, Shaw et al. (1999) found that higher levels of therapist competence were associated with better outcome on one of the three outcome measures they included in the study. In addition, results indicated that the positive finding was driven largely by the CTS items that assess the therapist's ability to structure the therapy session (i.e., setting an agenda, pacing, and assigning and reviewing homework). Kingdon et al. (1996) reported that on some measures, and at some time points, patients whose therapists were deemed "competent" based on CTS scores exhibited better outcomes than patients of therapists' categorized as showing "uncertain competence." More recently, Trepka et al. (2004) found a positive relation between therapist competence and outcomes. After accounting for the quality of therapeutic alliance, however, this relationship was attenuated. Further work on the importance of competence to outcome in CT is needed, both to refine the theory of change in CT, and to provide guidance to efforts to disseminate CT.

In contrast to the CTS as a measure of therapist competence, the CSPRS focuses on the extent or amount of the therapist behavior of interest (i.e., therapist "adherence"). Also, whereas the CTS is designed to be used by experts, the CSPRS can be used by observers with little or no clinical expertise or experience, if these observers are trained to identify the relevant behaviors. Raters are instructed not to judge the quality of the interventions they rate, but to focus instead on the amount of time and effort spent by the therapist in a certain domain, such as helping the patient attend to the thoughts experienced while in an unpleasant emotional state. CT-relevant behavior is covered by 28 of the 96 CSPRS items (the other 68 items are designed to assess behavior relevant to other forms of therapy, such as interpersonal therapy and pharmacotherapy, as well as aspects of therapist behavior that cut across schools of therapy, such as "facilitative conditions"). DeRubeis and Feeley (1990) factor-analyzed the 28 CT items and found that they separated into two factors. One factor, "CT–Concrete," represents the symptom-focused, active CT methods. A prototypical item from this factor asks the rater to indicate the extent to which the therapist "asked the patient to record (his or her) thoughts." The other factor, "CT–Abstract," represents less focused discussions about therapy processes and the like (e.g., "Did the therapist explain the cognitive therapy rationale?" and "Did the therapist explore underlying assumptions?").

In two separate studies, DeRubeis and his colleagues found that higher scores on CT–Concrete observed in session 2 were associated with greater change in BDI scores from that point until the end of therapy (Feeley, DeRubeis, & Gelfand, 1999), or until the 12th week (DeRubeis & Feeley, 1990). These findings support the hypothesis that theory-specified CT techniques play an important role in subsequent symptom change. In a recent study, Webb et al. (2009) also found that the CT–Concrete factor, assessed at session 3, was a significant predictor of subsequent symptom change.

Cognitions

Theories of change that are meant to explain both the short- and long-term benefits of CT can be examined by testing whether expected cognitive and behavioral changes occur during successful treatment, and whether these changes are related to symptom reduction or the prevention of relapse (or recurrence) in a manner that suggests a mediational role. Pragmatically, findings from such research can help inform CT practice by indicating what kinds of cognitive or behavioral change therapists should attempt to maximize to produce the greatest therapeutic benefit.

Hollon, Evans, and DeRubeis (1985) proposed three kinds of changes that might occur in CT and account for symptom reduction during treatment. The first two kinds of change, deactivation and accommodation, refer to changes that occur in the patients' schemas. Change in a depressive schema is said to occur when the patient comes to use a nondepressive schema in responding to potentially upsetting events. At the beginning of therapy, when he or she is depressed, a patient's depressive schemas are said to be activated. So, for example, the patient may react to a message from an acquaintance who says that she cannot join a dinner party the patient was organizing with the inference, "She doesn't like me." As an indication that the deactivation or accommodation of the schema has occurred, the patient upon receiving similar news following therapy, would conclude, "It's too bad. It would have been good if she had been able to join us." According to this view, the difference between deactivation and accommodation is that following deactivation, the depressive schema is simply suppressed, and thus liable to become active again, whereas following accommodation, the change is in the schema itself, and is thus more enduring.

The third kind of change described by Hollon, Evans, and DeRubeis (1985) is the development of compensatory skills. Insofar as acquisition and use of compensatory skills are responsible for change, one would expect to find that even after therapy, patients are still liable to respond to potentially upsetting events by making depressive inferences immediately, but that they then apply the skills they have learned during CT. Each of the aforementioned change processes is a candidate mechanism for the short- and long-term changes produced by CT. The difficulties lie in developing measures that tap schematic versus compensatory processes, and in applying those measures in the relevant studies of therapeutic change.

In comparison to the therapist competence and adherence literature, a greater number of studies have examined patient cognitive processes in CT. For example, numerous studies have now shown that CT is associated with reductions of negative cognitions (e.g., Barber & DeRubeis, 2001; DeRubeis et al., 1990; Jacobson et al., 1996; Jarrett, Vittengl, Doyle, & Clark, 2007; Kolko, Brent, Baugher, Bridge, & Birmaher, 2000; Kwon & Oei, 2003; Oei & Sullivan, 1999; Tang & DeRubeis, 1999a; Tang, DeRubeis, Beberman, & Pham, 2005; Whisman, Miller, Norman, & Keitner, 1991). Garratt, Ingram, Rand, and Sawalani (2007) concluded in their review that the empirical literature is generally consistent with the hypothesis that CT results in cognitive changes that in turn predict reductions in depressive symptom severity. However, they noted that none of the studies they reviewed met each of the four cognitive mediation criteria put forth by DeRubeis et al. (1990). Indeed, although the research designs and statistical techniques employed in most of these studies are appropriate for testing whether reductions in depressive symptoms and negative cognitions covary during CT, they do not allow for rigorous tests of the causal relations between symptoms and cognitions (cf. Haaga, 2007; Kazdin, 2007; Jarrett et al., 2007). Notably, relatively few studies have included multiple assessments of both symptoms and plausible mediators, such as patient cognitions. A more comprehensive examination of process variables and depressive symptoms across multiple time points would allow a more accurate picture of how these variables change and relate to symptom improvement over the course of therapy. Moreover, the use of more sophisticated and powerful multivariate statistical techniques, such as structural equation modeling, may also help to clarify the mechanisms of change in CT and disentangle underlying causal relationships between process variables and symptoms. In summary, given the research designs and data-analytic strategies employed in the majority of studies to date, only tentative conclusions can be drawn from the literature regarding the role of cognition in mediating therapeutic improvement in CT.

Garratt et al. (2007) also examined studies of the "specificity" of cognitive change in CT. Namely, they reviewed the literature addressing whether CT is associated with greater reductions in negative cognitions in comparison to other, "noncognitive" treatment modalities, typically pharmacotherapy. The authors noted that findings have been mixed, but that the research designs have been limited in their ability establish the direction of causality between cognitive and symptom changes.

There are several ways to interpret the results of studies that report similar improvements in negative cognitions following CT and pharmacotherapy (Hollon, DeRubeis, & Evans, 1987). For example, it may be that reductions in negative cognitions following pharmacotherapy are more likely to be the *consequence*, rather than the cause, of depressive symptom improvement. In contrast, the reverse may be the case in CT. It may also be that the cognitive changes seen in pharmacotherapy and other "noncognitive" interventions are somewhat "superficial" relative to those occurring during successful CT. Indeed, the aforementioned prophylactic benefits of CT relative to pharmacotherapy may be partially a result of the "deeper" and more long-term changes that CT produces in patients. Perhaps the measures and methodologies within many of the aforementioned studies are not well-suited to reveal important differences between CT and pharmacotherapy in terms of cognitive change.

Miranda and Persons (1988) suggested that standard cognitive measures are unlikely to uncover schematic content in a person who has recovered from depression, because the depressive schema may have become latent. They developed a negative mood induction procedure that is to be given prior to administering the Dysfunctional Attitude Scale (DAS). Segal, Gemar, and Williams (1999) utilized such a method with two samples of patients who were successfully treated for depression. Following a negative mood induction, patients who had received pharmacotherapy exhibited greater increases in DAS scores than those treated with CT, suggesting that the pharmacotherapy-treated patients possessed more underlying negative (depressive) schemas than did the CT-treated patients. Moreover, Segal et al. found that scores on the mood-induced DAS at posttreatment predicted relapse (or recurrence) during the 30-month period when they followed these patients. In a replication of this study, Segal et al. (2006) once again found that patients who had responded to pharmacotherapy exhibited significantly greater cognitive reactivity in comparison to those in CT. Similarly, patients with greater levels of cognitive reactivity were at increased risk of relapse relative to those exhibiting lower levels of reactivity.

Whereas the DAS and the Attributional Style Questionnaire (ASQ) have been used or proposed as measures of schema change, the measurement of change in compensatory skills has received less attention. The construct "coping" is very close to that of compensatory skills, and there exist several validated coping measures. However, most measures and studies of coping strategies have grown out of interests other than CT. Lazarus and his colleagues have developed a series of measures that assess coping from their point of view (Folkman & Lazarus, 1980; Lazarus & Folkman, 1984). Pearlin and Schooler (1979) have also developed a measure of coping. Although these measures have not been obtained from depressed patients who have gone through a course of CT, it would be expected that given the nature of CT, patients would change their manner of coping relative to both major stressful events and minor annoyances or "hassles" (DeLongis, Coyne, Dakof, Folkman, & Lazarus, 1982).

Standard coping measures are limited in their utility as measures of change during CT. Patients rate the degree to which they have used a variety of coping strategies in response to recent stressful events. Patients can fairly easily recognize those coping skills that they "should" have (but perhaps did not) implement, especially if they have been through a course of CT. For this reason, a method is needed that would require the patient to produce rather than recognize the cognitive coping skills he or she would use in a given situation. Such measures would need to employ a free response format and a system that turns these free responses into coping categories.

Barber and DeRubeis's (1992) Ways of Responding (WOR) scale presents stressful scenarios, followed by initial negative thoughts to which patients are asked to respond. The WOR assesses the degree to which patients have developed the compensatory or metacognitive skills taught in CT. In addition, the scale assesses many cognitive techniques specifically encouraged in CT but not assessed in typical coping skills inventories, such as generating alternative explanations and evaluating negative beliefs based on evidence. The scale has been shown to have good internal consistency and high interrater reliability. Barber and DeRubeis (2001) have shown that WOR scores improve significantly over the course of therapy, and that these changes are associated with decreases in depressive symptoms.

Although the WOR assesses competence in the skills taught by cognitive therapists, it does not assess the extent to which patients actually apply these skills in their daily lives. To fill this void, Strunk, DeRubeis, Chui, and Alvarez (2007) developed the Performance of CT Strategies (PCTS), a measure used by observers of therapy sessions to assess the degree to which patients either exhibit in session or report using between sessions the cognitive and behavioral skills taught in CT. Strunk et al. reported that among CT patients who responded to treatment, reduced risk of relapse in the year following treatment was observed for patients who scored higher on either the WOR or the PCTS. In addition, integrating the findings from DeRubeis and colleagues (DeRubeis & Feeley, 1990; Feeley et al., 1999; Strunk et al., 2007). Webb et al. (2009) found that PCTS scores mediated the relationship between therapist delivery of CT–Concrete techniques and subsequent symptom change.

Tang and DeRubeis (1999a) developed the Patient Cognitive Change Scale (PCCS), a measure designed to assess changes in beliefs as they occur within

CT sessions. The scale is used by a rater who listens to (or reads transcripts from) a therapy session. The rater indicates how frequently changes in belief are explicitly acknowledged by the patient during the session. The PCCS was first designed to be used with audiotape recordings, and it yielded moderate levels of interrater reliability. Tang et al. (2005) subsequently developed a version requiring raters to use the audiotape recordings alongside the transcripts of the therapy sessions, and found this modified version to have very good interrater reliability. The validity of the PCCS has been demonstrated by its ability to distinguish "critical sessions" of CT (the session just before a large, sudden symptom improvement) from control sessions.

Tang and DeRubeis (1999a) observed that many individual patients' depressive symptoms improved suddenly and substantially in a single between-session interval. They named these sudden and substantial symptom improvements "sudden gains" and developed a set of quantitative criteria to identify them. The sudden gains occurred among 39% of the patients, and the magnitude of these sudden gains accounted for more than 50% of these patients' total symptom improvements. Sudden gains also appeared to represent a stable short-term symptom improvement, since depression only infrequently bounced back after the sudden gain. In addition, their outcomes were significantly better than those of the patients who did not experience sudden gains during two of the three assessments in the 18-month follow-up period.

The sudden gains phenomenon has been observed in several subsequent studies involving CT (Busch, Kanter, Landes, & Kohlenberg, 2006; Gaynor et al., 2003; Hardy et al., 2005; Kelly, Roberts, & Ciesla, 2004; Stiles et al., 2003; Tang et al., 2005; Tang, DeRubeis, Hollon, Amsterdam, & Shelton, 2007; Vittengl, Clark, & Jarrett, 2005).[1] Results from these studies have generally been consistent with those originally reported by Tang and DeRubeis (1999a). For example, similar to the Tang and DeRubeis study, several of these studies found that sudden gains predicted better posttreatment outcomes (Hardy et al., 2005; Tang et al., 2005; Vittengl et al., 2005). Other researchers reported that sudden gains occurring earlier (but not later) in therapy predict better outcomes (Busch et al., 2006; Kelly et al., 2004; Stiles et al., 2003), suggesting that the timing of gains may be an important factor to consider in future research.

Tang et al. (2007) recently examined the relationship between sudden gains and depression relapse/recurrence rates. Treatment responders who exhibited sudden gains evidenced a 67% lower risk of relapse and recurrence relative to responders who had not had sudden gains over the study's 2-year follow-up phase. In contrast, in a similar study, Vittengl et al. (2005) reported no difference in the relapse/recurrence rates between sudden gain responders and responders who had not evidenced a sudden gain. However, Vittengl and his colleagues utilized different sudden gains criteria than those originally described by Tang and DeRubeis (1999a). For example, rather than using

---

[1] Three of these studies involved cognitive therapy and additional treatment modalities (Gaynor et al., 2003; Stiles et al., 2003; Vittengl et al., 2005).

session-by-session BDI scores for each patient, Vittengl et al. (2008) used BDI scores from every other session for the first 16 sessions of their study. Moreover, they effectively excluded all sudden gains before session 5. Indeed, in the sample where Tang et al. (2007) found that sudden gains strongly predicted relapse/recurrence, they also found that if they used the same criteria as Vittengl et al. (2005), then the identified sudden gains did not predict relapse/recurrence.

A few studies have explored factors that may trigger sudden gains. Consistent with CT theory, Tang and DeRubeis (1999a) found that patients experienced substantial cognitive changes (as assessed by the PCCS) in the therapy session preceding the sudden gain (the pregain session), but very few cognitive changes in sessions selected to control for depression severity. This finding was replicated by Tang et al. (2005) in an independent dataset. Moreover, Hardy et al. (2005) found that sudden gains were not attributable to life events outside of therapy. These findings suggest that sudden gains may be triggered by cognitive changes that occur in the pregain sessions, offering support for the notion that cognitive changes play an important role in contributing to symptom improvements in CT.

Therapist–Patient Alliance

The "therapeutic alliance" refers to the collaborative relationship between the therapist and patient. Research in the early 1980s showed that the therapeutic alliance is positively related to change in various types of psychotherapy (cf. Morgan, Luborsky, Crits-Christoph, Curtis, & Solomon, 1982). A vast body of research has examined the relationship between therapeutic alliance and outcome across a variety of treatment modalities and mental health problems. In general, reviews of the literature indicate that a stronger therapeutic alliance is associated with better treatment outcomes (Horvath & Bedi, 2002; Martin, Garske, & Davis, 2000).

As DeRubeis and his colleagues (DeRubeis & Feeley, 1990; Feeley et al., 1999) noted, however, many of the studies reporting a significant alliance–outcome association do not control statistically for symptom change preceding the assessment of the alliance (e.g., Castonguay, Goldfried, Wiser, Raue, & Hayes, 1996; Gaston, Thompson, Gallagher, Cournoyer, & Gagnon, 1998). Thus, in such studies, a significant alliance–outcome correlation may in part reflect the influence of prior symptom improvement on the therapeutic alliance. Indeed, DeRubeis and Feeley (1990) and Feeley et al. (1999) found that the alliance was not a significant predictor of *subsequent* therapeutic change. In addition, they found that in the latter half of therapy, the level of therapeutic alliance was predicted by the amount of prior symptom improvement. In other words, these two studies found that good therapeutic alliance early on did not predict good outcome, but that good outcome early on predicted good therapeutic alliance later. This point is underscored by Tang and DeRubeis's (1999a) investigation of sudden gains. They found that in the therapy session before the sudden gains, the therapeutic alliance was not significantly better than that observed in the control sessions, but that therapeutic alliance increased significantly in the therapy session *after* the sudden gain. These results raise questions concerning past findings on the positive correlation between alliance and psychotherapy outcome. Most such studies have used the average alliance score from several or all treatment sessions, and show a relation between this average score and symptom change. It is possible that the correlations reported in some studies reflect the impact of good outcome on the alliance rather than any causal effect of the alliance on symptom improvement.

FUTURE DIRECTIONS

Although an impressive set of published findings has attested to the benefits of CT, there is much more to be learned about (1) the extent of those benefits; (2) the scope and limits of the applicability of CT; (3) its ability to be learned by therapists and applied faithfully outside the context of carefully controlled, carefully monitored clinical trials; and (4) its essential elements and processes. In the following, we call for research that builds on the accrued knowledge about CT since the first research reports on it appeared in the 1970s.

Outcome studies that cast doubt on the potency of CT with more severe forms of depression (Elkin et al., 1995) have had a substantial and sustained impact on how researchers and policymakers in the United States view the benefits of CT. However, recently completed large-scale efficacy studies (e.g., DeRubeis et al., 2005; Dimidjian et al., 2006; Jarrett et al., 1999) have employed the design features that caused the field to give such credence to the TDCRP findings. Also, policymakers in other countries now recognize that the TDCRP represents an anomaly to the major patterns of results in the field. There is no reason to continue to grant TDCRP findings the preeminent status they were accorded in the 1990s.

It may be argued that carefully conducted CT efficacy studies, from the first one (Rush et al., 1977) to that by Dimidjian et al. (2006), tell us about the benefits of CT under optimal conditions, such that they are likely to yield overestimates of the benefit patients can expect in mental health clinics and the like. We note that it has also been argued, to the contrary, that such efficacy studies may *underestimate* the benefits generally achieved by a treatment (see Seligman, 1995). The fact that it is not known whether outcome studies overestimate or underestimate the effects that CT can achieve in private practices and mental health centers indicates that studies of the generalizability of CT are sorely needed. This is beginning to happen, as funding agencies such as the National Institute of Mental Health have made "effectiveness" research a clear priority. Characteristically, in CT efficacy research, therapists (and patients) are carefully selected, and extensive resources are allocated to the training and monitoring of therapists, with the aim of testing the effects of high-quality therapy that adheres to the description provided in a CT manual (e.g., Beck et al., 1979). One way to view the efficacy studies conducted to date is that their findings tell us what may be achieved in the future if typi-cal therapist training programs were to produce trainees who provide high-quality therapy that adheres to the principles of CT. But it is nonetheless vital that pragmatic answers be obtained to the question: How well does CT, as it is currently delivered by mental health practitioners, reduce (and prevent) problems with depression?

Other questions that are relevant to the effectiveness of interventions should also be addressed in relation to CT. In particular, the long-term bene-fits of CT must be more carefully documented. Thus far, research has focused primarily on the ability of CT to prevent relapse in the months following treatment termination. Studies with longer follow-ups are needed to provide estimates of both the relapse prevention (medium term) and recurrence pre-vention (longer term) effects of CT.

Policymakers, managed care companies, and insurers are becoming more interested in, and sophisticated about, pragmatic issues in the delivery of men-tal health care. CT, because it is a relatively short-term treatment with impres-sive evidence of efficacy behind it, has been considered to be well-suited to the present climate of cost-consciousness. The field needs large-scale, sophis-ticated efforts to estimate the costs and benefits of CT, as well as other treat-ments, such as the more widely used antidepressant medications. Even though CT is somewhat more expensive than antidepressant medications in the short run, cost–benefit analyses to date have indicated that it pays for itself within a short time following treatment termination considering its potential to confer resistance to relapse and recurrence (Antonuccio, Thomas, & Danton, 1997; Dobson et al., 2008; Hollon et al., 2005).

Most investigations of therapeutic processes and mechanisms in CT have used correlational analyses (but see Jacobson et al., 1996, for a notable excep-tion). A variable (M) is suspected to be an important mechanism; M is then measured at a particular time, and its correlation with outcome (O) is cal-culated. This approach is subject to the two usual problems of correlational analysis: the ambiguity of the causal direction, and the possibility that a third variable caused both M and O. There is a straightforward solution to the problem of ambiguity of causal direction. If M is measured earlier than O, then the possibility that O caused M can be ruled out. In an example of this approach (Feeley et al., 1999), process variables were assessed in the second therapy session, then correlated with subsequent symptom improvement.

Outcome occurs not just at end of treatment but begins to accumulate relatively early in therapy (Ilardi & Craighead, 1994; Tang & DeRubeis, 1999b). Thus, to apply this method, it is not enough to just measure variable M before the end of treatment. Rather, suspected causal variables need to be evaluated early in treatment. However, this solution does not resolve the sec-ond problem with correlational analyses: the possibility that third variables affect both therapeutic processes and the outcomes of therapy. Third-variable causality cannot be resolved without random assignment to experimental and control conditions, which is often difficult or impossible in research on therapeutic mechanisms. However, there are alternative ways to conduct correlation analyses that tackle the third-variable problem from different angles. If diverse methods all point to the same causal relationship, our confidence in the relationship can be much higher, even if no single method is sufficient.

However, since the initial tests of the efficacy of CT, there have been few, if any, research-based, or research-tested, improvements of CT. This stands in contrast to research efforts in the pharmaceutical industry, on which vast resources are spent to improve the efficacy and side effect profiles of antidepressant medications. Eventually, a new generation of antidepressants might come along that is significantly more effective than today's CT. To better serve our patients, and to ensure that the progress of CT keeps pace with alternative treatments, researchers need to improve and refine CT and the training of cognitive therapists, so that more patients can benefit from it. To do so, we need first to understand better how CT achieves its effects.

REFERENCES

American Psychiatric Association. (2000). Practice guideline for the treatment of patients with major depressive disorder (revision). *American Journal of Psychiatry, 157*, 1–45.

Antonuccio, D. O., Thomas, M., & Danton, W. G. (1997). A cost-effectiveness analysis of cognitive behavior therapy and fluoxetine (Prozac) in the treatment of depression. *Behavior Therapy, 28*, 187–210.

Barber, J. P., & DeRubeis, R. J. (1992). The Ways of Responding: A scale to assess compensatory skills taught in cognitive therapy. *Behavior Assessment, 14*, 93–115.

Barber, J. P., & DeRubeis, R. J. (2001). Change in compensatory skills in cognitive therapy for depression. *Journal of Psychotherapy Practice Research, 10*, 8–13.

Barlow, D. H., Rapee, R. M., & Brown, T. A. (1992). Behavioral treatment of generalized anxiety disorder. *Behavior Therapy, 23*, 551–570.

Beck, A. T. (1961). A systematic investigation of depression. *Comprehensive Psychiatry, 2*, 305–312.

Beck, A. T. (1963). Thinking and depression. *Archives of General Psychiatry, 9*, 324–333.

Beck, A. T. (1964). Thinking and depression: 2. Theory and therapy. *Archives of General Psychiatry, 10*, 561–571.

Beck, A. T. (1972). *Depression: Causes and treatment*. Philadelphia: University of Pennsylvania Press.

Beck, A. T. (2005). The current state of cognitive therapy: A 40–year retrospective. *Archives of General Psychiatry, 62*, 953–959.

Beck, A. T., Emery, G., & Greenberg, R. L. (1985). *Anxiety disorders and phobias*. New York: Basic Books.

Beck, A. T., & Greenberg, R. L. (1974). *Coping with depression*. New York: Institute for Rational Living.

Beck, A. T., & Hurvich, M. (1959). Psychological correlates of depression. *Psychosomatic Medicine, 21*, 50–55.

Beck, A. T., Rush, A. J., Shaw, B. F., & Emery, G. (1979). *Cognitive therapy of depression*. New York: Guilford Press.

Beck, A. T., Steer, R. A., & Brown, G. K. (1996). *Manual for the Beck Depression Inventory* (2nd ed.). San Antonio, TX: Psychological Corporation.

Beck, A. T., & Ward, C. H. (1961). Dreams of depressed patients: Characteristic themes in manifest content. *Archives of General Psychiatry, 5,* 462–467.

Beck, J. (1995). *Cognitive therapy: Basics and beyond.* New York: Guilford Press.

Blackburn, I. N., Bishop, S., Glen, A. I. M., Whalley, L. J., & Christie, J. E. (1981). The efficacy of cognitive therapy in depression: A treatment trial using cognitive therapy and pharmacotherapy, each alone and in combination. *British Journal of Psychiatry, 139,* 181–189.

Blackburn, I. M., Eunson, K. M., & Bishop, S. (1986). A two-year naturalistic follow-up of depressed patients treated with cognitive therapy, pharmacotherapy and a combination of both. *Journal of Affective Disorders, 10,* 67–75.

Blackburn, I. M., & Moore, R. G. (1997). Controlled acute and follow-up trial of cognitive therapy in out-patients with recurrent depression. *British Journal of Psychiatry, 171,* 328–334.

Bockting, C. L. H., Schene, A. H., Spinhoven, P., Koeter, M. W. J., Wounters, L. F., Huyser, J., et al. (2005). Preventing relapse/recurrence in recurrent depression using cognitive therapy. *Journal of Consulting and Clinical Psychology, 73,* 647–657.

Bockting, C. L. H., Spinhoven, P ., Koeter, M. W. J., Wounters, L. F., Visser, I ., & Schene, A. H. (2006). Differential predictors of response to preventive cognitive therapy in recurrent depression: A 2–year prospective study. *Psychotherapy and Psychosomatics, 75,* 229–236.

Busch, A. M., Kanter, J. W., Landes, S. J., & Kohlenberg, R. J. (2006). Sudden gains and outcome: A broader temporal analysis of cognitive therapy for depression. *Behavior Therapy, 37,* 61–68.

Castonguay, L. G., Goldfried, M. R., Wiser, S., Raue, P. J., & Hayes, A. M. (1996). Predicting the effect of cognitive therapy for depression: A study of unique and common factors. *Journal of Consulting and Clinical Psychology, 64,* 497–504.

Chambless, D. L., & Gillis, M. M. (1993). Cognitive therapy of anxiety disorders. *Journal of Consulting and Clinical Psychology, 61,* 248–260.

Clark, D. M. (1996). Panic disorder: From theory to therapy. In P. M. Salkovskis (Ed.), *Frontiers of cognitive therapy* (pp. 318–344). New York: Guilford Press.

Clark, D. M. (1999). Anxiety disorders: Why they persist and how to treat them. *Behaviour Research and Therapy, 37,* S5–S27.

Clark, D. M., Salkovskis, P. M., & Chalkley, A. J. (1985). Respiratory control as a treatment for panic attacks. *Journal of Behavior Therapy and Experimental Psychiatry, 16,* 23–30.

Compas, B. E., Haaga, D. A. F., Keefe, F. J., & Leitenberg, H. (1998). Sampling of empirically supported psychological treatments from health psychology: Smoking, chronic pain, cancer, and bulimia nervosa. *Journal of Consulting and Clinical Psychology, 66,* 89–112.

Cooper, J. M. (Ed.). (1997). *Plato: Complete works.* Indianapolis: Hackett.

Deacon, B. J., & Abramowitz, J. S. (2004). Cognitive and behavioral treatments for anxiety disorders: A review of meta-analytic findings. *Journal of Clinical Psychology, 60,* 429–441.

DeLongis, A., Coyne, J. C., Dakof, G., Folkman, S., & Lazarus, R. S. (1982). Relationship of daily hassles, uplifts, and major life events to health status. *Health Psychology, 1,* 119–136.

DeRubeis, R. J., & Crits-Christoph, P. (1998). Empirically supported individual and group psychological treatments for adult mental disorders. *Journal of Consulting and Clinical Psychology, 66,* 37–52.

DeRubeis, R. J., & Feeley, M. (1990). Determinants of change in cognitive therapy for depression. *Cognitive Therapy and Research, 14,* 469–482.

DeRubeis, R. J., Gelfand, L. A., Tang, T. Z., & Simons, A. (1999). Medications versus cognitive behavioral therapy for severely depressed outpatients: Mega-analysis of four randomized comparisons. *American Journal of Psychiatry, 156,* 1007–1013.

DeRubeis, R. J., Hollon, S. D., Amsterdam, J. D., Shelton, R. C., Young, P. R., Salomon, R. M., et al. (2005). Cognitive therapy vs medications in the treatment of moderate to severe depression. *Archives of General Psychiatry, 62,* 409–416.

DeRubeis, R. J., Hollon, S. D., Evans, M. D., Garvey, M. J., Grove, W. M., & Tuason, V. B. (1990). How does cognitive therapy work?: Cognitive change and symptom change in cognitive therapy and pharmacotherapy for depression. *Journal of Consulting and Clinical Psychology, 58,* 862–869.

Dimidjian, S., Hollon, S. D., Dobson, K. S., Schmaling, K. B., Kohlenberg, R. J., Addis, M., et al. (2006). Randomized trial of behavioral activation, cognitive therapy, and antidepressant medication in the acute treatment of adults with major depression. *Journal of Consulting and Clinical Psychology, 74,* 658–670.

Dobson, D. J. G., & Dobson, K. S. (2009). *Evidence-based practice of cognitive-behavioral therapy.* New York: Guilford Press.

Dobson, K. S. (1989). A meta-analysis of the efficacy of cognitive therapy for depression. *Journal of Consulting and Clinical Psychology, 57,* 414–419.

Dobson, K. S., Hollon, S. D., Dimidjian, S., Schmaling, K. B., Kohlenberg, R. J., Gallop, R., et al. (2008). Randomized trial of behavioral activation, cognitive therapy, and antidepressant medication in the prevention of relapse and recurrence in major depression. *Journal of Consulting and Clinical Psychology, 76,* 468–477.

Durham, R. C., Murphy, T., Allan, T., Richard, K., Treliving, L. R., & Fenton, G. W. (1994). Cognitive therapy, analytic psychotherapy, and anxiety management training for generalized anxiety disorder. *British Journal of Psychiatry, 165,* 315–323.

Elkin, I., Gibbons, R. D., Shea, M. T., & Shaw, B. F. (1996). Science is not a trial (but it can sometimes be a tribulation). *Journal of Consulting and Clinical Psychology, 64,* 92–103.

Elkin, I., Gibbons, R. D., Shea, M. T., Sotsky, S. M., Watkins, J. T., Pilkonis, P. A., et al. (1995). Initial severity and differential treatment outcome in the National Institute of Mental Health Treatment of Depression Collaborative Research Program. *Journal of Consulting and Clinical Psychology, 63,* 841–847.

Elkin, I., Shea, M T., Watkins, J. T., Imber, S. D., Sotsky, S. M., Collins, J. F., et al. (1989). National Institute of Mental Health Treatment of Depression Collaborative Research Program: General effectiveness of treatments. *Archives of General Psychiatry, 46,* 971–982.

Ellis, A. (1984). Rational-emotive therapy. In R. J. Corsini (Ed.), *Current psychotherapies* (pp. 196–238). Itasca, IL: Peacock.

Ellis, A., & Harper, R. A. (1975). *A new guide to rational living.* North Hollywood, CA: Wilshire.

Evans, M. D., Hollon, S. D., DeRubeis, R. J., Piasecki, J., Grove, W. B., & Tuason,

V. B. (1992). Differential relapse following therapy and pharmacotherapy for depression. *Archives of General Psychiatry, 49,* 802–808.

Fava, G. A., Grandi, S., Zielezny, M. C., & Canestrari, R. (1996). Four-year outcome for cognitive behavioral treatment of residual symptoms in major depression. *American Journal of Psychiatry, 153,* 945–947.

Fava, G. A., Grandi, S., Zielezny, M., Canestrari, R., & Morphy, M. A. (1994). Cognitive behavioral treatment of residual symptoms in primary major depressive disorder. *American Journal of Psychiatry, 151,* 1295–1299.

Fava, G. A., Rafanelli, C., Grandi, S., Canestrari, R., & Morphy, M. A. (1998a). Six year outcome for cognitive behavioral treatment of residual symptoms in major depression. *American Journal of Psychiatry, 155,* 1443–1445.

Fava, G. A., Rafanelli, C., Grandi, S., Conti, S., & Belluardo, P. (1998b). Prevention of recurrent depression with cognitive behavioral therapy. *Archives of General Psychiatry, 55,* 816–820.

Fava, G. A., Ruini, C., Rafanelli, C., Finos, L., Conti, S., & Grandi, S. (2004). Six-year outcome of cognitive behavior therapy for prevention of recurrent depression. *American Journal of Psychiatry, 161,* 1872–1876.

Feeley, M., DeRubeis, R. J., & Gelfand, L. (1999). The temporal relation of adherence and alliance to symptom change in cognitive therapy for depression. *Journal of Consulting and Clinical Psychology, 67,* 578–582.

Folkman, S., & Lazarus, R. S. (1980). An analysis of coping in a middle-aged community sample. *Journal of Health and Social Behavior, 21,* 219–239.

Frank, J. D. (1973). *Persuasion and healing.* Baltimore: Johns Hopkins University Press.

Freud, S. (1957). Mourning and melancholia. In J. Strachey (Ed.), *The complete psychological works of Sigmund Freud* (Vol. 14, pp. 239–258). London: Hogarth. (Original work published 1917)

Garratt, G., Ingram, R. E., Rand, K. L., & Sawalani, G. (2007). Cognitive processes in cognitive therapy: Evaluation of the mechanisms of change in the treatment of depression. *Clinical Psychology: Science and Practice, 14,* 224–239.

Gaston, L., Thompson, L., Gallagher, D., Cournoyer, L., & Gagnon, R. (1998). Alliance, technique, and their interactions in predicting outcome of behavioral, cognitive, and brief dynamic therapy. *Psychotherapy Research, 8,* 190–209.

Gaynor, S. T., Weersing, V. R., Kolko, D. J., Birmaher, B., Heo, J., & Brent, D. A. (2003). The prevalence and impact of large sudden improvements during adolescent therapy for depression. *Journal of Consulting and Clinical Psychology, 71,* 386–393.

Gould, R. A., Otto, M. W., Pollack, M. H. (1995). A meta-analysis of treatment outcome for panic disorder. *Clinical Psychology Review, 15,* 819–844.

Haaga, D. A. F. (2007). Could we speed this up?: Accelerating progress in research on mechanisms of change in cognitive therapy of depression. *Clinical Psychology: Science and Practice, 14,* 240–243.

Hardy, G. E., Cahill, J., Stiles, W. B., Ispan, C., Macaskill, N., & Barkham, M. (2005). Sudden gains in cognitive therapy for depression: A replication and extension. *Journal of Consulting and Clinical Psychology, 73,* 59–67.

Horvath, A. O., & Bedi, R. P. (2002). The alliance. In J. C. Norcross (Ed.), *Psychotherapy relationships that work: Therapists contributions and responsiveness to patients* (pp. 37–69). New York: Oxford University Press.

Hollon, S. D. (1999). Rapid early response in cognitive behavior therapy: A commentary. *Clinical Psychology: Science and Practice, 6,* 305–309.

Hollon, S. D., & Beck, A. T. (1979). Cognitive therapy of depression. In P. E. Kendall & S. D. Hollon (Eds.), *Cognitive-behavioral interventions: Theory, research, procedures* (pp. 153–203). New York: Academic Press.

Hollon, S. D., DeRubeis, R. J., & Evans, M. D. (1987). Causal mediation of change in treatment for depression: Discriminating between nonspecificity and noncausality. *Psychological Bulletin, 202,* 139–149.

Hollon, S. D., DeRubeis, R. J., Evans, M. D., Wiemer, M. J., Garvey, M. J., Grove, W. M., et al. (1992). Cognitive therapy and pharmacotherapy for depression: Singly and in combination. *Archives of General Psychiatry, 49,* 774–781.

Hollon, S. D., DeRubeis, R. J., Shelton, R. C., Amsterdam, J. D., Salomon, R. M., O'Reardon, J.P., et al. (2005). Prevention of relapse following cognitive therapy versus medications in moderate to severe depression. *Archives of General Psychiatry, 62,* 417–422.

Hollon, S. D., Emerson, M., & Mandell, M. (1982). *Psychometric properties of the Cognitive Therapy Scale.* Unpublished manuscript, University of Minnesota and the St. Paul–Ramsey Medical Center, Minneapolis–St. Paul.

Hollon, S. D., Evans, M. D., Auerbach, A., DeRubeis, R. J., Elkin, I., Lowery, A., et al. (1985). *Development of a system for rating therapies for depression: Differentiating cognitive therapy, interpersonal psychotherapy, and clinical management pharmacotherapy.* Unpublished manuscript, University of Minnesota and the St. Paul–Ramsey Medical Center, Minneapolis–St. Paul.

Hollon, S. D., Evans, M. D., & DeRubeis, R. J. (1985). Preventing relapse following treatment for depression: The cognitive-pharmacotherapy project. In N. Schneiderman & T. Fields (Eds.), *Stress and coping* (Vol. 2, pp. 227–243). New York: Erlbaum.

Hollon, S. D., & Kriss, M. R. (1984). Cognitive factors in clinical research and practice. *Clinical Psychology Review, 4,* 35–76.

Hollon, S. D., Shelton, R. C., & Loosen, P. T. (1991). Cognitive therapy and pharmacotherapy for depression. *Journal of Consulting and Clinical Psychology, 59,* 88–99.

Ilardi, S. S., & Craighead, W. E. (1994). The role of nonspecific factors in cognitive-behavior therapy for depression. *Clinical Psychology: Science and Practice, 1,* 138–156.

Jacobson, N. S., Dobson, K. S., Truax, P. A., Addis, M. E., Koerner, K., Gollan, J. K., et al. (1996). A component analysis of cognitive-behavioral treatment for depression. *Journal of Consulting and Clinical Psychology, 64,* 295–304.

Jacobson, N. S., & Gortner, E. T. (2000). Can depression be de-medicalized in the 21st century: Scientific revolutions, counter-revolutions and the magnetic field of normal science. *Behaviour Research and Therapy, 8,* 103–117.

Jacobson, N. S., & Hollon, S. D. (1996a). Cognitive-behavior therapy versus pharmacotherapy: Now that the jury's returned its verdict, it's time to present the rest of the evidence. *Journal of Consulting and Clinical Psychology, 64,* 74–80.

Jacobson, N. S., & Hollon, S. D. (1996b). Prospects for future comparisons between drugs and psychotherapy: Lessons from the CBT vs. pharmacotherapy exchange. *Journal of Consulting and Clinical Psychology, 64,* 104–108.

Jarrett, R. B., Basco, M. R., Risser, R., Ramanan, J., Marwill, M., Kraft, D., et al. (1998). Is there a role for continuation phase cognitive therapy for depressed outpatients? *Journal of Consulting and Clinical Psychology, 66,* 1036–1040.

Jarrett, R. B., Schaffer, M., McIntire, D., Witt-Browder, A., Kraft, D., & Risser, R.

C. (1999). Treatment of atypical depression with cognitive therapy or phenelzine. *Archives of General Psychiatry, 56,* 431–437.

Jarrett, R., Vittengl, J., Doyle, K., & Clark, L. (2007) Changes in cognitive content during and following cognitive therapy for recurrent depression: Substantial and enduring, but not predictive of change in depressive symptoms. *Journal of Consulting and Clinical Psychology, 75,* 432–446.

Kazdin, A. E. (2007). Mediators and mechanisms of change in psychotherapy research. *Annual Review of Clinical Psychology, 3,* 1–27.

Kelly, M. A. R., Roberts, J. E., & Ciesla, J. A. (2004). Sudden gains in cognitive behavioral treatment for depression: When do they occur and do they matter? *Behaviour Research and Therapy, 43,* 703–714.

Kingdon, D., Tyrer, P., Seivewright, N., Ferguson, B., & Murphy, S. (1996). The Nottingham Study of Neurotic Disorder: Influence of cognitive therapists on outcome. *British Journal of Psychiatry, 169,* 93–97.

Klein, D. F. (1996). Preventing hung juries about therapy studies. *Journal of Consulting and Clinical Psychology, 64,* 81–87.

Kolko, D. J., Brent, D. A., Baugher, M., Bridge, M., & Birmaher, B. (2000). Cognitive and family therapies for adolescent depression: Treatment specificity, mediation, and moderation. *Journal of Consulting and Clinical Psychology, 68,* 603–614.

Kovacs, M., Rush, A. J., Beck, A. T., & Hollon, S. D. (1981). Depressed outpatients treated with cognitive therapy or pharmacotherapy: A one-year follow-up. *Archives of General Psychiatry, 38,* 33–39.

Kuyken, W., & Tsivrikos, D. (2009). Therapist competence, co-morbidity and cognitive-behavioral therapy for depression. *Psychotherapy and Psychosomatics, 78,* 42–48.

Kwon, S., & Oei, T. P. S. (2003). Cognitive change processes in a group cognitive behavior therapy of depression. *Journal of Behavior Therapy and Experimental Psychiatry, 34,* 73–85.

Lazarus, R. S., & Folkman, S. (1984). *Stress, appraisal, and coping.* New York: Springer.

Ma, S. H., & Teasdale, J. D. (2004). Mindfulness-based cognitive therapy for depression. *Journal of Consultant and Clinical Psychology, 72,* 31–40.

Martin, D., Garske, J. P., & Davis, K. (2000). Relation of the therapeutic alliance with outcome and other variables: A meta-analytical review. *Journal of Consulting and Clinical Psychology, 68,* 438–450.

Meichenbaum, D. (1972). *Cognitive-behavior modification.* New York: Plenum Press.

Meterissian, G. B., & Bradwejn, J. (1989). Comparative studies on the efficacy of psychotherapy, pharmacotherapy, and their combination in depression: Was adequate pharmacotherapy provided? *Journal of Clinical Psychopharmacology, 9,* 334–339.

Miranda, J., & Persons, J. B. (1988). Dysfunctional attitudes are mood-state dependent. *Journal of Abnormal Psychology, 97,* 76–79.

Morgan, R., Luborsky, L., Crits-Christoph, P., Curtis, H., & Solomon, J. (1982). Predicting the outcomes of psychotherapy by the Penn Helping Alliance Rating Method. *Archives of General Psychiatry, 39,* 397–402.

Murphy, G. E., Simons, A. D., Wetzel, R. D., & Lustman, P. J. (1984). Cognitive therapy and pharmacotherapy: Singly and together in the treatment of depression. *Archives of General Psychiatry, 41,* 33–41.

Nisbett, R., & Ross, L. (1980). *Human inference: Strategies and shortcomings of social judgment.* Englewood Cliffs, NJ: Prentice-Hall.

Oei, T. P. S., & Sullivan, L. M. (1999). Cognitive changes following recovery from depression in a group cognitive-behaviour therapy program. *Australian and New Zealand Journal of Psychiatry, 33,* 407–415.

Overholser, J. C. (1993a). Elements of the Socratic method: I. Systematic questioning. *Psychotherapy, 30,* 67–74.

Overholser, J. C. (1993b). Elements of the Socratic method: II. Inductive reasoning. *Psychotherapy, 30,* 75–85.

Paykel, E. S., Scott, J., Cornwall, P. L., Abbott, R., Crane, C., Pope, M., et al. (2005). Duration of relapse prevention after cognitive therapy in residual depression: Follow-up of controlled trial. *Psychological Medicine, 35,* 59–68.

Paykel, E. S., Scott, J., Teasdale, J. D., Johnson, A. L., Garland, A., Moore, R., et al. (1999). Prevention of relapse in residual depression by cognitive therapy. *Archives of General Psychiatry, 56,* 829–835.

Pearlin, L. I., & Schooler, C. (1979). The structure of coping. *Journal of Health and Social Behavior, 19,* 337–356.

Persons, J. B. (1989). *Cognitive therapy in practice: A case formulation approach.* New York: Norton.

Rush, A. J., Beck, A. T., Kovacs, J. M., & Hollon, S. D. (1977). Comparative efficacy of cognitive therapy and pharmacotherapy in outpatient depressives. *Cognitive Therapy and Research, 1,* 17–37.

Salkovskis, P. M. (1985). Obsessional–compulsive problems: A cognitive behavioral analysis. *Behaviour Research and Therapy, 23,* 571–583.

Salkovskis, P. M. (1996). The cognitive approach to anxiety: Threat beliefs, safety-seeking behavior, and the special case of health anxiety and obsession. In P. M. Salkovskis (Ed.), *Frontiers of cognitive therapy* (pp. 48–74). New York: Guilford Press.

Salkovskis, P. M., Clark, D. M., Hackmann, A., Wells, A., & Gelder, M. (1999). An experimental investigation of the role of safety-seeking behaviours in the maintenance of panic disorder with agoraphobia. *Behaviour Research and Therapy, 37,* 559–574.

Segal, Z. V., Gemar, M., & Williams, S. (1999). Differential cognitive response to a mood challenge following successful cognitive therapy or pharmacotherapy for unipolar depression. *Journal of Abnormal Psychology, 108,* 3–10.

Segal, Z. V., Kennedy, S., Gemar, M., Hood, K., Pedersen, R., & Buis, T. (2006). Cognitive reactivity to sad mood provocation and the prediction of depressive relapse. *Archives of General Psychiatry, 63,* 749–755.

Seligman, M. E. P. (1995). The effectiveness of psychotherapy: The Consumer Reports study. *American Psychologist, 50,* 965–974.

Shaw, B. F., Elkin, I., Yamaguchi, J., Olmstead, M., Vallis, T. M., Dobson, K. S., et al. (1999). Therapist competence ratings in relation to clinical outcome in cognitive therapy of depression. *Journal of Consulting and Clinical Psychology, 67,* 837–846.

Shea, M. T., Elkin, I., Imber, S. D., Sotsky, S. M., Watkins, J. T., Collins, J. F., et al. (1992). Course of depressive symptoms over follow-up: Findings from the National Institute of Mental Health Treatment of Depression Collaborative Research Program. *Archives of General Psychiatry, 49,* 782–787.

Simons, A. D., Murphy, G. E., Levine, J. L., & Wetzel, R. D. (1986). Cognitive therapy and pharmacotherapy for depression: Sustained improvement over one year. *Archives of General Psychiatry, 43*, 43–48.

Stiles, W. B., Leach, C., Barkham, M., Lucock, M., Iveson, S., Shapiro, D. A., et al. (2003). Early sudden gains in psychotherapy under routine clinic conditions: Practice-based evidence. *Journal of Consulting and Clinical Psychology, 71*, 14–21.

Strunk, D. R., DeRubeis, R. J., Chui, A., & Alvarez, J. A. (2007). Patients' competence in and performance of cognitive therapy skills: Relation to the reduction of relapse risk following treatment for depression. *Journal of Consulting and Clinical Psychology, 75*, 523–530.

Tang, T. Z., & DeRubeis, R. J. (1999a). Sudden gains and critical sessions in cognitive behavioral therapy for depression. *Journal of Consulting and Clinical Psychology, 67*, 894–904.

Tang, T. Z., & DeRubeis, R. J. (1999b). Reconsidering rapid early response in cognitive behavioral therapy for depression. *Clinical Psychology: Science and Practice, 6*, 283–288.

Tang, T. Z., DeRubeis, R. J., Beberman, R., & Pham, T. (2005). Cognitive changes, critical sessions, and sudden gains in cognitive-behavioral therapy for depression. *Journal of Consulting and Clinical Psychology, 73*, 168–172.

Tang, T. Z., DeRubeis, R. J., Hollon, S. D., Amsterdam, J., & Shelton, R. (2007). Sudden gains in cognitive therapy of depression and depression relapse/recurrence. *Journal of Consulting and Clinical Psychology, 75*, 404–408.

Teasdale, J. D., Segal, Z. V., Williams, J. M. G., Ridgeway, V. A., Soulsby, J. M., & Lan, M. A. (2000). Prevention of relapse/recurrence in major depression by mindfulness-based cognitive therapy. *Journal of Consultant and Clinical Psychology, 68*, 615–623.

Trepka, C., Rees, A., Shapiro, D. A., Hardy, G. E., & Barkham, M. (2004). Therapist competence and outcome of cognitive therapy for depression. *Cognitive Therapy and Research, 28*, 143–157.

Van Oppen, P., de Haan, E., Van Balkom, A. J. L. M., Spinhoven, P., Hoogduin, K., & Van Dyck, R. (1995). Cognitive therapy and exposure *in vivo* in the treatment of obsessive compulsive disorder. *Behaviour Research and Therapy, 33*, 379–390.

Vittengl, J. R., Clark, L. A., & Jarrett, R. B. (2005). Validity of sudden gains in acute phase treatment of depression. *Journal of Consulting and Clinical Psychology, 73*, 172–182.

Webb, C. A., DeRubeis, R. J., Gelfand, L. A., Amsterdam, J. D., Shelton, R. C., Hollon, S. D., et al. (2009). *Mechanisms of change in cognitive therapy for depression: Therapist adherence, symptom change and the mediating role of patient skills.* Manuscript in preparation.

Whisman, M. A., Miller, I. W., Norman, W. H., & Keitner, G. I. (1991). Cognitive therapy with depressed inpatients: Speci?c effects on dysfunctional cognitions. *Journal of Consulting and Clinical Psychology, 59*, 282–288.

Young, J., & Beck, A. T. (1980). *The development of the Cognitive Therapy Scale.* Unpublished manuscript, Center for Cognitive Therapy, Philadelphia, PA.

CHAPTER 10

Schema Therapy

Rachel Martin
Jeffrey Young

"Schema therapy" (Young, 1990) is an integrative therapy approach and theoretical framework used to treat clients with personality disorders, characterological issues, some chronic Axis I diagnoses, and various other difficult individual and couples' problems. Schema therapy evolved from Beck's cognitive therapy (Beck, Rush, Shaw, & Emery, 1979) to integrate aspects of cognitive therapy, behavioral therapy, object relations, Gestalt therapy, constructivism, attachment models, and psychoanalysis. Schema therapy targets the chronic and characterological aspects of a disorder rather than the acute psychiatric symptoms.

The Young Schema Questionnaire (YSQ) and Schema Mode Inventory (SMI) have been developed and validated as measures of schemas and modes, respectively. Schema therapy offers a flexible framework for treatment, targeting maladaptive schemas, coping strategies, and/or modes as appropriate to each client. Therapy is usually of intermediate or long-term duration and is often conducted in conjunction with other modalities. Current research shows empirical support for schema therapy, and there are ongoing efficacy studies under way around the globe.

ORIGINS OF SCHEMA THERAPY

Schema therapy developed from the cognitive-behavioral practices and clinical experiences of Jeffrey Young, who recognized the need for a broader life issues perspective to address long-standing patterns of behavior and emotional problems (Young, Klosko, & Weishaar, 2003). Effective cognitive-behavioral treatments exist for many Axis I disorders (Barlow, 2001), but these treatments are ineffective for many clients. Although cognitive-behavioral therapy (CBT) is typically brief and present-focused, some clients have chronic and persistent dysfunction or characterological features that complicate and expand the course of treatment. For example, as many as 40% of depressed clients do not respond successfully to treatment, and approximately 30% of treatment responders experience relapse within 1 year (Young, Weinberger, & Beck, 2001).

Clients with underlying personality disorders often fail to respond to traditional CBT (Beck, Freeman, & Associates, 1990) and may encounter a variety of difficulties in traditional CBT therapeutic work. These clients often have ambivalent or complicated motivations for therapy, and may be unwilling or unable to comply with therapeutic procedures. Clients with characterological problems habitually engage in cognitive, affective, and behavioral avoidance, and may therefore be unwilling or unable to observe and report their thoughts and feelings. Such clients may lack the psychological flexibility necessary for short-term modification of entrenched and enduring maladaptive thoughts and behaviors. Note that rigidity is a hallmark feature of personality disorders (DSM-IV; American Psychiatric Association, 1994, p. 633). Chronic disturbances with significant others are another signature feature of personality disorders (Millon, 1981), and the fundamental interpersonal difficulties of clients with characterological issues may be reflected in difficulties engaging in a therapeutic alliance. Some clients become overly absorbed with having the therapist meet their emotional needs and cease to work independently, whereas other clients may be too disengaged or hostile to form a working alliance with the therapist. Finally, clients with characterological problems often present with problems that are vague, chronic, and pervasive, relating to dissatisfaction in love, work, or play. These themes can be difficult to concretize and operationalize as targets of treatment for the standard CBT approach.

Schema therapy, which originally emerged for treating personality disorders, has since been shown to be useful in treatment of chronic anxiety and depressive disorder, eating disorders, couple problems, long-standing difficulties maintaining satisfying intimate relationships, and relapse in substance use disorders. Schema therapy is indicated when the presenting problem is chronic and long term; when a person with an Axis I disorder relapses chronically or is nonresponsive to therapy; when the presenting problem is vague yet pervasive; when there are long-term relationship problems; when the client is highly avoidant, shows rigid patterns of thought and behavior, or is unusually needy, demanding, or feels entitled.

DIFFERENTIATION OF SCHEMA THERAPY

Schema therapy emerged from a foundation of cognitive therapy to stand as a unique theory and approach to treatment. It diverges from traditional CBT, however, in its greater emphasis on the developmental origins of psychological problems, on lifelong patterns of psychosocial functioning, and on entrenched core themes of maladaptive cognition and behavior. Schema therapy also expands the areas of functioning typically associated with CBT, to emphasize affective states and emotive techniques, coping styles, and interpersonal aspects of the therapeutic relationship. As such, schema therapy integrates aspects of cognitive, behavioral, object relations, Gestalt, constructivist, attachment, and psychoanalytic approaches into a unified conceptual model. The techniques employed in schema therapy are diverse and incorporate cognitive, behavioral, experiential, and interpersonal methods.

The Schema Therapy Model

Schema therapy targets the chronic and characterological aspects of a disorder rather than the acute psychiatric symptoms. The schema therapy model describes three main constructs: "schemas" are core psychological themes; "coping styles" are characteristic behavioral responses to schemas; and "modes" are the schemas and coping styles operating at a given moment. Emotional difficulties arise predominantly from unmet core needs in childhood and adolescent development, which lead to maladaptive schemas and coping styles (Young et al., 2003).

Schemas

"Schemas" are internal phenomena that influence external behavior through the development of coping styles. Early maladaptive schemas (EMSs) are broad, self-defeating, pervasive patterns that begin in childhood and repeat throughout a person's life. By definition, EMSs comprise memories, emotions, cognitions, and bodily sensations. They incorporate how one conceptualizes oneself and one's relationships with others. They develop during childhood and adolescence, are elaborated throughout one's lifetime, and may be dysfunctional to a significant degree. Indeed, the dysfunctional or maladaptive schemas are the focus of schema therapy. For convenience, the terms "early maladaptive schemas" and "schemas" are used interchangeably here.

EMSs are dimensional; they vary in their degree of intensity, pervasiveness, and frequency of activation. EMSs can interfere significantly with a client's ability to meet core needs for autonomy, connection, and self-expression. They are capable of producing high levels of disruptive affect, extremely self-defeating consequences, and even significant harm to others. There are positive and negative schemas, as well as early and later schemas. Early maladaptive schemas are the focus of schema therapy, although some authors have proposed that certain adaptive schemas correspond to each EMS (see Elliott's polarity theory; Elliott & Lassen, 1997). Similarly, there are healthy and unhealthy coping styles and modes. The "Healthy Adult" is a positive mode that we describe later in this chapter.

The earliest and central schemas typically originate in the nuclear family. As the child matures, other influences (e.g., peers, school, community groups, and culture) become increasingly important and may also contribute to schema development. However, later schemas are generally not as pervasive or as powerful as early schemas. The origins of EMSs are often traumatic, or at least destructive, and many are caused by repeated harmful experiences throughout childhood and adolescence. The noxious effects of these repetitive, related experiences accumulate, leading to emergence of a schema. The most damaging schemas usually involve childhood experiences of abandonment, abuse, neglect, or rejection.

Early schemas begin as reality-based representations of the child's environment. They develop from an interaction of the child's innate temperament and specific unmet, core childhood needs. Five postulated core emotional needs in childhood are (1) secure attachments to others (includes safety, stability, nurturance, and acceptance); (2) autonomy, competence, and sense of identity; (3) freedom to express valid needs and emotions; (4) spontaneity and play; and (5) realistic limits and self-control.

Four types of early life experiences may foster the acquisition of EMSs. The first, "toxic frustration of needs," occurs when the child experiences deficits in the early environment (in stability, understanding, or love), and acquires schemas such as Emotional Deprivation or Abandonment. The second type of early life experience is "traumatization," which occurs when the child is harmed, criticized, controlled, or victimized, and develops schemas such as Mistrust/Abuse, Defectiveness, or Subjugation. In the third type, the child is provided with "too much of a good thing" (something that, in moderation, would be healthy for a child), which leads to schemas such as Dependence or Entitlement. The fourth type of life experience that creates schemas is "selective internalization or identification" with significant others, which occurs when the child selectively identifies with, and internalizes, the parent's thoughts, feelings, experiences, and schemas. Internalization/identification appears to be a common origin for the Vulnerability schema. Innate temperament is a major determinant of child identification with, and internalization of, parent characteristics.

Temperament interacts with childhood events in schema development. A considerable body of literature supports the biological underpinnings, presence in infancy, and temporal stability of temperamental traits and personality (e.g., Kagan, Reznick, & Snidman, 1998). Some dimensions of emotional temperament that might be innate and relatively unchangeable through psychotherapy alone include Labile ↔ nonreactive; dysthymic ↔ optimistic; anxious ↔ calm; obsessive ↔ distractible; passive ↔ aggressive; irritable ↔ cheerful; and shy ↔ sociable. Different temperaments differentially expose children to certain life circumstances. For example, a violent parent might be more likely to abuse an aggressive child than a placating, passive child. In addition, different temperaments cause children to react differently to similar life circumstances. A shy child may become increasingly withdrawn and dependent on a neglectful mother, whereas a sociable child of the same mother may develop independence and make other, more positive connections. The interaction of temperament and early life events produces different coping styles in each child. Table 10.1 lists the 18 schemas, grouped into five broad categories of unmet emotional needs called "schema domains."

Although schemas originate as reality-based representations of the childhood environment, they are perpetuated into adulthood, where they may no longer be accurate or adaptive, and their dysfunctional nature becomes apparent. Adult schemas are triggered by life events that the person perceives as similar to the toxic childhood events. When a schema is triggered, the person experiences strong negative emotions, such as grief, shame, fear, or rage. More severe schemas are activated by a greater number of situations, and generally provoke more intense and longer-lasting negative affect. For example, an individual who faced extreme and frequent criticism from both parents in childhood may have a Defectiveness schema that is strongly activated by contact with almost anyone. In contrast, an individual who experienced only occasional mild criticism from his or her father may have a Defectiveness schema triggered only by negative interactions with demanding male authority figures.

Schemas are a major determinant of how individuals think, feel, behave, and interact socially. Schemas are generally accepted as a priori truths and are outside of awareness, despite their influence on the processing of experiences. Furthermore, schemas are familiar and comfortable. Individuals are drawn to people who trigger their schemas—a phenomenon called "schema chemistry." The schema is known and feels "right," even though it actually causes suffering.

"Schema perpetuation" describes all that an individual does internally or behaviorally to maintain a schema, including thoughts, feelings, actions, and interactions. Consider, for example, a woman with a Mistrust/Abuse schema who lends money to her boyfriend. When he is slightly late in paying her back, she thinks that he is deliberately misleading and using her, because he does not truly care for her, and she feels humiliated and enraged. When she expresses her strong emotions and accuses her boyfriend of trying to "rip her off," he is alarmed by her behavior and breaks up with her. The woman concludes that she cannot trust men; thus, her cognitive distortions, extreme emotional reactions, and self-defeating behaviors have served to perpetuate her schema. In contrast, in "schema healing," the goal of schema therapy, the intensity and influence of a schema are diminished, and clients learn to replace maladaptive coping styles with more adaptive patterns of behavior.

Coping Styles

Various strategies are utilized to cope with a schema. Note that a schema contains memories, emotions, bodily sensations, and cognitions, and is differentiated from behavior, which is part of the coping response. Coping styles

(text continues on p. 326)

TABLE 10.1. Maladaptive Schemas, Grouped by Schema Domain of Unmet Core Needs

<u>Disconnection and Rejection</u>

(Expectation that one's needs for security, safety, stability, nurturance, empathy, sharing of feelings, acceptance, and respect will not be met in a predictable manner. Typical family origin is detached, cold, rejecting, withholding, lonely, explosive, unpredictable, or abusive.)

Abandonment/ Instability	Perceived *instability* or *unreliability* of those available for support and connection. Involves the sense that significant others will not be able to continue providing emotional support, connection, strength, or practical protection because they are emotionally unstable and unpredictable (e.g., angry outbursts), unreliable, or erratically present; because they will die imminently; or because they will abandon the patient in favor of someone "better."
Mistrust/Abuse	Expectation that others will hurt, abuse, humiliate, cheat, lie, manipulate, or take advantage. Usually involves perceptions that the harm is intentional or the result of unjustified and extreme negligence. May include the sense of always being cheated or disadvantaged relative to others.
Emotional Deprivation	Expectation that others will not adequately meet one's desire for a normal degree of emotional support. Major forms of deprivation are [A] *Deprivation of nurturance*: Absence of attention, affection, warmth, or companionship; [B] *Deprivation of empathy*: Absence of understanding, listening, self-disclosure, or mutual sharing of feelings from others; [C] *Deprivation of protection*: Absence of strength, direction, or guidance from others.
Defectiveness/ Shame	Feeling that one is defective, bad, unwanted, inferior, or invalid in important respects; or that one would be unlovable to significant others if exposed. May involve hypersensitivity to criticism, rejection, and blame; self-consciousness, comparisons, and insecurity around others; or a sense of shame regarding one's perceived flaws. These flaws may be *private* (e.g., selfishness, angry impulses, unacceptable sexual desires) or *public* (e.g., undesirable physical appearance, social awkwardness).
Social Isolation/ Alienation	Feeling that one is isolated from the rest of the world, different from other people, and/or not part of any group or community.

<u>Impaired Autonomy and Performance</u>

(Expectations about oneself and the environment that interfere with one's perceived ability to separate, survive, function independently, or perform successfully. Typical family origin is enmeshed, undermining of the child's confidence, overprotective, or fails to reinforce the child for performing competently outside the family.)

Dependence/ Incompetence	Belief that one is unable to handle one's *everyday responsibilities* in a competent manner, without considerable help from others (e.g., take care of oneself, solve daily problems, exercise good judgment, tackle new tasks, make good decisions). Often presents as helplessness.

(cont.)

TABLE 10.1. *(cont.)*

Vulnerability to harm or illness	Exaggerated fear that *imminent* catastrophe will strike at any time and that one will be unable to prevent it. Fears focus on one or more of the following: [A] *Medical catastrophes* (e.g., heart attacks, AIDS); [B] *Emotional catastrophes* (e.g., going crazy); [C] *External catastrophes* (e.g., elevators collapsing, victimized by criminals, airplane crashes, earthquakes).
Enmeshment/ Undeveloped Self	Excessive emotional involvement and closeness with one or more significant others (often parents) at the expense of full individuation or normal social development. Often involves the belief that at least one of the enmeshed individuals cannot survive or be happy without the constant support of the other. May also include feelings of being smothered by, or fused with, others *or* having insufficient individual identity. Often experienced as a feeling of emptiness and floundering, having no direction or, in extreme cases, questioning one's existence.
Failure	The belief that one has failed, will inevitably fail, or is fundamentally inadequate relative to one's peers, in areas of *achievement* (school, career, sports, etc.). Often involves beliefs that one is stupid, inept, untalented, ignorant, lower in status, less successful than others, and so forth.

Impaired Limits

(Deficiency in internal limits, responsibility to others, or long-term goal orientation. Leads to difficulty respecting the rights of others, cooperating with others, making commitments, or setting and meeting realistic personal goals. Typical family origin is characterized by permissiveness, overindulgence, lack of direction, or a sense of superiority—rather than appropriate confrontation, discipline, and limits in relation to taking responsibility, cooperating in a reciprocal manner, and setting goals. In some cases, the child may not have been pushed to tolerate normal levels of discomfort, or may not have been given adequate supervision, direction, or guidance.)

Entitlement/ Grandiosity	The belief that one is superior to other people; entitled to special rights and privileges; or not bound by the rules of reciprocity that guide normal social interaction. Often involves insistence that one should be able to do or have whatever one wants, regardless of what is realistic, what others consider reasonable, or the cost to others; *or* an exaggerated focus on superiority (e.g., being among the most successful, famous, wealthy) in order to achieve *power* or *control* (not primarily for attention or approval). Sometimes includes excessive competitiveness toward, or domination of, others: asserting one's power, forcing one's point of view, or controlling the behavior of others in line with one's own desires—without empathy or concern for others' needs or feelings.

(cont.)

TABLE 10.1. *(cont.)*

Insufficient Self-control/Self-discipline	Pervasive difficulty or refusal to exercise sufficient self-control and frustration tolerance to achieve one's personal goals, or to restrain the excessive expression of one's emotions and impulses. In its milder form, the patient presents with an exaggerated emphasis on *discomfort avoidance*: avoiding pain, conflict, confrontation, responsibility, or overexertion—at the expense of personal fulfillment, commitment, or integrity.

Other-Directedness

(An excessive focus on the desires, feelings, and responses of others at the expense of one's own needs—in order to gain love and approval, maintain one's sense of connection, or avoid retaliation. Usually involves suppression and lack of awareness regarding one's own anger and natural inclinations. Typical family origin is based on conditional acceptance: Children must suppress important aspects of themselves in order to gain love, attention, and approval. In many such families, the parents' emotional needs and desires—for social acceptance and status—are valued more than the unique needs and feelings of each child.)

Subjugation	Excessive surrendering of control to others because one feels *coerced*—usually to avoid anger, retaliation, or abandonment. The two major forms of subjugation are [A] *subjugation of needs*: suppression of one's preferences, decisions, and desires; and [B] *subjugation of emotions*: suppression of emotional expression, especially anger. Usually involves the perception that one's own desires, opinions, and feelings are not valid or important to others. Frequently presents as excessive compliance, combined with hypersensitivity to feeling trapped. Generally leads to a buildup of anger, manifested in maladaptive symptoms (e.g., passive–aggressive behavior, uncontrolled outbursts of temper, psychosomatic symptoms, withdrawal of affection, "acting out," substance abuse).
Self-sacrifice	Excessive focus on *voluntarily* meeting the needs of others in daily situations, at the expense of one's own gratification. The most common reasons are to prevent causing pain to others; to avoid guilt from feeling selfish; or to maintain the connection with others perceived as needy. Often results from an acute sensitivity to the pain of others. Sometimes leads to a sense that one's own needs are not being adequately met and to resentment of those who are taken care of. (Overlaps with concept of codependency.)
Approval seeking/ Recognition seeking	Excessive emphasis on gaining approval, recognition, or attention from other people, or fitting in, at the expense of developing a secure and true sense of self. One's sense of esteem is dependent primarily on the reactions of others rather than on one's own natural inclinations. Sometimes includes an overemphasis on status, appearance, social acceptance, money, or achievement—as means of gaining *approval, admiration,* or *attention* (not primarily for power or control). Frequently results in major life decisions that are inauthentic or unsatisfying; or in hypersensitivity to rejection.

(cont.)

TABLE 10.1. *(cont.)*

Overvigilance and Inhibition

(Excessive emphasis on suppressing one's spontaneous feelings, impulses, and choices, or on meeting rigid, internalized rules and expectations about performance and ethical behavior—often at the expense of happiness, self-expression, relaxation, close relationships, or health. Typical family origin is grim, demanding, and sometimes punitive: Performance, duty, perfectionism, following rules, hiding emotions, and avoiding mistakes predominate over pleasure, joy, and relaxation. There is usually an undercurrent of pessimism and worry—that things could fall apart if one fails to be vigilant and careful at all times.)

Negativity/ Pessimism	A pervasive, lifelong focus on the negative aspects of life (pain, death, loss, disappointment, conflict, guilt, resentment, unsolved problems, potential mistakes, betrayal, things that could go wrong, etc.), while minimizing or neglecting the positive or optimistic aspects. Usually includes an exaggerated expectation—in a wide range of work, financial, or interpersonal situations—that things will eventually go seriously wrong, or that aspects of one's life that seem to be going well will ultimately fall apart. Usually involves an inordinate fear of making mistakes that might lead to financial collapse, loss, humiliation, or being trapped in a bad situation. Because potential negative outcomes are exaggerated, these patients are frequently characterized by chronic worry, vigilance, complaining, or indecision.
Emotional inhibition	The excessive inhibition of spontaneous action, feeling, or communication— usually to avoid disapproval by others, feelings of shame, or losing control of one's impulses. Common areas of inhibition involve: [A] inhibition of *anger* and aggression; [B] inhibition of *positive impulses* (e.g., joy, affection, sexual excitement, play); [C] difficulty expressing *vulnerability* or *communicating* freely about one's feelings, needs, and so forth; or [D] excessive emphasis on *rationality*, while disregarding emotions.
Unrelenting standards/ hypercriticalness	The underlying belief that one must strive to meet very high *internalized standards* of behavior and performance, usually to avoid criticism. Typically results in feelings of pressure or difficulty slowing down, and in hypercriticalness toward oneself and others. Must involve significant impairment in pleasure, relaxation, health, self-esteem, sense of accomplishment, or satisfying relationships. Unrelenting standards typically present as [A] *perfectionism*, inordinate attention to detail, or an underestimation of how good one's own performance is relative to the norm; [B] *rigid rules* and "shoulds" in many areas of life, including unrealistically high moral, ethical, cultural, or religious precepts; or [C] preoccupation with *time and efficiency*, so that more can be accomplished.
Punitiveness	The belief that people should be harshly punished for making mistakes. Involves the tendency to be angry, intolerant, punitive, and impatient with those people (including oneself) who do not meet one's expectations or standards. Usually includes difficulty forgiving mistakes in oneself or others, because of a reluctance to consider extenuating circumstances, allow for human imperfection, or empathize with feelings.

are usually adaptive, healthy, survival mechanisms in childhood, but they may become maladaptive over time if they perpetuate an EMS, even when conditions change and more adaptive coping strategies and/or schemas are available. Most patients use a combination of coping responses and styles. Whereas a schema remains stable over time, coping styles are used variably to cope with the schema in different situations and at different stages of life. Thus, coping behaviors are not intrinsic to specific schemas. Furthermore, an individual can exhibit different coping styles with different schemas. Temperament also plays a considerable role in determining coping styles. Individuals with passive temperaments are probably more likely to surrender or to avoid, whereas those with active or aggressive temperaments may tend to overcompensate.

There are three basic maladaptive coping styles (see Table 10.2): surrender, avoidance, and overcompensation. When an individual surrenders to a schema, that schema is accepted as true. The individual does not try to avoid or to fight the schema, and he or she directly feels the emotional consequences of the schema. Schema-driven patterns are repeated, so that childhood experiences that created the schema are relived, and sometimes even strengthened, in adulthood. Individuals who surrender to their schemas typically choose partners who are likely to treat them as the "offending" parent did, then relate to these partners in ways that exacerbate the situation. In the therapy relationship, these clients may enact the schema with the therapist in the role of this same parent. Surrender coping styles include compliance and dependence.

Some individuals arrange their lives to avoid activating the schema. Thoughts, feelings, and behaviors connected to the schema are avoided, and avoidance behaviors may be extreme or excessive. Situations that trigger the schema are avoided, such as intimate relationships, work challenges, or even entire areas of life in which an individual feels vulnerable. These clients may avoid engagement in therapy; they may "forget" to complete homework assignments, arrive late to sessions, address only superficial issues at shallow levels of exploration, or terminate therapy prematurely. Avoidance coping styles include social and psychological withdrawal, excessive autonomy, compulsive stimulation seeking, addictive self soothing, and substance use or abuse.

Individuals who use the coping style of overcompensation resist the schema by going to the opposite extreme. When the schema is triggered, they counterattack vigorously. Overcompensation may originate as a healthy impulse to combat the schema, but it becomes disproportionate to the situation, may disregard the feelings of others, and is unlikely to lead to a desirable outcome. Overcompensation develops because it offers a means of escape from childhood feelings of helplessness and vulnerability, and an alternative to the effects of the schema. Adults with this coping style try to differentiate themselves from their childhood selves who acquired the schema. However, overcompensation typically develops into a rigid coping style, involving excessive, insensitive, or unproductive behavior. Strategies include aggression, hostility, dominance, excessive self-assertion, recognition seeking, status seeking,

TABLE 10.2. Examples of Maladaptive Behaviors Associated with Schemas and Coping Styles

Early maladaptive schema	Examples of surrender	Examples of avoidance	Examples of overcompensation
Abandonment/ Instability	Selects partners who cannot make a commitment, and remains in the relationships	Avoids intimate relationships; drinks when alone	Clings to and "smothers" to the point of pushing partner away; vehemently attacks partner for even minor separations
Mistrust/Abuse	Selects abusive partners and permits abuse	Avoids becoming vulnerable and trusting anyone; keeps secrets	Uses and abuses others ("get others before they get you")
Emotional deprivation	Selects emotionally depriving partners and does not ask to get needs met	Avoids intimate relationships altogether	Acts emotionally demanding with partners and close friends
Defectiveness/ Shame	Selects critical and rejecting friends; puts self down	Avoids expressing true thoughts and feelings, and letting others get close	Criticizes and rejects others, while seeming to be perfect oneself.
Social isolation	At social gatherings, focuses exclusively on one's differences rather than one's similarities to others	Avoids social situations and groups	Becomes a chameleon to fit into groups
Dependence/ Incompetence	Asks significant others (parents, spouse) to make all of one's financial decisions	Avoids taking on new challenges, such as learning to drive	Becomes so self-reliant that one does not ask anyone for anything ("counterdependent")
Vulnerability to harm and illness	Obsessively reads about catastrophes in newspapers and anticipates them in everyday situations	Avoids going places that do not seem totally "safe"	Acts recklessly, without regard to danger ("counterphobic")
Enmeshment/ Undeveloped Self	Tells one's mother everything, even as an adult; lives through partner	Avoids intimacy; stays independent	Tries to become the opposite of significant others in all ways

(cont.)

TABLE 10.2. *(cont.)*

Failure	Does tasks in a half-hearted or haphazard manner	Avoids work challenges completely; procrastinates tasks	Becomes an "overachiever" by ceaselessly driving oneself
Entitlement/ Grandiosity	Bullies others to get one's way, brags about one's accomplishments	Avoids situations where one is average, not superior	Attends excessively to the needs of others
Insufficient Self-control/ Self-discipline	Gives up easily on routine tasks	Avoids employment or accepting responsibility	Becomes overly self-controlled or self-disciplined
Subjugation	Lets the other individual control situations and make choices	Avoids situations that might involve conflict with another individual	Rebels against authority
Self-sacrifice	Gives a lot to others and asks for nothing in return	Avoids situations involving giving or taking	Gives as little to others as possible
Approval seeking/ Recognition seeking	Acts to impress others	Avoids interacting with those whose approval is coveted	Goes out of one's way to provoke the disapproval of others; stays in the background
Negativity/ Pessimism	Focuses on the negative; ignores the positive; worries constantly; goes to great lengths to avoid any possible negative outcome	Drinks to blot out pessimistic feelings and unhappiness	Is overly optimistic ("Pollyanna-ish"); denies unpleasant realities
Emotional Inhibition	Maintains a calm, emotionally flat demeanor	Avoids situations where people discuss or express feelings	Awkwardly tries to be the "life of the party," even though it feels forced and unnatural
Unrelenting standards	Spends inordinate amounts of time trying to be perfect	Avoids or procrastinates situations and tasks in which performance will be judged	Does not care about standards at all—does tasks in a hasty, careless manner
Punitiveness	Treats self and others in harsh, punitive manner	Avoids others for fear of punishment	Behaves in an overly forgiving way

manipulation, exploitation, passive–aggressiveness, rebellion, excessive order-liness, and obsessiveness.

Modes

The term "modes" describe the schemas and coping styles that are active at a given moment. Whereas schemas and coping styles are client traits, modes are client states, as an individual may shift between modes based on the activation of different sets of schemas or coping styles. Modes are activated when specific schemas or coping responses burgeon into overwhelming emotions or rigid coping styles. They are often triggered by life situations to which a client is oversensitive ("emotional buttons").

The concept of modes originated from work with clients with borderline personality disorder (BPD). The schema model was difficult to apply, because clients with BPD often have numerous complex and dynamic schemas. The concept of "modes," developed as a different unit of analysis, grouped schemas together to make them more manageable to treat. Furthermore, the affective lability of clients with BPD seemed to be better represented with a state model, which involved modes as the primary construct as opposed to more enduring trait constructs, such as schemas and coping styles. The concept of modes is now applied to many other diagnostic categories and to clients with different levels of functioning.

Four main types of modes are proposed, and each is associated with certain schemas and coping styles (see Table 10.3). These four mode types are the Child modes, the Maladaptive Coping modes, the Dysfunctional Parent modes, and the Healthy Adult mode. The child modes are the Vulnerable Child, the Angry Child, the Impulsive/Undisciplined Child, and the Contented Child. The three maladaptive coping modes are the Compliant Surrenderer, the Detached Protector, and the Overcompensator, which correspond, respectively, to coping styles of surrender, avoidance, and overcompensation. The two dysfunctional parent modes, the Punitive Parent and the Demanding Parent, are prominent in clients with borderline and narcissistic disorders, respectively.

The Healthy Adult mode serves an "executive" or parental function to the self. The Healthy Adult serves three basic functions: (1) to nurture, affirm, and protect the Vulnerable Child; (2) to set limits for the Angry Child and the Impulsive/Undisciplined Child; and (3) to combat or moderate the Maladaptive Coping and Dysfunctional Parent modes. The effectiveness of the Healthy Adult mode differentiates between higher- and lower-functioning individuals. Although every person has a Healthy Adult mode, it is activated more strongly and frequently in psychologically healthy individuals. Furthermore, the Healthy Adult mode in psychologically healthy people can more effectively moderate dysfunctional modes. Strengthening the client's Healthy Adult mode is an overarching goal of mode work in schema therapy.

TABLE 10.3. Schema Modes, Grouped by Modal Type

Child modes

Vulnerable Child	Individual feels lonely, isolated, sad, misunderstood, unsupported, defective, deprived, overwhelmed, incompetent, doubtful about self, needy, helpless, hopeless, frightened, anxious, worried, victimized, worthless, unloved, unlovable, lost, directionless, fragile, weak, defeated, oppressed, powerless, left out, excluded, and/or pessimistic.
Angry Child	Individual feels intensely angry, enraged, infuriated, frustrated, and/or impatient, because the core needs of the Vulnerable Child are not being met.
Impulsive/ Undisciplined Child	Individual acts on noncore desires or impulses in a selfish or uncontrolled manner to get his or her own way and often has difficulty delaying short-term gratification. Individual often feels intensely angry, enraged, infuriated, frustrated, and/or impatient when desires or impulses cannot be met. Individual may appear "spoiled."
Contented Child	Individual feels loved, contented, connected, satisfied, fulfilled, protected, accepted, praised, worthwhile, nurtured, guided, understood, validated, self-confident, competent, appropriately autonomous or self-reliant, safe, resilient, strong, in control, adaptable, included, optimistic, and/or spontaneous.

Maladaptive Coping Modes

Compliant Surrenderer	Individual acts in a passive, subservient, submissive, approval-seeking, or self-deprecating way around others out of fear of conflict or rejection; tolerates abuse and/or bad treatment; does not express healthy needs or desires to others; selects people or engages in other behavior that directly maintains the self-defeating schema-driven pattern.
Detached Protector	Individual cuts off needs and feelings; detaches emotionally from people and rejects their help; feels withdrawn, spacey, distracted, disconnected, depersonalized, empty, and/or bored; pursues distracting, self-soothing, or self-stimulating activities in a compulsive way or to excess; may adopt a cynical, aloof, or pessimistic stance to avoid investing in people or activities.
Overcompensator	Individual feels and behaves in an inordinately grandiose, aggressive, dominant, competitive, arrogant, haughty, condescending, devaluing, overcontrolled, controlling, rebellious, manipulative, exploitive, attention-seeking, or status-seeking way. These feelings or behaviors must originally have developed to compensate for or gratify unmet core needs.

Maladaptive Parent modes

Punitive Parent	Individual feels that self or others deserve punishment or blame, and often acts on these feelings by being blaming, punishing, or abusive toward self or others. This mode describes the *style* with which rules are enforced rather than the *nature* of the rules.

(cont.)

TABLE 10.3. *(cont.)*

Demanding/ Critical Parent	Individual feels that it is ideal and desirable to be perfect or to achieve at a very high level, to keep everything in order, to strive for high status, to be humble, to put others' needs before one's own, or to be efficient or avoid wasting time; or the individual feels that it is wrong to express feelings or act spontaneously. This mode describes the *nature* of the internalized high standards and rules rather than the *style* with which these rules are enforced. These rules are not compensatory in their function.

Healthy Adult mode

Healthy Adult	This mode nurtures, validates, and affirms the Vulnerable Child mode; sets limits for the Angry and Impulsive Child modes, promotes and supports the Healthy Child mode; combats and eventually replaces the Maladaptive Coping modes; neutralizes or moderates the Maladaptive Parent modes. This mode performs appropriate adult functions such as working, parenting, taking responsibility, and committing. This mode also pursues healthy pleasurable adult activities such as sex; intellectual, esthetic and cultural interests; health maintenance; and athletic activities.

Each client exhibits certain characteristic modes; indeed, some Axis II diagnoses are readily described in terms of their typical modes (Young et al., 2003). Clients with borderline personality disorder usually shift rapidly among four modes: the Abandoned Child, who experiences pain from schemas; the Angry Child, who expresses rage over unmet needs; the Punitive Parent, who punishes the child for the expression of needs and emotions; and the Detached Protector, who blocks emotions and detaches from people. Clients with narcissistic personality disorder typically exhibit overcompensation for Emotional Deprivation and Defectiveness schemas, with typical modes of the Self-Aggrandizer, the Detached Self-Soother, and the Lonely Child.

Some personality disorders are best conceptualized in terms of the original model of schemas and coping styles (Young et al., 2003). For example, the Mistrust/Abuse schema is related to paranoid personality disorder, and the Defectiveness schema and an avoidant coping style may underlie avoidant personality disorder. In contrast, obsessive–compulsive personality disorder is explained by the Unrelenting Standards schema, whereas compulsive behavior and dependent personality disorder are related to the Dependence/Incompetence schema. There is no one-to-one correspondence between the schema and mode models and DSM-IV personality disorders, however. Rather, these models offer an alternative system for conceptualizing characterological problems and personality disorders within the therapeutic setting. As part of the schema healing process, therapy clients are encouraged and assisted to switch from a dysfunctional mode to a healthy mode.

ASSESSMENT IN SCHEMA THERAPY

The assessment phase of schema therapy begins with the identification of clients' schemas and an attempt to understand their possible developmental origins. Next, maladaptive coping styles (surrender, escape, and counterattack) are identified and evaluated as mechanisms for perpetuating clients' schemas. Finally, primary modes are identified, and the shifts between modes are observed. Assessment is multifaceted and multimodal. Assessment techniques typically include a life history interview, behavioral observation, self-monitoring assignments, and imagery exercises designed to activate schemas and to clarify emotional links between current problems and past experiences.

The goal of assessment in schema therapy is to develop a complete schema-focused case conceptualization. Case conceptualization incorporates Axis I symptoms or diagnoses, current major problems, developmental origins of problems, possible temperamental or biological contributors, core childhood memories and unmet needs, major schemas and current schema triggers, coping behaviors (including surrender, avoidance, and counterattack styles), primary schema modes, core cognitions and distortions, and the quality of the therapeutic relationship.

Young Schema Questionnaire

The Long Form of the Young Schema Questionnaire, third edition (YSQ-L3; Young & Brown, 2003a) is a 232–item measure that asks respondents to rate the accuracy of self-descriptive statements on a Likert-type scale ranging from 1 (*Completely untrue of me*) to 6 (*Describes me perfectly*). Sample statements include "I have not had someone who really listens to me, understands me, or is tuned into my true needs and feelings" and "I feel that there is constant pressure for me to achieve and get things done." Items were written to capture each of the 18 schemas, and cutoff values are provided to evaluate scores on each schema as low, medium, high, or very high. A Short Form of the YSQ (YSQ-S3; Young & Brown, 2003b) also measures the 18 schemas using only 90 rated self-descriptive statements. The YSQ has been translated into most major languages, including French, Spanish, German, Portuguese, Italian, Dutch, Turkish, Japanese, Korean, Finnish, and Norwegian.

The psychometric properties of the YSQ were first studied by Schmidt, Joiner, Young, and Telch (1995), who reported that the schemas demonstrated high test–retest reliability and internal consistency. The YSQ also demonstrated good convergent and discriminant validity with measures of psychological distress, self-esteem, cognitive vulnerability to depression, and personality disorder symptomatology. Factor analysis supported the schema structure of the YSQ in both clinical and nonclinical populations. The investigators replicated these results in a second sample from the same population. A replication by Lee, Taylor, and Dunn (1999), using an Australian clinical population, also supported the schema domains detailed in the YSQ. This factor-analytic study reported 16 primary components, including 15 of the 16 schemas proposed in the original schema therapy model. Correlations have been reported between EMSs and measures of both adult attachment and childhood trauma (Cecero, Nelson, & Gillie, 2004).

The YSQ-S3 has also been shown to have good internal consistency, a supported factor structure, and solid construct validity (Welburn, Coristine, Dagg, Pontefract, & Jordan, 2002). Results of an unpublished study suggest that the YSQ-S3 has a validated factor structure and good internal consistency when used with adolescents as well as adults, although it does not appear to be viable for use with individuals under 12 years of age (Waller, Meyer, Beckley, Stopa, & Young, 2004). A comparison of the short and long forms of the YSQ indicates that both versions have similar internal consistency, parallel forms reliability and concurrent validity, and that the short form can be used in clinical and research applications with reasonable confidence (Stopa, Thorns, Waters, & Preston, 2001).

Schema Mode Inventory

The Schema Mode Inventory (SMI; Young et al., 2007) asks respondents to rate the frequency with which they would endorse 186 self-descriptive statements, using a Likert-type scale ranging from 1 (*Never or almost never*) to 6 (*Almost all of the time*). Sample self-descriptive statements include, for example, "I don't feel connected to other people" and "I'm trying to do my best at everything I try." Arntz, Klokman, and Sieswerda (2004) studied modes in clients with borderline personality disorder (BPD), using the SMI. Compared to normal subjects, these clients were significantly more likely to score high on all four characteristic borderline modes (Abandoned Child, Detached Protector, Angry Child, and Punitive Parent). Clients with BPD scored lowest on the Healthy Adult mode. Examination of the correlations among different modes and personality disorders revealed unique patterns of modes for different personality disorders (Lobbestael, Van Vreeswijk, & Arntz, 2008). Results suggested that the combination of mode scores, rather than the score on any particular mode, best defined each specific mode. Although mode construct validity was supported, the high number of correlations for some personality disorders may indicate a need for increased specificity of the modes.

TREATMENT IN SCHEMA THERAPY

Emotional difficulties arise predominantly from unmet core needs in childhood and adolescent development that lead to maladaptive schemas and behavioral coping patterns. The schema therapy model holds that psychologically healthy individuals can get their core emotional needs met by adaptive means. In therapy, clients learn to identify and change the maladaptive schemas, coping styles, and modes that block them from getting their needs met. Then clients explore and adopt more adaptive means of meeting their own core needs.

Schema therapy offers a flexible framework that can be used to target schemas, coping styles, modes, or any combination thereof, depending on the needs of the client. The overarching goal of schema therapy is schema healing, which is accomplished with cognitive, behavioral, experiential, and interpersonal interventions. Schema therapy reduces the intensity of the memories, emotions, bodily sensations, and maladaptive cognitions associated with maladaptive schemas. Behavioral change is another component of schema healing, as clients learn more adaptive behavioral patterns to replace their maladaptive coping styles. Schema healing renders schemas more difficult to activate, which reduces their impact and enhances recovery from negative experiences. Over the course of healing, clients begin to develop self-esteem and select more caring interpersonal relationships.

Schemas are deeply entrenched beliefs that are learned early and repeated throughout life. They can be highly resistant to change. Furthermore, they provide clients with a sense of predictability and security. Schema healing requires that clients be willing to confront schemas directly, with the support and alliance of the therapist. Clients must systematically become aware of their schema and practice new ways of thinking, feeling, and behaving. This process requires discipline and commitment to regular practice. Whether therapy targets schemas, coping styles, or modes, the therapist–client relationship comprises a fundamental component of schema therapy. Client schemas, coping styles, and modes are assessed and addressed as they arise in the therapeutic relationship. The therapist models a Healthy Adult mode for the client to internalize to fight maladaptive schemas and pursue emotional fulfillment by healthy means. The therapist uses the therapeutic stance of "empathic confrontation" to highlight the reasons for client change, while maintaining empathy for the client's schemas and coping styles. Finally, the therapist uses "limited reparenting" within appropriate therapeutic boundaries to satisfy partially the client's unmet childhood needs.

Schema therapy work begins with an assessment and identification of the client's core needs and central schemas. Schemas are then linked to the client's presenting problems and life history patterns. The therapist triggers client schemas through imagery and discussion, and the client begins to experience emotions associated with the schemas. Coping styles, characteristic modes, and patterns in the therapy relationship are observed and identified. At this stage, the case conceptualization is developed and should be shared with the client for feedback.

Cognitive interventions are used to test schemas empirically and rationally, and to challenge their validity. Patterns from the past and present are identified and reframed to discredit the schemas. Cognitive interventions include schema flashcards, a schema diary, and "schema dialogues," client enactment of imaginal dialogues between schemas and the Healthy Adult.

Experiential techniques use imagery and dialogues to explore and synchronize the link between emotions and cognitive changes. Expression of appropriate emotions related to memories is encouraged and coached, if necessary. Experiential exercises include "empty chair" imaginal dialogues, and expressive letter writing to parents and significant others (although, in most cases, the letters are not sent).

Behavioral interventions help clients to identify maladaptive coping responses and to rehearse alternative behaviors. Problem behaviors are assessed for patterns and linked to the underlying schema. Graduated homework assignments expose client to different life situations and interpersonal interactions. Flashcards, imagery, contingency management, and schema mode work may be used to overcome obstacles. Finally, the schema therapy model advocates for the involvement of loved ones in the recovery process, if such involvement is possible, appropriate, and adaptive. If appropriate, clients are encouraged and assisted to forgive their parents toward the end of treatment process, through a developed understanding of their parents' schemas and coping styles.

Schema therapy suggests specific therapeutic goals for addressing different schemas (see Table 10.4). Mode work in schema therapy has the ultimate goal of strengthening the client's Healthy Adult mode, so that it can work more adaptively with the client's other modes. Initially, the therapist serves as the Healthy Adult, sets limits, and models adaptive behavior when the client is unable to do so. Over the course of therapy, the client gradually internalizes the therapist's thoughts, feelings, and behavior into his or her own Healthy Adult mode and takes over this role.

Although mode work developed from clinical experience with clients with BPD, mode work is applicable to a wider range of clients. Mode work may be indicated when a client demonstrates a rigid, avoidant coping style; a rigid, compensatory coping style; strongly self-punitive, self-critical tendencies; internal confusion or apparently unresolvable internal conflicts; or frequent fluctuations in mood and coping styles.

Mode work in schema therapy may take many different forms depending on the needs of the client. In general, however, a sequence of seven broad steps is defined:

1. Identify and label the client's modes as they arise, both in therapy and outside the session.
2. Explore the origin and function of each mode.
3. Link maladaptive modes to current problems and symptoms to provide rationale for change.
4. Demonstrate the advantages of modification or abandonment of dysfunctional modes, if they interfere with access to another mode or create dysfunction in other ways.

(text continues on p. 343)

TABLE 10.4. Therapeutic Goals for Addressing Specific Schemas

Early maladaptive schema	Therapeutic goals
Abandonment/ Instability	*Cognitive:* • Alter exaggerated view that others will eventually leave, withdraw, or behave unpredictably. • Alter unrealistic expectations that significant others should always be consistent and available. • Reduce exaggerated focus on making sure partner is there. *Experiential:* • Use imagery to reexperience memories of unstable, unpredictable, or absent parent. • Express anger toward unstable parent. • Help client nurture his or her inner abandoned child. *Behavioral:* • Choose partners who are stable and committed. • Don't push partners away through excessive jealousy, clinging, etc. • Learn to tolerate being alone gradually, and to tolerate stable secure environments. *Therapy relationship:* • Therapist becomes transitional source of safety and stability. • Correct distortions about likelihood of abandoning client and promoting acceptance of any therapist unavailability.
Mistrust/Abuse	*Cognitive:* • Reduce hypervigilance to abuse or mistreatment. • Alter exaggerated view of others as badly intentioned, abusive, manipulative, or dishonest. • Alter view of self as to blame for abuse. • Label abuse accurately and do not make excuses for the abuser. • Alter view of self as helpless against abuse. • Teach spectrum of mistreatment; shades of gray versus right–wrong. *Experiential:* • Recall memories of abuse or humiliation. • Express anger verbally and physically; confront abuser in imagery. • Find a safe place away from the abuser. *Behavioral:* • Gradually trust people, at increasing levels of intimacy. • Join a support group for other victims and share "secrets" and memories. • Choose nonabusive partners. • Don't abuse others. • Set limits with abusive people. • Be less punitive when others make mistakes.

(cont.)

TABLE 10.4. *(cont.)*

	Therapy relationship:
	• Therapist is completely honest and genuine with client.
	• Ask regularly about in-session trust, intimacy, and vigilance toward therapist.
	• If needed, hold off on experiential work while trust is built up.

Emotional Deprivation

Cognitive:
• Change exaggerated sense that all people act selfishly or are depriving the client.
• Teach shades of gray with levels of deprivation.
• Learn what emotional needs are not being met.

Experiential:
• Express anger and pain at depriving parents in imagery.
• Ask to have needs met by parents in imagery.

Behavioral:
• Choose nurturing partners.
• Ask appropriately to have needs met by partners.
• Don't react to levels of deprivation with anger.
• Don't withdraw or isolate when hurt by others.

Therapy relationship:
• Therapist provides nurturing atmosphere of empathy, guidance, and attention.
• Help client accept feelings of deprivation, without overreacting or remaining silent.
• Help client accept therapist's limitations, while appreciating nurturing that is given.
• Link relationship with early memories.

Defectiveness/ Shame

Cognitive:
• Alter view of self as bad, unlovable or flawed by focusing on assets and minimizing flaws.

Experiential:
• Vent anger at critical parents and dialogue with critical schema, in imagery.

Behavioral:
• Choose accepting partners.
• Don't overreact to criticism.
• Self-disclose more, to overcome shame.
• Don't overcompensate (e.g., with excessive emphasis on status).

Therapy relationship:
• Therapist creates a nonjudgmental, accepting environment.
• Share minor weaknesses of therapist.
• Compliment client appropriately.

(cont.)

TABLE 10.4. *(cont.)*

Social isolation/ Alienation	*Cognitive:* • Alter view of self as socially undesirable by focusing on assets and altering exaggerated negative view of appearance and social skills. • Minimize differences and heighten similarities with other people. *Experiential:* • Use imagery of memories of rejection or alienation, and allow venting toward rejecting group. • Use imagery of an accepting adult group. *Behavioral:* • Overcome avoidance. • Participate in group therapy. • Improve social skills. • Gradually develop circle of friends and ties to community. *Therapy Relationship:* • Confront avoidance of social situations and praise positive social attributes.
Dependence/ Incompetence	*Cognitive:* • Alter view that client is unable to function without constant assistance from others. • Alter view that client cannot trust his or her own decisions or judgment in everyday situations. *Experiential:* • Express anger at parents, in imagery, for overprotecting client and undermining judgment. *Behavioral:* • Use gradual exposure to a hierarchy of everyday tasks to handle alone, without assistance from others. *Therapy relationship:* • Therapist resists client attempts to take on dependent role. • Encourage client to make his or her own decisions and choices; praise judgment and progress.
Vulnerability to harm or illness	*Cognitive:* • Challenge exaggerated perceptions of harm and danger in areas of criminal danger, financial ruin, medical illness, and mental illness. *Experiential:* • Dialogue with phobic, overprotective parents in imagery. • Visualize safe outcomes in everyday situations.

(cont.)

TABLE 10.4. *(cont.)*

	Behavioral: • Use gradual exposure to a hierarchy of feared/avoided situations. *Therapy relationship:* • Confront avoidance and provide calm, rational reassurance. • Enmeshment/Undeveloped self
Enmeshment/ Undeveloped self	*Cognitive:* • Alter view that client or parent cannot survive without continual contact with the other. *Experiential:* • Use imagery of separating from parents. • Use dialogue in imagery between two sides to overcome obstacles to establishing separate identity. *Behavioral:* • Identify personal preferences and natural inclinations in everyday situations, in order to act on one's own preferences and disentangle from expectations of others. • Select appropriate partners who do not encourage fusion or enmeshment. *Therapy relationship:* • Therapist sets appropriate boundaries; neither too close nor too distant.
Failure	*Cognitive:* • Challenge view that client is inherently inept or stupid, and reattribute failure to schema maintenance. • Highlight successes and skills. • Set realistic expectations. *Experiential:* • Access memories of critical or nonsupportive adults, of comparisons with siblings, or of unrealistic expectations. • Use imagery to overcome avoidance of performance/achievement. *Behavioral:* • Use gradual exposure to a hierarchy of new challenges. • Set limits and create structure to overcome procrastination and teach self-discipline. *Therapy relationship:* • Support success. • Set realistic expectations. • Provide structure and limits.

(cont.)

TABLE 10.4. *(cont.)*

Entitlement/ Grandiosity	*Cognitive:* • Challenge view of being special with special rights. • Encourage empathy for others and consider reciprocity. • Highlight negative consequences of entitlement or grandiosity. *Experiential:* • Access vulnerability and underlying schemas. *Behavioral:* • Stop acting entitled. • Learn to balance own needs with needs of others. • Follow the rules. *Therapy relationship:* • Confront entitlement and set limits. • Support vulnerability, but not status/grandiosity, etc.
Insufficient Self-control/Self- discipline	*Cognitive:* • Teach about value of long-term versus short-term gratification. *Experiential:* • Explore deeper schemas and affect through imagery. *Behavioral:* • Teach self-discipline through structured tasks. • Teach techniques for self-control of emotions. *Therapy relationship:* • Be firm and set limits.
Subjugation	*Cognitive:* • Challenge exaggerated negative consequences of expressing needs. *Experiential:* • Express anger and assert rights with controlling parents through imagery. *Behavioral:* • Select noncontrolling partners. • Gradually assert needs with others. • Learn natural inclinations and act on them. *Therapy relationship:* • Don't overcontrol. • Encourage client to make choices. • Point out deferential choices and identify anger.

(cont.)

TABLE 10.4. *(cont.)*

Self-sacrifice	*Cognitive:* • Change exaggerated perception of how needy others are. • Increase awareness of one's own needs. • Highlight imbalance of give–get ratio. *Experiential:* • Access resentment over emotional deprivation and imbalance with parents, in imagery. *Behavioral:* • Ask to have needs met. • Don't choose needy partners. • Set limits on giving to others. *Therapy relationship:* • Therapist models appropriate boundaries and right to own needs. • Discourage client from taking care of therapist. • Encourage client to rely on therapist and validate dependency needs.
Approval-seeking/ Recognition-seeking	*Cognitive:* • Explore the perceived negative consequences of acting in a genuine way. • Identify disadvantages of working so hard to please others. *Experiential:* • Dialogue with significant others from whom the client is trying to gain approval or recognition. • Visualize reactions of others when the client is direct and honest, and expresses own needs. *Behavioral:* • Practice behaving in a genuine, authentic manner with others. *Therapy relationship:* • Therapist confronts client empathically when he or she appears to be "too pleasing" or too focused on the therapist's reactions and approval.
Negativity/ Pessimism	*Cognitive:* • Stop exaggerating negatives, and instead focus on positives in life. • Consider illusory glow versus depressive realism. *Experiential:* • Dialogue with negative parent. • Dialogue between negative and positive sides. • Access possible emotional deprivation, anger, or loss.

(cont.)

TABLE 10.4. *(cont.)*

Behavioral:
- Ask to have needs met in relationships.
- Do things for fun and enjoyment.

Therapy relationship:
- Therapist avoids falling into the "Pollyanna" role, and instead encourages the client to play the positive role.

Emotional
inhibition

Cognitive:
- Highlight advantages of showing emotions.
- Minimize feared consequences of acting on emotion and impulse.

Experiential:
- Access and express unacknowledged emotions in imagery.
- Dialogue in imagery with inhibited parent.

Behavioral:
- Discuss and express feelings more.
- Be more spontaneous: dance, sex, aggression, etc.
- Use gradual exposure to a hierarchy of tasks letting go of control.

Therapy relationship:
- Model and encourage more expression of affect and spontaneity.

Unrelenting
standards/
Hypercriticalness

Cognitive:
- Reduce unrealistic standards, by teaching a continuum of standards and using cost–benefit analysis.
- Highlight advantages and disadvantages of unrelenting standards.
- Reduce perceived risks of imperfection.

Experiential:
- Dialogue with parents with high expectations.

Behavioral:
- Gradually reduce standards.
- Increase time spent relaxing and having fun.

Therapy relationship:
- Model balanced standards in approach to therapy and in own life.

Punitiveness

Cognitive:
- Weigh advantages and disadvantages of acting toward oneself or others in a punishing manner.
- Discuss the fact that punishment is not an effective long-term strategy for behavior change.

(cont.)

TABLE 10.4. *(cont.)*

Experiential:
- Get angry at punitive parental figures in imagery.
- Practice dialogues between the Punitive Parent mode and the Healthy Adult.

Behavioral:
- Practice talking and behaving in a forgiving tone toward self and others.

Therapy relationship:
- Therapist models forgiving response when client behaves in a punitive manner during sessions.

---

5. Access the Vulnerable Child through imagery, while providing the voice of the Healthy Adult.
6. Gradually draw other modes into dialogues using imagery. Encourage the Healthy Adult mode to solve problems arising in the dialogue among modes.
7. Help the client generalize mode work to life situations outside therapy sessions.

SCHEMA THERAPY
FOR BORDERLINE PERSONALITY DISORDER

Schema therapy for BPD helps the client to develop and fortify a Healthy Adult mode, modeled after the therapist. First, client schemas, coping styles, and characteristic modes are identified, and their origins and functions are explored. The therapist empathizes with current client problems, outlines therapy goals and rationales, and educates the client about schemas, coping styles, and modes.

Clients with BPD often shift rapidly among several schema modes. The phenomenon of flipping modes is linked to the definitive borderline feature of affective and interpersonal instability and reactivity. The characteristic modes of BPD are the Abandoned Child, the Detached Protector, the Punitive Parent, the Angry Child, the Impulsive Child, and the Healthy Adult. Given the client's tendency to flip modes, schema therapists must take care to enforce appropriate limits and boundaries. Treatment begins with therapist–client bonding to establish an empathic and nurturing therapeutic relationship that will facilitate limited reparenting. The Abandoned Child mode is healed through limited reparenting, validation of needs and feelings, development of a nurturing and stable base, and confidence-building through direct praise.

The Detached Protector is bypassed with the use of experiential observation and imaginal dialogue.

As the client begins to learn coping skills, techniques such as flashcards, schema diaries, and assertiveness skills are introduced. Schema mode change initially uses education, cognitive reattribution, self-esteem building, and experiential techniques to combat the Punitive Parent mode. Next, the Angry Child and Impulsive Child modes are rechanneled, so that anger is directed toward the parental figure. The client learns to practice appropriate assertion and affective expression. Limits are explored with the client around extreme expression of emotions, the amount of outside therapeutic contact, suicidal crisis management, and destructive impulsive behavior.

The final stages of schema therapy for BPD focus on client autonomy. The development of healthy intimacy and individuation is facilitated by empathic confrontation, imagery, and behavioral rehearsal in therapy and in real life. Clients discover their natural inclinations, and begin to select stable and appropriate interpersonal relationships. Over time, frequency of therapeutic contact is reduced, and clients achieve gradual independence.

EMPIRICAL SUPPORT FOR SCHEMA THERAPY

Empirical support for the effectiveness of schema therapy is accumulating. A multicenter study in Holland (Giesen-Bloo et al., 2006) followed 88 clients with borderline personality disorder over 3 years of biweekly treatment with either schema-focused therapy (SFT) or psychodynamically oriented transference-focused therapy (TFT). Treatment effectiveness was evaluated with multiple measures, including a psychometrically validated, semistructured clinical interview based on DSM-IV diagnostic criteria for BPD. Other measures included quality-of-life questionnaires and various other measures of relevant constructs, such as general psychopathology, social functioning, the therapeutic relationship, and biases in information processing. The results demonstrated that both therapy approaches were effective at reducing psychopathology and dysfunction, and improving quality of life. Notably, schema therapy was more effective than TFT across all measures, and had significantly reduced risk of dropout over the course of treatment. Furthermore, a subsequent economic analysis by these authors determined that schema therapy was more cost-effective than TFT (Van Asselt et al., 2008).

Although the results of the Giesen-Bloo et al. (2006) study are positive, it is clear that more research is needed to evaluate the results of schema therapy. Further outcome studies are in progress around the world, and the results of these studies will be informative in this regard. There is a concomitant need for process research related to schema therapy, to evaluate the actual mechanisms of treatment and to relate these methods to outcome. As the field progresses, it may also be possible to evaluate the comparative efficacy of schema therapy and other approaches to targets of intervention.

CONCLUSION

This chapter has presented the conceptual framework, primary methods, and early support for schema therapy (Young, 1990), which integrates aspects of cognitive, behavioral, experiential, Gestalt, and psychodynamic schools of thought into a unifying theory and treatment approach. Schema therapy is used to treat clients with chronic disorders and underlying characterological problems, such as personality disorders, chronic depression and anxiety, and other difficult problems. It targets the chronic and characterological aspects of a presenting problem and may be conducted simultaneously with other treatment modalities. The schema therapy model describes three main constructs: "schemas" are core psychological themes; "coping styles" are characteristic behavioral responses to schemas; and "modes" are the schemas and coping styles operating at a given moment. Schema therapy offers a flexible treatment framework that targets maladaptive schemas, coping strategies, and/or modes as needed (Young et al., 2003). Empirical support for schema therapy is emerging, as research is ongoing into this innovative approach.

REFERENCES

American Psychiatric Association. (1994). *Diagnostic and statistical manual of mental disorders* (4th ed.). Washington, DC: Author.

Arntz, A., Klokman, J., & Sieswerda, S. (2004). An experimental test of the schema mode model of borderline personality disorder. *Journal of Behavior Therapy and Experimental Psychiatry, 36,* 226–239.

Barlow, D. H. (Ed.). (2001). *Clinical handbook of psychological disorders: A step-by-step treatment manual* (3rd ed.). New York: Guilford Press.

Beck, A. T., Freeman, A., & Associates. (1990). *Cognitive therapy of personality disorders.* New York: Guilford Press.

Beck, A. T., Rush, A. J., Shaw, B. F., & Emery, G. (1979). *Cognitive therapy of depression.* New York: Guilford Press.

Cecero, J. J., Nelson, J. D., & Gillie, J. M. (2004). Tools and tenets of schema therapy: Toward the construct validity of the Early Maladaptive Schema Questionnaire— Research Version (EMSQ-R). *Clinical Psychology and Psychotherapy, 11,* 344–357.

Elliott, C. H., & Lassen, M. K. (1997). A schema polarity model for case conceptualization, intervention, and research. *Clinical Psychology: Science and Practice, 4,* 12–28.

Giesen-Bloo, J., van Dyck, R., Spinhoven, P., van Tilburg, W., Dirksen, C., Van Asselt, T., et al. (2006). Outpatient psychotherapy for borderline personality disorder: Randomized trial of schema-focused therapy vs transference-focused psychotherapy. *Archives of General Psychiatry, 63,* 649–658.

Kagan, J., Reznick, J. S., & Snidman, N. (1988). Biological bases of childhood shyness. *Science, 240,* 167–171.

Lee, C. W., Taylor, G., & Dunn, J. (1999). Factor structures of the Schema Questionnaire in a large clinical sample. *Cognitive Therapy and Research, 23,* 421–451.

Lobbestael, J., Van Vreeswijk, M. F., & Arntz, A. (2008). An empirical test of schema mode conceptualizations in personality disorders. *Behaviour Research and Therapy, 46,* 854–860.

Millon, T. (1981). *Disorders of personality.* New York: Wiley.

Schmidt, N. B., Joiner, T. E., Young, J. E., & Telch, M. J. (1995). The Schema Questionnaire: Investigation of psychometric properties and the hierarchical structure of a measure of maladaptive schemata. *Cognitive Therapy and Research, 19,* 295–321.

Stopa, L., Thorns, P., Waters, A., & Preston, J. (2001). Are the short and long forms of the Young Schema Questionnaire comparable and how well does each version predict psychopathology scores? *Journal of Cognitive Psychotherapy, 15,* 253–272.

Van Asselt, A. D. I., Dirksen, C. D., Arntz, A., Giesen-Bloo, J. H., van Dyck, R., Spinhoven, P., et al. (2008). Outpatient psychotherapy for borderline personality disorder: Cost-effectiveness of schema-focused therapy v. transference-focused psychotherapy. *British Journal of Psychiatry, 192,* 450–457.

Waller, G., Meyer, D., Beckley, R., Stopa, L., & Young, J. E. (2004). *Psychometric validation of the short form of the Young Schema Questionnaire and norms for non-clinical adolescents and adults.* Unpublished manuscript, University of Southhampton, UK.

Welburn, K., Coristine, M., Dagg, P., Pontefract, A., & Jordan, S. (2002). The Schema Questionnaire—Short Form: Factor analysis and relationship between schemas and symptoms. *Cognitive Therapy and Research, 26,* 519–530.

Young, J. E. (1990). *Cognitive Therapy for Personality Disorders.* Sarasota, FL: Professional Resources Press.

Young, J. E., Arntz, A., Atkinson, T., Lobbestael, J., Weishaar, M. E., van Vreeswijk, M. F., et al. (2007). *The Schema Mode Inventory.* New York: Schema Therapy Institute.

Young, J. E., & Brown, G.(2003a). The Young Schema Questionnaire—Long Form. Retrieved January 27, 2009, from *www.schematherapy.com/id53.htm.*

Young, J. E., & Brown, G.(2003b). The Young Schema Questionnaire—Short Form. Retrieved January 27, 2009, from *www.schematherapy.com/id55.htm.*

Young, J. E., Klosko, J., & Weishaar, M. E. (2003). *Schema therapy: A Practitioner's guide.* New York: Guilford Press.

Young, J. E., Weinberger, A. D., & Beck, A. T. (2001). Cognitive therapy for depression. In D. Barlow (Ed.), *Clinical handbook of psychological disorders: A step-by-step treatment manual* (3rd ed., pp. 264–308). New York: Guilford Press.

CHAPTER 11

Mindfulness and Acceptance Interventions in Cognitive-Behavioral Therapy

Alan E. Fruzzetti
Karen R. Erikson

The use of acceptance and mindfulness interventions in cognitive-behavioral therapy (CBT) has become common in recent years and continues to expand (Baer, 2003; Dimidjian & Linehan, 2003; Roemer & Orsillo, 2003; Kabat-Zinn, 2003). Moreover, increased interest in research on both the inclusion of these concepts within a therapeutic context and the nature of mindfulness and acceptance as clinical applications has brought mindfulness and acceptance into CBT's empirical tradition. In this chapter we present the concepts and definitions of acceptance and mindfulness, and discuss the ways that mindfulness and acceptance interventions have been integrated into CBT. Prominent among these approaches are dialectical behavior therapy, mindfulness-based relapse prevention, acceptance and commitment therapy, mindfulness-based cognitive therapy, mindfulness-based stress reduction, and integrative behavioral couple therapy, all of which incorporate essential mindfulness and acceptance strategies, and have data to support their utility. We conclude with a description of several core clinical mindfulness and acceptance strategies and interventions, illustrated by brief clinical examples.

DEFINITIONS AND THE CONCEPTUALIZATION OF MINDFULNESS AND ACCEPTANCE

It is important to define the terms "mindfulness" and "acceptance," and to see how they are used in CBT. The terms "mindfulness" and "acceptance" are often used in conjunction with one another or even interchangeably. Mindfulness has been described as "bringing one's complete attention to the present experience on a moment-to-moment basis" (Marlatt & Kristeller, 1999, p. 68) and as "the awareness that emerges through paying attention on purpose, in the present moment, and non-judgmentally to the unfolding of experience moment by moment" (Kabat-Zinn, 2003). Baer (2003) suggests that mindfulness can include bringing one's attention to internal experiences, such as thoughts, feelings, or bodily sensations, or to the external environment, such as sights and sounds. Thus, mindfulness includes being aware, being nonjudgmental, and accepting present experience. "Acceptance," furthermore, has been defined as being open to experience, or willing to experience the reality of the present moment (Roemer & Orsillo, 2002). This definition is similar to the definition of "mindfulness" as nonjudgmental awareness, and includes actively or purposefully allowing experiences (thoughts, emotions, desires, urges, sensations, etc.) to occur, without attempting to block or suppress them. Similarly, Hayes and Wilson (2003) emphasize that acceptance focuses on increased "contact" with previously avoided private events, again focusing on the essential role of awareness of experience. Clearly, mindfulness and acceptance are overlapping constructs in CBT.

Many of the interventions associated with CBT focus on change of either the situation or of the client's reactions to situations. Many of the CBT approaches emphasize the development of problem lists and the use of change to solve these problems over the course of treatment. Acceptance becomes relevant in the CBT treatment context when highly desired change is difficult, impossible, or at least not imminent. Because change is highly desired, the first step of acceptance, which involves not putting energy into change, is not necessarily an easy or obvious alternative, and the client likely will resist giving up on desired outcomes (acceptance). Because neither change nor acceptance are occurring, the client may be considered stuck in a situation of "nonacceptance/nonchange." Either actual change or acceptance of the reality that change will not occur in the imminent future provides avenues for the client to get "unstuck" and move on, with diminished suffering. Acceptance and mindfulness interventions provide an alternative way to reduce suffering, and to help clients let go of their "stuck" situations when change is not immediately available.

Mindfulness and acceptance may be considered to be adaptive responses or skills that replace maladaptive behaviors. In these situations, mindfulness activities and skills are operants that are negatively reinforced by decreased suffering. Or mindfulness and acceptance-oriented activities may be considered stimulus control strategies: Rather than change the situation itself, when change is either undesirable or impossible, the stimulus properties of the situation are changed significantly, allowing a new meaning of the situation to be created, and new cognitive, emotional, and overt responses, to emerge. In both of these ways mindfulness can function to augment exposure (habituation, extinction), or be considered an exposure strategy (a subtype of stimulus control). To the extent that mindfulness also, at times, involves reappraisal (e.g., "The situation is what it is" rather than "The situation is awful"), these strategies may also be considered a part of the set of cognitive restructuring strategies or skills.

Mindfulness has its roots in both Eastern religious traditions and some Western spiritual, philosophical, and psychological practices. Kabat-Zinn (2003) reviewed mindfulness as it relates to its spiritual foundation, and noted that mindfulness was developed and articulated within a Buddhist tradition over a 2,500-year period. It is often called the "heart" of Buddhist meditation. Within this tradition, mindfulness has never been a "stand-alone" practice, but rather is nested within a larger framework oriented toward nonharm. Teasdale, Segal, and Williams (2003) state that mindfulness has always been only one of a number of components of a much wider path.

Some Western contemplative practices also employ elements of mindfulness, and existential philosophy and psychology developed in Europe in the 20th century included essential elements of mindful practice. For example, Binswanger (1963) described "Being-In-the-World" as having three elements: (1) being in the natural or physical world (*umwelt*); (2) being in the relational world (the "with world," or *mitwelt*); and (3) being in the world with oneself ("I world," or *eigenwelt*). In each case the emphasis is on mindful engagement in the world, in the moment, with full awareness and participation.

The incorporation of mindfulness into CBT in recent years has often had an Eastern influence, albeit independent of its religious origins (Baer, 2003). The secularization of mindfulness was pragmatic, in the effort to make the treatment accessible to as many individuals as possible (Dimidjian & Linehan, 2003). The goal of mindfulness training in CBT is not to teach Buddhism; mindfulness intervention must be free of cultural, religious, and ideological factors (Kabat-Zinn, 2003). Yet Dimidjian and Linehan (2003) suggest that it is possible that something is lost when mindfulness is separated from its roots. To maintain the integrity of mindfulness interventions, they suggest that Western researchers maintain dialogue with spiritual teachers of mindfulness to prevent the "reinvention of the wheel" and to guide researchers in their efforts to "identify the core qualities of therapist competence" (p. 167). Indeed, several of the prominent CBT approaches that incorporate mindfulness and acceptance have accentuated the spiritual origins of mindfulness.

There are challenges inherent in the incorporation of a historically spiritual or religious practice into a scientific practice, even after modification. Hayes and Wilson (2003) suggest that because mindfulness and acceptance have spiritual and religious origins, they start out as "prescientific." However, as integrated parts of treatment, they must be specified and evaluated, and thereby become incorporated into the realm of science.

One consequence of mindfulness and acceptance in psychotherapy beginning as "prescientific" is a lack of consistency within the field, which includes the multiple definitions and conceptualizations that are present today. Dimidjian and Linehan (2003) suggest that the lack of a clear and consistently employed operational definition has contributed to ambiguity in the field and hindered research. Bishop et al. (2004) also noted that it is not possible to investigate the mechanisms of action of mindfulness without an operational definition. Indeed, mindfulness is at times considered a technique or strategy, and at other times a collection of techniques or strategies, a psychological process or mechanism of change that leads to specified outcomes, and the desired outcome of intervention. For example, Bishop and colleagues (2004) considered mindfulness as a mode of awareness, which emphasizes that mindfulness is a psychological process. However, they acknowledge that other related constructs, such as insight and self-awareness, likely reflect the outcome of practicing mindfulness. Teasdale et al. (2003) noted that mindfulness was "never seen as an end in itself, but as one part of a comprehensive, multifaceted path to resolve a clearly formulated problem" (p. 158). Given the ways that mindfulness is defined and applied, each of these approaches may be quite sensible in context.

In response to the ambiguity concerning the definition and conceptualization of mindfulness, Bishop and colleagues (2004) proposed a consensus, two-component, operational definition. Their definition characterizes mindfulness "as a process of regulating attention in order to bring a quality of nonelaborative awareness to current experience and a quality of relating to one's experience within an orientation of curiosity, experiential openness, and acceptance" (p. 234). Thus, this definition emphasizes both an attentional control component of mindfulness and an awareness with nonreactivity, or acceptance, component. It is similar to the definition offered by Brown and Ryan (2003), which also emphasizes purposeful attention control and broad awareness of reality in the present moment. Adoption of a consistent operational definition will facilitate the study of mindfulness.

However, even if a consistent or consensual operational definition of mindfulness can be formulated, it is not clear whether, or how, mindfulness relates to the prevention or remediation alleviation of psychopathology. Hayes and Wilson (2003) suggest a strong test for mechanisms of change: It is not enough for a procedure to be useful when appropriately applied; eventually, the procedure must enter into a scientific account of psychopathology and its remediation. In other words, is an increase in mindfulness and acceptance a legitimate mechanism of change? Roemer and Orsillo (2003) maintain that mindfulness is multifaceted, and that any or all of the elements of mindfulness may contribute to its clinical effectiveness. Similarly, Baer (2003) provides a comprehensive summary of the proposed mechanisms of change associated with mindfulness, including exposure, cognitive change, self-management, relaxation, and acceptance. These putative mechanisms of change are next reviewed briefly.

Baer (2003) suggested that a mindful stance facilitates exposure and response prevention to internal emotional and psychological states. Similarly, Linehan (1993a) suggested that mindfulness practice may be helpful for individuals who are afraid of their own emotions. She stated, "In its entirety, mindfulness is an instance of exposure to naturally arising thoughts, feelings, and sensations" (p. 354), and that through the process of *observing* that these sensations come and go, fear of emotions can be reduced. This process is dialectical: *Acceptance leads to change* in situations of prior "nonacceptance" (escape, avoidance, severe reactivity, etc.), and as exposure operates arousal is reduced, and this *change leads to further acceptance*. Acceptance in many situations *is* change and may alleviate suffering (Fruzzetti & Fruzzetti, 2008). Baer (2003) suggested that the beneficial effects of mindfulness-based stress reduction (MBSR; Kabat-Zinn, 1982) may be due to exposure. Specifically, the exposure to pain in the absence of catastrophic consequences may lead to desensitization, a reduction in the suffering and distress associated with chronic pain, and an increase in functionality and quality of life.

Within traditional cognitive therapy, the primary focus is often on the identification and modification of the content of irrational thoughts. However, in a mindfulness approach, observing the thought as a thought, or observing that a certain stimulus elicits the thought, or observing the emotion associated with either the stimulus or the thought (or both), all help a person to reduce his or her emotional reactivity to the situation and the thought (Fruzzetti, Crook, Erikson, Lee, & Worrall, 2008). In addition, the practice of mindfulness may lead to changes in *attitudes* about one's thoughts (Baer, 2003). Roemer and Orsillo (2003) summarize this difference: "Cognitive therapy typically focuses on changing the *content* of cognitions. On the other hand, mindfulness approaches focus on changing one's *relationship* to one's thoughts and feelings, encouraging the viewing of thoughts as thoughts rather than as reality" (p. 173). Similarly, Segal, Teasdale, and Williams (2004) suggest that mindfulness-based cognitive therapy (MBCT) may effectively prevent depressive relapse due to the "decentering" effects of mindfulness, as occurs when patients see their thoughts and feelings as passing events and not as valid reflections of reality. This concept is similar in acceptance and commitment therapy (ACT; Hayes, Strosahl, & Wilson, 1999), in which an important therapeutic component is to "deliteralize" thoughts. It is also similar to the "observing" and "describing" mindfulness skill in dialectical behavior therapy (DBT; Linehan, 1993b), in which a person discriminates between the "facts" of a thought (i.e., that the person is thinking it, that thinking it is associated with certain emotional reactions and/or action urges) and the literality of the content of the thought, which may be present or not.

Although mindfulness may be used in the service of relaxation or mood management, mindfulness approaches are not these techniques per se (Bishop et al., 2004; Fruzzetti et al., 2008). In fact, the evidence suggests that mindfulness practice may lead to improvements in many areas, including pain, stress, anxiety, depressive relapse, and disordered eating (Baer, 2003). Given these impressive results, mindfulness as a technique might be applied to varied clinical problems. Teasdale et al. (2003) caution against the use of mindfulness as a generic technique applied across a range of disorders, though, stating that attempts to apply mindfulness training indiscriminately "as if it were simple, general purpose technology" (p. 157) is unlikely to yield positive results. Rather, mindfulness is most useful with practitioners "who have adequately formulated views of the disorders that they seek to treat and ways that mindfulness training can be helpful to clients with those disorders" (p. 157). From a scientific standpoint, the relevance of mindfulness to a particular problem must be fully formulated.

Furthermore, Teasdale et al. (2003) suggest that mindfulness and acceptance may be legitimate mechanisms of change, along with more traditional CBT strategies, such as exposure, cognitive modification, self-management, and relaxation. They stated that the impact of mindfulness training can be enhanced if the relative emphasis given to different components reflects the relative importance of the psychopathological process they target. Thus, researchers and clinicians need to have a clear conceptualization of how mindfulness and acceptance are related to their conceptualization of psychopathology and its remediation.

HISTORY AND CLINICAL ROOTS OF MINDFULNESS AND ACCEPTANCE INTERVENTIONS IN COGNITIVE-BEHAVIORAL THERAPY

Hayes (2004) maintained that behavior therapy has experienced two "generations" and is now progressing into the third generation of behavior therapy, or the "third wave." The first generation rejected the dominant clinical theories and practices, and in particular psychoanalytic theories. It adopted first-order, direct change strategies that had an emphasis on overt behaviors as both treatment targets and outcomes. Subsequently, the first generation was transformed with the addition of cognitive intervention methods in the second generation, or "cognitive revolution." This revolution allowed for first-order change of cognitive content and the alleviation of suffering through a combination of cognitive and behavior change strategies. The third generation of behavior therapy has abandoned an emphasis on first-order change, and has adopted mindfulness and acceptance as "radical additions" that "challenge the universal applicability of first-order change strategies" (Hayes, 2004, p. 5). In other words, behavior change may be accomplished by addressing targets other than the problematic behavior itself. This approach includes changing the function of behavior as a treatment target.

There is disagreement within CBT about whether the "third wave" is truly a difference in epistemology that includes models for behavior, behavior change, and clinical interventions, or merely the result of a slow and assimilative process that can integrate acceptance and mindfulness strategies with traditional change strategies. For example, Hofmann and Asmundson (2008) have suggested that acceptance strategies are response-focused emotion-regulation strategies, whereas traditional CBT strategies are more antecedent-focused, but both share common ultimate change goals, such as the regulation of emotion and improvement in quality of life. They further note that key developers of acceptance-oriented treatments, such as Marsha Linehan and Adrian Wells, consider their treatments to reside entirely within CBT rather than being part of a distinct "third wave."

Whether the developments associated with mindfulness and acceptance are profound enough to be considered a third wave, or are the result of long and sustained integration and evolution, important shifts in both epistemology and clinical emphasis are now recognizable. The roots of mindfulness and acceptance in scientific psychology and in CBT are long-standing, even if they did not become mainstream until recently. For example, the Melbourne Academic Mindfulness Group (2006) stated that interest in meditative practices in the scientific community began in the 1970s, with work such as Wallace and Benson's classic paper "The Physiology of Meditation" (1972). Wallace and Benson coined the phrase "wakeful hypometabolic state" to describe subjects who practiced transcendental meditation (Wright, 2006). Wright describes transcendental meditation as a simple mantra meditation. In contrast, virtually all of the mindfulness applications in CBT use focused awareness rather than a mantra. Marlatt et al. (2004) describe various meditation practices as one method to practice and develop mindfulness. Meditation can be a spiritual practice, or more of a psychological or behavioral practice, and therefore a form of "global desensitization" in which meditative practice acts as a form of counterconditioning to pathological processes (Marlatt et al., 2004).

DIFFERENT MINDFULNESS AND ACCEPTANCE STRATEGIES

Despite the adoption of mindfulness and acceptance practices into humanistic therapy after World War II, it took longer for the Eastern Buddhist and Western existential influences (e.g., Binswanger, 1956; 1963) of acceptance and mindfulness to have much impact on CBT (Dryden & Still, 2006). Moreover, in part because they developed from different sources, the ways that mindfulness and acceptance strategies and concepts were integrated into different forms of CBT varied extensively. We now explore different facets of mindfulness and acceptance by explicating their role in cognitive and behavioral therapies that have integrated fully various mindfulness and acceptance strategies with traditional change strategies.

Rational Emotive Behavior Therapy

Albert Ellis was influential in the introduction of acceptance into Western psychotherapy through his work in rational emotive therapy, and later rational emotive behavior therapy (REBT; Ellis, 1961, 1962). Although REBT does not use formal mindfulness or meditation practice, it does attend to thinking in a manner that is similar to more formal mindfulness approaches given its emphasis on observing but not literalizing thoughts, and on the rational acceptance of reality (Ellis, 2006). REBT maintains that irrational thinking causes distress for individuals (Ellis, 2006), and that emotional and behavioral dysfunction is largely correlated with rigid and inflexible insistencies rather than flexible preferences (Ellis, 2005).

Ellis (2006) stated that REBT seeks to help clients "(1) become aware of and (2) to *change* thinking, feeling, and behavioral distortions" (pp. 66–67). Although the focus on changing thought content is more consistent with traditional CBT than other acceptance-based approaches, REBT also places significant focus on acceptance. Ellis states, "REBT especially teaches its clients, among other things, non-judging, patience, non-compulsive striving, and acceptance, and has been doing so since the 1950s" (p. 68). Specifically, REBT promotes unconditional self-acceptance, other-acceptance, and life-acceptance, within a context of commitment to change in goal-directed and valued directions (Ellis, 2006). Ellis stated, "You fully accept your self *whether or not* you succeed at important tasks and *whether or not* your are approved by significant people ... you fully accept (although not necessarily *like*) all other humans ... *whether or not* they act fairly and competently ... you fully accept life *whether or not* it is fortunate or unfortunate" (2005, p. 158). Thus, although REBT maintains a focus on changing the content of thought, its emphasis on acceptance is clear and similar to more recent "third-wave" approaches.

However, acceptance in REBT often has a rational emphasis to promote acceptance and nonreactivity. For example, through statements like "Life is not fair" and "So what if life is not fair?", REBT fosters acceptance of reality, in part through exposure to cognitive stimuli that had elicited strong negative reactions, as noted earlier. Ellis (2006) suggested that mindfulness-based interventions, particularly MBSR, are "remarkably close to REBT theory and practice in many ways, because although the techniques of these two systems seem to be far apart, the *philosophies* that they teach through their methods have much in common" (p. 78).

Mindfulness-Based Stress Reduction

Jon Kabat-Zinn has been called "the most influential teacher of mindfulness meditation in America" (Ellis, 2006, p. 63), and his influence can be seen in a variety of mindfulness-based treatments (cf. Ellis, 2006; Teasdale, Segal, & Williams, 1995). The Melbourne Academic Mindfulness Group (2006) noted that the work of Kabat-Zinn "has brought attention to the clinical and psychotherapeutic applications of mindfulness" (p. 286). Mindfulness-based stress reduction (MBSR; Kabat-Zinn, 1982) was developed within a behavioral medicine setting for patients who deal with chronic pain and stress-related disorders, and has substantial empirical support (cf. Baer, 2003). The purposes in developing MBSR were twofold: (1) to establish effective training of medical patients in relatively intensive mindfulness meditation and its immediate application to stress, pain, and illness; and (2) to serve as a model for other hospitals and medical centers (Kabat-Zinn, 2003). This program was originally designed to serve as a referral site to which physicians sent patients who had not responded to traditional treatment, and was intended as a complement to medical treatment (Kabat-Zinn, 2003). Training in mindfulness was intended to allow patients "a degree of responsibility for their own well-being and [to] participate more fully in their own unique movement toward greater levels of health by cultivating and refining our innate capacity for paying attention and a for a deep, penetrative seeing/sensing of the interconnectedness of apparent separate aspects of experience" (Kabat-Zinn, 2003, p. 149).

Mindfulness is not about "getting anywhere" or "fixing anything" in MBSR, which is consistent with a Buddhist approach (cf. Nhat Hanh, 2007). Rather, it is "an invitation to allow oneself to be where one already is and to know the inner and outer landscape of the direct experience of the moment" (Kabat-Zinn, 2003, p. 148). This invitation can create a paradox, as clients often come to treatment with specific treatment goals. Kabat-Zinn states that the teacher must reconcile the client's goals with a mindful stance of nonstriving and nondoing. As this is not a simple task, MBSR emphasizes that teachers must have a foundation of personal practice.

MBSR is based on traditional meditation practices, including motionless sitting. This practice includes maintaining a position even if painful sensations arise. Participants learn to notice these sensations and observe them nonjudgmentally. The focus is on acceptance of the experience, tolerance, redirection of attention, and the ability to focus on other things despite the pain, rather than not being able to engage in these activities because of the pain. The ability to notice pain, without judgments and without trying to escape it, may reduce both cognitive and emotional reactivity (and other secondary responses) associated with pain, and thus reduces distress associated with pain. Thus, the person's "relationship" with pain is changed, and in this respect MBSR may function partially due to the effects of exposure (Baer, 2003).

Relapse Prevention

Relapse prevention was developed in the 1980s by Alan Marlatt and colleagues (Marlatt & Gordon, 1985; Marlatt & Donovan, 2005) as a cognitive-behavioral treatment to prevent substance abuse relapse. The program is based on a cognitive-behavioral model of addiction (cf. Witkiewitz, Marlatt, & Walker, 2005), and includes a focus on the precipitants of substance use, including situational, social, affective, and cognitive precipitants and cues. The model of relapse is based on a linear progression of response in high-risk situations (Witkiewitz et al., 2005). Effective coping is believed to increase self-efficacy, which in turn results in a reduced response to cues and a consequent decrease in substance use. Substance use or relapse follows the perceived effects of a substance and the attributions a person makes that may increase or decrease subsequent misuse and relapse. For example, if a person views the substance use as a learning opportunity, he or she is less likely to use again.

However, the "abstinence violation effect" states that if an individual views the substance use an uncontrollable or as a failure, he or she is more likely to use again. Therefore, the critical predictor of relapse within the relapse prevention model is the use of effective coping strategies to deal with high-risk situations (Marlatt & Donovan, 2005; Witkiewitz et al., 2005).

Relapse prevention combines behavioral skills training with cognitive interventions, including acceptance strategies (Marlatt & Donovan, 2005). Mindfulness is included as a key skill to cope with urges to use substance. For example, clients are taught to "urge-surf" by imagining their urges as waves that grow and then gradually subside. Marlatt (1994) noted that mindfulness involves acceptance of the constantly changing experiences of the present moment. In contrast, addiction may be understood as an inability to accept the present moment, so that the person instead persistently seeks escape and avoidance of reality in the next "high." The experience of craving can be addressed successfully by helping clients either to restructure or to accept maladaptive cravings. In addition, self-monitoring techniques lead to increased self-awareness or increased awareness of the present moment. If people become more aware of their cravings, and the cues for their cravings, then they will have more opportunities to respond (accept or change) in an effective manner, and therefore reduce the likelihood of relapse.

Marlatt (2002) proposed coping with substance use urges specifically based on the Buddhist concept of "skillful means," yet explained it in behavioral terms as negative reinforcement: "Giving into the urge when it peaks only serves to further reinforce the addictive behavior. Not acting on the urge, on the other hand, weakens the addictive conditioning and strengthens acceptance and self-efficacy" (p. 47). Marlatt et al. (2004, p. 269) expanded on the rationale for using mindfulness meditation in the treatment of addiction:

> Craving responses that are common in addiction create a complex system composed of environmental cues and rigid cognitive responding (subjective experience of craving), increased outcome expectancies for the desired effects of the substance (positive reinforcement) and/or increased motivation for engaging in the addictive behavior to provide a reduction in negative affect or withdrawal symptoms (negative reinforcement). Mindfulness meditation may disrupt this system by providing heightened awareness and acceptance of the initial craving response, without judging, analyzing, or reacting. By interrupting this system, meditation may act as a form of counterconditioning, in which a state of meta-cognitive awareness and relaxation replaces the positive and negative reinforcement previously associated with engaging in the addictive behavior. In this sense, mindfulness may serve as a "positive addiction" (Glasser, 1976). Therefore, mindfulness is more than a coping strategy for dealing with urges and temptations; it could also be a gratifying replacement or substitute for addictive behavior.

Witkiewitz et al. (2005) have proposed that mindfulness-based relapse prevention (MBRP) may be a "new" cognitive-behavioral intervention for substance use disorders, and they provide early data to complement existing data from earlier acceptance-oriented relapse prevention approaches. The goals of

MBRP are to develop awareness and acceptance of thoughts, feelings, and sensations through mindfulness, and to utilize these coping skills in the face of high-risk situations. Clients form an association between being mindful and the application of relapse prevention skills. Mindfulness provides clients with a new way to process situational cues and monitor their own reaction to environmental contingencies (cf. Baer, 2003), which provides another reason to consider that mindfulness may be, in large measure, a stimulus control strategy. In traditional CBT, stimulus control most often involves control of access to a stimulus, and sometimes reconditioning a stimulus. With mindfulness, the properties of the stimulus are not reconditioned; the relationship between the stimulus and prior learned responses is altered by the use of mindfulness practices. Specifically, in the presence of substance use cues, mindfulness leads to a broadening of awareness to include context, goals, and other cues rather than a narrowing of awareness to include only the cues for substance use.

Dialectical Behavior Therapy

DBT was developed in the 1970s as a treatment for suicidality, self-harm, and borderline personality disorder (BPD; Linehan, 1993a, 1993b). Robins, Schmidt, and Linehan (2004) described this treatment as an application of standard behavior therapy for individuals with multiple suicide attempts. The aim of treatment is to create a life worth living. Over time, it became apparent that a focus on either change or acceptance would not work: "From either therapeutic stance, an exclusive focus on change or on acceptance, clients experienced their therapist as invalidating not only specific behaviors but also the client as a whole" (Robins et al., 2004, p. 31). More recently, DBT has been applied successfully to a variety of related problems, including depression, substance abuse, eating disorders, and couple and family problems (Feigenbaum, 2007; Robins & Chapman, 2004).

DBT is founded on a dialectical worldview, in which apparent opposites (thesis and antithesis) are tolerated and eventually forged into a new synthesis, in a continuous process of change and evolution (Fruzzetti & Fruzzetti, 2008). The primary dialectic in DBT is between acceptance and change: To facilitate change, a client must be aware of, and able to tolerate, the pain associated with the problem, at least temporarily (Fruzzetti et al., 2008). In contrast, the inability to accept problems, experiences, situations, and so forth, prohibits change.

Acceptance is considered both an outcome and an activity in DBT (Robins et al., 2004), and a core treatment strategy. Acceptance can be likened to radical truth: "Acceptance is experiencing something without the haze of what one wants and does not want it to be" (p. 39). Thus, acceptance is critical in work with impulsive, sensitive, and reactive clients, and includes focusing on the current moment, seeing reality as it is without "delusions," and accepting reality without judgment.

DBT is based on a biosocial theory or transactional model, which holds that BPD is primarily a dysfunction of the emotion regulation system (Fruzzetti, Shenk, & Hoffman, 2005; Linehan, 1993a). Emotion dysregulation results from high emotional vulnerability, which is characterized by high sensitivity to emotional stimuli, emotional intensity, and slow return to baseline, as well as invalidating social and family responses. DBT teaches clients skills they can use to modulate emotional reactions, solve problems, and tolerate suffering, then generalize further to increase nonjudgmental awareness, improve relationships, and engage in important activities (with or without emotional pain).

Mindfulness is the core skill in DBT (Linehan, 1993b), and it lays the foundation for emotion regulation, distress tolerance, and interpersonal effectiveness skills. Thus, mindfulness is conceptualized as a set of psychological skills, which includes intentional processes, used in a nonjudgmental manner in the moment, and with effectiveness. Specifically, "what" a person does when being mindful (observe, describe, or participate) is practiced, as opposed to nonmindful alternatives, such as dissociation, distraction, or being reactive. Similarly, "how" a person practices is important, because practice is ideally nonjudgmental, with one thing at a time, and with a focus on what works or is effective to achieve long-term goals (Linehan, 1993b).

Mindfulness is not just taught as a skill to the client in DBT, but it is strengthened and generalized, both in therapy sessions and in daily life, and is used by the client, the therapist, and the treatment team. Problem solving involves helping clients to replace nonmindful, reactive, judgmental, and other problematic behaviors with more mindful ones. Because self-judgments lead to shame, and judgments of others promote anger (and excesses of both shame and anger are common in people with BPD), helping clients become more aware, more descriptive, and less judgmental is an example of how pervasively mindfulness is employed in DBT.

Mindfulness may work as a form of exposure and/or to increase self-management in DBT. However, mindfulness is used to create a context conducive to learning other skills and developing more adaptive patterns. For example, exposure to emotions may demonstrate to clients that even painful emotions are temporary and not catastrophic per se, which may help clients to learn skills to modulate those emotions, or problem-solving skills to improve situations, so that they elicit fewer painful negative emotions. Furthermore, awareness and acceptance of important longer-term goals, combined with the ability to tolerate and not react to short-term discomfort, can lead to change. Thus, mindfulness and practice in DBT synthesize acceptance and change, and promote the creation of, and full engagement in, a higher quality of life.

Acceptance and Commitment Therapy

Acceptance and commitment therapy (ACT; Hayes et al., 1999) emerged from behavior analysis and has contextual behavioral roots (Hayes, 2004). "Contextualism" conceptualizes psychological events as sets of ongoing interactions between organisms and their historically and situationally defined contexts. Like traditional behavior therapy, contextualism is concerned primarily with the function of behavior: In ACT "there is a conscious posture of openness and acceptance toward psychological events, even if they are formally 'negative,' irrational,' or 'psychotic.' What determines whether an event will be targeted for change is not form but function" (Hayes, 2004, p. 9).

ACT is also based on a theory of language and cognition called relational frame theory (RFT), which is concerned with the derivation and relationships of language, and provides a "contextually focused explanation for why normal verbal/cognitive processes undermine 'attention to the present moment' and 'an attitude of acceptance'" (Hayes & Shenk, 2004, p. 251). RFT holds that it is the process of language and its dominance over direct experience that promote much of human suffering (Hayes & Wilson, 2003), for example, the idea that the importance and legitimacy of avoiding psychological pain is built into the normal function of human language, and that this process of avoidance can cause harm (Hayes & Shenk, 2004). Specifically, ACT proposes that many forms of psychopathology can be thought of as forms of experiential avoidance, "the phenomenon that occurs when a person is unwilling to remain in contact with particular private experiences (e.g., bodily sensations, emotions, thoughts, memories, behavior predisposition) and takes steps to alter the form or frequency of these events and the contexts that occasion them, event when doing so causes life harm" (Hayes & Wilson, 2003, p. 162). In addition, because literal, evaluative language strategies (called "cognitive fusion" in ACT) dominate human behavior, inflexibility in some domains develops, which in turn prevents people from engagement in more effective behaviors.

A primary goal of ACT is to create psychological flexibility, which is accomplished through acceptance and mindfulness skills, and commitment and behavior change skills (similar to the acceptance and change dialectic in DBT). Acceptance is distinguished from tolerance, and means "to take what is offered," or the "active nonjudgmental embracing of experience in the here and now. Acceptance involves undefended 'exposure' to thoughts, feelings, and bodily sensations as they are directly experienced to be" (Hayes, 2004, p. 21). Mindful awareness of thoughts as thoughts is fundamental, as in other acceptance and mindfulness approaches in CBT. Mindfulness facilitates the deliberate and nonjudgmental/nonevaluative engagement of the person with his or her experience, in the present moment, and thus plays a key role in ACT.

By increasing mindfulness and acceptance-oriented repertoires, individuals come into contact with previously avoided private events and experiences. An evolved ability to be in the here and now in turn reduces the literal and evaluative functions of language (Hayes & Wilson, 2003). However, according to ACT, the important process/outcome is not the reduction of the literal and evaluative functions of language per se, but the resulting increase in the range and flexibility of responses (see Hayes, Luoma, Bond, Masuda, & Lillis, 2006). The focus on the present moment may facilitate adaptive, flexible responding as opposed to more rigid, rule-governed behavior, which is often neither based in current circumstances nor particularly adaptive (Hayes et al., 1999). In addition, meditation temporarily puts the literal, temporal, and evaluative functions of language on extinction, and creates a context in which a much broader range of stimulus events can enter awareness and become relevant (Hayes & Shenk, 2004).

Mindfulness-Based Cognitive Therapy

MBCT was developed by Teasdale, Segal, and Williams (1995) as an integration of CBT and acceptance-based approaches. MBCT was developed to reduce the risk of relapse after successful completion of CBT for depression (Segal, Williams, & Teasdale, 2001). Treatment components are delivered sequentially, and the intervention includes components of traditional CBT, as well as DBT, MBSR, and ACT. MBCT focuses on changing awareness of, and relationships to, thoughts, feelings, and bodily sensations. This process includes many of the "decentering" approaches found in CBT (Segal et al., 2001, 2004). Growing evidence suggests that MBCT is successful (e.g., Teasdale et al., 2003).

According to Segal and colleagues (2001), depressive relapse is due to the reactivation of negative, self-critical, hopeless thinking that is characteristic of major depression. The reactivation of these patterns is elicited by dysphoria, and people maintain and intensify dysphoria through cycles of ruminative cognitive processing. Therefore, a central focus of relapse prevention is to prevent these ruminative patterns during periods of vulnerability to relapse. In this model, it is "a whole, integrated, configuration of information processing, or 'mode of mind' that gets 'wheeled in' in states of dysphoria in depression-prone individuals. This mode represents both negative cognitive *content* and a maladaptive cognitive *process* (ruminative thought patterns)" (Teasdale, 1997, p. 50, as cited in Segal et al., 2004). Furthermore, depressed individuals may think about negative aspects of the self or situation to resolve the problem, but this thinking likely will perpetuate a depressive state. Mindfulness training diminishes these ruminative processes. Because ruminative thinking requires attentional resources, "it follows that the intentional deployment of conscious awareness, which is a defining characteristic of mindfulness, will require limited attentional resources and reduce their availability for the processing configurations that might otherwise support the relapse process" (Segal et al., 2004, p. 52).

Ruminative thinking may also be described as a "doing" mode, with a goal of reducing the depressive state. Alternatively, mindfulness may establish a different cognitive mode, described as a "being" mode (Segal et al., 2004). Mindfulness allows individuals to switch out of goal-based processing and into an alternative mode of processing that is not inherently goal based (Teasdale et al., 2003). Finally, mindfulness is introduced as a way to counter emotional and experiential avoidance. People may divert their attention away from early signs of relapse because these sensations cause distress (both because they include "negative" emotions and may be associated with more severe depressive states). Unfortunately, avoidance prevents individuals from taking effective early action that may allay the exacerbation of depression. Mindfulness training provides a repertoire to reduce avoidance and to increase awareness of early depressive cues, and therefore increases the chance that individuals can respond effectively to prevent relapse.

Integrative Behavioral Couple Therapy

Integrative behavioral couple therapy (IBCT; Jacobson & Christensen, 1996) was developed as an alternative to traditional behavioral couple therapy (TBCT). Whereas TBCT focuses on purposeful change of behaviors that contribute to relationships distress, IBCT helps partners accept aspects of their partners that were previously considered unacceptable. IBCT emphasizes mindfulness and acceptance within the context of the relationship (Christensen, Sevier, Simpson, & Gattis, 2004). Evidence suggests improvements beyond those achieved by TBCT (Jacobson, Christensen, Prince, Cordova, & Eldridge, 2000; Christensen, Atkins, et al., 2004). TBCT conceptualizes relationship problems in terms of specific behaviors. In contrast, IBCT focuses on a broader unit of analysis (Christensen, Sevier, et al., 2004). For example, instead of a focus on a specific behavior exchange, such as doing things to please the partner, IBCT may focus on a broader response class (i.e., enhancing closeness). IBCT also differs from TBCT in its treatment goals. While TBCT focuses on the primary goal of behavior change, IBCT emphasizes acceptance. Acceptance targets in IBCT include each partner's emotional reactions to the other, the conditions that elicit them, and the impact they have (Christensen, Sevier, et al., 2004). Emotional reactions are discussed in a nonjudgmental, empathic way to help people become more mindful of their own and the partners' reactions, to become mindful of each other, and consequently to develop less negative reactivity within the relationship. This process may also help to change partners' cognitive interpretations of each other's actions (Christensen, Sevier, et al., 2004). Acceptance within the context of a relationship requires acceptance of one's own emotional responses to one's partner (Fruzzetti, 2006). Thus, in some ways, acceptance of undesired partner behaviors in a couple therapy context provides a special case of acceptance, so all of the other mindfulness and acceptance strategies used in CBT can also be employed in a couple context. Understandably, dangerous and destructive behaviors, such as physical violence and substance abuse, should not be the focus of acceptance interventions.

Other Acceptance and Mindfulness Approaches in Cognitive-Behavioral Therapy

The prevalence of the use of mindfulness and acceptance in CBT is far greater than that of the treatments described earlier, and other applications with empirical support also exist. For example, mindfulness and acceptance have been integrated with CBT for the treatment of eating disorders (Wilson, 2004), as well as anxiety disorders (Borkovec & Sharpless, 2004; Orsillo, Roemer,

Block Lerner, & Tull, 2004; Roemer & Orsillo, 2002), trauma (Follette, Palm, & Rasmussen Hall, 2004), and couple and family problems (Carson, Carson, Gil, & Baucom, 2004; Fruzzetti & Iverson, 2004; Hoffman, Fruzzetti, & Buteau, 2007). Although each application is novel, the interventions employed are similar to those already described. Thus, this review is not comprehensive in terms of all applications of mindfulness and acceptance, but it provides an introduction to the use of these concepts and strategies within CBT. We now turn our attention to elaboration of several clinical strategies and applications of mindfulness and acceptance in CBT.

CLINICAL APPLICATIONS
OF MINDFULNESS AND ACCEPTANCE

A variety of specific protocols employ mindfulness and acceptance strategies across several different subtypes of CBT, and they have many common themes. We describe the core intervention strategies in mindfulness and acceptance. Although some strategies or practices are more specific or more common in some treatments than in others, they are all interrelated, and all are variants of core mindfulness and acceptance practices of nonjudgmental awareness, attention control, and/or allowing the experience of present reality.

Mindfulness as a Skill

Linehan specified the components of mindfulness as a psychological practice, and how to teach these components as skills (Linehan, 1993b). Based on the mindfulness work of Thich Nhat Hanh (1975), the mindfulness skills in DBT include many of the components utilized by a variety of CBT approaches. Linehan has broken these skills into two parts. The first set of mindfulness skills involves *what* activity a person is doing while being mindful, and includes observing, describing, and participating. The idea is that the person can do one of these at any time: observe, describe, or participate in an activity. The second set involves *how* the person engages in those activities, and includes engaging in activities (cognitively, emotionally, or overtly) in a nonjudgmental manner, doing one thing at a time in the present moment, and choosing activities that in fact effectively achieve a life worth living (Linehan, 1993b). The idea is that the person would do all of these simultaneously.

Observing

Observing provides the foundation for awareness. Observing, or simply noticing, is the act of becoming aware, and includes self-conscious awareness. There are many choices in terms of what to observe or notice; thus, this particular skill is far more sophisticated than may be immediately apparent. For example, in a conversation, being mindful involves noticing or observing what the other person is saying, other dimensions of his or her communication, the context for the conversation, how what the other person is saying or doing affects one (thoughts, desires, emotions, urges), and so on. In addition, nascent awareness often leads to other behaviors that may be more or less mindful. For example, awareness that the other person wants something that one does not want to provide may elicit awareness of anxiety or fear, or judgments about the other person. Another facet of observing is that it involves attention control. It requires open attention to notice something, especially if its stimulus properties do not elicit strong reactions. Attention is related to awareness, but it includes the ability to focus to become aware of a stimulus.

Describing

Describing is the process of applying nonjudgmental words to events, objects, and situations. There are no good or bad sweaters or cars or people in a mindful world. There are sweaters, cars, and people that we like or do not like, sweaters that are red or have holes, or fit snugly or are uncomfortable, and cars that need repair or are broken, or have better or worse fuel efficiency, and so on. In part because describing takes the judgment out of the equation, it may contribute to nonreactivity, which is another core component of mindfulness and acceptance. Describing also has an attention control component: Without focused attention, descriptions would be very limited or include only superficial descriptive properties.

Participating

It is possible to be mindful, without narrowly focused awareness and a lot of language and cognitive activity, but instead with a kind of deep awareness that is absent in a lot of thinking. For example, most people have had the experience of "losing themselves" in an activity, such as singing, playing a sport, dancing, playing an instrument, or hiking. In these cases there is deep, noncognitive attention and awareness. In sports, people may say that a player is "unconscious" to capture the idea that his or her performance was not affected by self-conscious awareness or evaluation. The person simply *is* the activity for a while. Thus, participation involves full engagement in the activity, without competing, self-conscious activities such as thinking, problem solving, or even self-awareness.

Nonjudgmental Stance

Making judgments is such a common activity that many clients have difficulty at first identifying them as such. For example, it is common for widely held judgments to be considered facts, such as when certain pieces of art are widely accepted as beautiful or ugly (which is a judgment). From a mindful perspective, we might instead say that we enjoy viewing the art or find it aesthetically pleasing. Then the descriptive properties of the art are understood to reside in the artwork (certain textures, colors, forms, patterns, etc.), and the reactions to the art (beautiful, ugly, etc.) are correctly seen to reside in the viewer.

Of clinical relevance is how clients react toward themselves and others. But the process is the same: From a mindfulness perspective, a person's behavior is neither good nor bad. Rather, the person does things that can be described, and the way we react to those behaviors can also be described. Thus, one person might do something that another person does not like, or that even may be against his or her values (e.g., be mean to a spouse, cheat at a game, or intentionally try to get something desired at the expense of another). Of course, we can also notice and describe our own behaviors, and our reactions to them. This nonjudgmental perspective fosters an awareness of the nature of reality, because reality can be described objectively, but judgments are not "real" in the same way, because they are subjective. As clients become aware that they engage in judgmental thinking, they begin to develop an alternative repertoire. Describing is a key antidote to judgmental thinking that clients can use once they become aware that they are indeed judging themselves or others.

One-Mindful Engagement

Doing one thing at a time may be decreasingly valued in a multitasking culture. However, the capacity for doing one thing mindfully, in the present moment, may be essential to engage a variety of other activities skillfully, such as problem solving, building relationships, driving a car safely, or learning any new task or skill. This aspect of mindfulness is primarily concerned with attention control, although awareness follows from one-mindful engagement as well.

Being Effective

In some ways, being effective is implied in other mindfulness skills. However, the explicit inclusion of effectiveness as a criterion for mindfulness helps to rule out behaviors that may be dangerous or counterproductive, but in which a client engages with full attention and awareness, and without judgment. For example, self-harm and aggression and violence toward others are activities in which clients engage that might be considered mindful if not for the fact that these activities are virtually always problematic.

The previously discussed set of skills can be learned in ways that are common in CBT. These methods include an acquisition phase, which involves instruction in the basics of the skills, the rationale for their use, and initial practice guided by instructions. Then, with continued practice and feedback, the skills may be strengthened. Finally, mindfulness is generalized when clients use any of these skills to replace a more dysfunctional behavior in their lives and doing so leads to improved outcomes (Linehan, 1993b). The idea is to practice mindfulness so as to be more mindful in daily life. Paradoxically, the more one "practices" in daily life, the less one is practicing *per se*, and the more one is simply mindfully engaged in his or her life. Practicing is a part of living mindfully, and living mindfully is robust practice.

Reducing Emotional Reactivity to Thoughts: Observing Thoughts as Thoughts

One of clients' key problems in the development of mindfulness is that certain thoughts elicit strong negative emotional reactions. Judgments (e.g., "I am a bad person") can be associated with not only strong negative emotional reactivity but also other kinds of thoughts, such as appraisals (e.g., "I did not do well in the interview"), and even some descriptive thinking (e.g., "My spouse wants a divorce") may be associated with specific emotional reactions. Although not all of these reactions are problematic, and some emotional reactions are useful and adaptive, when consistently strong and painful negative reactions become overlearned, there may be value in disentangling the emotional reactions from their antecedent thoughts.

One way to begin to disentangle and reduce these problematic emotional reactions is to observe the thought as a thought; that is, the thought is a product of a brain, with a given biology, a certain history and in a specific situation. The content of the thought may reflect objective reality (e.g., "I can't find my car in the parking lot") or may not (e.g., "I'm such an idiot ... I can't even find my car" or "Someone must have stolen my car while I was in the mall!"). The observation that the thought is simply a thought, however, can lead to awareness of the circumstances or context in which that kind of thought is likely to be produced. For example, noticing and tolerating frustration may help a person to recognize that he or she is frantically looking for the car but not mindfully doing so, and that frantic behavior is counterproductive. Subsequently, the person may become more aware of the present circumstances, retrace his or her steps, or recall the level on which the car is parked.

The central idea in being mindful is to change the overall reaction to thinking, to slow down and discontinue dysfunctional cognitive–emotional action patterns. Different therapies use different practices to help clients learn this process. For example, DBT clients are given instructions in specific practices, such as to observe thinking. Irreverence may be used to augment this type of practice; the therapist might tell the client to think an obviously false or ridiculously silly thought, to demonstrate that the client can have thoughts that do not reflect objective reality, for example, "I am the star of the Olympic basketball team" or "I don't care at all whether my friends respect me." In ACT, a variety of metaphors are employed to help "deliteralize" thoughts, and in a variety of CBT approaches basic exposure may be employed. For example, repetition of a disturbing thought, until it becomes untangled from its cognitive–emotional action pattern, is a common strategy in obsessive thinking.

Observing Emotional Experiences and Their Context

One of the components of many forms of psychological distress is the suffering associated with secondary emotional reactions (Fruzzetti et al., 2008). In essence, "primary" emotions are the more universal, natural, unlearned, and authentic reactions to given situations, and they are unencumbered by interpretations or judgments (Greenberg & Safran, 1989). For example, in situations of loss, the primary emotions are sadness, disappointment, and/or grief. When faced with uncertain and possibly undesirable outcomes, such as situations that may be dangerous to ourselves, our loved ones, or important aspects of our lives, we feel anxiety or fear. When we have acted inconsistently with our values, or have the urge to do so, we feel guilty or ashamed. However, we can sometimes learn to react to our primary emotions, or have reactions to reactions, and these "secondary" emotions become the main response to given situations. For example, instead of feeling sad or hurt when put down by someone we care about, we might instead feel ashamed or angry, which is actually a secondary response to the primary emotional reaction of being hurt. Primary emotional responses tend to be more adaptive and healthy than secondary emotions, because secondary responses are often less authentic emotional reactions. The expression of secondary emotions may also be confusing to others, because the natural connection between the situation or stimulus and the emotional response is not always obvious.

From a mindfulness perspective, judgments and lack of awareness in the present are the main causes of secondary emotional reactions. Judgments about ourselves typically lead to shame, whereas judgments about others typically lead to anger. Similarly, not wanting or being able to tolerate a situation and its accompanying primary emotion may lead to escape conditioning, or secondary emotional reactions. In contrast, simply being aware of a situation allows the person to react naturally with authentic and primary emotion. These reactions are typically more understandable to others and may facilitate more soothing, supportive, and validating responses (Fruzzetti et al., 2008). Thus, the person accepts both the reality of the situation and his or her primary emotional response, and it is easier for others similarly to be more accepting.

A shift toward primary emotional responses and away from secondary ones can be facilitated by mindfulness practice. For example, noting negative emotions or judgmental thinking can become the cue to stop and reorient one's attention back to the situation, and to use observing and describing skills to become aware of primary emotional responses. In this way, nascent secondary emotions can become signals to stop "participating" in those responses and instead to divert attention back to the situation, thus allowing more authentic emotions to occur in response to awareness of the situation. Perception and acceptance of primary emotions thus contrast with avoidance or escape situations and emotions, which in extreme cases can involve dysfunctional behaviors such as substance use, self-harm, withdrawal, and/ or aggression.

Allowing: Accepting and Tolerating Distressing Experiences

When faced with intense suffering or pain, most people desire change. Mindfulness can facilitate change in a variety of ways, including early awareness of pain, awareness of the links between certain situations or behaviors and the likelihood of painful outcomes, and awareness of empathy toward others. However, pain and suffering cannot always be alleviated, and certainly may not be alleviated quickly in many situations. When change is not immediately available through healthy and adaptive means, some people act impulsively and attempt to achieve short-term reductions in suffering without regard for the long-term consequences. Substance use, suicide, compulsive behaviors, bingeing or purging, and a variety of other severe clinical problems have a common theme of avoidance of painful emotions through escape behaviors. Individuals may even maintain that they will stop the dysfunctional behavior once the pain goes away, but these escape behaviors paradoxically contribute significantly to the pain, so that the alternative rarely becomes available. Instead, more dysfunctional escape follows, which leads to increased pain and diminished life satisfaction.

The ability to allow one's experience to be what it is, to have it unfold naturally and neither avoid nor escape present reality are the critical features of mindfulness and the cornerstones to reduce impulsive and destructive behaviors. This process involves (1) tolerating painful experience at least temporarily and sometimes over the long term (see Linehan, 1993b, on "distress tolerance"); (2) mindful awareness of long-term goals, and a purposeful shift of attention from the immediate relief associated with avoidance and escape to the satisfaction and joy associated with a life that is consistent with goals and values; and (3) the ability to recontextualize the meaning of the suffering; rather than to say "I can't stand this" or "This is awful," to acknowledge that the situation involves necessary pain, to tolerate or even to welcome that pain as integral to living in an authentic, valued, and satisfying way.

Genuine and mindful awareness of the stimulus, even while tolerating its learned secondary emotional responses, is the hallmark of desensitization, exposure, and response prevention strategies. The ability to respond to situations without escape or numbing allows the person to choose activities meaningfully to build a satisfying life and to discontinue other activities. Mindful awareness of a situation can also facilitate awareness of "positive," enjoyable, or satisfying emotional reactions that can be useful whether the situation has "negative" stimulus properties from prior learning or is a novel situation. Thus, mindfulness and allowing whatever responses may occur rather than avoidance, impulsive action, or escape, are also core components of successful behavioral activation (Fruzzetti et al., 2008).

Acceptance and Validation of Self and Others

Other people are key "stimuli" in our daily lives, and we can learn to respond to others as a way to avoid or to preclude certain potential emotional reactions. However, mindfulness in relationships simply applies all of the prior mindfulness and acceptance strategies to the special case in which another person's activities are the essence of the situation or stimulus (Fruzzetti &

Iverson, 2004). Thus, being aware of the other leads to a deep understanding and forms the basis for acceptance of him or her. This process requires awareness and self-acceptance, especially of whatever primary emotions one experiences. A person's articulation of this understanding and acceptance of others validates and helps to soothe and support them, which in turn helps them become more descriptive, and helps them validate that person as well (Fruzzetti, 2006). This process is key in all close relationships and may be similarly beneficial in developing an effective therapeutic relationship.

Radical Acceptance

Acceptance is relatively easy when it is pleasant. "Radical acceptance" is the ability to welcome into our experience those things in life that are hard, unpleasant, or even apparently impossibly painful. If it were not difficult, it would not be "radical." The idea is that all of the mindfulness and acceptance strategies already noted can be brought to bear in situations of intense suffering, or in the face of highly undesirable circumstances. Rather than focus on the undesirable or painful aspects of the situation, however, one embraces the experience as part of life, even if a less desirable or painful part. Thus, reality is truly fully embraced, even welcomed, without judgment or escape, delusion or rationalization, and without rigid attachment to nonreality or wishful thinking, and attempts to change reality in the present moment. The saying "Things are as they should be" recognizes that reality is inevitable, that whatever happens *should* happen. This is not a moral or hortatory "should," but rather a reflection of the recognition that reality sits in the present moment. The current moment is a necessary part of an ongoing process, and if something happens, it must and it should happen, because everything that happened before it actually happened. Radical acceptance is associated with less lamentation of the past and effort to escape the reality of the present, and therefore may lead to more success at meaningful living in the present, and a more valued and satisfying future.

Therapist Mindfulness and Acceptance

Although these various mindfulness and acceptance strategies have been oriented toward clients, therapists need to engage in some form of mindfulness and acceptance practice to develop these skills, in order to effectively help clients. Different therapies approach therapist mindfulness quite differently. For example, practicing daily mindfulness meditation is expected of therapists in MBCT and MBSR, but not in most of the other therapies described. In general, it makes sense that the prescribed practice of the therapist reflect the kind of practice the therapy also prescribed for clients, as therapists must demonstrate and teach the same practices. Mindfulness and acceptance are experiential practices, and therefore require experiential practice of the therapist. Intellectual understanding is likely not sufficient.

CONCLUSIONS

Mindfulness and acceptance interventions in CBT have become mainstream after following a long developmental course over the past 30 to 40 years. Although they differ in form, the many and various approaches to mindfulness and acceptance practices in CBT share the same foundations and overlap in functional practice. Virtually all CBT applications of mindfulness and acceptance employ acceptance of reality, nonjudgmental awareness, being in the present, allowance for experiences to occur and unfold naturally, and an ability to focus the attention on what works and is effective. The data suggest that mindfulness and acceptance interventions have salutary effects on both treatment outcomes and relapse prevention, although much work remains to understand the mechanisms of change and their optimal utilization in CBT. However, after decades on the periphery, acceptance and mindfulness are now part of the empirical traditions of CBT. We should expect that research in the coming years will help us to understand the psychological roles of mindfulness and acceptance in well-being, and how best to employ them as part of effective CBT interventions.

REFERENCES

Baer, R. (2003). Mindfulness training as a clinical intervention: A conceptual and empirical review. *Clinical Psychology: Science and Practice, 10,* 125–143.

Binswanger, L. (1956). Existential analysis and psychotherapy. In E. Fromm-Reichmann & J. L. Moreno (Eds.), *Progress in psychotherapy* (pp. 144–168). New York: Grune & Stratton.

Binswanger, L. (1963). *Being-in-the-world: Selected papers of Ludwig Binswanger* (J. Needleman, Trans.). New York: Basic Books.

Bishop, S., Lau, M., Shapiro, S., Carlson, L., Anderson, N., Carmody, J., et al. (2004). Mindfulness: A proposed operational definition. *Clinical Psychology: Science and Practice, 11,* 230–241.

Borkovec, T. D., & Sharpless, B. (2004). Generalized anxiety disorder: Bringing cognitive-behavioral therapy into the valued present. In S. C. Hayes, V. M. Follette, & M. M. Linehan (Eds.), *Mindfulness and acceptance: Expanding the cognitive-behavioral tradition* (pp. 209–242). New York: Guilford Press.

Brown, K. W., & Ryan, R. M. (2003). The benefits of being present: Mindfulness and its role in psychological well-being. *Psychological Science, 14,* 822–848.

Carson, J. W., Carson, K. M., Gil, K. M., & Baucom, D. H. (2004). Mindfulness-based relationship enhancement. *Behavior Therapy, 35,* 471–494.

Christensen, A., Atkins, D. C., Berns, S., Wheeler, J., Baucom, D. H., & Simpson, L. E. (2004). Traditional versus integrative behavioral couple therapy for significantly and chronically distressed married couples. *Journal of Consulting and Clinical Psychology, 72,* 176–191.

Christensen, A., Sevier, M., Simpson, L., & Gattis, K. (2004). Acceptance, mindfulness, and change in couple therapy. In S. C. Hayes, V. M. Follette, & M. M. Linehan (Eds.), *Mindfulness and acceptance: Expanding the cognitive-behavioral tradition* (pp. 288–309). New York: Guilford Press.

Dimidjian, S., & Linehan, M. (2003). Defining an agenda for future research on the clinical application of mindfulness practice. *Clinical Psychology: Science and Practice, 10,* 166–171.

Dryden, W., & Still, A. (2006). Historical aspect of mindfulness and self-acceptance in psychotherapy. *Journal of Rational-Emotive and Cognitive-Behavior Therapy, 24,* 3–28.

Ellis, A. (2006). Rational emotive behavior therapy and the mindfulness based stress reduction training of Jon Kabat-Zinn. *Journal of Rational-Emotive and Cognitive-Behavior Therapy, 24,* 63–78.

Ellis, A. (2005). Can rational-emotive behavior therapy (REBT) and acceptance and commitment therapy (ACT) resolve their differences and be integrated? *Journal of Rational-Emotive and Cognitive-Behavior Therapy, 23,* 153–168.

Ellis, A. (1961). *A guide to rational living.* Englewood Cliffs, NJ: Prentice-Hall.

Ellis, A. (1962). *Reason and emotion in psychotherapy.* Secaucus, NJ: Citadel.

Feigenbaum, J. (2007). Dialectical behaviour therapy: An increasing evidence base. *Journal of Mental Health, 16,* 51–68.

Follette, V. M., Palm, K. M., & Rasmussen Hall, M. L. (2004). Acceptance, mindfulness, and trauma. In S. C. Hayes, V. M. Follette, & M. M. Linehan (Eds.), *Mindfulness and acceptance: Expanding the cognitive-behavioral tradition* (pp. 192–208). New York: Guilford Press.

Fruzzetti, A. E. (2006). *The high conflict couple: A dialectical behavior therapy guide to finding peace, intimacy, and validation.* Oakland, CA: New Harbinger Press.

Fruzzetti, A. E., Crook, W., Erikson, K., Lee, J., & Worrall, J. M. (2008). Emotion regulation. In W. T. O'Donohue & J. E. Fisher (Eds.), *Cognitive behavior therapy: Applying empirically supported techniques in your practice* (2nd ed.). New York: Wiley.

Fruzzetti, A. R., & Fruzzetti, A. E. (2008). Dialectics. In W. T. O'Donohue & J. E. Fisher (Eds.), *Cognitive behavior therapy: Applying empirically supported techniques in your practice* (2nd ed.). New York: Wiley.

Fruzzetti, A. E., & Iverson, K. M. (2004). Mindfulness, acceptance, validation and "individual" psychopathology in couples. In S. C. Hayes, V. M. Follette, & M. M. Linehan (Eds.), *Mindfulness and acceptance: Expanding the cognitive-behavioral tradition* (pp. 168–191). New York: Guilford Press.

Fruzzetti, A. E., Shenk, C., & Hoffman, P. D. (2005). Family interaction and the development of borderline personality disorder: A transactional model. *Development and Psychopathology, 17,* 1007–1030.

Greenberg, L. S., & Safran, J. D. (1989). Emotion in psychotherapy. *American Psychologist, 44,* 19–29.

Hayes, S. (2004). Acceptance and commitment therapy and the new behavior therapies: Mindfulness, acceptance, and relationship. In S. C. Hayes, V. M. Follette, & M. M. Linehan (Eds.), *Mindfulness and acceptance: Expanding the cognitive-behavioral tradition* (pp. 1–29). New York: Guilford Press.

Hayes, S. C., Luoma, J. B., Bond, F. W., Masuda, A., & Lillis, J. (2006). Acceptance and commitment therapy: Model, processes and outcomes. *Behaviour Research and Therapy, 44,* 1–25.

Hayes, S. C., & Shenk, C. (2004). Operationalizing mindfulness without unnecessary attachments. *Clinical Psychology: Science and Practice, 11,* 249–254.

Hayes, S. C., Strosahl, K. D., & Wilson, K. G. (1999). *Acceptance and commitment therapy: An experiential approach to behavior change.* New York: Guilford Press.

Hayes, S. C., & Wilson, K. (2003). Mindfulness: Method and process. *Clinical Psychology: Science and Practice, 10,* 161–165.

Hoffman, P. D., Fruzzetti, A. E., & Buteau, E. (2007). Understanding and engaging families: An education, skills and support program for relatives impacted by borderline personality dsorder. *Journal of Mental Health, 16,* 69–82.

Hoffman, S., & Asmundson, G. (2008). Acceptance and mindfulness-based therapy: New wave or old hat? *Clinical Psychology Review, 28,* 1–16.

Jacobson, N., & Christensen, A. (1996). *Acceptance and change in couple therapy: A therapist's guide to transforming relationships.* New York: Norton.

Jacobson, N. S., Christensen, A., Prince, S. E., Cordova, J., & Eldridge, K. (2000). Integrative behavioral couple therapy: An acceptance-based, promising new treatment for couple discord. *Journal of Consulting and Clinical Psychology, 68,* 351–355.

Kabat-Zinn, J. (1982). An outpatient program in behavioral medicine for chronic pain patients based on the practice of mindfulness meditation: Theoretical considerations and preliminary results. *General Hospital Psychiatry, 4,* 33–47.

Kabat-Zinn, J. (2003). Mindfulness-based interventions in context: Past, present and future. *Clinical Psychology: Science and Practice, 10,* 144–156.

Linehan, M. M. (1993a). *Cognitive-behavioral treatment of borderline personality disorder.* New York: Guilford Press.

Linehan, M. M. (1993b). *Skills training manual for treating borderline personality disorder.* New York: Guilford Press.

Marlatt, G. A. (1994). Addiction, mindfulness, and acceptance. In S. C. Hayes, N. S. Jacobson, V. M. Follette, & M. J. Dougher (Eds.), *Acceptance and change: Content and context in psychotherapy* (pp. 175–197). Reno, NV: Context Press.

Marlatt, G. A. (2002). Buddhist psychology and the treatment of addictive behavior. *Cognitive and Behavioral Practice, 9,* 44–49.

Marlatt. G. A., & Donovan, D. M. (2005). *Relapse prevention: Maintenance strategies e treatment of addictive behaviors* (2nd ed.). New York: Guilford Press.

Marlatt, G. A., & Gordon, J. R. (1985). *Relapse prevention: Maintenance strategies in the treatment of addictive behaviors.* New York: Guilford Press.

Marlatt, G. A., & Kristeller, J. (1999). Mindfulness and meditation. In W. R. Miller (Ed.), *Integrating spirituality into treatment* (pp. 67–84). Washington, DC: American Psychological Association.

Marlatt, G. A., Witkiewitz, K., Dillworth, T. M., Bowen, S. W., Parks, G. A., Macpherson, L. M., et al. (2004). Vipassana meditation as a treatment for alcohol and drug use disorders. In S. C. Hayes, V. M. Follette, & M. M. Linehan (Eds.), *Mindfulness and acceptance: Expanding the cognitive-behavioral tradition* (pp. 261–287). New York: Guilford Press.

Melbourne Academic Mindfulness Group. (2006). Mindfulness-based psychotherapies: A review of conceptual foundations, empirical evidence and practical considerations. *Australian and New Zealand Journal of Psychiatry, 40,* 285–294.

Nhat Hanh, T. (1975). *The miracle of mindfulness: A manual on meditation.* Boston: Beacon Press.

Nhat Hanh, T. (2007). *Nothing to do, nowhere to go: Waking up to who you are.* Berkeley, CA: Parallax Press.

Orsillo, S. M., Roemer, L., Block Lerner, J. B., & Tull, M. T. (2004). Acceptance, mindfulness, and cognitive-behavioral therapy: Comparisons, contrasts, and application to anxiety. In S. C. Hayes, V. M. Follette, & M. M. Linehan (Eds.), *Mindfulness and acceptance: Expanding the cognitive-behavioral tradition* (pp. 66–95). New York: Guilford Press.

Robins, C. J., & Chapman, A. L. (2004). Dialectical behavior therapy: Current status, recent developments, and future directions. *Journal of Personality Disorders, 18,* 73–89.

Robins, C. J., Schmidt, H., & Linehan, M. M. (2004). Dialectical behavior therapy: Synthesizing radical acceptance with skillful means. In S. C. Hayes, V. M. Follette, & M. M. Linehan (Eds.), *Mindfulness and acceptance: Expanding the cognitive-behavioral tradition* (pp. 30–44). New York: Guilford Press.

Roemer, L., & Orsillo, S. (2002). Expanding our conceptualization of and treatment for generalized anxiety disorder: Integrating mindfulness/acceptance-based approaches with existing cognitive-behavioral models. *Clinical Psychology: Science and Practice, 9,* 54–68.

Roemer, L., & Orsillo, S. (2003). Mindfulness: A promising intervention strategy in need of further study. *Clinical Psychology: Science and Practice, 10,* 172–178.

Segal, Z. V., Teasdale, J. D., & Williams, J. M. G. (2004). Mindfulness-based cognitive therapy: Theoretical rationale and empirical status. In S. C. Hayes, V. M. Follette, & M. M. Linehan (Eds.), *Mindfulness and acceptance: Expanding the cognitive-behavioral tradition* (pp. 45–65). New York: Guilford Press.

Segal, Z. V., Williams, J. M. G., & Teasdale, J. D. (2001). Mindfulness-based cognitive therapy for depression: A new approach to preventing relapse. New York: Guilford Press.

Teasdale, J. D. (1997). The relationship between cognition and emotion: The mind inplace in mood disorders. In D. M. Clark & G. C. Fairburn (Eds.), *Science and practice of cognitive behaviour therapy* (pp. 67–93). Oxford, UK: Oxford University Press.

Teasdale, J. D., Segal, Z. V., & Williams, J. M. G. (1995). How does cognitive therapy prevent depressive relapse and why should attentional control (mindfulness) training help? *Behaviour Research and Therapy, 33,* 25–39.

Teasdale, J. D., Segal, Z. V., & Williams, J. M. G. (2003). Mindfulness training and problem formulation. *Clinical Psychology: Science and Practice, 10,* 157–160.

Wallace, R., & Benson, H. (1972). The physiology of meditation. *Scientific American, 226,* 84–90.

Wilson, G. T. (2004). Acceptance and change in the treatment of eating disorders: The evolution of manual-based cognitive-behavioral therapy. In S. C. Hayes, V. M. Follette, & M. M. Linehan (Eds.), *Mindfulness and acceptance: Expanding the cognitive-behavioral tradition* (pp. 243–260). New York: Guilford Press.

Witkiewitz, K., Marlatt, G., & Walker, D. (2005). Mindfulness-based relapse prevention for alcohol and substance use disorders. *Journal of Cognitive Psychotherapy: An International Quarterly, 19,* 211–228.

Wright, L. (2006). Meditation: A new role for an old friend. *American Journal of Hospice and Palliative Medicine, 23,* 323–327.

PART IV

APPLICATIONS TO
SPECIFIC POPULATIONS

CHAPTER 12

Cognitive-Behavioral Therapy with Youth

Sarah A. Crawley
Jennifer L. Podell
Rinad S. Beidas
Lauren Braswell
Philip C. Kendall

Cognitive-behavioral therapies (CBTs) with children and adolescents use enactive, performance-based procedures, as well as cognitive interventions to produce changes in thinking, feeling, and behavior. Various forms of CBT have a common goal to help the child develop a constructive worldview and a problem-solving attitude. The problem-solving orientation can also be referred to as a "coping template." Through the provision of carefully planned experiences, CBT helps the child and family build an adaptive, problem-solving perspective.

CBT with children and adolescents continues to experience expansion and refinement. A number of edited volumes, meta-analyses, treatment manuals, and research studies have informed readers of the potentially beneficial gains associated with CBT for youth (e.g., Hibbs & Jensen, 2005; Kendall, 2006; Weisz, McCarty, & Valeri, 2006; Kendall & Hedtke, 2006a, 2006b; Pediatric OCD [Obsessive–Compulsive Disorder] Treatment Study Team, 2004). The outcome literature on CBT with youth has breadth and depth, and continues to be developed (e.g., Kendall, Choudhury, Hudson, & Webb, 2002). Yet despite this excellent growth, questions remain. There is a need for carefully executed outcome studies with children if the field is to develop a more truly evidence-based approach to practice. In the sections that follow, the differences between working with youth and with adults are considered.

The major components in CBT with children are then described, and applications of CBT to specific childhood disorders are discussed. The chapter concludes with a consideration of CBT for special populations, current issues within CBT research, and questions for future research.

DEVELOPMENTALLY INFORMED DIFFERENTIATIONS IN TREATMENT

There are differences that must be taken into consideration when treating children and adolescents compared to adults. Treatment must be implemented in a developmentally appropriate fashion to be effective. Factors that are particularly relevant to how one conducts CBT with youth include (1) recognition of how young clients come to treatment, (2) use of age-appropriate modes of delivery, (3) sensitivity to the client's cognitive and affective development, (4) awareness of the social context in which the youth is embedded, and (5) clarity about the therapist's role and expectations for therapy.

Entry into Therapy

The referral source has important clinical implications, because seeking help for oneself is very different than being sent for services by someone else. Other individuals, such as parents or teachers, typically initiate psychological services for children and adolescents. Children and adolescents are not known for their eagerness or even willingness to sit and talk about problems with an adult. Quite the contrary may be true: Children and adolescents may be impulsive, limited in their self-reflection, or nondisclosing in conversations with adults. It is essential that efforts be made to create a pleasant affective environment, so that children and adolescents may come to enjoy the experience and want to be in treatment.

Value of Age-Appropriate Modes of Delivery

One way to implement psychological treatments that include verbal exchanges, learning, working collaborations, and sharing of emotional experiences with youth involves the use of play-related activities in treatment. As stated by Kendall, Chu, Gifford, Hayes, and Nauta (1998), the effective therapist can both teach in a playful manner and play in a way that teaches. Being able to make skillful use of age-appropriate play activities accomplishes three important objectives: (1) It fosters a positive therapeutic relationship; (2) it can create a window for more direct observation of the child's operating expectations and beliefs; and (3) these activities can be vehicles to introduce and develop more adaptive behavior and more constructive thinking about issues that are troubling to the child. Pragmatically, this work can be done by incorporating games and fun activities into the treatment, such as role plays, charades, various art activities, and selected board games. With young children, the use of puppets or dolls can be a useful precursor to more direct dramatic role plays of targeted situations.

Attention to Level of Cognitive, Emotional, and Social Development

In addition to making developmentally sensitive choices in the use of play methods, consideration must also be given to the youth's cognitive and affective development, including memory and attention capacities, verbal fluency and comprehension, and the capacity for conceptual reasoning. Cognitive strategies that may be appropriate for adult clients may not be fully understood and managed by young clients, and it is essential that material be presented to the child in a developmentally appropriate fashion. For example, although a child may not have the cognitive maturity to distinguish between rational and irrational thoughts, he or she may be able to understand that certain events are more or less likely to happen. Children can be coached to collect evidence for the possibility that the event they are thinking about will actually happen. Through this exercise they may be able to determine the likelihood of the event occurring and conceptually come to understand the difference between rational and irrational thoughts.

A central issue concerning cognitive processing is the differentiation between cognitive deficiency and cognitive distortion in processing. Processing "deficiencies" refer to the absence of thinking (i.e., lacking careful information processing where it would be beneficial), whereas "distortion" refers to dysfunctional thinking. Youth with externalizing problems show deficiencies in processing, whereas those with internalizing problems tend to have more maladaptive, distorted processing. This distinction can help the clinician to target the specific nature of the dysfunction or work to identify the distortion. It is also important to recognize the role of processes, such as expectations, attributions, self-statements, beliefs, and schemas, in the development of emotional and behavioral patterns. Effective programs for children and adolescents intentionally plan and capitalize on creating behavioral experiences with intense positive emotional involvement, while paying attention to the anticipatory and after-the-fact cognitive activities of the participants. The therapist guides the child's attributions about prior behavior and emotions, and his or her expectations for future behavior and emotions, which allows the child to acquire a cognitive structure for future events.

Awareness of psychosocial development is important, because children and adolescents face different issues. Academic matters become important and stressful for adolescents, and dating and interpersonal relations take on increasing importance. These themes must be laced into treatment to address the teen's growing need for autonomy from parents. Treatment programs must be designed accordingly.

Therapist's Role and Expectations

The cognitive-behavioral therapist who works with children fulfills multiple roles, including diagnostician, consultant, and educator, often to both child and parent (Kendall, 2000). As diagnostician, the therapist integrates data about a particular client from a variety of sources and combines this information with knowledge of normal child developmental processes and psychopathology to create a problem formulation. As a consultant, the therapist shares the problem formulation and the knowledge of the costs and expected benefits of different treatment options with the family to prioritize treatment goals and make choices about treatment strategies. Depending on the treatment options selected, the therapist then provides education about the child's disorder and training in the needed skills areas to the child and/or parents. In general, the cognitive-behavioral therapist can be likened to a "coach" for the child and/or the family (Kendall, 2000). The coaching analogy helps the child understand that the therapist may be intensively involved with him or her for a given period of time and except in more unusual cases, is unlikely to be part of the family's support system for years to come.

In addition to managing the child's expectations regarding the therapist's role, therapists who work with youth must take special care in their own treatment expectations. Reasonable therapist expectations include the belief that interventions will help the child move toward successful adjustment, and that the child who acquires skills in therapy will at some time experience the benefit of those skills. It is not reasonable to expect that any child, with any problem, can be "fixed" using CBT or other psychotherapies. It is reasonable for the therapist to hold that therapy does not "cure" maladaptation, but it helps with the management of psychopathology. Child clients also do not always display their newly acquired skills right away. Sometimes, children act as if they were right all along, and do not want the therapist to know they have learned from their therapeutic interactions, or benefited from therapy. It is important for therapists to recognize that this behavior may be developmentally appropriate.

Recognition of the Social Context of Treatment

All clients function in a social context, but since children and adolescents are not capable of full independence, it is critical to consider the child's contextual influences. The recognition of the role of parents and other powerful people in the child's life, and the inclusion of these individuals in some aspect of the intervention process, is often crucial for the successful treatment of a young client. Parents can serve as "consultants" when they provide information about the child's behaviors, "collaborators" when they assist in the implementation of program requirements, and because parents often contribute to or maintain some aspect of the child's problem, they can be involved as "coclients" in the treatment itself (Kendall, 2000).

The nature and benefits of including parents in the treatment of youth with behavioral and emotional problems vary across child problems and with development. Parents of youth with conduct disorders often monitor their children's activities a lot, whereas parents of anxious youth are less vigilant in overseeing their children. Improvements in children's adjustment and symptoms may increase when parents are included in sessions, or when parents are intentionally separated from their children (Barmish & Kendall, 2005). Younger children may benefit more when parents are included as part of the treatment from the beginning, whereas an adolescent may benefit more when the parent is not included in treatment sessions. Further research is needed to inform the ideal involvement of parents and to examine the different parent roles relative to factors such as the child's age and principal disorder.

COMMON TREATMENT COMPONENTS

CBT varies according to the age of the child and the presenting problem, but several strategies are common in this approach to treatment (Kendall, 1993). In this next section, we discuss problem solving, cognitive restructuring, self-regulation, affective education, relaxation training, modeling/role playing, and behavioral contingencies. Following these discussions, we consider the applications of the strategies to specific childhood disorders.

Problem Solving

Problem solving, a key component of CBT, is common across different types of childhood disorders. Problem-solving training has a rich history of applications with both children and adults. During the 1970s, there were dramatic increases in attempts to formulate problem solving as a set of relevant skills for clinical endeavors (e.g., D'Zurilla & Goldfried, 1971; Mahoney, 1977; D'Zurilla & Nezu, 1999). Spivack, Platt, and Shure (1976) hypothesized that effective interpersonal, cognitive problem solving demands a number of sub-skills, such as sensitivity to human problems, the ability to generate alternative solutions, the capacity to conceptualize, the means to achieve a given solution, and sensitivity to consequences and cause–effect relationships in human behavior (Shure & Spivack, 1978; Spivack et al., 1976).

Teaching them how to solve problems allows children to gain confidence in their ability to resolve daily struggles that once may have seemed hopeless. For example (see Figure 12.1), with an anxious child, the first step in problem solving is to examine a non-anxiety-provoking situation, such as not being able to find one's shoes in the morning before school. The child works with the therapist to come up with a number of solutions (e.g., go to school barefoot, walk on one's hands to school, not go to school, wear slippers); then the child can evaluate each option before picking one. Once the child is able to implement problem-solving skills in a non-anxiety-provoking situation, he or she

Now list some of the possible things you could do. Ask yourself: "What can I do to make this situation less fearful?"

1. _____

2. _____

3. _____

Next you need to choose the best ideas for you. Focus on each possibility. Ask yourself:

"What might happen if I choose the first idea?" _____

_____

_____

"How would I feel?" _____

_____

_____

Now we'll go through the same process with your second and third possibilities. Ask yourself:

_____

_____

_____

"What might happen if I chose the second idea?" _____

_____

_____

"How would I feel?" _____

_____

_____

Ask yourself: "What might happen if I chose the third solution?" _____

_____

_____

"How would I feel?" _____

_____

_____

Now you have thought about each possibility.

Which one do you think might be the best one for you?

_____

FIGURE 12.1. Problem-Solving Worksheet. From Kendall and Hedtke (2006b). Copyright 2006 by Workbook Publishing. Reprinted by permission.

can practice problem solving for a feared situation (e.g., public speaking for a socially phobic youth).

Problem-solving training approaches have attained positive outcomes when used as a component in the treatment of difficulties experienced by children and adolescents, including anxiety (Kleiner, Marshall, & Spevack, 1987). Problem solving with a child who displays aggression might focus on the determination of appropriate ways to communicate anger and to acquire desired objects from others in a prosocial way (Lochman, Powell, Whidby, & Fitzgerald, 2006). With depressed children, problem-solving training might be used to help the youth take action to change distressing situations that lead to unpleasant affect (Stark et al., 2006).

In addition to differences in the kinds of problems experienced by children who manifest different disorders, different disorders are associated with certain difficulties with the problem-solving process. For example, children who are prone to aggression or acting-out difficulties may need training and support in the problem formulation phase due to their tendency to misperceive the intentions of others and overperceive hostility in their social environment (Dodge, 1985). They may also need help to slow themselves down during the alternative generation phase, so they can generate nonaggressive alternatives to address the problem situation. Children who are depressed may need special encouragement to use problem solving, because negative thinking may interfere with the application of problem-solving skills (e.g., "Why do this, since nothing is going to change anyway?"). Problem-solving training is conceptualized as a flexible vehicle that can be easily adapted to the needs of individual clients and their families.

Cognitive Restructuring

Research suggests that children who display emotional and behavioral concerns engage in various forms of negative cognition about the self (Crick & Dodge, 1994; Kendall, Stark, & Adam, 1990; Rabian, Peterson, Richters, & Jensen, 1993). Cognitive-based therapies aim to ameliorate these negative cognitions by identifying and testing maladaptive thoughts. Cognitive restructuring methods (e.g., Beck, Rush, Shaw, & Emery, 1979; Ellis & Harper, 1975) were developed to address these negative cognitive representations in adults, including expectations, beliefs, and self-statements. When using these techniques, therapists first help the client become aware of self-statements, expectancies, or beliefs that reflect unhelpful ways of thinking about the self, the world, and/or the future, then guide the client to consider the connection between these negative thoughts and the client's emotional experience. Finally, therapist and client collaborate in various ways to identify, create, and test more adaptive ways of thinking.

When working with children or adolescents, the basic elements of cognitive restructuring are similar to those used with adult clients, but with careful consideration of the developmental level of the child. Harter (1982) noted that children younger than 5 or 6 years of age are usually not interested or capable of reflection upon, or metacognition about, their thoughts and/or thinking processes. Over the elementary school years, this capacity for self-reflection develops as children examine thoughts about issues that are highly salient and current in their lives. It is probably not until adolescence that clients can fully examine thoughts as examples of broader schemas that have developed over time and as a result of specific experiences.

When conducting cognitive restructuring with children, therapists often introduce the notion of examining one's thinking by having the child fill in "thought bubbles" over the heads of cartoon characters facing various scenarios (e.g., filling in the thought for a cartoon child who has just spilled a lunch tray; see Kendall & Hedtke, 2006a, 2006b; see Figure 12.2). When the child understands that thoughts accompany actions and feeling states, the therapist may then ask the child to keep a simple diary of a particular kind of thought, such as a self put-down or other type of negative self-statement relevant to the child's presenting concerns. The therapist then guides the child to consider the connection between these negative thoughts and unpleasant emotions, perhaps having the child conduct mood ratings in connection with his or her thought monitoring. Through guided questioning, and designing and conducting behavioral experiments, the clinician then introduces the possibility that one could choose to think differently about the matter at hand, and

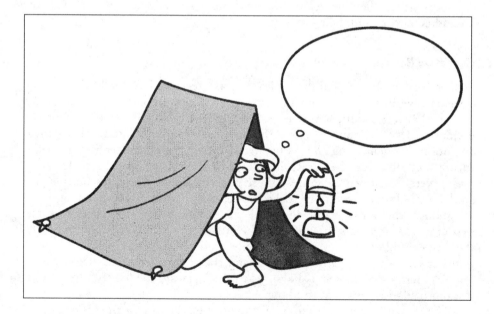

FIGURE 12.2. Example of a thought bubble. From Kendall and Hedtke (2006b). Copyright 2006 by Workbook Publishing. Reprinted by permission.

that thinking differently could lead to feeling differently. This process helps children pull themselves out of negative thoughts, or the "negative muck" (Stark et al., 2006).

In addition to uniquely child-focused examples of cognitive restructuring, efforts more like those associated with Beck's cognitive therapy for depression have also been employed with children and adolescents (Dudley, 1997; Stark, 1990; Wilkes, Belsher, Rush, & Frank, 1994). The therapist elicits negative self-statements in various ways, and the child and therapist then collaborate to examine the evidence that supports or refutes this negative interpretation. The question "What's the evidence to support this view?" is a basic tool of cognitive restructuring. With a second question, "Is there another way to look at this observation?", the therapist helps the child explore alternative explanations that could account for his or her troubling observations (e.g., a friend did not say hello in the hallway). A third common question used in cognitive restructuring involves asking "What if ... " or, put another way, "Even if the observation is true and there's not an alternative explanation, is this really so terrible?" (e.g., "Your friend didn't say hello. She is mad at you but, even so, is that the worst thing ever?"; Stark et al., 2006). Beyond these standard questions, the therapist may also help the child formulate a behavioral experiment to gather evidence for or against a particular viewpoint. For example, if a child is worried that other children will make fun of her, she may survey others to test the belief that she is the only person being targeted. The targets of cognitive restructuring tend to vary with the presenting difficulties of the child. For example, in anxiety disorders, the therapist is likely to explore maladaptive expectations or worries related to upcoming events, with the goals of removal of misinterpretations of environmental events, and the development of coping strategies. These goals allow youth to view formerly distressing situations through the lens of coping strategies rather than the previous misperceptions (Kendall & Suveg, 2006). With depressed clients, there is more of a tendency to ruminate and form misattributions about past events. Thus, the therapist helps to identify the child's core beliefs, and directly and indirectly challenges negative thoughts to help replace them with more realistic and positive thoughts (Stark et al., 2006).

Affective Education

Although affective education has implicitly been a part of most CBT programs, more recently there has been an explicit focus on the role of emotions in child and adult psychopathology treatment (see Kendall & Suveg, 2007). An important component of CBT is therefore to help children and teens learn how to recognize, label, and express emotional experiences accurately. CBT prevention and treatment programs for youth benefit from the inclusion of direct affective education (Suveg, Southam-Gerow, Goodman, & Kendall, 2007). In some cases, children may be keenly aware of their emotional state but need help to develop a vocabulary to discuss these experiences, or as

Southam-Gerow and Kendall (2000) reported, they need help to recognize that emotions are modifiable. They may also need information to understand and normalize the physiological symptoms that accompany the experience of strong emotions. Other children need help to understand the range and intensity of emotional expression. These children often need to learn to recognize the early physiological cues of emotional distress, so they can respond to the problem creating this distress while their emotions are still at relatively low intensity, rather than wait until they experience some type of emotional "meltdown." Still other children need help in understanding the connection between thoughts and feelings, and benefit from learning how self-talk has the potential to increase or decrease the intensity of one's emotional response.

As part of affective education, the cognitive-behavioral therapist may explain that strong emotions have a disorganizing effect on thinking in both children and adults, which makes it difficult to exhibit new learning or behavior patterns, unless these behavioral responses have been well-practiced. Ideally, practice first occurs in a nonthreatening context that provides support to attempt new behavior, as in therapy, then in challenging environments. Sports or coaching analogies can be useful to communicate this concept. The therapist can explain that learning a new self-management skill is much like trying out a new soccer or basketball move. First, the child must work on the skill in practice and receive a lot of coaching, then try out in the moves in scrimmages, and finally use the new move in a game situation.

Relaxation Training

Relaxation training has been a key element in the behavioral treatment of internalizing difficulties in children (Barrios & O'Dell, 1989; Morris & Kratochwill, 1983), and teaching children more effective ways to relax is a major component of cognitive-behavioral treatment for a variety of childhood concerns. Rather than viewing relaxation as an alternative conditioned response, however, cognitive-behavioral therapists present relaxation as a coping skill to be developed and purposely enacted whenever needed. Relaxation training is an important element in the treatment of children and adolescents with anger management difficulties (Feindler & Ecton, 1986; Lochman, White, & Wayland, 1991). Stark (1990) has cautioned that children may not understand the rationale for relaxation training as well as adult clients. Children may feel intimidated by the procedures, so it is important for the clinician to provide adequate information to both the parents and child about the purpose and appropriate uses of relaxation methods.

Relaxation training has been implemented in many forms. Both Stark (1990) and Kendall et al. (1992) have recommended the use of Ollendick and Cerny's (1981) modification of deep muscle relaxation training, in which children learn to tense and relax various muscle groups and become more adept at perceiving the physiological indicators of muscle tension. Children can use this awareness to respond to early cues of muscle tension and enact their relaxation procedures. Koeppen (1974) created a series of guided images to help school-age children to tense and relax various muscle groups, and modifications of relaxation procedures have been developed for children with special needs (Cautela & Groden, 1978).

There are a number of simple relaxation training procedures that clinicians can use with preschool and school-age children. For example, Kendall and Braswell (1993) describe the robot–ragdoll game, in which the therapist and child first move around the room like robots, making their arms and legs very stiff and tense. Upon the therapist's signal, the child is then instructed to flop gently in a nearby chair and allow his or her arms and legs to be relaxed and loose. The therapist then contrasts these two bodily states. Children can also be taught brief inductions to slow deep breathing, such as when a child holds her index finger in front of her mouth as though it were a candle. The child is told to take a deep breath and hold it, and then let it out so slowly that an imaginary candle flame on the end of her finger will flicker but not be extinguished. Other methods include backwards counting or the use of calm self-talk. It is usually advised to present different options to relax, then have the child select and practice the methods he or she prefers. After relaxation skills have been taught and practiced in the session, the therapist can create an audiotape of the child's preferred methods for use at home. Although relaxation training is typically employed as one component in a multifaceted treatment plan, Kahn, Kehle, Jenson, and Clark (1990) reported that relaxation training alone was as effective as cognitive-behavioral treatment involving self-monitoring, cognitive restructuring, and problem solving in decreasing depressive symptomatology and increasing self-esteem.

Modeling/Role Playing

Modeling and role playing are two important components of CBT for youth. Humans often learn by observing others in a form of learning that is referred to as "observational learning" or "modeling." Modeling derives its conceptual roots from the social learning paradigm (Bandura, 1969, 1986), in which certain behaviors are demonstrated in a situation to illustrate appropriate responses for the child. Modeling has been used to reduce behavioral deficits and excessive fears, to facilitate social behavior (Bandura, 1969, 1971; Rosenthal & Bandura, 1978), and to teach desired coping skills. Variations of modeling include filmed, live, and participant modeling. In filmed modeling, for example, an anxious child might watch a videotape of a model coping with an anxious situation. The model (therapist) interacts with the child in participant modeling and guides his or her approach to the feared stimulus. Regular corrective feedback and reinforcement for effort and success are required to help the child match the performance of the model (Ollendick & Francis, 1988).

Modeling has received significant research attention. A learner's response to modeling is influenced by at least three classes of factors: features of the model, features of the learner, and consequences associated with the modeled behavior (Goldstein, 1995). For example, models who verbalize their thoughts and actions while engaging in the behavior generate superior learning relative to models who do not verbalize (Meichenbaum, 1971). Verbalization demonstrates how the learner can think through a particular situation and provides both auditory and visual cues. Providing labels for actions may be particularly important, since young children tend to have greater difficulty differentiating central from peripheral information, and they may miss important contextual cues. Like adults, children are more likely to imitate behavior of similar models, or of someone they admire and respect. Youth can be helped to create their own models as well. As part of the treatment of anxious youth, Kendall, Chu, Pimentel, and Choudhury (2000) recommended having children imagine how their favorite cartoon or movie character might handle a feared situation.

"Coping models" may be superior to "mastery models" for some types of learning. A coping model demonstrates task performance that includes mistakes. The model may display some discomfort or distress, yet he or she is able to perform the task with persistent effort. Coping modeling shows the client how to execute the necessary behaviors, and also how to cope with thoughts, emotions, and behaviors that might interfere with task performance. A mastery model, in contrast, demonstrates successful performance without indications of anxiety or difficulty. The CBT clinician also works with parents and teachers to help them become more conscious models of the skills they wish to develop in the young clients.

Like modeling, role playing is used in CBT as a means to provide the client with performance-based learning experiences. Role playing also serves as a vehicle to assess the extent to which the client can produce the newly learned skills. Role plays in session typically involve the client and the therapist acting out various responses to problematic situations, which allows the child to be actively involved in the session and gives him or her the opportunity to model coping behaviors. Role plays can also serve as good practice for exposures, in which the young client is placed in a distressing situation and has to use newly acquired skills.

Behavioral Contingencies/Contingent Reinforcement

Shaping, positive reinforcement, and extinction are some of the most frequently used contingency management procedures. Behavioral contingencies within CBT are effective when their choice is guided by considerations of the youth's disorder and stage of development. Rewards tend to be tangible for younger children and connote social approval. Mastery incentives become increasingly important for older children, such as when rewards signify that the child has achieved some type of goal. Younger children may also require more frequent tangible rewards, whereas older children enjoy earning points toward a larger reward. Rewards and contingencies must also be sensitive to features of the child's disorder. For example, youth with attention-deficit/hyperactivity disorder (ADHD) exhibit a need for stimulation and quick satiation; such youth tend to respond best in reward conditions with frequent rewards (Zentall, 1995).

It is important to consider the implementation of rewards and other contingencies away from the therapist's office. Parents need to use rewards in a consistent manner in the home setting. They must understand what constitutes a reward for a child. For example, many parents are unaware of the reinforcing power of their attention. A parent may not realize that if the child acts out and he or she yells, this negative attention could actually reinforce the child's behavior. Parents can be primed to use their attention to encourage of more desirable behaviors. Charts and graphs can help to guide the implementation of behavioral methods to support change on the part of children and/ or parents.

APPLICATIONS WITH SPECIFIC CHILDHOOD DISORDERS

Although common elements might suggest that CBT is uniform in its application, this is not the case. Treatments are designed for specific disorders, and strategies are used differentially to be consistent with the nature of the disorder and the child's unique needs. In this section we describe some disorder-specific programs and related research findings.

Anxiety Disorders

The experience of fear and anxiety is part of normal development for most children. As children develop, the content of their anxieties and fears tends to reflect changes in their perceptions of reality. Children's fears tend to begin with content that is more global, imaginary, uncontrollable, and powerful (e.g., the "boogie man" that lurks in the dark), and over time fears become more specific, differentiated, and realistic (e.g., worries about peer acceptance and school performance; Bauer, 1976). Anxiety becomes a disorder when the experience is exaggerated beyond what would be expected in a given situation, or when it interferes with the youth's functioning. Treatment may be indicated when the severity and duration of the fears impinge on a child's accomplishment of key developmental tasks, such as making friends, attending school, and tolerating age-appropriate separation. Without treatment, it appears that anxiety disorders in childhood and adolescence have a chronic course and are associated with comorbid psychopathology in adulthood (anxiety, depression, substance use; Aschenbrand, Kendall, Webb, Safford, & Flannery-Schroeder, 2003; Woodward & Fergusson, 2001).

CBT for anxiety disorders in youth integrates the demonstrated efficiencies of the behavioral approach (e.g., exposure, relaxation training, role plays) with an added emphasis on the cognitive information-processing factors associated with each individual's anxiety. The goals of treatment are to teach children to recognize the signs of anxious arousal, and to let these signs serve as cues for the use of anxiety management techniques. A 16-session child-focused manualized treatment program for anxious youth called the Coping Cat Program (or C.A.T. Project for teens; Kendall, 1992) has been translated into many languages. The program is broken into two treatment segments: skills training (the first eight sessions) and skills practice (the last eight sessions). The skills training sessions focus on building four basic skills areas: awareness of bodily reactions to feelings and physical symptoms specific to anxiety; recognition and evaluation of anxious "self-talk"; problem-solving skills (see Table 12.1), including modifying anxious self-talk and developing plans for coping; and self-evaluation and reward. During the skills practice segment of

TABLE 12.1. Problem-Solving Steps for Adolescents and Parents

  I. Define the problem.
    A. You each tell the others what they are doing that bothers you and why.
      1. Be brief.
      2. Be positive, not accusing.
    B. You each repeat the others' statements of the problem to check out your understanding of what they said.

  II. Generate alternative solutions.
    A. You take turns listing possible solutions.
    B. You follow three rules for listing solutions:
      1. List as many ideas as possible.
      2. Don't evaluate the ideas.
      3. Be creative; suggest crazy ideas.
    C. You won't have to do it just because you say it.

  III. Evaluate/decide upon the best idea.
    A. You take turns evaluating each idea.
      1. Would this idea solve the problem for you?
      2. Would this idea solve the problem for others?
      3. Rate the idea "plus" or "minus" on a worksheet.
    B. You select the best idea.
      1. Look for ideas rated "plus" by all.
        a. Select one such idea.
        b. Combine several such ideas.
      2. If none was rated "plus" by all, see where you came closest to agreement and negotiate a compromise. If two parents are participating, look for ideas rated "plus" by one parent and the teenager.

  IV. Plan to implement the selected solution.
    A. You decide who will do what, when, where, and how.
    B. Plan reminders for task completion.
    C. Plan consequences for compliance or noncompliance.

Note. From A. L. Robin (personal communication, January 5, 2000). Copyright 2000 by The Guilford Press. Reprinted by permission.

treatment, youth practice the learned skills in actual anxiety-provoking situations.

This CBT program presents the main principles of anxiety management using the FEAR acronym (see Table 12.2): (1) recognizing bodily symptoms of anxiety (i.e., Feeling frightened?), (2) identifying anxious cognitions (i.e., Expecting bad things to happen), (3) developing a repertoire of coping strategies (i.e., Actions and attitudes that can help), and (4) Results and rewards (i.e., contingency management). The child learns the FEAR plan during the skills training portion of treatment and then applies these steps during the skills practice portion (see Table 12.3).

Variations on Kendall's child-focused CBT include group (Flannery-Schroeder & Kendall, 2000; Mendlowitz et al., 1999), family (Howard, Chu, Krain, Marrs-Garcia, & Kendall, 2000), and group school-based treatment (Masia-Warner, Nangle, & Hansen, 2006). Albano and Barlow (1996) also developed CBT groups for socially anxious teenagers (cf. Heimberg et al., 1990). The program components include cognitive restructuring to identify and change cognitive distortions that perpetuate anxiety, social skills training to address areas of deficit, and problem-solving training. Silverman, Ginsburg, and Kurtines (1995) have developed a CBT approach for children with phobias and other anxiety disorders that is similar to the approach presented by Kendall et al. (1992) but that includes separate and conjoint child and parent sessions. Recently, investigators have augmented child-focused with parent and family involvement (Barrett, Dadds, & Rapee, 1996; Cobham, Dadds, & Spence, 1998; Wood, Piacentini, Southam-Gerow, Chu, & Sigman, 2006), but the benefits of parental involvement relative to child-focused CBT are mixed. There is a need for future research in this area.

The literature supports the efficacy of CBT for anxiety disorders in youth. Reviewers (e.g., Kazdin & Weisz, 1998; Ollendick & King, 1998) have indicated that, using the criteria for empirically supported treatment (Chambless & Hollon, 1998), CBT can be considered to have demonstrated efficacy. Liter-

---

TABLE 12.2. FEAR Plan for Use with Anxious Youth

1. Feeling nervous?
   Are you feeling nervous? How can you tell?
2. Expecting bad things to happen?
   Tune into your self-talk. What is it that is worrying you in this situation?
3. Attitudes and actions can help.
   What are some others ways to think about this situation? What are some actions I can take to make this situation better?
4. Results and rewards.
   How did I do? Was I able to help myself take action and feel better? Way to go!

Note. From Kendall (1992). Copyright 1992 by Workbook Publishing. Reprinted by permission.

TABLE 12.3. Sample FEAR Plan

Situation: Ordering for myself at a restaurant

1. *Feeling frightened?*
   a. My hands are sweating and my stomach hurts.
2. *Expecting bad things to happen?*
   a. What if I forget what to say? What if the waiter laughs at me?
3. *Attitudes and actions that can help.*
   a. I can do this. The waiter looks like a nice person and he probably won't laugh at me. Besides, what's the worst thing that can happen?
4. *Results and rewards.*
   a. I did it! I ordered my own pizza and, wow, was it delicious! My dad will be so proud of me.

ature involving potential mechanisms associated with change is also receiving much needed attention. Kendall and Treadwell (2007) found that children's anxious, but not positive or depressed, self-statements predicted anxiety in children and mediated treatment gains. Research programs are utilizing a broader array of assessment tools that allow for the examination of self-talk, self-perceptions, coping abilities, and level of treatment satisfaction of children experiencing anxiety disorders.

Obsessive–Compulsive Disorder

There is an emerging literature on the efficacy of both CBT and pharmacological interventions for the treatment of obsessive–compulsive disorder (OCD) in youth. Findings from studies comparing CBT to pharmacological interventions in children (de Haan, Hoogduin, Buitelaar, & Kejers, 1998; Pediatric OCD Treatment Study Team, 2004), with regard to efficacy, safety, and durability of response have led to the consensus recommendation that CBT be considered the initial treatment choice for OCD across the age span (Albano, March, & Piacentini, 1999; March, Frances, Carpernter, & Kahn, 1997).

An efficacious cognitive-behavioral treatment for youth with OCD was developed by March and colleagues (March, 1995; March & Mulle, 1998; March, Mulle, & Herbel, 1994). This program uses traditional behavioral approaches of exposure, response prevention, and extinction, coupled with anxiety management components that include relaxation and cognitive restructuring. The behavioral conceptualization of OCD views obsessions as intrusive, unwanted thoughts, images, or urges that trigger a significant and rapid increase in anxiety, and views compulsions as overt behavior or cognition designed to reduce these negative feelings (Albano et al., 1999). Based on learning theory, compulsions are negatively reinforced over time by their ability to reduce the obsession-triggered distress. The more successfully that compulsive behaviors reduce distress, the more powerful they become. Each time a child carries out a compulsion, the reduction in distress strengthens the compulsive behavior.

March and colleagues' CBT program for youth with OCD includes a variety of treatment strategies, such as psychoeducation, creation of a symptom hierarchy, exposure and response prevention (ERP), addressing obsessions, and contingency management (March & Mulle, 1998). During the psychoeducation phase, the therapist educates the patient and the family about OCD, within a cognitive-behavioral conceptualization. The creation of the symptom hierarchy provides a template to design individual exposure tasks and determine the implementation sequence. During ERP the child remains in contact with feared stimuli and resists related rituals or other anxiety-reducing actions. Therapists model adaptive coping strategies to reduce anticipatory anxiety and enhance coping self-talk before and during ERP. Family factors are also important in the treatment of OCD in youth. Recent studies corroborate observations from substantial clinical experience and attest to the impact of family context on OCD expression and the impact of the child's symptoms on family functioning (Piacentini & Langely, 2004; Waters & Barrett, 2000). Youth who present for treatment of OCD likely will have a parent or other immediate family member who is similarly affected. Family functioning may also be an important predictor of both initial response to treatment and long-term outcome. High emotional reactivity and negative family perceptions about OCD have been associated with worse treatment response in adults, and further research is needed to determine whether this applies to youth (Livingston-Van Noppen, Rasmussen, Eisen, & McCartney, 1990).

Aggressive Behavior

Aggressive behavior is a pattern of severe, chronic, and frequent interpersonal interactions (i.e., verbal and physical behavior) that are destructive to others (Bandura, 1971). This pattern of behavior in children and adolescents is the leading cause of referral for mental health services in the United States (Achenbach & Howell, 1993; Lochman et al., 2006). Children with chronic, severe, and frequent aggressive behavior are frequently diagnosed with oppositional defiant disorder and conduct disorder.

The social-cognitive model proposes that the maladaptive behavior of an aggressive child is due to the child's perception and appraisal of a distressing event (Crick & Dodge, 1994). Specifically, these youth experience a misattribution of intentionality: Aggressive youth see negative outcomes from ambiguous situations that involve others as having been intentional and provocative, and thereby justifying retaliation (Dodge, 1985). The three components of this model suggest that perception and appraisal, arousal, and social problem solving contribute to the child's aggressive response (Lochman et al., 2006). CBT for aggressive children aims to address these distorted perceptions, misattributions of intentionality, overreliance on nonverbal solutions, and underreliance on verbal solutions (Lochman et al., 2006). A review of the literature suggests that aggressive children are responsive to CBT interventions, with success in both school- and clinic-based interventions for children who exhibit aggressive behavior.

School-based treatments have a long tradition, which includes the "turtle technique" (Robin & Schneider, 1974; Robin, Schneider, & Dolnick, 1976). The Lochman group program (Lochman et al., 2006; Lochman, Burch, Curry, & Lampron, 1984; Lochman & Curry, 1986; Lochman, Lampron, Gemmer, Harris, & Wyckoff, 1989) includes training and practice in the use of problem-solving steps, training in the recognition of physiological cues of arousal, and practice in the use of self-calming talk during provocation situations. The addition of behavioral goal setting has further improved treatment impact. In this circumstance, the goal setting involved having the child state a goal in group, while the classroom teacher monitored progress on the goal on a daily basis, with contingent reinforcement for successful goal attainment. In a 3-year follow-up of boys treated in the Anger Coping Program, Lochman (1992) reported lower rates of drug and alcohol involvement and higher levels of social problem-solving skills and self-esteem relative to untreated controls. The groups were equivalent, however, in rates of reported delinquent behavior, which led Lochman to suggest the need for interventions of greater intensity that also permit more parental involvement.

The Coping Power Program is an adaptation of Lochman's Anger Coping Program is (see Lochman, Wells, & Murray, 2007). This school-based treatment for fourth through sixth graders utilizes a 34-session group treatment for children, along with a 16-session parent component. The program focuses on social-cognitive difficulties in aggressive youth (Lochman et al., 2006). In addition to the components mentioned earlier, this treatment includes a parent component to improve on the dyadic relationship and to help teach effective parenting (Lochman et al., 2006). Other important aspects of treatment include self-control exercises and social perspective-taking skills. Self-control exercises put the child in an anger-provoking situation under controlled and supportive circumstances, whereas social perspective-taking skills allow the child to engage in both cognitive and affective perspective taking in others (Lochman et al., 2006). Evidence supports the program's efficacy on child social information-processing and parenting practices, because youth who received the intervention showed significant reductions in self-reported delinquency, parent-reported substance use, and teacher-reported behavioral problems at 1-year follow-up, particularly in youth who received the parent and child components of the treatment (Lochman & Wells, 2004).

Cognitive-behavioral interventions have also been successful with more severely impaired samples, as illustrated by the work of Kazdin and colleagues (Kazdin, 2005; Kazdin, Bass, Siegel, & Thomas, 1989; Kazdin, Esveldt-Dawson, French, & Unis, 1987a, 1987b; Kazdin, Siegel, & Bass, 1992) with 7- to 13-year-old children hospitalized for severe aggressive and destructive behavior. The cognitive-behavioral treatment emphasized problem-solving training, and treatment effects were improved by the addition of more *in vivo* opportunities for skills practice and by behavioral child management training for the parents. The combination of problem-solving training and parent management training was most successful at moving children from clinical to normative levels of functioning, as assessed by rating scale measures. Kazdin and Crowley (1997) observed that children with greater academic dysfunction and more symptoms at study outset across a range of different diagnostic categories appeared to benefit less from CBT. In addition, parent, family, and contextual factors, such as economic disadvantage, parent history of antisocial behavior, and poor child rearing practices, were associated with poorer outcomes. Kazdin and Whitley (2006) investigated th effect of comorbidity and case complexity on treatment outcome in youth referred for disruptive behavior. The authors found that neither comorbidity nor case complexity produced any significant differences on treatment outcome. This result suggests that this treatment can remediate complex and comorbid presentations of disruptive behavior.

A CBT intervention developed to prevent aggressive behavior in high-risk children has also been found to be effective at periods up to a 2-year follow-up (Families and Schools Together [FAST]; McDonald, 1993; McDonald et al., 2006). This school-based collaborative program for families, youth, and schools is an effort to reach elementary school children who have been identified by teachers as having behavioral problems.

Attention-Deficit/Hyperactivity Disorder

The evolution in thinking about the usefulness of CBT in the treatment of attention-deficit/hyperactivity disorder (ADHD) provides an interesting example in the cycle of science (Braswell, 2007; Hinshaw, 2006). Often a new approach is enthusiastically greeted, widely applied, then found to be less useful than was originally believed. Children who are diagnosed with ADHD have levels of inattention, impulsivity, and, in some cases, hyperactivity that exceed normative standards for their age and cognitive level. Because cognitive deficiencies are associated with ADHD-type behavior (August, 1987; see also Kendall & McDonald, 1993), there seems to be a match between the goals of certain types of CBT, such as problem-solving approaches, and the needs of children with ADHD. In their meta-analytic review of the cognitive-behavioral outcome literature with impulsive children, Baer and Nietzel (1991) concluded that CBT was associated with improvements of approximately one-third to three-quarters of a standard deviation relative to untreated controls, but the targeted groups had scores that fell close to comparison group means, both before and after treatment. Thus, the severity of the behavioral issues of these children must be questioned, and the efficacy of CBT with impulsiveness may not generalize to youth with ADHD.

Consistent with a concern about efficacy, researchers who conducted interventions with children who met full criteria for ADHD (or its diagnostic equivalent at the time of each study) generally did not achieve success on either social or academic outcome measures (see reviews by Abikoff, 1985, 1991; Kendall & Braswell, 1993). In addition, when CBT was combined with psychostimulant medication treatment, there was little evidence of effects beyond those achieved with medication alone (Abikoff et al., 1988; Brown, Borden, Wynne, Schleser, & Clingerman, 1986; Brown, Wynne, & Medenis, 1985). Braswell et al. (1997) evaluated the effects of a 2-year school-based child group training program that targeted children selected by parents and teachers on the basis of their disruptive behavior. Two-thirds of this sample met DSM-III-R criteria for ADHD. Treated children participated in 28 training groups over a 2-year period, and their parents and teachers participated in information and behavior management groups. The results of this multicomponent intervention were compared to those of a control condition in which parents and teachers received information, but the children received no direct service. Both conditions displayed improvement at posttest, but subsequent follow-up data indicated no significant difference in the functioning of the two groups. Thus, despite initial enthusiasm for the use of these methods, the results of other teams and our own compel the conclusion that problem-solving training efforts should not be considered a treatment for the primary symptoms of ADHD. Children with ADHD appear to need interventions at the point of performance rather than interventions that train skills in one setting and provide few or no prompts and reinforcements for skills use in the target environment (Goldstein & Goldstein, 1998).

Although cognitive problem-solving approaches may not be the most appropriate interventions for the primary symptoms of ADHD, these approaches may be suitable for adjunctive issues, such as parent–child conflict, and for coexisting concerns, such as aggressive behavior, anxiety, and depression. In a 14-month randomized trial, the Multimodal Treatment Study of Children with Attention-Deficit/Hyperactivity Disorder (MTA Cooperative Group, 1999a), carefully titrated medications appeared to have the greatest positive impact on the core symptoms of ADHD, while combined medication and intensive behavioral intervention demonstrated additional positive effect on coexisting issues, including oppositional and defiant disorder behavior, internalizing symptoms, and parent–child relationship concerns. Behavioral treatment without medication only outperformed community care for children who manifested ADHD and symptoms of anxiety (MTA Cooperative Group, 1999b). This study suggests that medication may be superior to behavioral interventions for ADHD.

This brief review leads to a question about the role of CBT in the treatment of ADHD. Hinshaw (2006) argues that although cognitive interventions do not provide meaningful change in clinical cases of ADHD, medication treatments are short-term and not curative. The combination of psychosocial and drug therapies has sometimes showed greater change than medication alone (Hinshaw, Klein, & Abikoff, 2002, Swanson, Kraemer, & Hinshaw, 2001). Thus, there may be a place for CBT interventions within the multimodal treatment of ADHD (Hinshaw, 2006). Hinshaw suggests that combining cognitive treatments for verbal mediation, along with contingencies and behavioral rehearsal, is an avenue for future research.

Depression

CBT has been labeled "possibly efficacious" for depressed children and "probably efficacious for depressed adolescents" (Kazdin & Weisz, 1998). More controlled outcome studies have been published, yet few studies have examined younger children and the research is somewhat diverse in terms of the CBT approaches that have been examined.

Lewinsohn and colleagues (Clarke et al., 2001; Lewinsohn, Clarke, Hops, & Andrews, 1990; Lewinsohn, Clarke, & Rohde, 1994; Lewinsohn, Clarke, Rohde, Hops, & Seeley, 1996) have conducted two randomized clinical trials of their cognitive-behavioral treatment with severely depressed adolescents, which have yielded evidence for change. The Adolescent Coping with Depression (CWD-A) group program trains skills that are emphasized in cognitive formulations of depression, such as learning to recognize depressogenic patterns of thinking and substituting more constructive cognitions, along with skills associated with more behavioral formulations, such as increasing client behaviors that elicit positive reinforcement and avoid negative reinforcement from the environment. This change in reinforcement patterns often requires the training of social and other coping skills, through structured group sessions that emphasize role playing, homework assignment, and rewards and contracts. A companion group education program for the parents of the depressed teens has also been developed (Lewinsohn, Rohde, Hops, & Clarke, 1991). Interestingly, adding parent group participation did not appear to yield outcomes significantly better than those achieved when only the adolescents participated in the program (Lewinsohn et al., 1990). Also, an attempt to clarify the most effective pattern of booster sessions following group completion did not yield results in favor of one pattern over another (Lewinsohn et al., 1994). Clarke, Rohde, Lewinsohn, Hops, and Seeley (1999) also demonstrated the effectiveness of CBT group treatment over a waiting-list control, with improvement rates not significantly different for the adolescent-only or adolescent plus parent group condition.

Brent and colleagues (Birmaher et al., 2000; Brent et al., 1997, 1998; Brent, Kolko, Birmaher, Baugher, & Bridge, 1999) compared the effectiveness of CBT with systemic behavioral family therapy and nondirective supportive therapy with depressed adolescents. CBT resulted in more rapid and complete relief of depressive symptoms than the other two treatments at the end of the 12-week acute treatment phase (Brent et al., 1997), and had a particular treatment advantage with patients' who were comorbid for anxiety (Brent et al., 1998). CBT's relative efficacy decreased in cases where maternal depression was present, however. Despite these superior results in the acute phase, patients in all conditions were equally likely to receive or be recommended for additional treatment during the 24-month follow-up period (Brent et al.,

1999). The need for follow-up treatment was best predicted by the continuing severity of depressive symptoms at the end of the acute phase, and the presence of disruptive behavior and family difficulties. Brent et al. speculated that CBT may be superior for initial symptom reduction, but approaches that provide some form of family involvement might be of greater value in addressing residual behavioral disruption and/or ongoing family conflicts.

The efficacy of CBT was evaluated in a large study of depressed youth, the Treatment for Adolescents with Depression Study (TADS; March, 2004), which compared medication (fluoxetine), CBT, medication plus CBT, and placebo in 351 adolescents with moderate to severe major depressive disorder. The TADS CBT program involved 12 weeks of treatment that included psychoeducation, goal setting, mood monitoring, increased activities, social problem solving, and cognitive restructuring. There were also modules that focused on social skills deficits and family sessions related to psychoeducation and parent–adolescent relationship concerns. The study found that although fluoxetine alone was effective, the combination of CBT and fluoxetine was the most effective for symptom reduction. Although the CBT in TADS was not itself as effective as in prior studies at posttreatment, a positive response to CBT was found at follow-up (TADS Team, 2007). At 18 months after treatment, response rates to CBT alone were equivalent to those of fluoxetine alone (both were effective), and at 3-year follow-up the response to CBT alone was equivalent to the combination of CBT and fluoxetine. It is also worth noting that the TDS study team reported that adolescents who received CBT, whether alone or in combination with fluoxetine, had lower rates of suicidal ideation and attempts in the 2 years following treatment.

Other treatment programs for depression have been developed, though more empirical data on these programs is needed. ACTION is a manual-based treatment program that is guided by individual case conceptualization (Stark et al., 2006), in which children are taught coping, problem solving, and cognitive restructuring skills. ACTION includes both parent training and teacher consultation components that encourage parents and teachers to modify their environments to support the application of the child's new skills. Research is still in progress, but preliminary results suggest that this intervention is effective (Stark et al., 2006).

Prevention or reduction of risk for relapse or recurrence of depression following successful treatment is also an important concern when working with children/adolescents. Kroll, Harrington, Jayson, Fraser, and Gowers (1996) conducted a pilot study of maintenance CBT for adolescents who had remitted from major depressive disorder. Adolescents in the maintenance CBT condition exhibited a lower cumulative risk of relapse over a 6-month period relative to controls (0.2 vs. 0.5). In contrast, Clarke et al. (1999) found that booster sessions did not reduce rates of recurrence during a 24-month follow-up period, although rates of recurrence were low for all conditions. Booster sessions did, however, appear to accelerate recovery for those adolescents who had continued symptoms of depression at the end of the acute treatment phase.

In a fascinating approach to school-based prevention, Clarke et al. (1995) identified ninth graders considered to be at risk but not yet experiencing an episode of depression, based on self-report measures and follow-up structured diagnostic interview. These students then participated in fifteen 45-minute afterschool groups, in which students were taught cognitive techniques for identifying and challenging unhelpful thinking that might increase feelings of depression. Using survival analysis, the investigators then examined how many cases of major depressive disorder or dysthymia emerged in the treated group versus a usual care control group of teens. At 12-month follow-up, rates of depression were 14.5% for the treated group compared to 25.7% for the control group.

As these studies indicate, CBT for depressed children and adolescents is a promising treatment. There is, however, a striking need for the treatment packages and treatment components within this domain to be carefully evaluated by research teams that are independent from the creators of these approaches.

Other Disorders

In addition to the research advancements in the previously discussed treatment areas, additional efficacy studies examining CBT have been published. For example, researchers have reported on outcomes associated with CBT for trauma and/or posttraumatic stress disorder, school refusal, adolescent suicidality, and eating disorders (for chapters on specific disorders, see Kendall, 2006).

SPECIAL ISSUES

Transportability/Dissemination

Two issues that face all of the empirically supported interventions are dissemination and implementation. There has been activity within the psychological community to advance the use of "empirically supported treatments" (ESTs), which are psychological interventions that have been evaluated scientifically (e.g., randomized controlled trials) and satisfy the Chambless and Hollon (1998) criteria (Kendall & Beidas, 2007). Examples of ESTs for children and adolescents can be found in (1) books and chapters (e.g., Hibbs & Jensen, 2005; Kazdin & Weisz, 2003; Kendall, 2006; Weisz, 2004; Chambless & Ollendick, 2001), (2) the results of reviews available on Web-based resources (Substance Abuse and Mental Health Services Administration [SAMHSA]-sponsored contract run by MANILA Consulting Group; available at *www.nationalregistry.samhsa.gov*), (3) lists generated by professional associations (e.g., Kettlewell, Morford, & Hoover, 2005), and (4) in journals (e.g., Herschell, McNeil, & McNeil, 2004; special issues of the *Journal of Consulting and Clinical Psychology* (Kendall & Chambless, 1998), and the *Journal of Clinical Child Psychology* (Lonigan & Ebert, 1998). Many of the listed ESTs for youth include CBT approaches. Illustrative examples of ESTs for various mental health disorders include Multisystemic Family Therapy (Henggeler & Borduin, 1990), Parent–Child Interaction Therapy (Brinkmeyer & Eyberg, 2003), Coping Power (Lochman et al., 2006), and Parent Management Training (Kazdin, 2005) for externalizing behavior in youth. For depressed youth, ESTs include the Taking Action Program (Stark et al., 2006). For anxious youth, ESTs include the Coping Cat Program (Kendall et al., 1997) and CBT for OCD (Pediatric OCD Team, 2004). Summary chapters and articles are also available that consider ESTs for the full range of childhood disorders (e.g., Ollendick, King, & Chorpita al., 2006; Herschell et al., 2004).

The bulk of the ESTs use treatment manuals to guide implementation and to help ensure treatment fidelity (i.e., treatment adherence). Treatment manuals have been critiqued as being too linear, as not applicable outside of a research setting, as cookbooks for therapy, and as reducing clinicians to technicians (Duncan & Miller, 2006; Lambert, 1998; Bohart, O'Hara, & Leitner, 1998; Westen, Novotny, & Thompson-Brenner, 2004). We suggest, however, that treatment manuals are not restrictive when done flexibly: *flexibility within fidelity* (Kendall & Beidas, 2007). To illustrate this point, the Coping Cat program (Kendall & Hedtke, 2006a), an EST for anxious youth, has been implemented flexibly but also with fidelity (Kendall & Chu, 2000). One component of the Coping Cat includes exposure tasks that challenge youth to face anxiety-provoking stimuli. All youth who go through the Coping Cat program complete exposure tasks, but these tasks are individualized. Treatment for social rejection in the classroom or for general worry about safety concerns includes and requires exposure tasks that are specific to the presenting problem (Kendall et al., 2005). For example, an exposure task for social anxiety might involve the child doing a survey or asking other children about classroom behavior. An exposure task for general distress about safety concerns might focus on an open discussion about health issues and a call to an expert to ask questions.

Computers are increasingly important in both dissemination and implementation. With regard to CBT for anxiety in youth, there is a dissemination DVD, entitled *CBT4CBT* (Computer-Based Training to be a Cognitive-Behavioral Therapist). *CBT4CBT* (Kendall & Khanna, 2008a) is organized in modules that are session-by-session guides for implementation. It includes video clips of therapy sessions, video examples of exposure tasks, "tips" from experienced therapists, and access to treatment materials. Users complete a "knowledge check" after each module before proceeding.

Also with regard to CBT for anxiety in youth, computers now facilitate implementation. There is a computer-assisted program called Camp Cope-A-Lot (Kendall & Khanna, 2008b). The program provides a 12-session interactive version of the empirically supported Coping Cat treatment for anxious youth. Along with other campers at Camp Cope-A-Lot, the user goes to an amusement park, puts on a talent show, meets someone new, speaks in public, and experiences other adventures that build confidence and teach ways to manage anxiety.

As discussed by Kazdin and Kendall (1998), demonstrating that CBT is efficacious is a first step. Dissemination and implementation comprise the next step in ensuring that CBT is transported to the community, as evidence-based practice is "the integration of the best available research with clinical expertise" (American Psychological Association, 2005, p. 5). It is unlikely however, that CBT will yield equivalent outcomes in community-based clinics, where features of the setting, therapists, and clients may be quite different. Recognition of this issue highlights the need for effectiveness treatment outcome research and experimental trials with clients whose severity levels and cultural backgrounds similar to those seen in community-based settings.

Comorbidity

Many, if not most, CBT treatments were originally developed to treat a specific disorder or set of disorders. In contrast, many disorders of childhood are highly comorbid with other disorders (Flannery-Schroeder, Suveg, Safford, Kendall, & Webb, 2004; Nock, Kazdin, Hiripi, & Kessler, 2007; Seligman & Ollendick, 1998). In the past, and with some exceptions (notably, treatments that are designed to treat multiple, similar disorders, such as the Coping Cat; Kendall & Hedke, 2006a), the approach to address comorbidity has been to make slight adaptations to the treatment for the primary disorder to accommodate these additional diagnoses. More recently, modular approaches have been developed to address some of these issues and to disseminate ESTs (Chorpita, 2007; Chorpita, Daleiden, & Weiz, 2005). The "modular approach" defines individualized ESTs for specific client problems and promotes flexible implementation of the core principles of CBT. A number of modules are considered core to the treatment, but these modules can be both selected and presented in varying sequences for each child. This approach allows for more *flexibility* and takes into account contextual factors of the child and the child's environment (e.g., family, school; Chorpita, 2007). At the same time, *structure* is still present, because the procedures are explicitly outlined within the manual and can be implemented with adherence (Chorpita, 2007).

There are a number of differences between modularized treatment (i.e., Chorpita, 2007) and standard manualized treatments (i.e., Kendall & Hedtke, 2006a). The frequency, parental involvement, duration of sessions, pace, setting, and skills taught are child-centered, meaning that they are more variable than in a standardized protocol (Chorpita, 2007). For example, a child who presents with a comorbid disruptive disorder, in addition to primary separation anxiety disorder, only needs specific modules that apply to his or her troubles, such as learning about anxiety, *in vivo* exposure, cognitive restructuring, and working with the parents on active ignoring, rewards, and time-out (Chorpita, 2007). Learning about social skills may not be necessary for this particular child's problem. However, another child with social phobia may need that social skills module and not the extra modules for disruptive behaviors. Modularized treatment allows for a variable and child-centered approach that individualizes the protocol for each child.

Cultural Considerations

Research on the efficacy of cognitive-behavioral treatments for youth has been conducted primarily with European American clients. To date, there is no uniform methodology or framework for adapting and modifying treatment interventions for ethnic/minority groups, or for widespread implementation of such adaptations (Hwang, Wood, & Lin, 2006). Culture can affect symptom expression, perception and etiology of the disorder, therapeutic alliance, and treatment compliance. It can also influence why and when a family seeks treatment, as well as how the family is organized, which in turn influences who takes part in the treatment.

Research has demonstrated many similarities in the expression of different disorders among children, but many cultural differences also exist, particularly with respect to how children report symptoms, respond to treatment, and even respond to the therapist (Ginsburg & Silverman, 1996). Sensitivity to these differences is critical to guide assessment and treatment strategies, and to optimize work with children and families from diverse backgrounds. The cultural sensitivity of cognitive-behavioral psychological interventions can be enhanced by the assessment of the client's worldview using culture-specific assessment instruments, including culture-specific rituals, and profiling contextual factors. Research is slowly emerging on culturally sensitive adaptations of ESTs.

CONCLUSIONS AND FUTURE DIRECTIONS

The field of child intervention has come a long way since the days when all we could offer children was well-meaning therapists with good intentions! Specific forms of cognitive-behavioral treatment can be now recommended with confidence as efficacious treatments for aggressive 7- to 13-year-olds, and anxious and/or depressed children and adolescents. Other reviews of the field have deemed several of these approaches as probably efficacious (Brestan & Eyberg, 1998; Kaslow & Thompson, 1998; Ollendick & King, 1998). Research questions and pragmatic concerns remain, however. The demonstration of the efficacy of a particular approach demands ever greater specificity, the refinement of research methods, and the integration of knowledge from related fields. Future treatment outcome research and practice will need to integrate existing and emerging knowledge from the domains of child development, education, psychopathology, and cross-cultural psychology.

REFERENCES

Abikoff, H. (1985). Efficacy of cognitive training interventions in hyperactive children: A critical review. *Clinical Psychology Review, 5,* 479–512.

Abikoff, H. (1991). Cognitive training in ADHD children: Less to it than meets the eye. *Journal of Learning Disabilities, 24,* 205–209.

Abikoff, H., Ganales, D., Reiter, G., Blum, C., Foley, C., & Klein, R. G. (1988). Cognitive training in academically deficient ADHD boys receiving stimulant medication. *Journal of Abnormal Child Psychology, 16,* 411–432.

Achenbach, T. M., & Howell, C. T. (1993). Are American children's problems getting worse?: A 13-year comparison. *Journal of the American Academy of Child and Adolescent Psychiatry, 32,* 1145–1154.

Albano, A. M., & Barlow, D. H. (1996). Breaking the vicious cycle: Cognitive-behavioral group treatment for socially anxious youth. In E. D. Hibbs & P. S. Jensen (Eds.), *Psychosocial treatments for child and adolescent disorders: Empirically based strategies for clinical practice* (pp. 43–62). Washington, DC: American Psychological Association.

Albano, A. M., March, J. S., & Piacentini, J. C. (1999). Obsessive–compulsive disorder. In R. T. Ammerman, M. Hersen, & C. G. Last (Eds.), *Handbook of prescriptive treatments for children and adolescents* (2nd ed., pp. 193–213). Needham Heights, MA: Allyn & Bacon.

American Psychological Association. (2005, August). *American Psychological Association policy statement on evidence-based practice in psychology.* Retrieved March 6th, 2006 from *www.apa.org/practice/ebpreport.pdf.*

Aschenbrand, S. G., Kendall, P. C., Webb, A., Safford, S. M., & Flannery-Schroeder, E. C. (2003). Is childhood separation anxiety disorder a predictor of adult panic disorder and agoraphobia?: A seven-year longitudinal study. *Journal of the American Academy of Child and Adolescent Psychiatry, 42,* 1478–1485.

August, G. (1987). Production deficiencies in free recall: A comparison of hyperactivity learning-disabled and normal children. *Journal of Abnormal Child Psychology, 15,* 429–440.

Baer, R. A., & Nietzel, M. T. (1991). Cognitive and behavioral treatment of impulsivity in children: A meta-analytic review of the outcome literature. *Journal of Clinical Child Psychology, 20,* 400–412.

Bandura, A. (1969). *Principles of behavior modification.* New York: Holt, Rinehart & Winston.

Bandura, A. (1971). Psychotherapy based upon modeling procedures. In A. Bergin & S. Garfield (Eds.), *Handbook of psychotherapy and behavior change.* New York: Wiley.

Bandura, A. (1986). Fearful expectations and avoidant actions as co-effects of perceived self-inefficacy. *American Psychologist, 41,* 1389–1391.

Barmish, A. J., & Kendall, P. C. (2005). Should parents be co-clients in cognitive-behavioral therapy for anxious youth? *Journal of Clinical Child and Adolescent Psychology, 34,* 569–581.

Barrett, P. M., Dadds, M. M., & Rapee, R. M. (1996). Family treatment of childhood anxiety: A controlled trial. *Journal of Consulting and Clinical Psychology, 64,* 333–342.

Barrios, B. A., & O'Dell, S. L. (1989). Fears and anxieties. In E. J. Mash & R. A. Barkley (Eds.), *Treatment of childhood disorders* (pp. 167–221). New York: Guilford Press.

Bauer, D. H. (1976). An exploratory study of developmental changes in children's fears. *Journal of Child Psychology and Psychiatry, 17,* 69–74.

Beck, A. T., Rush, A. J., Shaw, B. F., & Emery, G. (1979). *Cognitive therapy of depression.* New York: Guilford Press.

Birmaher, B., Brent, D. A., Kolko, D., Baugher, M., Bridge, J., Holder, D., et al. (2000). Clinical outcome after short-term psychotherapy for adolescents with major depressive disorder. *Archives of General Psychiatry, 54,* 877–885.

Bohart, A., O'Hara, M., & Leitner, L. (1998). Empirically violated treatments: Disenfranchisement of humanistic and other psychotherapies. *Psychotherapy Research, 8,* 141–157.

Braswell, L. (2007). Meeting the treatment needs of children with ADHD: Can cognitive strategies make a contribution? In R. W. Christner, J. L. Stewart, & A. Freeman (Eds.), *Handbook of cognitive behavior group therapy with children and adolescents: Specific settings and presenting problems* (pp. 317–322). New York: Routledge/Taylor & Francis.

Braswell, L., August, G., Bloomquist, M. L., Realmuto, G. M., Skare, S., & Crosby, R. (1997). School-based secondary prevention for children with disruptive behavior: Initial outcomes. *Journal of Abnormal Child Psychology, 25,* 197–208.

Brent, D. A., Holder, D., Kolko, D. A., Birmaher, B., Baugher, M., & Bridge, J. (1997). A clinical psychotherapy trial for adolescent depression comparing cognitive, family, and supportive treatments. *Archives of General Psychiatry, 54,* 877–885.

Brent, D. A., Kolko, D. J., Birmaher, B., Baugher, M., & Bridge, J. (1999). A clinical trial for adolescent depression: Predictors of additional treatment in the acute and follow-up phases of the trial. *Journal of the American Academy of Child and Adolescent Psychiatry, 38,* 263–271.

Brent, D. A., Kolko, D. J., Birmaher, B., Baugher, M., Bridge, J., Roth, C., et al. (1998). Predictors of treatment efficacy in a clinical trial of three psychosocial treatments for adolescent depression. *Journal of the American Academy of Child and Adolescent Psychiatry, 37,* 906–914.

Brestan, E. V., & Eyberg, S. M. (1998). Effective psychosocial treatments of conduct disordered children and adolescents: 29 years, 82 studies, and 5,272 kids. *Journal of Clinical Child Psychology, 27,* 180–189.

Brinkmeyer, M. Y., & Eyberg, S. M. (2003). Parent–child interaction therapy for oppositional children. In A. E. Kazdin & J. R. Weisz (Eds.), *Evidence-based psychotherapies for children and adolescents.* New York: Guilford Press.

Brown, R. T., Borden, K. A., Wynne, M. E., Schleser, R., & Clingerman, S. R. (1986). Methylphenidate and cognitive therapy with ADD children: A methodological reconsideration. *Journal of Abnormal Child Psychology, 13,* 69–87.

Brown, R. T., Wynne, M. E., & Medenis, R. (1985). Methylphenidate and cognitive therapy: A comparison of treatment approaches with hyperactive boys. *Journal of Abnormal Child Psychology, 13,* 69–87.

Cautela, J. R., & Groden, J. (1978). *Relaxation: A comprehensive manual for adults, children, and children with special needs.* Champaign, IL: Research Press.

Chambless, D., & Hollon, S. (1998). Defining empirically supported therapies. *Journal of Consulting and Clinical Psychology, 66,* 7–18.

Chambless, D., & Ollendick, T. (2001). Empirically supported psychological interventions: Controversies and evidence. *Annual Review of Psychology, 52,* 685–716.

Chorpita, B. F. (2007). *Modular cognitive-behavioral therapy for childhood anxiety disorders.* New York: Guilford Press.

Chorpita, B. F., Daleiden, E., & Weisz, J. (2005). Modularity in the design and application of therapeutic interventions. *Applied and Preventive Psychology, 11,* 141–156.

Clarke, G. N., Hawkins, W., Murphy, M., Sheeber, L. B., Lewinsohn, P. M., & Seeley, J. R. (1995). Targeted prevention of unipolar depressive disorder in an at-risk sample of high school adolescents: A randomized trial of group cognitive intervention. *Journal of Child and Adolescent Psychiatry, 32,* 312–321.

Clarke, G. N., Rohde, P., Lewinsohn, P. M., Hops, H., & Seeley, J. R. (1999). Cognitive-behavioral treatment of adolescent depression: Efficacy of acute group treatment and booster sessions. *Journal of the American Academy of Child and Adolescent Psychiatry, 38,* 272–279.

Clarke, G. N., Hornbrook, M., Lynch, F., Plen, M., Gale, J., Beardslee, W., et al. (2001). A randomized trial of a group cognitive intervention for preventing depression in adolescent offspring of depressed parents. *Archives of General Psychiatry, 58,* 1127–1134.

Cobham, V. E., Dadds, M., & Spence, S. H. (1998). The role of parental anxiety in the treatment of childhood anxiety. *Journal of Consulting and Clinical Psychology, 66,* 893–905.

Crick, N., & Dodge, K. (1994). A review and reformulation of social information-processing mechanisms in children's social adjustment. *Psychological Bulletin, 115,* 74–101.

de Haan, E., Hoogduin, K. A., Buitelaar, J., & Kejers, G. (1998). Behavior therapy versus clomipramine for the treatment of obsessive–compulsive disorder. *Journal of the American Academy of Child and Adolescent Psychiatry, 37,* 1022–1029.

Dodge, K. (1985). Attributional bias in aggressive children. In P. C. Kendall (Ed.), *Advances in cognitive-behavioral research and therapy* (Vol. 4). New York: Academic Press.

Duncan, B., & Miller, S. (2006). Treatment manuals do not improve outcomes. In J. C. Norcross, L. E. Butler, & R. F. Levant (Eds.), *Evidence-based practices in mental health.* Washington, DC: American Psychological Association.

D'Zurilla, T. J., & Goldfried, M. R. (1971). Problem-solving and behavior modification. *Journal of Abnormal Psychology, 78,* 107–126.

D'Zurilla, T. J., & Nezu, A. M. (1999). *Problem-solving therapy: A social competence approach to clinical intervention.* (2nd ed.). New York: Springer.

Ellis, A., & Harper, R. (1975). *A new guide to rational living.* New York: Wilshire.

Feindler, E. L., & Ecton, R. B. (1986). *Adolescent anger control: Cognitive-behavioral techniques.* Elmsford, NY: Pergamon Press.

Flannery-Schroeder, E., Suveg, C., Safford, S., Kendall, P. C., & Webb, A. (2004). Comorbid externalizing disorders and child anxiety treatment outcomes. *Behaviour Change, 21,* 14–25.

Flannery-Schroeder, E. C., & Kendall, P. C. (2000). Group and individual cognitive-behavioral treatments for youth with anxiety disorders: A randomized controlled trial. *Cognitive Therapy and Research, 24,* 251–278.

Ginsburg, G. S., & Silverman, W. K. (1996). Gender role orientation and fearfulness in children with anxiety disorders. *Journal of Anxiety Disorders, 14,* 57–67.

Goldstein, S. (1995). *Understanding and managing children's classroom behavior.* New York: Wiley.

Goldstein, S., & Goldstein, M. (1998). *Managing attention deficit hyperactivity disorder in children: A guide for practitioners.* New York: Wiley.

Harter, S. (1982). A developmental perspective on some parameters of self-regulation in children. In P. Karoly & F. H. Kanfer (Eds.), *Self-management and behavior change: From theory to practice* (pp. 165–204). New York: Pergamon Press.

Heimberg, R. G., Dodge, C. S., Hope, D. A., Kennedy, C. R., Zollo, L. J., & Becker, R. J. (1990). Cognitive behavioral group treatment for social phobia: Comparison with a credible placebo control. *Cognitive Therapy and Research, 14,* 1–23.

Henggeler, S., & Borduin, C. (1990). *Family therapy and beyond: A multisystemic approach to treating the behavior problems of children and adolescents.* Pacific Grove, CA: Brooks/Cole.

Herschell, A., McNeil, C., & McNeil, D. (2004). Clinical child psychology's progress in disseminating empirically supported treatments. *Clinical Psychology: Science and Practice, 11,* 267–288.

Hibbs, E. D., & Jensen, P. S. (Eds.). (2005). *Psychosocial treatments for child and adolescent disorders: Empirically based strategies for clinical practice* (2nd ed.). Washington, DC: American Psychological Association.

Hinshaw, S. P. (2006). Treatment for children and adolescents with attention-deficit/hyperactivity disorder. In P. Kendall (Ed.), *Child and adolescent therapy: Cognitive-behavioral procedures* (3rd ed., pp. 82–113). New York: Guilford Press.

Hinshaw, S., Klein, R., & Abikoff, H. (2002). Nonpharmacologic treatments and their combination with medication. In P. E. Nathan & J. M. Gorman (Eds.), *A guide to treatments that work* (2nd ed., pp. 3–23). New York: Oxford University Press.

Howard, B., Chu, B. C., Krain, A. L., Marrs-Garcia, M. A., & Kendall, P. C. (2000). *Cognitive-behavioral family therapy for anxious children: Therapist manual* (2nd ed.). Ardmore, PA: Workbook Publishing.

Hwang, W. C., Wood, J. J., & Lin, K. H. (2006). Cognitive-behavioral therapy with Chinese Americans: Research, theory, and clinical practice. *Cognitive and Behavioral Practice, 13,* 293–303.

Kahn, J. S., Kehle, T. J., Jenson, W. R., & Clark, E. (1990). Comparison of cognitive-behavioral, relaxation, and self-modeling interventions for depression among middle-school students. *School Psychology Review, 19,* 196–208.

Kaslow, N. J., & Thompson, M. P. (1998). Applying the criteria for empirically supported treatments to studies of psychosocial interventions for child and adolescent depression. *Journal of Clinical Child Psychology, 27,* 146–155.

Kazdin, A. (2005). *Parent management training: Treatment for oppositional, aggressive, and antisocial behavior in children and adolescents.* New York: Oxford University Press.

Kazdin, A. E., Bass, D., Siegel, T., & Thomas, C. (1989). Cognitive-behavioral therapy and relationship therapy in the treatment of children referred for antisocial behavior. *Journal of Consulting and Clinical Psychology, 57,* 522–535.

Kazdin, A. E., & Crowley, M. J. (1997). Moderators of treatment outcome in cognitively based treatment of antisocial children. *Cognitive Therapy and Research, 21,* 185–207.

Kazdin, A. E., Esveldt-Dawson, K., French, N. H., & Unis, A. S. (1987a). Effects of parent management training and problem-solving skills training combined in the treatment of antisocial child behavior. *Journal of the American Academy of Child and Adolescent Psychiatry, 26,* 416–424.

Kazdin, A. E., Esveldt-Dawson, K., French, N. H., & Unis, A. S. (1987b). Problem-solving skills training and relationship therapy in the treatment of antisocial child behavior. *Journal of Consulting and Clinical Psychology, 55,* 76–85.

Kazdin, A. E., & Kendall, P. C. (1998). Current progress and future plans for developing effective treatments: Comments and perspectives. *Journal of Clinical Child Psychology, 27,* 217–226.

Kazdin, A. E., Siegel, T. C., & Bass, D. (1992). Cognitive problem-solving skills training and parent management training in the treatment of antisocial behavior in children. *Journal of Consulting and Clinical Psychology, 60,* 733–747.

Kazdin, A. E., & Weisz, J. R. (1998). Identifying and developing empirically supported child and adolescent treatments. *Journal of Consulting and Clinical Psychology, 66,* 19–36.

Kazdin, A. E., & Weisz, J. R. (Eds.). (2003). *Evidence-based psychotherapies for children and adolescents.* New York: Guilford Press.

Kazdin, A. E., & Whitley, M. (2006). Comorbidity, case complexity, and effects of evidence-based treatment for children referred for disruptive behavior. *Journal of Consulting and Clinical Psychology, 74,* 455–467.

Kendall, P. C. (1992). *Coping Cat workbook.* Ardmore, PA: Workbook Publishing.

Kendall, P. C. (1993). Cognitive-behavioral therapies with youth: Guiding theory, current status, and emerging developments. *Journal of Consulting and Clinical Psychology, 61,* 235–247.

Kendall, P. C. (Ed.). (2000). *Child and adolescent therapy: Cognitive-behavioral procedures* (2nd ed.). New York: Guilford Press.

Kendall, P. C. (Ed.). (2006). *Child and adolescent therapy: Cognitive-behavioral procedures* (3rd ed.). New York: Guilford Press.

Kendall, P. C., & Beidas, R. S. (2007). Smoothing the trail for dissemination of evidence-based practices for youth: Flexibility within fidelity. *Professional Psychology: Research and Practice, 38,* 13–20.

Kendall, P. C., & Braswell, L. (1993). *Cognitive behavioral therapy for impulsive children* (2nd ed.) New York: Guilford Press.

Kendall, P. C., & Chambless, D. (Eds.). (1998). Empirically supported psychological therapies, *Journal of Consulting and Clinical Psychology, 66* [Special issue].

Kendall, P. C., Chansky, T. E., Kane, M., Kane, R., Kortlander, E., Ronan, K., et al. (1992). *Anxiety disorders in youth: Cognitive-behavioral interventions.* Needham Heights, MA: Allyn & Bacon.

Kendall, P. C., Choudhury, M. S., Hudson, J. L., & Webb, A. (2002). *The C.A.T. Project Manual: Manual for the individual cognitive-behavioral treatment of adolescents with anxiety disorders.* Ardmore, PA: Workbook Publishing.

Kendall, P. C., & Chu, B. C. (2000). Retrospective self-reports of therapist flexibility in a manual-based treatment for youths with anxiety disorders. *Journal of Clinical Child Psychology, 29,* 209–220.

Kendall, P. C., Chu, B., Gifford, A., Hayes, C., & Nauta, M. (1998). Breathing life into a manual. *Cognitive and Behavioral Practice, 5,* 177–198.

Kendall, P. C., Chu, B. C., Pimentel, S. S., & Choudhury, M. (2000). Treating anxiety disorders in youth. In P. C. Kendall (Ed.), *Child and adolescent therapy: Cognitive-behavioral procedures* (2nd ed., pp. 235–290). New York: Guilford Press.

Kendall, P. C., Flannery-Schroeder, E., Panichelli-Mindel, S. M., Southam-Gerow, M., Henin, A., & Warman, M. J. (1997). Therapy for youth with anxiety disorders: A second randomized clinical trial. *Journal of Consulting and Clinical Psychology, 65*, 366–380.

Kendall, P. C., & Hedtke, K. (2006a). *Cognitive-behavioral therapy for anxious children: Therapist manual* (3rd ed.). Ardmore, PA: Workbook Publishing.

Kendall, P. C., & Hedtke, K. (2006b). *The Coping Cat Workbook* (2nd ed.). Ardmore, PA: Workbook Publishing.

Kendall, P. C., & Khanna, M. (2008a). *CBT4CBT: Computer-based training to be a cognitive-behavioral therapist (for anxiety in youth)*. Ardmore, PA: Workbook Publishing.

Kendall, P. C., & Khanna, M. (2008b). *Camp Cope-A-Lot: The Coping Cat CD.* Ardmore, PA: Workbook Publishing.

Kendall, P. C., & McDonald, J. P. (1993). Cognition in the psychopathology of youth and implications for treatment. In K. S. Dobson & P. C. Kendall (Eds.), *Psychopathology and cognition* (pp. 387–427). San Diego: Academic Press.

Kendall, P. C., Robin, J., Hedtke, K., Suveg, C., Flannery-Schroeder, E., & Gosch, E. (2005). Considering CBT with anxious youth?: Think exposures. *Cognitive and Behavioral Practice, 12*, 136–148.

Kendall, P. C., Stark, K. D., & Adam, T. (1990). Cognitive deficit or cognitive distortion in childhood depression. *Journal of Abnormal Child Psychology, 18*, 255–270.

Kendall, P. C., & Suveg, C. (2006). Treating anxiety disorders in youth. In P. Kendall (Ed.), *Child and adolescent therapy: Cognitive-behavioral procedures* (3rd ed., pp. 243–294). New York: Guilford Press.

Kendall, P. C., & Suveg, C. (Eds.). (2007). *Clinical Psychology: Science and Practice, 14* [Special issue].

Kendall, P. C., & Treadwell, K. (2007). The role of self-statements as a mediator in treatment for youth with anxiety disorders. *Journal of Consulting and Clinical Psychology, 75*, 380–389.

Kettlewell, P., Morford, M. E., & Hoover, H. (2005). *Evidence-based treatment: What is it and how can it help children* [Pennsylvania Child and Adolescent Service System Program]. Pennsylvania State University.

Kleiner, L., Marshall, W., & Spevack, M. (1987). Training in problem-solving and exposure treatment for agoraphobics with panic attacks. *Journal of Anxiety Disorders, 1*, 219–238.

Koeppen, A. S. (1974). Relaxation training for children. *Elementary School Guidance and Counseling, 9*, 14–26.

Kroll, L., Harrington, R., Jayson, D., Fraser, J., & Gowers, S. (1996). Pilot study of continuation cognitive-behavioral therapy for major depression in adolescent psychiatric patient. *Journal of the American Academy of Child and Adolescent Psychiatry, 35*, 1156–1161.

Lambert, M. (1998). Manual-based treatment and clinical practice: Hangman of life or promising development? *Clinical Psychology: Science and Practice, 5*, 391–395.

Lewinsohn, P. M., Clarke, G. N., Hops, H., & Andrews, J. (1990). Cognitive-behavioral group treatment of depression in adolescents. *Behavior Therapy, 21*, 385–401.

Lewinsohn, P. M., Clarke, G. N., & Rohde, P. (1994). Psychological approaches to the treatment of depression in adolescents. In W. M. Reynolds & H. F. Johnston (Eds.), *Handbook of depression in children and adolescents* (pp. 309–344). New York: Plenum Press.

Lewinsohn, P. M., Clarke, G. N., Rohde, P., Hops, H., & Seeley, J. R. (1996). A course in coping: A cognitive-behavioral approach to the treatment of adolescent depression. In E. D. Hibbs & P. S. Jensen (Eds.), *Child and adolescent disorders: Empirically based strategies for clinical practice* (pp. 109–135). Washington, DC: American Psychological Association.

Lewinsohn, P. M., Rohde, P., Hops, H., & Clarke, G. (1991). *Leader's manual for parent groups: Adolescent coping with depression.* Eugene, OR: Castalia Press.

Livingston-Van Noppen, B., Rasmussen, S. I., Eisen, J., & McCartney, L. (1990). Family function and treatment in obsessive–compulsive disorder. In M. A. Jenike, L. Baer, & W. E. Minichiello (Eds.), *Obsessive–compulsive disorders: Theory and management* (pp. 118–131). Littleton, MA: Year Book Medical Publishers.

Lochman, J. E. (1992). Cognitive-behavioral intervention with aggressive boys: Three-year follow-up and preventive effects. *Journal of Consulting and Clinical Psychology, 60,* 426–434.

Lochman, J. E., & Burch, P. R., Curry, J. F., & Lampron, L. B. (1984). Treatment and generalization effects of cognitive-behavioral and goal-setting interventions with aggressive boys. *Journal of Consulting and Clinical Psychology, 52,* 915–916.

Lochman, J. E., & Curry, J. F. (1986). Effects of social problem-solving training and self-instruction training with aggressive boys. *Journal of Consulting and Clinical Psychology, 5,* 159–164.

Lochman, J. E., Lampron, L. B., Gemmer, T. C., Harris, R., & Wyckoff, G. M. (1989). Teacher consultation and cognitive-behavioral interventions with aggressive boys. *Psychology in the Schools, 26,* 179–188.

Lochman, J. E., Powell, N. R., Whidby, J. M., & Fitzgerald, D. P. (2006). Aggressive children: Cognitive-behavioral assessment and treatment. In P. Kendall (Ed.), *Child and adolescent therapy: Cognitive-behavioral procedures* (3rd ed., pp. 33–81). New York: Guilford Press.

Lochman, J., & Wells, K. (2002). The Coping Power Program at the middle-school transition: Universal and indicated prevention effects. *Psychology of Addictive Behaviors, 16,* S40–S54.

Lochman, J., & Wells, K. (2004). The Coping Power Program for preadolescent aggressive boys and their parents: Outcome effects at the 1-year follow-up. *Journal of Consulting and Clinical Psychology, 72,* 571–578.

Lochman, J., Wells, K., & Murray, M. (2007). The Coping Power Program: Preventative intervention at the middle school transition. In P. Tolan, J. Szapocznik, & S. Sambrano (Eds.), *Preventing substance abuse: 3 to 14* (pp. 185–210). Washington, DC: American Psychological Association.

Lochman, J. E., White, K. J., & Wayland, K. K. (1991). Cognitive-behavioral assessment and treatment with aggressive children. In P. C. Kendall (Ed.), *Child and adolescent therapy: Cognitive-behavioral procedures* (pp. 25–65). New York: Guilford Press.

Lonigan, C., & Elbert, J. (Eds.). (1998). Empirically-supported psychosocial interventions for children [Special issue]. *Journal of Clinical Child Psychology, 27.*

Mahoney, M. J. (1977). Reflections in the cognitive-learning trend in psychotherapy. *American Psychologist, 32,* 5–18.

March, J. (1995). Behavioral psychotherapy for children and adolescents with obsessive–compulsive disorder: A review of the literature and recommendation for treatment. *Journal of the American Academy of Child and Adolescent Psychiatry, 34,* 7–18.

March, J. (2004). The Treatment for Adolescents with Depression Study (TADS): Short-term effectiveness and safety outcomes. *Journal of the American Medical Association, 292,* 807–820.

March, J. S., Frances, A., Carpenter, D., & Kahn, D. (1997). The expert consensus guidelines series: Treatment of obsessive–compulsive disorder. *Journal of Clinical Psychiatry, 58*(Suppl. 4), 1–72.

March, J. S., & Mulle, K. (1998). *OCD in children and adolescents: A cognitive-behavioral treatment manual.* New York: Guilford Press.

March, J., Mulle, K., & Herbel, B. (1994). Behavioral psychotherapy for children and adolescents with obsessive–compulsive disorder: An open trial of a new protocol-driven treatment package. *Journal of the American Academy of Child and Adolescent Psychiatry, 33,* 333–341.

Masia-Warner, C., Nangle, D. W., & Hansen, D. J. (2006). Bringing evidence-based child mental health services to the schools: General issues and specific populations. *Education and Treatment of Children, 29,* 165–172.

McDonald, L. (1993). Families and Schools Together (FAST). Final Report. Washington, DC: U.S. Department of Health and Human Services, Office of Human Development Services, Administration for Children and Families.

McDonald, L., Moberg, D. P., Brown, R., Rodriguez-Espiricueta, I., Flores, N. I., Burke, M. P., et al. (2006). After-school multifamily groups: A randomized controlled trial involving low-income, urban, Latino children. *Children and Schools, 28*(1), 25–34.

Meichenbaum, D. (1971). Examination of model characteristics in reducing avoidance behavior. *Journal of Personality and Social Psychology, 17,* 298–307.

Mendlowitz, S. L., Manassis, K., Bradley, S., Scapillato, D., Miezitis, S., & Shaw, B. F. (1999). Cognitive-behavioral group treatments in childhood anxiety disorders: The role of parental involvement. *Journal of the American Academy of Child and Adolescent Psychiatry, 38,* 1223–1229.

Morris, R. J., & Kratochwill, T. R. (1983). *Treating children's fears and phobias: A behavioral approach.* New York: Pergamon Press.

MTA Cooperative Group. (1999a). A 14-month randomized clinical trial of treatment strategies for attention-deficit/hyperactivity disorder. *Archives of General Psychiatry, 56,* 1073–1086.

MTA Cooperative Group. (1999b). Moderators and mediators of treatment response for children with attention-deficit/hyperactivity disorder. *Archives of General Psychiatry, 56,* 1088–1096.

Nock, M. K., Kazdin, A. E., Hiripi, E., & Kessler, R. C. (2007). Lifetime prevalence, correlates, and persistence of oppositional defiant disorder: Results from the National Comorbidity Survey Replication. *Journal of Child Psychology and Psychiatry, 48,* 703–713.

Ollendick, T. H., & Cerny, J. A. (1981). *Clinical behavior therapy with children.* New York: Plenum Press.

Ollendick, T. H., & Francis, G. (1988). Behavioral assessment and treatment of childhood phobias. *Behavior Modification, 12,* 165–204.

Ollendick, T. H., & King, N. (1998). Empirically supported treatments for children with phobic and anxiety disorders: Current status. *Journal of Clinical Child Psychology, 27,* 156–167.

Ollendick, T. H., King, N. J., & Chorpita, B. F. (2006). Empirically supported treatments for children and adolescents. In P. C. Kendall (Ed.), *Child and adolescent therapy* (3rd ed., pp. 492–520). New York: Guilford Press.

Pediatric OCD Treatment Study Team. (2004). Cognitive-behavioral therapy, sertraline, and their combination for children and adolescents with obsessive–compulsive disorder: The Pediatric OCD Treatment Study (POTS) randomized controlled trial. *Journal of the American Medical Association, 292,* 1969–1976.

Piacentini, J. C., & Langely, A. K. (2004). Cognitive-behavioral therapy for children who have obsessive–compulsive disorder. *Journal of Clinical Psychology, 60,* 1181–1194.

Rabian, B., Peterson, R., Richters, J., & Jensen, P. (1993). Anxiety sensitivity among anxious children. *Journal of Clinical Child Psychology, 22,* 441–446.

Robin, A. L., & Schneider, M. (1974). *The turtle technique: An approach to self-control in the classroom.* Unpublished manuscript, State University of New York, Stony Brook.

Robin, A. L., Schneider, M., & Dolnick, M. (1976). The turtle technique: An extended case study of self-control in the classroom. *Psychology in the Schools, 13,* 449–453.

Rosenthal, T., & Bandura, A. (1978). Psychological model: Theory and practice. In S. L. Garfield & A. E. Bergin (Eds.), *Handbook of psychotherapy and behavior change* (2nd ed.). New York: Wiley.

Seligman, L. D., & Ollendick, T. H. (1998). Comorbidity of anxiety and depression in children and adolescents: An integrative review. *Clinical Child and Family Psychology Review, 1,* 125–144.

Shure, M. B., & Spivack, G. (1978). *Problem-solving techniques in childrearing.* San Francisco: Jossey-Bass.

Silverman, W. K., Ginsburg, G. S., & Kurtines, W. M. (1995). Clinical issues in treating children with anxiety and phobic disorders. *Cognitive and Behavioral Practice, 2,* 93–117.

Southam-Gerow, M. A., & Kendall, P. C. (2000). Emotion understanding in youth referred for treatment of anxiety disorders. *Journal of Clinical Child Psychology,*

Spivack, G., Platt, J. J., & Shure, M. B. (1976). *The problem-solving approach to adjustment.* San Francisco: Jossey-Bass.

Stark, K. D. (1990). *Childhood depression: School-based intervention.* New York: Guilford Press.

Stark, K. D., Hargrave, J., Sander, J., Custer, G., Schnnoebelen, S., Simpson, J., et al. (2006). Treatment of childhood depression: The ACTION treatment program. In P. Kendall (Ed.), *Child and adolescent therapy: Cognitive-behavioral procedures* (pp. 169–216). New York: Guilford Press.

Swanson, J., Kraemer, H. C., & Hinshaw, S. P. (2001). Clinical relevance of the primary findings of the MTA: Success rates based on severity of ADHD and ODD symptoms at the end of treatment. *Journal of the American Academy of Child and Adolescent Psychiatry, 40,* 168–179.

Suveg, C., Southam-Gerow, M., Goodman, K., & Kendall, P. C. (2007). The role of emotion theory and research in child therapy development. *Clinical Psychology: Science and Practice, 14,* 358–372.

TADS Team. (2007). The treatment for adolescents with depression study (TADS): Long term effectiveness and safety outcomes. *Archives of General Psychiatry, 64*, 1132–1144.

Waters, T. L., & Barrett, P. M. (2000) The role of the family in childhood obsessive-compulsive disorder. *Clinical Child and Family Psychology Review, 3*, 173–184.

Weiner, B. (1979). A theory of motivation of some classroom experience. *Journal of Educational Psychology, 71*, 3–25.

Weisz, J. (2004). *Psychotherapy for children and adolescents: Evidence-based treatments and case examples*. New York: Cambridge University Press.

Weisz, J., McCarty, C., & Valeri, S. (2006). Effects of psychotherapy for depression in children and adolescents: A meta-analysis. *Psychological Bulletin, 132*, 132–249.

Westen, D., Novotny, C., & Thompson-Brenner, H. (2004). The empirical status of empirically supported psychotherapies: Assumptions, findings, and reporting in controlled clinical trials. *Psychological Bulletin, 130*, 631–663.

Wilkes, T. C. R., Belsher, G., Rush, A. J., & Frank, E. (1994). *Cognitive therapy for depressed adolescents*. New York: Guilford Press.

Wood, J. J., Piacentini, J. C., Southam-Gerow, M. A., Chu, B. C., & Sigman, M. (2006). Family cognitive behavioral therapy for child anxiety disorders. *Journal of American Academy of Child and Adolescent Psychiatry, 45*(3), 314–321.

Woodward, L. J., & Fergusson, D. M. (2001). Life course outcomes of young people with anxiety disorders in adolescence. *Journal of the American Academy of Child and Adolescent Psychiatry, 40*, 1086–1093.

Zentall, S. S. (1995). Modifying classroom tasks and environments. In S. Goldstein (Ed.), *Understanding and managing children's classroom behavior* (pp. 356–374). New York: Wiley.

CHAPTER 13

Cognitive-Behavioral Couple Therapy

Donald H. Baucom
Norman B. Epstein
Jennifer S. Kirby
Jaslean J. LaTaillade

Cognitive-behavioral couple therapy (CBCT) emerged in the early 1980s, although it had roots in therapeutic approaches and research traditions with longer histories. The primary precursor for CBCT was behavioral couple therapy (BCT), which developed during the late 1960s as couple therapists applied learning principles to understanding and treating distressed relationships. Stuart (1969) applied the social exchange theory (Thibaut & Kelley, 1959) concept that in satisfying relationships, the ratio of positive behaviors that partners reciprocally exchange relative to negative behaviors tends to be high. In contrast, distressed couples tend to exchange relatively few positive behaviors relative to the negative behaviors that occur. Stuart also used operant conditioning principles to help partners reinforce positive acts. To create a more favorable ratio of positive to negative behavior between partners, Stuart (1969) asked each individual to generate a list of positive behaviors that he or she desired from the partner and coached partners to reach an agreement to reward each other with tokens for enacting the desired behaviors. Subsequently, behavioral couple therapists substituted written contracts for such a "token economy" to institute changes in behavioral exchanges between partners, and they also added communication and problem-solving skills training (Jacobson & Margolin, 1979; Stuart, 1980).

Liberman (1970) emphasized an extensive behavioral analysis of the interactional patterns associated with the presenting problems of distressed couples and families, such as unintentional reinforcement of an individual's undesirable behavior. Based on social learning principles (Bandura & Walters, 1963), Liberman (1970) also added the strategies of therapist modeling of alternative interpersonal communication patterns and client rehearsal of new role behaviors to the treatment of dysfunctional couple and family relationships (Falloon, 1991).

Operant conditioning research, and associated treatments to modify children's behavior, also contributed to the development of BCT. Patterson (1974) conducted studies of "coercive family systems," in which both parents and children use aversive behavior to try to influence each other's actions. They taught parents to use reinforcers and punishers selectively to increase a child's desired behaviors and decrease negative behavior. Weiss, Hops, and Patterson (1973) applied these learning-based principles and methods to the treatment of distressed couples. They also established a tradition of empiricism in BCT that involves systematic collection of data concerning couples' behavioral strengths and problems, as well as data regarding the degree to which partners' specific behaviors change as a function of treatment.

The first BCT treatment manuals based on social exchange and learning principles were published in the late 1970s and early 1980s (Jacobson & Margolin, 1979; Stuart, 1980). On the one hand, they emphasized increasing partners' relationship satisfaction through behavioral contracts that involve agreements to increase specific desired behaviors and decrease specific negative acts. On the other hand, they emphasized improving partners' skills for interacting in ways that generate feelings of intimacy, provide mutual social support, and resolve conflicts through constructive communication.

The BCT model involves an idiographic functional analysis of the patterns of reciprocal and circular sequences that have developed in each couple's relationship and are operating currently. The influences of each individual's prior learning experiences (e.g., in family-of-origin relationships) are considered. The emphasis in BCT tends to be on a functional analysis of partners' current interaction patterns, however, and the use of specific actions to improve and assess behavioral change (LaTaillade & Jacobson, 1995).

Numerous outcome investigations have found that BCT is effective (Baucom, Shoham, Mueser, Daiuto, & Stickle, 1998; Hahlweg, Baucom, & Markman, 1988), although some studies have indicated that increases in partners' exchanges of positive behavior and improved communication skills have had limited impact on relationship satisfaction (Halford, Sanders, & Behrens, 1993; Iverson & Baucom, 1988). In addition, other couple therapy approaches that do not emphasize the modification of behavioral exchanges and skills training have been found to be as efficacious as BCT in alleviating marital distress, suggesting that behavioral interventions may not be necessary or sufficient for effective treatment of relationship problems (Baucom, Epstein, & Gordon, 2000; Baucom et al., 1998). Furthermore, that research has indicated marked discrepancies between partners' perceptions of the relationship behaviors highlights the subjectivity of individuals' experiences (Fincham, Bradbury, & Scott, 1990). It became clear that a behavioral skills deficit model was limited in the treatment of couple distress. Therefore, an approach that included partners' subjective cognitions about their own and each other's behavior was needed (Baucom & Epstein, 1990; Epstein & Baucom, 2002; Fincham et al., 1990). It was this recognition that helped to set the stage for the development of CBCT.

Influences of Cognitive Therapies on the Development of Cognitive-Behavioral Couple Therapy

A second major influence on CBCT was the development of cognitive models for understanding and treating individual psychopathology (Beck, Rush, Shaw, & Emery, 1979; Ellis, 1962; Meichenbaum, 1977). These models emphasize that an individual's emotional and behavioral responses to life events often are mediated by idiosyncratic interpretations that may be distorted or inappropriate. Cognitive therapists began to apply their model to relationship problems, and in turn behavioral couple therapists began to integrate cognition into the BCT model (Epstein, 1982; Margolin & Weiss, 1978). Cognitive therapists whose roots were primarily in individual therapy (e.g., Beck, 1988; Dattilio & Padesky, 1990; Ellis, Sichel, Yeager, DiMattia, & DiGiuseppe, 1989) have employed some BCT concepts and methods, such as communication skills training, but their versions of CBCT tend to emphasize cognitive restructuring with each partner much more than targeting the dyad's problematic behavioral interaction patterns and emotional responses on which we focus in our approach.

CBCT has evolved, and cognitions, behaviors, and emotions are given attention in assessment and intervention (Baucom & Epstein, 1990; Epstein & Baucom, 2002; Rathus & Sanderson, 1999). Consequently, CBCT therapists help couples become more active observers and evaluators of their own cognitions, work to modify negative behavioral interactions to foster more positive cognitions and emotions about each other, and address partners' problems with either inhibited or unregulated emotional experiences to create a more satisfying atmosphere within the couple relationship (Epstein & Baucom, 2002). Thus, CBCT has developed a systemic quality in which the mutual impacts of two partners' cognitions, behaviors, and emotions are assessed and targeted for change to improve relationship quality.

Influences of Social Cognition Research on Cognitive-Behavioral Couple Therapy

CBCT also has been shaped by information-processing and social cognition research (Baldwin, 2005; Fiske & Taylor, 1991; Fletcher & Fitness, 1996; Noller, Beach, & Osgarby, 1997). There has been a focus on the *attribu-*

tions that individuals make about determinants of positive and negative events in their relationships and relatively stable *schemas* (e.g., the concept of a "caring spouse") that individuals develop from past relationship experiences but then apply to understand current relationship events. Evidence from research regarding information-processing errors also has had great relevance for understanding the sources of relationship distress. During the 1980s and 1990s, couple therapists increasingly assessed and intervened with the forms of cognition that emerged from research as important influences on couples' relationship adjustment (Baucom, Epstein, & Rankin, 1995; Epstein & Baucom, 2002).

Recent Enhancements of Cognitive-Behavioral Couple Therapy

CBCT recently has been expanded to include other phenomena concerning intimate relationships. First, we now emphasize broad "macro" level interaction patterns and core relationship themes, such as differences between partners' desired levels of closeness and intimacy, in addition to discrete "micro" relational events (Epstein & Baucom, 2002). Second, in addition to a focus on a couple's cognitive processing and behavioral interactions, our enhanced CBCT also addresses personality, motives, and other more stable individual characteristics that each partner brings to the couple relationship, and examines how these factors influence partners' behavior and interpretations of events in their relationship. Because both normative individual differences and psychopathology influence relationship satisfaction and functioning (e.g., Christensen & Heavey, 1993; Karney & Bradbury, 1995), they have been incorporated into enhanced CBCT.

Third, enhanced CBCT has also been influenced by systems and ecological models of relationship functioning (e.g., Bronfenbrenner, 1989) to focus on external and environmental stressors (e.g., demands of work and children; racial discrimination) that place significant pressure on a couple's ability to adapt, or that can be enlisted to a facilitate couple's adaptation to demands (Epstein & Baucom, 2002). Fourth, whereas emotions in BCT were given secondary status and viewed as the result of partners' relationship behaviors and cognitions, enhanced CBCT directly addresses both the difficulties that some partners have in experiencing and/or expressing emotions and others' problems with regulating negative emotions. This emphasis on emotion is consistent with the recent trend toward focusing on emotional processes in couple therapy (Fruzzetti, 2006; Johnson, 2004; Johnson & Denton, 2002; Kirby & Baucom, 2007a, 2007b). Fifth, whereas CBCT traditionally has focused on the assessment and modification of negative behavior, cognition, and emotion, enhanced CBCT places greater emphasis on efforts to increase positives, such as mutual social support (Cutrona, 1996; Pasch, Bradbury, & Davila, 1997), to help couples experience optimum fulfillment from their relationships.

THE HEALTHY/WELL-FUNCTIONING
VERSUS THE DYSFUNCTIONAL COUPLE RELATIONSHIP

In contrast to traditional BCT and CBCT foci on the couple as the unit of analysis in defining the couple's well-being, enhanced CBCT takes a broader contextual perspective that considers characteristics of the individual partners, the couple, and the couple's environment (Baucom, Epstein, LaTaillade, & Kirby, 2008; Baucom, Epstein, & Sullivan, 2004; Epstein & Baucom, 2002). A healthy relationship contributes to the growth and well-being of both partners; the partners interact constructively as a dyad, and the couple adapts effectively to demands from the physical and social environment.

A healthy couple relationship fosters each partner's growth, development, well-being, and needs fulfillment. The relationship should serve as a source of both instrumental and emotional support to individual partners (Cutrona, Suhr, & MacFarlane, 1990; Pasch, Bradbury, & Sullivan, 1997). Partners in a healthy relationship generally perceive each other in positive ways and contribute to the well-being of the relationship by working together to communicate and resolve problems effectively, develop and maintain intimacy, engage in mutually pleasurable activities, and reciprocate positive behavior (Epstein & Baucom, 2002). They adapt to both normative (e.g., pregnancy and childbirth) and non-normative (e.g., unemployment) stressors through collaborative efforts. Their constructive coping is aided by their positive connections to sources of support in their social and physical environment, such as their families and extended kin networks, community agencies, and social institutions (Baucom et al., 2004). In turn, the partners may strengthen their own relationship by contributing to their community or broader society; for example, by working for a charitable organization (Baucom et al., 2008).

As noted earlier, the health and development of a couple's relationship depends on their ability to adapt to normative and non-normative demands (e.g., transitioning to parenthood; Carter & McGoldrick, 1999). On the one hand, adaptation to life demands can be compromised, and the quality of the relationship can deteriorate as a result of vulnerabilities at the individual level (e.g., clinical depression) and couple level (e.g., a tendency to avoid discussions of problems). On the other hand, the partners' individual, dyadic, and environmental resources can result in maintenance or enhancement of their relationship quality in the face of stressors (Epstein & Baucom, 2002).

Predictors of Relationship Distress

The expanded CBCT model of relationship discord draws on research from a number of sources. For example, research indicates that compared to happy couples, distressed couples are characterized by a high frequency of reciprocal negative or punishing exchanges between partners, a relative scarcity of positive outcomes that each partner provides for the other, and deficits in communication and problem-solving skills (Gottman, 1994; Jacobson & Margolin, 1979; Karney & Bradbury, 1995; Weiss & Heyman, 1997). Research has also demonstrated that partners in distressed relationships are more likely to notice selectively or "track" each other's negative behavior (Jacobson, Waldron, & Moore, 1980), make negative attributions about the determinants of such behavior (e.g., that the partner has malicious intent; Baucom & Epstein, 1990; Fincham et al., 1990), hold unrealistic beliefs about intimate relationships (Eidelson & Epstein, 1982), and be dissatisfied with the ways that their personal standards for the relationship (e.g., regarding the amount of time and effort that they should put into their relationship) are met (Baucom, Epstein, Rankin, & Burnett, 1996). Furthermore, Weiss (1980) described a process of "sentiment override," in which partners develop global negative evaluations and emotions toward each other over time as they continue to behave destructively toward each other. Once established, sentiment override can contribute to partners' negative expectancies or predictions that the other person will engage in negative acts, and it can increase the likelihood that they will behave negatively toward each other (Baucom & Epstein, 1990). These negative behavioral, cognitive, and affective patterns can lead distressed couples into a self-maintaining process of discord.

Enhanced CBCT recognizes that both the *process* of the interactions between members of a couple and the themes in the *content* of couple conflicts influence relationship quality. Relationship discordant themes often involve differences between two partners' personal needs and motives. Epstein and Baucom (2002) identified several needs and motives that often become sources of conflict and distress in couples' relationships. "Communally oriented," or relationship-focused needs, include *affiliation* with other people to share activities; *intimacy,* or deep sharing of personal experiences with one's partner; *altruism* toward one's partner and others; and *succorance,* or being nurtured by one's partner. "Individually oriented," needs include *autonomy,* or the freedom to make choices and function on one's own; *control* over one's life and environment, and *achievement.* All of these communally and individually oriented needs can serve as sources of personal satisfaction. Differences in partners' needs, even between two emotionally healthy individuals, contributes to relationship distress (Epstein & Baucom, 2002).

For example, partners who differ in their need for intimacy might make negative attributions about each other (e.g., "She doesn't like to share her personal feelings with me because she doesn't love me"), behave negatively toward each other (he pressures her for self-disclosure and she consequently withdraws), and become emotionally upset with each other. The enhanced CBCT model refers to the distress that occurs when individuals' needs are unmet as "primary distress." When partners respond to each other in maladaptive ways in response to their unmet needs (e.g., by withdrawing or verbally abusing each other), these negative interaction patterns can create "secondary distress" and become relationship problems that may require therapeutic intervention (Baucom et al., 2004; Epstein & Baucom, 2002).

Psychopathology or long-term, unresolved individual issues in one or both partners also can create stress within a couple's relationship by interfering with needs fulfillment. For example, one partner's major depression can limit the couple's opportunities for intimacy. Similarly, if a member of a couple was abandoned in a prior relationship, he or she may experience chronic unmet needs for succorance, or make frequent requests for attention and reassurance from a partner that can result in conflict and secondary relationship distress. Finally, enhanced CBCT assesses how an accretion of environmental stressors can overwhelm a couple's coping and result in a relationship crisis that involves disorganized functioning and severe distress (Schlesinger & Epstein, 2007).

The Impact of Gender and Cultural Factors on Relationship Functioning

Partners' gender, ethnicity, and cultural backgrounds can influence the effects of individual, couple, and environmental factors on the couple's relationship. For example, distressed couples commonly exhibit a pattern in which one partner pursues the other for interaction, while the other partner withdraws (Christensen, 1988; Christensen & Heavey, 1990, 1993). Females are more likely to be in the demanding role, whereas males more often withdraw, perhaps due to females' tendency to be more oriented than males toward achieving intimacy through mutual self-disclosure, as well as females' attempts to achieve equity in relationships in which males frequently have more power (Prager & Buhrmester, 1998). There also is a gender difference in partners' processing of information about their relationship; whereas females are more likely than males to consider both partners' contributions to couple interaction patterns ("relationship schematic processing"), males are more likely to focus on linear effects that each partner has on the relationship ("individual schematic processing") (Baucom, 1999; Rankin, Baucom, Clayton, & Daiuto, 1995; Sullivan & Baucom, 2005).

Although gender differences have been addressed increasingly in CBCT, the potential effects of racial, ethnic, and cultural issues on relationship functioning and treatment have received little attention. Different rates of divorce across ethnic groups have been attributed to stressors that disproportionately affect ethnic/minority couples, including economic instability, joblessness, exposure to poverty and violence, and continued experiences of racism and discrimination (LaTaillade, 2006). Couples' exposure to such stressors tends to be associated with both concurrent relationship distress and longitudinal declines in marital quality (Bradbury & Karney, 2004). For example, ethnic/minority couples may turn their frustration with racism and other social stressors against each other, blame each other for relationship problems, and feel powerless to effect change. The contextual focus of enhanced CBCT prevents adoption of a "value and culture free" approach to assessment and treatment, and instead identifies themes that characterize conflict in ethnically diverse couple relationships (e.g., balancing power and respect), and empowers couples to build on their strengths and resources (Kelly, 2006; Kelly & Iwamasa, 2005; LaTaillade, 2006).

THE PRACTICE OF COUPLE THERAPY

The Structure of the Therapy Process

CBCT has evolved over time and is practiced somewhat differently by various practitioners. The following description of the implementation of CBCT is presented within the context of our approach, which emphasizes recent enhancements described earlier. CBCT tends to be implemented as a brief therapy approach, with a range from several to over 20 weekly sessions, although the therapist may schedule "booster" sessions to help partners maintain skills for adaptive behavioral interactions, cognitions, and expression of emotions. The length of treatment varies depending on the severity of functional problems in the individuals (e.g., a personality disorder or severe psychopathology) and/or couple (e.g., infidelity) (Epstein & Baucom, 2002; Snyder, Baucom, & Gordon, 2007). The therapist and couple set goals at both the "micro" level (e.g., instituting a weekly "date night" for the couple) and "macro" level (e.g., increasing the couple's overall level of intimacy). They also collaborate in designing homework assignments that the partners are to complete between sessions to replace ingrained dysfunctional interaction patterns with new constructive ones through repeated rehearsal. The therapist attempts to reduce the couple's noncompliance through an exploration of cognitions that the partners may have about the homework (e.g., that it is too time-consuming or contrived).

Joining with the Couple and Establishing a Treatment Alliance

Joining simultaneously with two members of a couple can involve some challenges that therapists do not face when conducting individual therapy (Epstein & Baucom, 2002, 2003). First, each partner may desire to convince the therapist that the other person is responsible for the couple's problems. It is important that the therapist demonstrate that he or she does not side with either member of the couple and takes each person's concerns seriously. Second, one or both partners may be concerned about the safety of participating in conjoint sessions, in anticipation of being verbally or physically attacked by their partner during or after sessions. Therapists must screen couples for ongoing or potential physical violence and forgo conjoint therapy if there is apparent risk. Therapists also establish behavioral guidelines for constructive couple interaction during sessions and intervene quickly to block aversive behavior (Epstein & Baucom, 2002, 2003). Third, partners may be concerned that therapy will change relationship patterns that have been reinforcing for them; for example, an individual may anticipate that his or her power in the relationship will be reduced if the couple moves toward egalitarian problem solving. The therapist must alleviate such concerns and help the couple to develop new rewards for the person to replace those that will be lost when the couple institutes the therapeutic changes (see Epstein & Baucom, 2002, 2003).

Sessions with Individual Partners and with the Couple

Assessments include both a couple interview focused on the couple's functioning and an individual interview with each partner. The individual assessment focuses on family-of-origin history, other significant relationship experiences, educational and employment history, areas of personal strength, and physical and mental health history (Epstein & Baucom, 2002). The therapist tells the partners that all information they provide will be kept confidential from each other, although he or she may encourage partners to share information with each other regarding past experiences that might influence the couple relationship. If an individual reports physical abuse by the current partner, the therapist typically does not share that information with the partner, in order to protect the individual from additional abuse. If the therapist judges that it is risky to conduct couple therapy, however, then he or she tells the couple that they are not ready for joint therapy and that each partner could benefit from individual sessions focused on conflict resolution, perhaps followed later by joint sessions. Protection of each individual's physical and psychological well-being is given top priority in the decision regarding the best modality for intervention (Epstein & Baucom, 2002; Holtzworth-Munroe, Marshall, Meehan, & Rehman, 2002). In contrast to our confidentiality regarding reports of physical abuse, we advise couples that we cannot share in a secret about ongoing infidelity, because to do so would result in therapist collusion in secrecy with the unfaithful partner.

Following the initial assessment, most CBCT sessions are conducted with both partners, because CBCT focuses on direct observation and modification of patterns *as they are occurring*. One or more individual sessions may be conducted with a member of a couple to address a problem that interferes with couple interventions, such as when an individual who has difficulty regulating his or her emotional responses in the partner's presence is coached in anger management strategies. It is important to counteract any perceptions that the therapist views one partner as "the problem" in the relationship. Thus, if an individual session is held with one partner, at times it is helpful to schedule an individual session with the other partner, or to focus on contributions both people can make in improving their relationship.

The Role of the Therapist

During the assessment and the early stages of therapy, the therapist takes a didactic role, guiding and collaborating with the couple in setting therapy goals, and using cognitive-behavioral strategies to achieve those goals (Epstein & Baucom, 2002). The therapist provides rationales for interventions and homework assignments, models adaptive social skills, and coaches the partners to practice these skills both within and outside of sessions. The therapist also collaborates with the couple to set the agenda for each session and monitors the use of time to follow that agenda efficiently. He or she creates a safe and supportive environment in which each member of the couple can address challenging issues, maintaining supportive but firm control of sessions, for example, by interrupting inappropriate behaviors (Epstein & Baucom, 2002). Across sessions, the therapist gradually decreases his or her directiveness, so that partners can assume more responsibility to resolve their concerns by using the skills learned in therapy, design their own homework, and so forth (Baucom, Epstein, & LaTaillade, 2002).

Assessment and Treatment Planning

The primary goals of assessment are to (1) identify the concerns for which a couple has sought therapy; (2) clarify characteristics of the individuals, couple, and environment that contribute to their concerns; and (3) determine whether CBCT is appropriate to address the concerns. In addition, the therapist determines each partner's level of motivation to continue the relationship. The first two or three sessions are devoted to assessment, unless the couple is in a state of crisis, such as responding to abusive behavior or a partner's affair (Epstein & Baucom, 2002; LaTaillade & Jacobson, 1995). If the couple and therapist decide that conjoint therapy is not the best alternative, then they devise an alternative plan, such as individual therapy for one or both partners. The assessment of relationship strengths, as well as problems, often draws partners' attention to the positive aspects of their relationship and may instill hope that they can overcome the difficulties (Epstein & Baucom, 2002).

Assessment of the Individual Partners, Their Relationship, and Their Environment

The therapist assesses characteristics of the individual partners that may influence their current concerns, such as personality styles, psychopathology, subclinical character traits, communally and individually oriented needs, and effects that experiences in prior significant relationships have on their responses within the present relationship. Dyadic factors assessed include macro-level patterns (e.g., a consistent demand–withdraw pattern), as well as degrees of difference between partners' personality characteristics, needs, and values. Interpersonal and physical environmental factors that need to be assessed include demands from nuclear and extended family members, work pressures, stresses from community violence, or broader societal factors, such as racial or sexual discrimination, and economic stresses.

Assessment Methods

The initial assessment in CBCT typically involves clinical interviews with both the couple and the individual partners, direct observation of the couple's interaction patterns, and self-report questionnaires. *Joint interviews* include a relationship history (e.g., how the partners met, how they developed a deeper commitment, life events that influenced their relationship positively or negatively, any prior therapy) (Baucom & Epstein, 1990; Epstein & Baucom, 2002). The therapist explores influences of race, ethnicity, religion, and other aspects of culture (Hardy & Laszloffy, 2002; LaTaillade, 2006), as well as any acculturative stress that a couple may have experienced due to immigration. In addition to historical factors, the therapist inquires about partners' current relationship concerns, including individual, dyadic, and environmental factors that contribute to the presenting issues. The therapist inquires about the partners' perceptions of the presenting problems, attributions for causes of the problems, personal standards for how the relationship should function, and behavioral and emotional responses to the problems (Baucom et al., 1995; Epstein & Baucom, 2002). The joint interviews, which commonly require two or three sessions, also focus on relationship strengths and the partners' history of solving problems together. The therapist gives the partners the opportunity to express their concerns during the assessment sessions and engages in crisis intervention as needed to control apparent destructive exchanges.

The *individual interviews* with each partner are conducted with the confidentiality guidelines described earlier. These interviews cover both the person's history (e.g., family-of-origin experiences, prior couple relationships, educational and job performance, physical health, psychopathology, prior therapy) and his or her current functioning. Personal strengths and successes are also covered.

During the joint interview, the therapist obtains a sample of the partners' communication skills by observing them while engaged in a structured discussion. The therapist may ask the partners to discuss an area of concern in their relationship, to observe how they make decisions; to share thoughts and feelings about themselves or the relationship, to assess their expressive and listening skills; or to provide each other with instrumental or expressive support (Epstein & Baucom, 2002).

Questionnaires can supplement interviews by efficiently surveying various characteristics of the individuals, the couple, and the environment, and identifying topics that the therapist can later explore during the interviews. Therapists can use scales selectively to assess (1) partners' satisfaction with areas of their relationship; (2) each partner's personality characteristics and needs; (3) types of environmental demands experienced by the partners individually and as a couple; (4) partners' cognitions regarding their relationship; (5) the couple's communication patterns; (6) symptoms of psychopathology; (7) physical and psychological abuse; and (8) strengths of the couple, such as mutual social support (Epstein & Baucom, 2002; see Table 13.1).

Although self-report scales are often used in research, individual and relationship functioning are assessed primarily through interviews and behavioral observation in clinical practice. Clinicians can use scales judiciously to conduct a thorough assessment and to identify topics for clinical interviews (Epstein & Baucom, 2002). If scales are used, it is helpful to have the members

TABLE 13.1. Assessment Areas and Potential Measures

Assessment area	Measure(s)
Relationship satisfaction	Dyadic Adjustment Scale (DAS; Spanier, 1976)
	Marital Satisfaction Inventory (MSI; Snyder, 1979; Snyder & Costin, 1994)
Desired direction and degree of change	Areas of Change Questionnaire (A-C; Weiss et al., 1973)
Individually oriented and communally oriented needs	Need Fulfillment Inventory (Prager & Buhrmester, 1998)
Normative and non-normative events	Family Inventory of Life Events and Changes (FILE; McCubbin & Patterson, 1987)
Forms of physically or psychologically abusive behaviors exhibited by partners	Revised Conflict Tactics Scale (CTS2; Straus, Hamby, Boney-McCoy, & Sugarman, 1996)
Psychologically abusive behavior	Multidimensional Measure of Emotional Abuse (MMEA; Murphy & Hoover, 2001)
Psychopathology	Brief Symptom Inventory (BSI; Derogatis & Spencer, 1982)
Partners' assumptions and standards regarding couple relationships	Relationship Belief Inventory (Eidelson & Epstein, 1982)
	Inventory of Specific Relationship Standards (Baucom, Epstein, Daiuto, & Carels, 1996; Baucom, Epstein, Rankin, et al., 1996)
Dyadic communication patterns	Communication Patterns Questionnaire (CPQ; Christensen, 1987, 1988)

of a couple complete inventories independently prior to their initial interview, so that the therapist can review them and identify areas for further exploration. We inform couples that, with few exceptions (e.g., responses regarding abuse), partners' questionnaire responses will not be kept confidential, and that they may be discussed during joint interviews.

Goal Setting and Feedback

Based on the initial assessment, the therapist presents his or her understanding of the couple, individual, and environmental factors that significantly influence the relationship, asks the partner whether this conceptualization matches their views of their difficulties, and collaborates with them to transform descriptions of problems into stated goals for positive changes in their relationship (Epstein & Baucom, 2002). CBCT therapists emphasize that partners need to take responsibility for their own behavior in the relationship. Helping partners understand the rationales for these tasks can increase the likelihood that they will complete the assignments. If members of the couple feel that the therapist has not addressed issues that are of concern to them, their motivation for therapy is likely to wane. In addition, for partners who experience secondary distress based on aversive responses to each other (e.g., mutual verbal attacks), the goal of decreasing high levels of negative interaction becomes a prerequisite for other work on the partners' central concerns about their relationship (Epstein & Baucom, 2002). Finally, relationship trauma or crisis (e.g., violence) takes priority over other goals of therapy.

Assessment continues throughout the course of CBCT as the therapist monitors the couple's progress toward treatment goals and refines the initial goals as needed (Baucom & Epstein, 1990). Goals for therapy often evolve over time, and the therapist helps the partners become aware of additional goals that they might pursue.

COMMONLY USED INTERVENTIONS
AND THE PROCESS OF THERAPY

A wide variety of cognitive-behavioral interventions have been developed to assist couples. Although differentiation among these interventions is possible, it is important to recognize that behavior, cognitions, and emotions are integrally related, and changes in one domain typically produce changes in the others. Thus, if a wife starts to think about her husband differently and interprets his behavior in a less condemning manner, she will likely have more positive emotional reactions to him and behave toward him more positively. Furthermore, an individual's subjective experience is typically a blend of cognitions and emotions that are not clearly differentiated from each other. Thus, although we discuss behavioral, cognitive, and emotional interventions, it is with some recognition that these distinctions are made partially for heuristic purposes, and that most interventions affect all of these domains of relationship functioning. Frequently, specific interventions focus on one of these domains, with the intention that other aspects of functioning will be altered simultaneously.

Interventions for Modifying Behavior

Early versions of CBCT focused on partners' behaviors, with little explicit attention to their cognitions and emotions. This approach was based on the logic that if partners behave more positively toward each other, they will think and feel more positively toward each other as well. A strong emphasis on helping members of couples behave in more constructive ways with each other continues in our current conceptualization as well. In fact, there are a large number of specific behavioral interventions that therapists might employ with couples; these interventions fall into two categories—guided behavior change and skills-based interventions (Epstein & Baucom, 2002).

Guided Behavior Change

"Guided behavior change" includes interventions that focus on behavioral exchanges but, in contrast to an explicit exchange of behaviors, these interventions ask both partners in a couple to commit to making constructive behavior changes irrespective of the other person's behavior (Halford, Sanders, & Behrens, 1994). Thus, we rarely emphasize the rule-governed behavior exchanges that were common in early days of BCT (Jacobson & Margolin, 1979). Instead, we help partners to develop a series of agreements on how they want to make changes in their relationship to meet the needs of both people, to help their relationship function effectively, and to interact constructively with their environment.

Guided behavior changes can be implemented for different reasons and at two levels of specificity. More generally, a couple and therapist might decide that they need to change the overall emotional tone of the relationship by decreasing the overall frequency and magnitude of negative behaviors and interactions, and increasing the frequency and magnitude of positive behaviors. To shift the overall ratio of positives to negatives, therapists may have each partner choose a "love day" or "caring day" on which they engage in positive behaviors to make the other person happier (e.g., washing dishes after dinner, giving their partner a backrub). In essence, these rather broad-based interventions are intended to help couples regain a sense of respectful, caring, and thoughtful relations. Guided behavior changes also can be used in a more focal manner, in which behavior changes are enacted around key themes and issues that have been associated with a couple's relationship distress. For example, if members of a couple complain about feeling disconnected, the therapist may instruct them to call or e-mail one another during the workday, so that they may feel closer when they are apart. Thus, rather than attempting to shift the overall balance of positives to negatives, more focal guided behavior change interventions can be designed around important needs that one or both people have noted as central to their well-being.

Skills-Based Interventions

Skills-based interventions typically involve instruction in the use of specific behavioral skills, through didactic discussions and/or other media, such as readings or videotapes. Following the instruction, couples practice these behaviors. Labeling these as skills-based interventions might suggest that the partners lack the knowledge or skills to behave constructively and effectively with each other, although this often is not the case. For example, some couples might only experience communication difficulties as stress increases (Bodenmann, 2005). Regardless of whether difficulties result from a skills deficit or a performance deficit, a discussion of guidelines for constructive communication can help partners to interact in positive ways.

We differentiate two major types of communication: couple conversations focused on sharing thoughts and feelings, and decision-making or problem-solving conversations (Baucom & Epstein, 1990; Epstein & Baucom, 2002). Tables 13.2 and 13.3 provide guidelines for these two types of communication. These guidelines are presented as recommendations and personalized to the couple's specific communication patterns, with a primary focus on the *process* of communicating, without particular attention to the content of conversations. Conceptualization of the primary content themes in the couple's

---

TABLE 13.2. Guidelines for Couple Discussions

Skills for sharing thoughts and emotions

1. State your views *subjectively*, as *your own* feelings and thoughts, not as absolute truths. Also, speak for yourself, what you think and feel, not what your partner thinks and feels.
2. Express your *emotions or feelings, not just your ideas.*
3. When talking about your partner, state your feelings about your partner, not just about an event or a situation.
4. When expressing negative emotions or concerns, also include any *positive feelings* you have about the person or situation.
5. Make your statement as *specific* as possible, both in terms of specific emotions and thoughts.
6. Speak in "paragraphs." That is, express one main idea with some elaboration, then allow your partner to respond. Speaking for a long time period without a break makes it hard for your partner to listen.
7. Express your feelings and thoughts with *tact* and *timing,* so that your partner can listen to what you are saying without becoming defensive.

Skills for listening to partner

Ways to respond while your partner is speaking
1. Show that you *understand* your partner's statements and accept his or her right to have those thoughts and feelings. Demonstrate this *acceptance* through your tone of voice, facial expressions, and posture.
2. Try to put yourself *in your partner's place* and look at the situation from his or her perspective to determine how the other person feels and thinks about the issue.

Ways to respond after your partner finishes speaking
3. After your partner finishes speaking, *summarize* and restate your partner's most important feelings, desires, conflicts, and thoughts. This is called a "reflection."
4. While in the listener role, *do not*:
   a. ask questions, except for clarification,
   b. express your own viewpoint or opinion,
   c. interpret or change the meaning of your partner's statements,
   d. offer solutions or attempt to solve a problem if one exits,
   e. make judgments or evaluate what your partner has said.

TABLE 13.3. Guidelines for Decision-Making Conversations

1. *Clearly and specifically state what the issue is.*
   a. Phrase the issue in terms of behaviors that are currently occurring or not occurring or in terms of what needs to be decided.
   b. Break down large, complex problems into several smaller problems, and deal with them one at a time.
   c. Make certain that both people agree on the statement of the problem and are willing to discuss it.

2. *Clarify why the issue is important and what your needs are.*
   a. Clarify why the issue is important to you and provide your understanding of the issues involved.
   b. Explain your needs that you would like to see taken into account in the solution; do not offer specific solutions at this time.

3. *Discuss possible solutions.*
   a. Propose concrete, specific solutions that take both people's needs and preferences into account. Do not focus on solutions that meet only your individual needs.
   b. Focus on solutions for the present and the future. Do not dwell on the past or attempt to attribute blame for past difficulties.
   c. If you tend to focus on a single or a limited number of alternatives, consider brainstorming (generating a variety of possible solutions in a creative way).

4. *Decide on a solution that is feasible and agreeable to both of you.*
   a. If you cannot find a solution that pleases both partners, suggest a compromise solution. If a compromise is not possible, agree to follow one person's preferences.
   b. State your solution in clear, specific, behavioral terms.
   c. After agreeing on a solution, have one partner restate the solution.
   d. Do not accept a solution if you do not intend to follow through with it.
   e. Do not accept a solution that will make you angry or resentful.

5. *Decide on a trial period to implement the solution if it is a situation that will occur more than once.*
   a. Allow for several attempts of the new solution.
   b. Review the solution at the end of the trial period.
   c. Revise the solution if needed, taking into account what you have learned thus far.

areas of concern needs to be developed, then taken into account while the couple engages in these conversations. For example, if a lack of being vulnerable with each other is a major issue for partners, their conversations might emphasize ways of taking some chances to open up by discussing more personal or intimate issues. In essence, the therapist should attend to both the process of communication and to important themes and issues that the partners need to address in their relationship.

A therapist might provide educational information to facilitate a couple's use of communication skills. For instance, the therapist might provide information about a variety of types of social support that individuals generally find to be helpful, if partners have discussed how they might be supportive to each other in addressing stressful and unrealistic demands at work. The partners can then discuss how this information applies to their relationship. Such an intervention represents an important shift within cognitive-behavioral approaches, providing a needed balance between addressing interactive processes and attending to the content of a couple's concerns.

Interventions That Address Cognitions

The behavior between intimate partners often has great meaning for both participants. These meanings can in turn evoke strong positive and negative emotional responses in each person. For example, individuals often have strong standards for how partners should behave toward each other in a variety of domains. If these standards are not met, the individual is likely to become upset and behave negatively toward the partner. Likewise, one person's level of satisfaction with the other's behavior can be influenced by the attributions that person makes about the reasons for the partner's actions. Thus, a husband might clean the house before his wife arrives at home, but whether she interprets this as a positive or negative behavior is likely to be influenced by her attribution or explanation for his behavior. If she concludes that he is attempting to be thoughtful and loving, she might experience his efforts to provide a clean house as positive. However, if she believes that he wishes to buy a new computer and is attempting to bribe her by cleaning the house, she might feel manipulated and experience the same behavior as negative. In essence, partners' behaviors in intimate relationships carry great meaning, and not considering these cognitive factors can limit the effectiveness of treatment. We have described a variety of cognitive variables that are important in understanding couples' relationships (Baucom & Epstein, 1990; Epstein & Baucom, 2002), including the following:

- Selective attention—what each person notices about the partner and the relationship.
- Attributions—causal and responsibility explanations about marital events.
- Expectancies—predictions of what will occur in the relationship in the future.
- Assumptions—how each person believes people and relationships actually function.
- Standards—how each person believes people and relationships *should* function.

These cognitions help to shape how each individual experiences the relationship. However, a therapist does not necessarily initiate cognitive restructuring simply because cognitions are negative. Instead, the therapist considers cognitive interventions if one or both partners seem to be processing information in a markedly *distorted* manner. For example, an individual might selectively attend to instances when a partner forgets to do household chores but pay little attention to other ways the partner succeeds with various tasks. Similarly, this individual might attribute the partner's failure to accomplish tasks to a lack of concern for the individual's preferences, or a lack of love. Typically, such cognitions will trigger negative emotions such as resentment or anger, which might then lead to retaliation and reciprocal negative behavior. Therefore, therapy at times will not focus on behavioral change but will help the partners reassess their cognitions about behaviors, so that they can be viewed in a more reasonable and balanced fashion. A wide variety of cognitive intervention strategies can be used, many of which are noted below (see Epstein & Baucom, 2002):

- Evaluate experiences and logic supporting a cognition.
- Weigh advantages and disadvantages of a cognition.
- Consider worst and best possible outcomes of situations.
- Provide educational minilectures, readings, and tapes.
- Use the inductive "downward arrow" method.
- Identify macro-level patterns from cross-situational responses.
- Identify macro-level patterns in past relationships.
- Increase relationship schematic thinking by pointing out repetitive cycles in couple interaction

These interventions can be grouped into two broad approaches: (1) Socratic questioning and (2) guided discovery.

Socratic Questioning

Cognitive therapy for individuals often has emphasized "Socratic questioning," which involves a series of questions to help an individual reevaluate the logic of his or her thinking, and understand underlying issues and concerns that are not at first apparent. Socratic questioning can also be employed with couples, but it should be used cautiously, because the context for individual therapy is different from that of couple therapy. In individual therapy, the individual meets alone with a caring, concerned therapist, with whom he or she can be open and honest in reevaluating cognitions. In couple therapy, however, the individual's partner is present in the session. Often the partner has told the individual that his or her thinking is distorted and blames the individual for their relationship problems. Therefore, if a therapist begins to question an individual's thinking in the presence of the partner, then these efforts might be unsuccessful or even be seen as supportive of the critical partner's thoughts, and so contribute to negative outcomes. With the partner present, an individual might become defensive and unwilling to acknowledge that his or her thinking has been distorted or unfairly slanted against the partner. If an individual acknowledges that his or her thinking was extreme or distorted, the partner might use this acknowledgment against the individual in the future. Therefore, Socratic questioning in the presence of a critical or hostile partner can arouse a person's defensiveness. Such interventions may be more successful with couples in which the partners are less hostile and hurtful toward each other.

Guided Discovery

"Guided discovery" includes a wide variety of treatment strategies to create insession experiences, so that one or both partners may begin to question their thinking and develop a different perspective of one another or the relationship. For example, if a woman has noticed her partner's withdrawal and interpreted it as his not caring about her, then the therapist could address this attribution in a variety of ways. First, the therapist could use Socratic questioning and ask her to think of a variety of interpretations for her partner's behavior. The therapist could then ask her to look for evidence that supports or refutes each of those possible interpretations. Alternatively, the therapist could structure an interaction in which the woman obtains additional information that might alter her attributions. For example, the therapist might ask the couple to have a conversation in which the man shares his thoughts and feelings at the time he withdrew. Through this conversation, the woman might learn that her partner withdrew because he felt hurt, rather than due to a lack of caring. This new understanding and experience might shift the woman's perspective, without the therapist questioning her thinking directly. Similarly, a man might develop an expectancy that his partner does not respect his perspective on a variety of issues. If, however, they agree to start having couple conversations on a weekly basis in which his partner solicits and listens to his opinions, his expectation may change.

An important set of cognitions involves each person's standards about how partners "should" behave in close relationships. Because standards are not based on logic, they are not evaluated in terms of logical reasoning. Rather, standards are best addressed with techniques that highlight their utility, or the advantages and disadvantages of living according to them. Standards might involve an individual's behavior, the ways that the partners interact with each other, or how to interact with the social environment. In general, we proceed through the following steps to address relationship standards:

- Clarify each person's existing standards.
- Discuss the advantages and disadvantages of existing standards.
- If standards need alteration, then help to define new, acceptable standards.
- Problem-solve how new standards will be expressed behaviorally.
- If partners' standards continue to differ, then discuss the acceptability of these differences.

We often discuss how any given standard usually has some positive and negative consequences. First, it is important to clarify each person's standards in a given domain of the relationship (e.g., having couple time vs. individual time). Once the partners are able to articulate their standards about time together and time alone, each partner is asked to describe the pros and cons of conducting a relationship according to those standards. We encourage each person to share both the positive and negative consequences of his or her standard, to avoid or to minimize polarization. Following a full discussion of their different standards regarding an aspect of their relationship, the partners are asked to develop a moderated standard that would be responsive to both partner's perspectives and acceptable to both. Given that individuals typically hold strongly to their standards and values, it is not likely that partners will give up their standards totally. Greater success occurs from slight alterations that make standards less extreme or more similar to the other person's standards. After the partners agrees on a newly evolved standard, they are asked to decide how this new standard will be regularly implemented in their relationship, through the identification of specific, concrete behaviors in which each partner will engage.

Interventions Focused on Emotions

Whereas many behavioral and cognitive interventions influence a couple's emotional experiences in a relationship, at times more direct attention needs to be given to emotional factors in the relationship. This focus is especially important when therapists treat couples in which one or both partners demonstrate either restricted or minimized emotions, or extreme emotional responses. Each of these broad domains includes specific difficulties that individuals experience with emotions, with particular interventions that are appropriate.

Restricted or Minimized Emotions

Many individuals in committed relationships appear to be uncomfortable with emotions in general or with specific emotions. For example, some partners have difficulty experiencing emotions in general or specific emotions, whereas other partners might experience both positive and negative emotions, but their levels of emotional experience are so muted that they do not find their relationship experiences very fulfilling. In addition, some partners might have stronger emotional experiences but be somewhat limited in their ability to differentiate among different emotions. Other partners might experience difficulty relating emotions to their internal and external experiences. Finally, some individuals avoid what Greenberg and Safran (1987) describe as "primary emotions" that are related to important needs and motives, such as anxiety associated with concern that a partner will fail to meet one's attachment needs. Because these emotions are seen as dangerous, individuals may avoid their experience or expression. Greenberg proposes that people, therefore, cover these primary emotions with secondary emotions that seem safer or less vulnerable. Consequently, rather than experiencing and expressing fear and anxiety to a critical partner, an individual might experience feelings such as anger, which are less threatening and help the individual to feel less vulnerable.

A number of strategies help individuals access and heighten emotional experience, many of which are drawn from emotionally focused couple therapy (Johnson & Greenberg, 1987). Several broad principles form the basis of these treatment strategies. First, the therapist works to establish a safe atmosphere by normalizing the experience and expression of both positive and negative emotions. The therapist also fosters this safe environment by encouraging the partner to respond to the individual in a caring and supportive manner when he or she expresses these emotions. Even so, an individual might try to avoid an emotion or escape once emotions become the focus of the session. In this situation, the therapist might refocus the individual to express an emotional experience; of course, this focus must be conducted with appropriate timing and moderation to avoid overwhelming the individual.

Once a safe environment is created, therapists may use a variety of treatment strategies to heighten emotional experience. The therapist could ask an individual to describe a particular incident in detail, in the hope of evoking the emotions within this experience. If direct discussion of emotions is difficult or frightening, a person could be encouraged to use metaphors and images as ways to express emotions. The therapist can also use questions, reflections, and interpretations to draw out primary emotions. By tailoring these interventions to the individual styles and needs of the partners in a given couple, the therapist works to help the individual enrich his or her emotional experience and expression, in a manner that is helpful to both the individual and couple. Deciding to work within this set of interventions should not be based on a therapist's own belief that a "healthy" person should have a full emotional life, as well as a wide range of emotional expression; instead, the choice to use these strategies should be grounded within a thorough assessment, and a conceptualization that restricted emotional experience or expression interferes with this particular couple's, or the partner's, well-being.

Containing the Experience/Expression of Emotions

In contrast to individuals who have trouble experiencing and expressing emotions, therapists may find themselves working with partners who have difficulty regulating their experience and expression of emotion. Frequently, the couple labels this pattern as a problem if one or both partners experience and express high levels of negative emotion, or express these emotions in situations or ways that create difficulty for the couple. The therapist may find such couples to be quite demanding, because the partners' lives appear to consist of a series of emotional crises, strong arguments, or extreme behaviors, potentially including spousal abuse, resulting from extreme negative emotions.

Several treatment strategies are helpful to work with couples in such circumstances. One technique is for the couple to schedule times to discuss issues that are upsetting to one or both partners. The goal of this intervention is to restrict or contain the frequency and settings in which the partners express strong emotions. If such times have not been set aside, then an individual with poor affect regulation is more likely to express strong feelings whenever they arise. Some people find that they can resist the expression of strong negative feelings if they know there is a time set aside to address their concerns. This intervention can create limits around the expression of strong negative affect, so that it does not intrude into other aspects of the couple's life. In particular, scheduling such discussions can help to ensure that strong negative expression does not occur at times that are likely to lead to increasing frustration for one or both persons (e.g., before one partner leaves for work in the morning, or just as guests arrive for a social engagement).

To assist individuals who have poor emotion regulation, Linehan (1993) has developed a treatment approach known as dialectical behavior therapy (DBT) that integrates cognitive-behavioral theory and strategies with acceptance. Although her interventions do not focus on strong affect in an interpersonal context, often they are applicable. Recently, Kirby and Baucom (2007a, 2007b) integrated principles from CBCT with such skills from DBT to assist couples experiencing chronic emotion dysregulation. For example, one of these interventions involves teaching individuals to observe when they feel a strong emotion while they are talking to their partners, to identify what that emotion may be and how it might influence their responses to their partner in that moment. With increased awareness of their feelings when they interact with each other, individuals can learn how to communicate more effectively with their partners. For example, some partners may learn how to stay engaged in a difficult but important conversation if they can label their feelings of anxiety and the urge to avoid the conversation. In contrast, other individuals who gain greater awareness of feeling angry and an urge to argue may become better able to respect their mutual decision to take a time-out from a heated argument.

An additional strategy may involve helping the couple seek alternative ways to communicate feelings and elicit support, perhaps from individuals outside of the relationship. For example, the individual may learn to rely on friends to express some concerns, or begin to keep a journal to express emotions. This approach is intended not as an alternative to addressing an individual's concerns with a partner, but as a means to modulate the frequency and intensity of emotional expression. These strategies and skills can be difficult or at times implausible to teach an individual in a couple context. Often, the other person serves as a strong negative stimulus to the individual who has difficulty regulating emotion, or there is insufficient time to address the individual's emotion regulation difficulties in addition to the couple's broader relationship concerns. In such cases, individual therapy for the person who has poor affect regulation should be considered as an important adjunct to couple therapy.

As can be seen, a wide variety of interventions can be employed in CBCT to work with relationship distress. Whereas the focus of the intervention is typically on one of the three domains of behavior, cognition, or emotion, the goal often is to impact all three spheres of functioning. Rather than routine or manualized application of these techniques, optimal treatment involves personalizing a detailed, integrated conceptualization and treatment plan to the couple's specific concerns.

EMPIRICAL SUPPORT AND TREATMENT APPLICABILITY

Cognitive interventions are rarely utilized in clinical practice without consideration of their behavioral effects; likewise, behavioral interventions that do not attend to cognitive and emotional interventions are rare. Given that current evidence suggests no significant differences between strictly behavioral couple therapy and a broader CBCT (Baucom & Lester, 1986; Baucom, Sayers, & Sher, 1990; Halford et al., 1993; Shadish & Baldwin, 2003), we discuss the empirical status of these interventions together as CBCT.

Efficacy of Cognitive-Behavioral Couple Therapy

CBCT, the most widely evaluated couple treatment, has been the focus of approximately 30 controlled treatment outcome studies. CBCT has been reviewed in detail in a number of previous publications, including findings from specific investigations (e.g., Alexander, Holtzworth-Munroe, & Jameson, 1994; Baucom & Epstein, 1990; Baucom & Hoffman, 1986; Baucom et al., 1998; Bray & Jouriles, 1995; Christensen & Jacobson, 1994; Jacobson & Addis, 1993; Snyder, Castellani, & Whisman, 2006) as well as meta-analyses (Baucom, Hahlweg, & Kuschel, 2003; Dunn & Schwebel, 1995; Hahlweg & Markman, 1988; Shadish & Baldwin, 2003, 2005). All of these reviews reached the same conclusion: CBCT is an efficacious intervention for distressed couples.

Research suggests that between one- to two-thirds of couples will be in the nondistressed range of marital satisfaction after receiving CBCT. Shadish and Baldwin (2005) conducted a meta-analysis of 30 randomized treatment outcome investigations involving distressed couples, contrasting CBCT with no-treatment control conditions. Across these 30 studies CBCT versus no treatment yielded a mean effect size of 0.59 (this mean dropped to 0.50 when corrected for the nonpublication of nonsignificant findings). This average effect size is somewhat smaller than the mean effect size presented in previous meta-analyses of CBCT. For example Shadish and Baldwin (2003) reported an average effect size of 0.84 for couple therapy pooled across theoretical approaches (with CBCT being at least as effective as other approaches). Shadish and Baldwin (2005) suggest that these smaller effect sizes result from the inclusion of unpublished dissertations, with smaller sample sizes and small or negative effect sizes, in their 2005 analysis that were not included in previous analyses.

Most couples appear to maintain the gains they receive from CBCT for short time periods (6–12 months); however, the long-term results are not as clear. For example, Jacobson, Schmaling, and Holtzworth-Munroe (1987) found that approximately 30% of couples who had recovered during therapy had subsequently relapsed during a 2-year follow-up of strictly BCT. In addition, Snyder, Wills, and Grady-Fletcher (1991) reported that 38% of couples who received BCT had divorced during a 4-year follow-up period. However, recent results are more encouraging and point to the complexity of changes over time. Over a 2 year follow-up, couples who received BCT showed a "hockey stick" pattern of change (Christensen, Atkins, Yi, Baucom, & George, 2006); that is, they showed deterioration immediately after the end of treatment, then reversed their course and began improving throughout the follow-up period. At 2 years posttreatment, 60% of couples who received BCT had obtained clinically significant improvements over the pretreatment level of satisfaction.

Isolating What Works: The Utility of Specific Cognitive-Behavioral Couple Therapy Interventions and Mechanisms of Change

CBCT includes a number of specific interventions, typically offered within a multicomponent approach to addressing relationship distress. Shadish and Baldwin (2005) evaluated whether specific components of CBCT were more related than others to treatment outcome (i.e., whether specific components predicted effect sizes comparing CBCT to no-treatment controls). The components they investigated included (1) communication/problem solving, (2) behavioral contracting, (3) behavioral exchange, (4) desensitization, (5) emotional expressiveness training, (6) cognitive restructuring, and (7) "other." Their results indicated that communication/problem solving was associated with larger effect sizes and cognitive restructuring with smaller effect sizes; however, when Bonferroni corrections were taken into account for multiple tests, these differences were no longer significant. Thus, there is not strong evidence that specific interventions within CBCT are more effective overall than others to decrease couple distress. It is important to recognize that this lack of differentiation among treatment techniques for distressed couples does not necessarily mean that a clinician should utilize random CBCT interventions. In the studies evaluated by Shadish and Baldwin (2005), couples were randomly assigned to treatment condition involving specific interventions, without any attempt to match treatment to couples' presenting complaints. Thus, the findings must be interpreted to mean that when specific concerns of a couple are not taken into account to select specific interventions, various CBCT interventions are equally effective overall. In almost all clinical settings, specific interventions within CBCT are selected according to the needs of a particular couple. Whereas clinicians assume that the selection of certain interventions for a given couple will lead to superior outcomes, no treatment-matching studies have been conducted to address this issue.

Even if specific CBCT interventions were more efficacious overall than others, such results still would not indicate what about those interventions was helpful to couples, merely that they were beneficial. CBCT has been predicated on the notion that both behavioral and cognitive change are central to the effectiveness of treatment. Whereas CBCT is efficacious overall, the mechanisms of change in CBCT have not been successfully isolated (Lebow, 2000; Snyder et al., 2006). For example, although CBCT leads to increases in both communication skills and relationship adjustment, the degree of improvement in communication is not correlated with level of improvement in relationship adjustment (Halford et al., 1993; Iverson & Baucom, 1990). Likewise, Baucom, Sayers, and Sher (1988) have demonstrated that cognitive restructuring techniques do indeed lead to cognitive changes among distressed couples, yet these cognitive changes do not account for the observed increases in relationship adjustment at the end of treatment. The difficulty in isolating the essential ingredients of change in couple therapy is not unique to CBCT; instead, it is difficult to isolate the specific mechanisms of change in any of the empirically supported couple therapies that currently exist (Snyder et al., 2006).

Cognitive-Behavioral Couple Therapy Compared to Other Theoretical Approaches

As noted earlier, the absolute efficacy of CBCT has been demonstrated across a number of investigations. It also is important to know whether CBCT is more efficacious than other theoretical approaches that have demonstrated empirical utility, such as emotion-focused couple therapy (Johnson & Greenberg, 1987) and insight-oriented couple therapy (Snyder & Wills, 1989). Based on their meta-analytic findings, Shadish and Baldwin (2003) concluded that overall differences in efficacy among these theoretical orientations are minor and nonsignificant. Christensen et al. (2004) conducted a clinical trial in which 134 seriously and chronically distressed couples were randomly assigned to strict BCT or integrative BCT, which places a major premium on acceptance, as well as behavior change. Although the two treatments showed different patterns of change over the course of the therapy sessions, they appeared relatively comparable in assisting distressed couples by the end of therapy. This overall comparability was maintained at 2-year follow-up (Christensen et al., 2006). Overall, there is little evidence at present that CBCT is a more efficacious treatment than other established models of couple therapy.

Common Factors and Principles of Change

The apparent comparability of different theoretical approaches to couple therapy and the difficulty of isolating specific mechanisms of change for a given approach raise the possibility that there are important common factors for all effective interventions (Baucom et al., 1998). Building on the work of Barlow and colleagues (Allen, McHugh, & Barlow, 2008; Barlow, Allen, & Choate, 2004) related to general principles of therapeutic change for individual psychopathology, Christensen (in press) suggests that all of the empirically supported couple therapies have five common elements: (1) alteration of cognitive distortions regarding the bases for relationship distress; (2) decreases in negative, destructive behaviors between partners; (3) increases in positive behaviors and an emphasis on strengths; (4) encouragement for couples to address difficult issues that they have avoided; and (5) teaching effective communication to assist in achieving these goals.

The employment of broad principles might contribute to an even more pervasive effect that cuts across different theoretical approaches. The previously mentioned principles might make couples more relationally attuned and aware, and provide them with novel ways to think about how to improve their relationship. As noted earlier, Sullivan and Baucom (2004, 2005) have addressed this issue from the perspective of "relationship schematic processing" (RSP), which refers to the degree to which an individual processes information in terms of relationship processes. An individual who is high on RSP thinks about his or her own behavior and its impact on the other person and the relationship, along with anticipating the other partner's needs and preferences, and balancing the partner's needs with one's own needs. Sullivan and Baucom (2004, 2005) proposed that increasing RSP might be a common mechanism of change that cuts across theoretical approaches, such that any effective couple therapy teaches individuals to think more appropriately in relationship terms. Consistent with this notion, they demonstrated (1) that CBCT does increase the quantity and quality of men's RSP, and (2) that women's increases in marital satisfaction in response to CBCT were correlated with the degree to which their male partners' RSP increased. Stated differently, women became more satisfied with the marriage when men learned to process more effectively in relationship terms. Likewise, they demonstrated that couples receiving insight-oriented couple therapy in Snyder's outcome study (Sullivan, Baucom, & Snyder, 2002) increased in RSP as well. Whether the education of couples to think more effectively in relationship terms or the use of principles suggested by Christensen (in press) turn out to be common mechanisms of change that are central to all efficacious forms of couple therapy is not known at present, but it is important to continue to explore whether specific interventions that therapists employ are the critical variables, or whether therapeutic change can be accounted for in other ways as well.

Applicability of Cognitive-Behavioral Couple Therapy to Various Populations

CBCT is applicable to a wide range of specific relationship concerns. A particular class of relationship distress involves couples who have experienced relationship trauma, such as infidelity or psychological and physical abuse (Baucom, Gordon, Snyder, Atkins, & Christensen, 2006; LaTaillade, 2006). Traumatic experiences within the marriage have been addressed successfully from a CBCT perspective but require additional consideration, as described by Gordon, Baucom, Snyder, and Dixon (2008). These CBCT principles have also been adapted to prevent distress and enhance relationship functioning, as demonstrated in the widely used Prevention and Relationship Education Program (PREP) developed by Markman, Renick, Floyd, Stanley, and Clements (1993).

Couple-based interventions that employ a cognitive-behavioral approach also have been used successfully to assist couples in which one partner has either psychopathology or health problems. Although these latter two applications are beyond the scope of this chapter, the results of investigations are promising (see Baucom et al., 1998; Hahlweg & Baucom, 2008; Schmaling & Sher, 2000; Snyder et al., 2006; Snyder & Whisman, 2002).

CONCLUSIONS

The evidence mirrors what clinicians experience; although relationship discord is a challenging clinical phenomenon to address, there are efficacious interventions that help a great number of couples. The provision of effective couple treatment is complex, because basic research indicates that relationship functioning is influenced by such a wide range of factors, including, individual, dyadic, and environmental factors. These factors are also dynamic, and they change over the course of a couple's relationship. Clinically sophisticated interventions must take all of these factors into account as potential contributors to the partners' experience of their current relationship. Clinicians must also recognize that factors that might help to alleviate relationship distress will not necessarily be the same factors that maximize optimal relationship functioning.

Over the past decades, our CBCT interventions have become increasingly varied attempts to take these empirically supported factors into account for specific couples. Perhaps even more encouraging is the recognition that the interventions originally developed for the treatment of "general marital distress" can be adapted and used successfully with couples in a variety of contexts, including relationship education, prevention, and enhancement; with couples who are devastated by relationship crises, such as infidelity;with couples confronting significant psychopathology in one or both partners; and with couples who experience a variety of health problems. The ongoing commitment to cognitive-behavioral conceptualizations of relationships that are grounded in basic research, and an insistence on empirical validation of treatments from those research-derived principles, will help to ensure that the field advances to maximally benefit couples who seek to alleviate distress and optimize their relationships.

REFERENCES

Alexander, J. F., Holtzworth-Munroe, A., & Jameson, P. B. (1994). The process and outcome of marital and family therapy: Research review and evaluation.. In A. E. Bergin & S. L. Garfield (Eds.), *Handbook of psychotherapy and behavior change* (4th ed., pp. 595–630). New York: Wiley.

Allen, L. B., McHugh, R. K., & Barlow, D. H. (2008). Emotional disorders: A unified protocol. In D. H. Barlow (Ed.), *Clinical handbook of psychological disorders* (4th ed.). New York: Guilford Press.

Baldwin, M. W. (2005). *Interpersonal cognition.* New York: Guilford Press.

Bandura, A., & Walters, P. (1963). *Social learning and personality development.* New York: Holt, Rinehart & Wilson.

Barlow, D. H., Allen, L. B., & Choate, M. L. (2004). Toward a unified treatment for emotional disorders. *Behavior Therapy, 35,* 205–230.

Baucom, D. H. (1999, November). *Therapeutic implications of gender differences in cognitive processing in marital relationships.* Paper presented at the 33rd annual meeting of the Association for the Advancement of Behavior Therapy, Toronto, Canada.

Baucom, D. H., & Epstein, N. (1990). *Cognitive-behavioral marital therapy.* New York: Brunner/Mazel.

Baucom, D. H., Epstein, N., Daiuto, A. D., & Carels, R. A. (1996). Cognitions in marriage: The relationship between standards and attributions. *Journal of Family Psychology, 10*(2), 209–222.

Baucom, D. H., Epstein, N., & Gordon, K. C. (2000). Marital therapy: Theory, practice, and empirical status. In C. R. Snyder & R. E. Ingram (Eds.), *Handbook of psychological change: Psychotherapy processes and practices for the 21st century* (pp. 280–308). New York: Wiley.

Baucom, D. H., Epstein, N., & LaTaillade, J. J. (2002). Cognitive-behavioral couple therapy. In A. S. Gurman & N. S. Jacobson (Eds.), *Clinical handbook of couple therapy* (3rd ed., pp. 26–58). New York: Guilford Press.

Baucom, D. H., Epstein, N., LaTaillade, J. J., & Kirby, J. S. (2008). Cognitive-behavioral couple therapy. In A. S. Gurman (Ed.), *Clinical handbook of couple therapy* (4th ed., pp. 31–72). New York: Guilford Press.

Baucom, D. H., Epstein, N., & Rankin, L. (1995, July). *The role of thematic content in couples' cognitions.* Paper presented at the 5th World Congress on Behavior Therapy, Copenhagen, Denmark.

Baucom, D. H., Epstein, N., Rankin, L., & Burnett, C. K. (1996). Understanding and treating marital distress from a cognitive-behavioral orientation. In K. S. Dobson & K. D. Craig (Eds.), *Advances in cognitive-behavioral therapy* (pp. 210–236). Thousand Oaks, CA: Sage.

Baucom, D. H., Epstein, N., & Sullivan, L. J. (2004). Brief couple therapy. In M. Dewan, B. Steenbarger, & R. P. Greenberg (Eds.), *The art and science of brief therapies* (pp. 189–227). Washington, DC: American Psychiatric Publishing.

Baucom, D. H., Gordon, K. C., Snyder, D. K., Atkins, D. C., & Christensen, A. (2006). Treating affair couples: Clinical considerations and initial findings. *Journal of Cognitive Psychotherapy, 20,* 375–392.

Baucom, D. H., Hahlweg, K., & Kuschel, A. (2003). Are waiting list control groups needed in future marital therapy outcome research? *Behavior Therapy, 34,* 179–188.

Baucom, D. H., & Hoffman, J. A. (1986). The effectiveness of marital therapy: Current status and application to the clinical setting. In N. S. Jacobson & A. S. Gurman (Eds.), *Clinical handbook of marital therapy* (pp. 597–620). New York: Guilford Press.

Baucom, D. H., & Lester, G. W. (1986). The usefulness of cognitive restructuring as an adjunct to behavioral marital therapy. *Behavior Therapy, 17*(4), 385–403.

Baucom, D. H., Sayers, S. L., & Sher, T. G. (1988, November). *Expanding behavioral marital therapy*. Paper presented at the 22nd annual meeting of the Association for the Advancement of Behavior Therapy, New York, NY.

Baucom, D. H., Sayers, S. L., & Sher, T. G. (1990). Supplementing behavioral marital therapy with cognitive restructuring and emotional expressiveness training: An outcome investigation. *Journal of Consulting and Clinical Psychology, 58*(5), 636–645.

Baucom, D. H., Shoham, V., Mueser, K. T., Daiuto, A. D., & Stickle, T. R. (1998). Empirically supported couples and family therapies for adult problems. *Journal of Consulting and Clinical Psychology, 66*, 53–88.

Beck, A. T. (1988). Cognitive approaches to panic disorder: Theory and therapy. In S. Rachman & J. D. Maser (Eds.), *Panic: Psychological perspectives* (pp. 91–109). Hillsdale, NJ: Erlbaum.

Beck, A. T., Rush, A. J., Shaw, B. F., & Emery, G. (1979). *Cognitive therapy of depression*. New York: Guilford Press.

Bodenmann, G. (2005). Dyadic coping and its significance for marital functioning. In T. Revenson, K. Kayser, & G. Bodenmann (Eds.), *Couples coping with stress: Emerging perspectives on dyadic coping* (pp. 33– 50). Washington, DC: American Psychological Association.

Bradbury, T. N., & Karney, B. R. (2004). Understanding and altering the longitudinal course of marriage. *Journal of Marriage and Family, 66*, 862–879.

Bray, J. H., & Jouriles, E. N. (1995). Treatment of marital conflict and prevention of divorce [Special issue: The effectiveness of marital and family therapy]. *Journal of Marital and Family Therapy, 21*(4), 461–473.

Bronfenbrenner, U. (1989). *Ecological systems theory* (Vol. 6). Greenwich, CT: JAI Press.

Carter, B., & McGoldrick, M. (Eds.). (1999). *The expanded family life cycle: Individual, family, and social perspectives* (3rd ed.). Boston: Allyn & Bacon.

Christensen, A. (1987). Detection of conflict patterns in couples. In K. Hahlweg & M. J. Goldstein (Eds.), *Understanding major mental disorder: The contribution of family interaction research* (pp. 250–265). New York: Family Process.

Christensen, A. (1988). Dysfunctional interaction patterns in couples. In P. Noller & M. A. Fitzpatrick (Eds.), *Perspectives on marital interaction: Monographs in social psychology of language* (No. 1, pp. 31–52). Clevedon, UK: Multilingual Matters.

Christensen, A. (in press). A "unified protocol" for couple therapy. In K. Hahlweg, M. Grawe-Gerber & D. H. Baucom (Eds.), *Couples in despair: Evidence-Based interventions for treatment and prevention*.

Christensen, A., Atkins, D., Berns, S., Wheeler, J., Baucom, D. H., & Simpson, L. (2004). Traditional versus integrative behavioral couple therapy for significantly and stably distressed married couples. *Journal of Consulting and Clinical Psychology, 72*, 176–191.

Christensen, A., Atkins, D., Yi, J., Baucom, D. H., & George, W. H. (2006). Couple and individual adjustment for two years following a randomized clinical trial comparing traditional versus integrative behavioral couple therapy. *Journal of Consulting and Clinical Psychology, 74,* 1180– 1191.

Christensen, A., & Heavey, C. L. (1990). Gender and social structure in the demand/ withdraw pattern of marital conflict. *Journal of Personality and Social Psychology, 59*(1), 73–81.

Christensen, A., & Heavey, C. L. (1993). Gender differences in marital conflict: The demand/withdraw interaction pattern. In S. Oskamp & M. Costanzo (Eds.), *Gender issues in contemporary society: Claremont Symposium on Applied Social Psychology* (Vol. 6, pp. 113–141). Newbury Park, CA: Sage.

Christensen, A., & Jacobson, N. S. (1994). Who (or what) can do psychotherapy: The status and challenge of nonprofessional therapies. *Psychological Science, 5*(1), 8–14.

Cutrona, C. E. (1996). Social support as a determinant of marital quality. In G. R. Pierce, B. R. Sarason & I. G. Sarason (Eds.), *Handbook of social support and the family* (pp. 173–194). New York: Plenum Press.

Cutrona, C. E., Suhr, J. A., & MacFarlane, R. (1990). Interpersonal transaction and the psychological sense of support. In S. Duck (Ed.), *Personal relationships and social support* (pp. 30–45). London: Sage.

Dattilio, F. M., & Padesky, C. A. (1990). *Cognitive therapy with couples.* Sarasota, FL: Professional Resource Exchange.

Derogatis, L. R., & Spencer, M. S. (1982). *The Brief Symptom Inventory (BSI): Administration, scoring, and procedures manual–1.* Baltimore: Johns Hopkins University School of Medicine, Clinical Psychometrics Research Unit.

Dunn, R. L., & Schwebel, A. I. (1995). Meta-analytic review of marital therapy outcome research. *Journal of Family Psychology, 9*(1), 58–68.

Eidelson, R. J., & Epstein, N. (1982). Cognition and relationship maladjustment: Development of a measure of dysfunctional relationship beliefs. *Journal of Consulting and Clinical Psychology, 50*(5), 715–720.

Ellis, A. (1962). *Reason and emotion in psychotherapy.* New York: Lyle Stuart.

Ellis, A., Sichel, J. L., Yeager, R. J., DiMattia, D. J., & DiGiuseppe, R. (Eds.). (1989). *Rational-emotive couples therapy.* Elmsford, NY: Pergamon Press.

Epstein, N. (1982). Cognitive therapy with couples. *American Journal of Family Therapy, 10*(1), 5–16.

Epstein, N., & Baucom, D. H. (2002). *Enhanced cognitive-behavioral therapy for couples: A contextual approach.* Washington, DC: American Psychological Association.

Epstein, N., & Baucom, D. H. (2003). Overcoming roadblocks in cognitive-behavioral therapy with couples. In R. L. Leahy (Ed.), *Overcoming roadblocks in cognitive therapy* (pp. 187–205). New York: Guilford Press.

Falloon, I. R. H. (1991). *Behavioral family therapy* (Vol. 2). New York: Brunner/ Mazel.

Fincham, F. D., Bradbury, T. N., & Scott, C. K. (1990). Cognition in marriage. In F. D. Fincham & T. N. Bradbury (Eds.), *The psychology of marriage: Basic issues and applications* (pp. 118–149). New York: Guilford Press.

Fiske, S. T., & Taylor, S. E. (1991). *Social cognition.* New York: McGraw Hill.

Fletcher, G. J. O., & Fitness, J. (Eds.). (1996). *Knowledge structures in close relationships: A social psychological approach.* Mahwah, NJ: Erlbaum.

Fruzzetti, A. E. (2006). *The high-conflict couple: A dialectical behavior therapy guide to finding peace, intimacy, and validation.* Oakland: Harbinger.

Gordon, K. C., Baucom, D. H., Snyder, D. K., & Dixon, L. J. (2008). Couple therapy and the treatment of affairs. In A. S. Gurman (Ed.), *Clinical handbook of couple therapy* (4th ed., pp. 429–458). New York: Guilford Press.

Gottman, J. M. (1994). *What predicts divorce?* Hillsdale, NJ: Erlbaum.

Greenberg, L. S., & Safran, J. D. (1987). *Emotion in psychotherapy: Affect, cognition, and the process of change.* New York: Guilford Press.

Hahlweg, K., & Baucom, D. H. (2008). *Partnerschaft und psychische Störung: Fortschritte der Psychotherapie* (Band 30) [Couples and individual functioning: The development of therapeutic interventions]. Göttingen: Hogrefe.

Hahlweg, K., Baucom, D. H., & Markman, H. J. (1988). Recent advances in therapy and prevention. In I. R. H. Falloon (Ed.), *Handbook of behavioral family therapy* (pp. 413–448). New York: Guilford Press.

Hahlweg, K., & Markman, H. J. (1988). Effectiveness of behavioral marital therapy: Empirical status of behavioral techniques in preventing and alleviating marital distress. *Journal of Consulting and Clinical Psychology, 56*(3), 440–447.

Halford, W. K., Sanders, M. R., & Behrens, B. C. (1993). A comparison of the generalisation of behavioral martial therapy and enhanced behavioral martial therapy. *Journal of Consulting and Clinical Psychology, 61*, 51–60.

Halford, W. K., Sanders, M. R., & Behrens, B. C. (1994). Self-regulation in behavioral couples' therapy. *Behavior Therapy, 25*(3), 431–452.

Hardy, K. V., & Laszloffy, T. A. (2002). Couple therapy using a multicultural perspective. In A. S. Gurman & N. S. Jacobson (Eds.), *Clinical handbook of couple therapy* (3rd ed., pp. 569–593). New York: Guilford Press.

Holtzworth-Munroe, A., Marshall, A. D., Meehan, J. C., & Rehman, U. (2002). Physical aggression. In D. K. Snyder & M. A. Whisman (Eds.), *Treating difficult couples: Helping clients with coexisting mental and relationship disorders* (pp. 201–230). New York: Guilford Press.

Iverson, A., & Baucom, D. H. (1988, November). *Behavioral marital therapy: The role of skills acquisition in marital satisfaction.* Paper presented at the 22nd annual meeting of the Association for the Advancement of Behavior Therapy, New York, NY.

Iverson, A., & Baucom, D. H. (1990). Behavioral marital therapy outcomes: Alternative interpretations of the data. *Behavior Therapy, 21*(1), 129–138.

Jacobson, N. S., & Addis, M. E. (1993). Research on couples and couple therapy: What do we know? Where are we going? [Special section: Couples and couple therapy]. *Journal of Consulting and Clinical Psychology, 61*(1), 85–93.

Jacobson, N. S., & Margolin, G. (1979). *Marital therapy: Strategies based on social learning and behavior exchange principles.* New York: Brunner/Mazel.

Jacobson, N. S., Schmaling, K. B., & Holtzworth-Munroe, A. (1987). Component analysis of behavioral marital therapy: Two-year follow-up and prediction of relapse. *Journal of Marital and Family Therapy, 13*(2), 187–195.

Jacobson, N. S., Waldron, H., & Moore, D. (1980). Toward a behavioral profile of marital distress. *Journal of Consulting and Clinical Psychology, 48*(6), 696–703.

Johnson, S. M. (2004). *The practice of emotionally focused marital therapy: Creating connection* (2nd ed.). New York: Routledge.

Johnson, S. M., & Denton, W. (2002). Emotionally focused couple therapy: creating secure connections. In A. S. Gurman & N. S. Jacobson (Eds.), *Clinical handbook of couple therapy* (3rd ed., pp. 221–250). New York: Guilford Press.

Johnson, S. M., & Greenberg, L. S. (1987). Emotionally focused marital therapy: An overview [Special Issue: Psychotherapy with families]. *Psychotherapy, 24*(3S), 552–560.

Karney, B. R., & Bradbury, T. N. (1995). The longitudinal course of marital quality and stability: A review of theory, methods, and research. *Psychological Bulletin, 118*(1), 3–34.

Kelly, S. (2006). Cognitive behavioral therapy with African Americans. In P. A. Hays & G. Y. Iwamasa (Eds.), *Culturally responsive cognitive-behavioral therapy: Assessment, practice, and supervision* (pp. 97–116). Washington DC: American Psychological Association.

Kelly, S., & Iwamasa, G. Y. (2005). Enhancing behavioral couple therapy: Addressing the therapeutic alliance, hope, and diversity. *Cognitive and Behavioral Practice, 12*, 102–112.

Kirby, J. S., & Baucom, D. H. (2007a). Integrating dialectical behavior therapy and cognitive-behavioral couple therapy: A couples skills group for emotion dysregulation. *Cognitive and Behavioral Practice, 14*, 394–405.

Kirby, J. S., & Baucom, D. H. (2007b). Treating emotional dysregulation in a couples context: A pilot study of a couples skills group intervention. *Journal of Marital and Family Therapy, 33*(3), 1–17.

LaTaillade, J. J. (2006). Considerations for treatment of African American couple relationships. *Journal of Cognitive Psychotherapy: An International Quarterly, 20*, 341–358.

LaTaillade, J. J., & Jacobson, N. S. (1995). Behavioral couple therapy. In M. Elkaim (Ed.), *Therapies familiales: Les principles approaches* [Family therapies: The principal approaches] (pp. 313–347). Paris: Editions du Seuil.

Lebow, J. L. (2000). What does the research tell us about couple and family therapies? *Journal of Clinical Psychology, 56*, 1083–1094.

Liberman, R. P. (1970). Behavioral approaches to family and couple therapy. *Journal of Orthopsychiatry, 40*, 106–118.

Linehan, M. M. (1993). *Cognitive-behavioral treatment of borderline personality disorder.* New York: Guilford Press.

Margolin, G., & Weiss, R. L. (1978). Comparative evaluation of therapeutic components associated with behavioral marital treatments. *Journal of Consulting and Clinical Psychology, 46*(6), 1476–1486.

Markman, H. J., Renick, M. J., Floyd, F. J., Stanley, S. M., & Clements, M. (1993). Preventing marital distress through communication and conflict management training: A 4- and 5-year follow-up [Special section: Couples and couple therapy]. *Journal of Consulting and Clinical Psychology, 61*(1), 70–77.

McCubbin, H. I., & Patterson, J. M. (1987). FILE: Family Inventory of Life Events and Changes. In H. I. McCubbin & A. I. Thompson (Eds.), *Family assessment inventories for research and practice* (pp. 81–98). Madison: University of Wisconsin–Madison, Family Stress Coping and Health Project.

Meichenbaum, D. (1977). *Cognitive-behavior modification.* New York: Plenum Press.

Murphy, C. M., & Hoover, S. A. (2001). Measuring emotional abuse in dating relationships as a multifactorial construct. In K. D. O'Leary & R. D. Maiuro (Eds.),

Psychological abuse in violent domestic relationships (pp. 3–28). New York: Springer.

Noller, P., Beach, S. R. H., & Osgarby, S. (1997). Cognitive and affective processes in marriage. In W. K. Halford & H. J. Markman (Eds.), *Clinical handbook of marriage and couples interventions* (pp. 43–71). Chichester, UK: Wiley.

Pasch, L. A., Bradbury, T. N., & Davila, J. (1997). Gender, negative affectivity, and observed social support behavior in marital interaction. *Personal Relationships, 4*(4), 361–378.

Pasch, L. A., Bradbury, T. N., & Sullivan, K. T. (1997). Social support in marriage: An analysis of intraindividual and interpersonal components. In G. R. Pierce, B. Lakey, I. G. Sarason, & B. R. Sarason (Eds.), *Sourcebook of theory and research on social support and personality* (pp. 229–256). New York: Plenum Press.

Patterson, G. R. (1974). Interventions for boys with conduct problems: Multiple settings, treatments, and criteria. *Journal of Consulting and Clinical Psychology, 42,* 471–481.

Prager, K. J., & Buhrmester, D. (1998). Intimacy and need fulfillment in couple relationships. *Journal of Social and Personal Relationships, 15,* 435–469.

Rankin, L. A., Baucom, D. H., Clayton, D. C., & Daiuto, A. D. (1995, November). *Gender differences in the use of relationship schemas versus individual schemas in marriage.* Paper presented at the 29th annual meeting of the Association for the Advancement of Behavior Therapy, Washington, DC.

Rathus, J. H., & Sanderson, W. C. (1999). *Marital distress: Cognitive behavioral interventions for couples.* Northvale, NJ: Aronson.

Schlesinger, S. E., & Epstein, N. B. (2007). Couple problems. In F. M. Dattilio & A. Freeman (Eds.), *Cognitive-behavioral strategies in crisis intervention* (3rd ed., pp. 300–326). New York: Guilford Press.

Schmaling, K. B., & Sher, T. G. (2000). *The psychology of couples and illness: Theory, research and practice.* Washington, DC: American Psychological Association.

Shadish, W. R., & Baldwin, S. A. (2003). Meta-analysis of MFT interventions. *Journal of Marital and Family Therapy, 29,* 547–570.

Shadish, W. R., & Baldwin, S. A. (2005). Effects of behavioral marital therapy: A meta-analysis of randomized controlled trials. *Journal of Consulting and Clinical Psychology, 73,* 6–14.

Snyder, D. K. (1979). Multidimensional assessment of marital satisfaction. *Journal of Marriage and the Family, 41*(4), 813–823.

Snyder, D. K., Baucom, D. H., & Gordon, K. C. (2007). *Getting past the affair: A program to help you cope, heal, and move on—together or apart.* New York: Guilford Press.

Snyder, D. K., Castellani, A. M., & Whisman, M. A. (2006). Current status and future directions in couple therapy. *Annual Review of Psychology, 57,* 317–344.

Snyder, D. K., & Costin, S. E. (1994). Marital Satisfaction Inventory. In M. E. Maruish (Ed.), *The use of psychological testing for treatment planning and outcome assessment* (pp. 322–351). Hillsdale, NJ: Erlbaum.

Snyder, D. K., & Whisman, M. A. (2002). Understanding psychopathology and couple dysfunction: Implications for clinical practice, training, and research. In D. K. Snyder & M. A. Whisman (Eds.), *Treating difficult couples: Managing emotional, behavioral, and health problems in couple therapy* (pp. 419–438). New York: Guilford Press.

Snyder, D. K., & Wills, R. M. (1989). Behavioral versus insight-oriented marital therapy: Effects on individual and interspousal functioning. *Journal of Consulting and Clinical Psychology, 57*(1), 39–46.

Snyder, D. K., Wills, R. M., & Grady-Fletcher, A. (1991). Long-term effectiveness of behavioral versus insight-oriented marital therapy: A 4-year follow-up study. *Journal of Consulting and Clinical Psychology, 59*(1), 138–141.

Spanier, G. B. (1976). Measuring dyadic adjustment: New scales for assessing the quality of marriage and similar dyads. *Journal of Marriage and the Family, 38,* 15–28.

Straus, M. A., Hamby, S. L., Boney-McCoy, S., & Sugarman, D. B. (1996). The Revised Conflict Tactics Scales (CTS2): Development and preliminary psychometric data. *Journal of Family Issues, 17*(3), 283–316.

Stuart, R. B. (1969). Operant interpersonal treatment for marital discord. *Journal of Consulting and Clinical Psychology, 33,* 675–682.

Stuart, R. B. (1980). *Helping couples change: A social learning approach to marital therapy.* New York: Guilford Press.

Sullivan, L. J., & Baucom, D. H. (2004). The relationship–schematic coding system: Behavioral manifestations of thinking in relationships terms. In P. K. Kerig & D. H. Baucom (Eds.), *Couple observational coding systems* (pp. 289–304). Mahwah, NJ: Erlbaum.

Sullivan, L. J., & Baucom, D. H. (2005). Observational coding of relationship-schematic processing. *Journal of Marital and Family Therapy, 31,* 31–43.

Sullivan, L. J., Baucom, D. H., & Snyder, D. K. (2002, November). *Relationship-Schematic Processing and Relationship Satisfaction Across Two Types of Marital Interventions.* Paper presented at the Annual Meeting of the Association for Advancement of Behavior Therapy, Reno, NV.

Thibaut, J. W., & Kelley, H. H. (1959). *The social psychology of groups.* New York: Wiley.

Weiss, R. L. (1980). Strategic behavioral martial therapy: Toward a model for assessment and intervention. In J. P. Vincent (Ed.), *Advances in family intervention, assessment and theory* (Vol. 1, pp. 229–271). Greenwich, CT: JAI Press.

Weiss, R. L., & Heyman, R. E. (1997). A clinical-research overview of couples interactions. In W. K. Halford & H. J. Markman (Eds.), *Clinical handbook of marriage and couples interventions* (pp. 39–41). Chichester, UK: Wiley.

Weiss, R. L., Hops, H., & Patterson, G. R. (1973). A framework for conceptualizing marital conflict, a technology for altering it, some data for evaluating it. In M. Hersen & A. S. Bellack (Eds.), *Behavior change: Methodology, concepts and practice* (pp. 309–342). Champaign, IL: Research Press.

CHAPTER 14

Cognitive-Behavioral Therapy with Diverse Populations

David W. Pantalone
Gayle Y. Iwamasa
Christopher R. Martell

Cognitive-behavioral therapy (CBT) is the leading theoretical orientation among health service providers in psychology in the United States; over one-third of psychologists endorse a cognitive or behavioral orientation (Norcross, Karg, & Prochaska, 1997). As established in previous chapters of this volume, as well as in countless empirical and theoretical articles published over the past 50 years, CBT has demonstrated efficacy for a variety of mental disorders, including anxiety, mood, eating, substance use, and personality disorders (e.g., Dobson, 2001), as well as other problems in living, such as marital problems (e.g., Snyder, Castellani, & Whisman, 2006). Although there are many topographical differences in these treatments, there remain certain invariant aspects as well. The competent practice of CBT requires that a therapist meaningfully consider the context of the client's life in all aspects of evaluation, assessment, intervention, and consultation, including social, political, historical, and economic contexts. In CBT, assessment of the topography, or specific features, of behavior is instructive, but attention to *function* and *context* is essential.

Given the nature of the idiographic case conceptualizations that are standard in behavioral assessment (Haynes & O'Brien, 2000), a focus on the importance of the client's context is unlikely to surprise readers. Throughout this volume, well-seasoned experts have discussed the theoretical underpinnings of various CBT treatments, as well as provided instruction and data about the empirical support for a variety of specific CBT techniques. In this chapter, we aim to elucidate both the *what* and the *how*—that is, the content and process knowledge—necessary for incorporating multiculturalism into the practice of standard CBT. To meet this goal, we first discuss terminology and provide a rationale for the importance of cultural competence in the practice of CBT. We then discuss what to do in practice when one encounters a client who is culturally different in any of a number of demographic areas. Although the techniques of CBT per se do not differ, certainly cultural norms that differ across groups are important to keep in one's awareness. Given the constraints of this chapter, we briefly review several elements and guide the reader to additional resources for further detail.

WHAT'S IN A NAME?: DEFINING TERMS RELATED TO DIVERSITY FOR THIS CHAPTER

When we speak of "diversity," what exactly do we mean? Are "diverse populations" the same as "special populations?" To avoid confusion, an explicit discussion of definitions is necessary. Without question, human beings are diverse. We come in different sizes and colors, speak a variety of languages, hold varied cultural values, and live in a multiplicity of circumstances. Diversity is inherent in the human experience. Unfortunately, when diversity is considered "special," the very definitions belie a cultural bias that one group is the norm and all other "diverse" groups are "different." As is true for the general psychological literature, much of the cognitive-behavioral literature is written from the perspective of middle-class, heterosexual, North Americans of European descent. Thankfully, at the time of this writing, that vantage point is no longer predominantly male, as it was only a few decades ago.

In using the term "diverse populations," we mean to consider the individual differences in the human population that, for the sake of simplicity, are broken into classifications of race, ethnicity, sexual orientation, gender identity, socioeconomic status, religion, age, and ability–disability status. We say "for the sake of simplicity" because, within these categories, there is enormous variability. Race is one example of the categories typically considered in a discussion of diversity. However, despite the fact that many people hold essentialist beliefs about race, empirical data from a number of sources—including the Human Genome Project itself—lends strong support to the idea that these differences are socially constructed, with culturally arbitrary boundaries (Anderson & Nickerson, 2005). When considering these broad group labels, it may be true that the within-group variability is greater than the between-group variability in some, or even most, cases. We must be sure to recognize that people are not simply an ethnicity, an age, or a sexual orientation. Thus, we consider diversity to include the heterogeneity of human experience that both fits and transcends categories, and differentiates individuals who are members of various groups. For example, Kim (2006) found diversity in mental health issues among Southeast Asian ethnic groups, arguing against the practice of considering Cambodians, Vietnamese, and Laotians as one homogenous group. "Diversity" is the general label given to the natural variation in experience, identity, and biology of humankind.

Mental health providers who successfully provide treatment to culturally different clients are considered to have some amount of "cultural competence." Here, again, we use the term "culture" broadly and functionally to include any number of areas of difference—not simply a focus on race, ethnicity, or any other unconcealed area of diversity. Although clearly topographical aspects of identity are important to consider (e.g., race, cultural norms), a sufficiently expansive definition of "difference" is necessary. Individuals can be impacted when they live in *any* environment that surrounds them with images and ideas to which they do not subscribe.

Volumes have been written about what cultural competence is and how one might achieve some measure of it. Here we posit that "cultural competence" includes the skill of holding two seemingly contradictory strategies at the forefront of one's practice. First, it is necessary to become knowledgeable about the sociocultural groups to which a client belongs, without asking the client to provide such education, a situation that can itself be a stressor for minority group members (e.g., Meyer, 2003). It is essential to use this knowledge to infuse one's cognitive-behavioral case conceptualization and to choose relevant intervention techniques. Simultaneously, however, one must acknowledge that a given individual's experience of the world is unique and not determined by group membership alone. People are members of sociocultural groups, but they are also uniquely individual. Culturally competent therapists embrace the inherent tension and meet it with informed curiosity and openness.

WHY IS CULTURAL COMPETENCE IMPORTANT?: AN ETHICAL RATIONALE

The importance of cultural competence in the practice of CBT mimics the importance of cultural considerations in the general practice of professional psychology. Overall, key arguments are based on ethical and empirical grounds (e.g., Whaley & Davis, 2007). Ethically, the U.S. Surgeon General has noted mental health providers' lack of effectiveness in providing culturally competent services to culturally diverse populations (U.S. Department of Health and Human Services, 1999). Eminent psychologists also have written considerably about past inadequacies in basic and intervention research with racial and ethnically diverse individuals (e.g., Sue, 2006). Mental health professions have increasingly realized that special attention must be paid to issues of training in cultural competency (e.g., Korman, 1974), and this realization has morphed over time from suggestions and recommendations to ethical obligations. Eventually, the ethical code of the American Psychological Association (1992) has come to include *Principle D: Respect of People's Rights and Dignity*, which in part states that "psychologists are aware of cultural, individual, and role differences, including those related to age, gender, race, ethnicity, and national origin" (p. 1598).

To the extent we agree that therapeutic skills addressing elements of human diversity are essential, then what follows is an *ethical imperative* to attain cultural competence. If, indeed, these are essential skills, then requiring provider competence is no different than requiring basic abilities in diagnostic assessment or clinical intervention. Indeed, it has been argued that "delivering mental health services outside of one's area of competence constitutes an ethical infraction" (Ridley, 1985, p. 613). Increasing cultural competence at a fundamental, ethical level is the right thing to do. However, there is another line of reasoning for prioritizing cultural competence in psychotherapy, and this one is based on data.

WHY IS CULTURAL COMPETENCE IMPORTANT?

Empirical Rationale 1: Our Clients Are Diverse

According to the *Guidelines on Multicultural Education, Training, Research, Practice, and Organizational Change for Psychologists,* published by the American Psychological Association (2003), an increasingly large percentage of the U.S. population comprises individuals who are ethnically or racially diverse, including those with a biracial, multiethnic, or multiracial heritage (U.S. Census Bureau, 2001). The largest population growth rates are in Asian Americans/Pacific Islanders and Latinos/Hispanics (Hobbs & Stoops, 2002). Overall, whites/European Americans continue to be the majority group, but in some U.S. states this is no longer the case. Thus, there exists a growing inevitability about working with culturally different clients. Furthermore, an expanding empirical literature shows that providers with higher levels of cultural competence have more favorable outcomes in terms of assessment and the psychotherapy process (e.g., Sue, 2001).

Psychologists are likely to confront other areas of diversity in the practice of psychotherapy. These include older adults, since the proportion of the population over 65 continues to grow (Gist & Hetzel, 2004), and people living in poverty. Despite the relative wealth of the United States, approximately 12% of the population report incomes below the poverty level. Furthermore, in a given 10-year period, fully 40% of the population experiences poverty in at least 1 year (Zweig, 2004). Increasingly, the number of diverse people who seek mental health services continues to grow; this includes sexual minorities, people living with physical disabilities, as well as individuals representing other areas of diversity. Thus, the diversity of the United States, determined by multiple criteria, is vast and only increasing.

Empirical Rationale 2: Providers Are Seemingly Less Diverse

Data culled from the American Psychological Association (2006) indicate that 85% of psychologists, and fully 94% of association members are of European American descent. The reality is that most doctoral-level psychologists are culturally homogenous. Data are not available for all areas of diversity; however, if the statistics related to ethnic and racial representation within psychology are indicative of other areas, psychology has a significant challenge in terms of shaping the profession to represent better the diversity of its clients. In examining rates of psychology bachelor's, master's, and doctoral degrees conferred, there is a precipitous drop in the proportion of degrees (from bachelor's to graduate degrees) awarded to members of diverse racial and ethnic groups compared to European Americans (American Psychological Association, 2003). In an analysis, Kite and colleagues (2001) reported that the number of ethnic/minority psychologists was too small even to break down by ethnicity. This difference is especially notable at the graduate level, which suggests that some structural factors may impede the entry of individuals of diverse backgrounds into psychology.

There are significant consequences of this dearth of diversity within the profession. First, it is likely that knowledge of other cultures is variable among European American psychologists, with some extremely knowledgeable individuals and others lacking such knowledge or experience. It is commonly understood that cultural competence is developed through ongoing personal or professional contact with individuals who are culturally different or, for psychologists whose routine contact is limited, based on engaging in additional training experiences. Some providers may lack an awareness of their cultural naivete, however. Indeed, all providers will have some "little vacuum packs of ignorance regarding various groups" (Hays, 2006, p. 8). Mental health providers with a culturally homogenous social and professional milieu may be forced to seek out such knowledge specifically via additional education and supervised practice. Indeed, Hall (1997) termed the inability to address effectively the weaknesses in one's professional skills and abilities as "cultural malpractice."

The discussion of cultural competence in this chapter is based on the premise that the United States is diverse and that its constituents—patients, clients, supervisees, students, research participants—come for assistance with various elements of diversity. If the goal is to provide competent CBT, as it ought to be, then it behooves providers to assess realistically their ability to address areas of diversity and multiculturalism as a first step toward increasing their skills.

DEFINING THE SCOPE OF DIVERSITY

This chapter details how CBT can be used with a variety of diverse populations. However, the danger of overgeneralizing about any group of people is ever-present. Thus, it is beyond the scope of this chapter to detail everything that must be considered when working with "diverse" individuals. However, a chapter on diversity requires that we point out some generalities that may distinguish particular groups' members from members of other groups, and that should be considered for potential inclusion in a cognitive-behavioral case conceptualization. Using the language of generalities should not be interpreted to imply that any individual who fits a particular classification into a "diverse" group will have the same needs, or will have had the same experiences, as others. General knowledge about a population should be used judiciously; remember that within-group differences may be greater than between-group differences on some key variables.

Consider an example of the misappropriation of generalities: A late-middle-aged, Catholic, Latino man reports that his current sexual partner is a man. Basing a case conceptualization on generalities, a therapist could assume that because the man has a male sexual partner, he identifies as gay. The therapist could assume that since he is Latino, he is likely to be the dominant partner in the relationship and not engage in "passive" or receptive sexual behaviors. Furthermore, the therapist may believe that since the man is Catholic, his sexual orientation is likely to conflict with the views of his church, and he probably harbors negative beliefs about himself, Catholicism, and all people with strong religious beliefs. *All* of these assumptions can be wrong, however. Not all people who have relationships with others of the same sex identify as gay, lesbian, or bisexual. Behavior and identity may not match. Not all Latino men conform to a culture of *machismo*. There is no single "Latino" grouping, for example, since Latino culture includes people from many different geographic locations. Many Catholics who hold beliefs on social issues that are markedly divergent from Church doctrine still consider themselves to be faithful. Thus, we comment on various groups with caution, acknowledging the insufficiency of the data and the all-too-human tendency to chunk information into simplistic categories that require little effort and quickly communicate that others are "like us" or "not like us."

COGNITIVE-BEHAVIORAL THERAPY AND MULTICULTURAL THERAPY ARE COMPATIBLE, BUT DIVERSE INDIVIDUALS ARE UNDERREPRESENTED IN THE COGNITIVE-BEHAVIORAL THERAPY LITERATURE

CBT and multicultural therapy in general are among the two fastest growing trends in psychotherapy (Norcross, Hedges, & Prochaska, 2002). Pamela Hays (2006) points out that CBT fits nicely within the framework of multicultural therapy. The two therapies share the premise that treatment must be based on an individualized case conceptualization. The bedrock of the therapeutic situation is that the specific issues addressed and techniques employed are based on the particular context of a given client. Also, both CBT and multicultural therapy endeavor to empower clients. CBT is collaborative, and the individual client is considered the expert regarding his or her life. Thus, treatment is not something that is *done to the client* by an expert; rather, it is a collaborative process in which the therapist assists the client in exploring the ways his or her particular beliefs and behaviors may contribute to heightened distress. The treatment is *done with the client* to develop a plan to examine and modify beliefs and behaviors as needed. A clinical example provided by Sue and Zane (1987) demonstrates how case formulation is not only culturally sensitive but also culturally consistent. Furthermore, both treatments direct attention to clients' strengths and the importance of social support as a key contextual variable.

Diversity is a complex topic and, although our standard lexicon of categories has inherent limitations, we can roughly divide underrepresented groups into six broad areas. These include individuals with a background or identity based on one or more of the following characteristics or identities: race or ethnic heritage; sexual orientation or gender identity/presentation; ability or disability; religious beliefs or lack thereof; age; and socioeconomic status. Many of these groups have been left out of discussions of psychotherapeutic processes.

Racial and ethnic groups that have been underrepresented in published reports of CBT outcome studies in the United States and Canada include Native Americans, Alaskan Natives, Latino/as, African Americans, Asian Americans, and Arab Americans. Lesbians, gay men, and bisexual and transgender individuals have also been underrepresented in treatment outcome literature or have been the focus of treatment that considers their sexual orientation or gender identity to be pathological (Martell, Safren, & Prince, 2004). Much of the literature excludes differently-abled individuals; thus, it is unclear how our treatment protocols apply to people other than the able bodied. Apart from trials by experts in the psychology of religion, psychologists rarely consider religion as a demographic variable expected to result in varied treatment outcomes. The majority of treatment outcome research is on adults, with less focus on children and youth below the age of 21 or, likewise, with senior citizens above age 65. Finally, research designed and conducted at major universities is often more accessible for people from middle or upper social classes, unless specifically designed to target a population from lower socioeconomic strata.

WHY ARE MULTICULTURAL INDIVIDUALS UNDERREPRESENTED?: WHAT DOES THAT MEAN FOR THE FIELD?

Some groups remain underrepresented in the treatment outcome literature, because individuals who consider themselves to be partially or completely part of these identity groups may approach psychotherapy with trepidation— and for good reason. Research on human subjects in general, and on certain groups in particular, has not always been conducted ethically. One need only reflect on the Tuskegee experiments (Jones, 1981) of the last century, when male African American research participants with syphilis were left untreated, without their consent, so that the federally funded researchers could better understand the natural history of the disease. Given these and other less egregious historical experiences, it is understandable that people from some ethnic or racial groups may not trust researchers. Interestingly, however, although there is evidence that Latino and African American individuals have a greater fear of participation in research than the majority, group members continue to participate in biomedical research at rates comparable to those of European Americans (Katz et al., 2007).

People from traditionally oppressed groups may also be particularly apprehensive about an approach to therapy that claims to "modify thoughts" or "change behavior." For example, part of the African American shared experience includes a history of oppression, racism, and systematic attempts to punish and eradicate African culture and heritage (Kelly, 2006). The history of CBT, especially, has not always been favorable toward oppressed groups. The past use of aversive conditioning techniques to change sexual orientation serves as a dramatic example. Descriptions of such "treatments" can be found in behavior therapy textbooks published as late as the early 1990s, despite the removal of homosexuality as a mental disorder from the American Psychiatric Association's *Diagnostic and Statistical Manual of Mental Disorders, Third Edition* (DSM-III) in 1980. Not only behaviorists but also cognitive therapists once put into practice their theories about how to "cure" homosexuality (Ellis & Cory, 1965). While many of these therapists changed their opinions following social and diagnostic changes, it is unsurprising that some lesbian, gay, or bisexual clients might be reticent to seek out CBT, even if their problem can be efficiently treated with a standard CBT protocol. Transgender individuals, who have often faced the roadblock of mental health professionals determining the course of their lives in evaluations for sex reassignment surgery, may be concerned about being judged, classified, or pathologized.

When evidence is based on populations of predominantly middle-class, heterosexual, white individuals, people from other groups may not recognize themselves in the description; thus, they may minimize or discount the research's applicability to their lives. Such discounting of the research could occur on the part of both consumers and providers who are skeptical of the degree of generalization from more mainstream samples to disenfranchised individuals. Without direct evaluation, the applicability of treatments to diverse group members will continue to be suspect—as it should be. As clinical scientists, we have long known that threats to external validity should be a chief concern for treatment development and dissemination efforts. We must always, therefore, ask, "Empirically supported treatments ... for whom?"

Furthermore, as a result of limited knowledge about, and experience with, dissemination of evidence-based therapies to diverse individuals and communities, their relevance and effectiveness should be questioned. Adapting evidence-based therapies for clients from various populations may be justified when contextual factors demonstrate the vulnerability of a specific group of people to specific problems for which there are established evidence-based therapies, or when specific resiliencies identified for a particular group would inform relevant modifications. Lau (2006) argues for a systematic approach to evaluation and dissemination of these therapies with diverse constituents. While the present chapter advocates for culturally appropriate adaptations of evidence-based therapies (see also Hall, 2001), little evidence has emerged about how to accomplish this task. A thorough discussion of the emergent issues is beyond the scope of this chapter, but readers are directed to Lau's excellent work (2006) for further elucidation of relevant issues.

TREATING INDIVIDUALS FROM DIVERSE BACKGROUNDS

There is a lack of agreement about how best to provide CBT for individuals from diverse backgrounds. Because these individuals are excluded from some of these groups in efficacy and effectiveness trials, whether (or how) to modify treatment protocols to best serve these clients is unclear. However, in the meantime, our offices and clinics continue to be populated by many diverse group members. So what should a clinician do to provide high-quality CBT? Based on the knowledge currently available, we recommend an approach that includes the following elements.

Honest Self-Assessment and Information Gathering

Therapists who work with people who are different from themselves must make an honest appraisal of their own biases and blind spots. It is naive to believe that anyone is completely without bias. Even when our biases are not ill-intentioned, we can still make errors. Take, for example, the simple assessment question "Are you married?" This question is biased against people who are in same-sex relationships, because for them marriage is illegal in nearly all states in the United States and most other parts of the world. A more appropriate question might be "Are you currently in a romantic relationship?" Without living within the culture of a particular client, it is easy to make stereotypical assumptions, and to remain unaware of the ways such assumptions bias our decisions. Thus, culturally competent CBT therapists must make a *lifelong commitment* to understand the breadth of cultural differences, and engage in introspection to recognize where their own cultural experiences blind them to the experiences of others.

Martell and colleagues (2004) suggest that therapists consider the questions provided in Table 14.1 when they work with lesbian, gay, or bisexual (LGB) clients. Most of these questions can be adapted for work with any client who is somehow different from the therapist. For example, therapists should ask themselves whether they are more likely to assume that ambiguous symptoms indicate psychopathology if a client is of a different ethnic or racial background. Does the therapist make personality disorder diagnoses more frequently for one gender or another, or without due regard to prevalence rates?

TABLE 14.1. Questions to Consider When Working with Lesbian, Gay, or Bisexual (LGB) Clients

1. Do I believe that LGB people are immoral or disordered simply because of their sexual orientation?
2. Am I anxious when I meet a client who exhibits gender-atypical behavior (e.g., a man with strongly feminine characteristics)?
3. Do I avoid asking clients about their sexual orientation?
4. When clients discuss dating or families, do I assume their partner is of the opposite sex?
5. Do I feel uncomfortable discussing sexual acts between two people of the same sex?
6. If I am uncomfortable with such discussion, do I make attempts to discourage clients from disclosing details of their sexual behavior?
7. Am I more likely to assume psychopathology if I know my client is LGB?
8. Do I diagnose personality disorders more frequently if my client is LGB?
9. Do I perceive LGB couples to have more problems than heterosexual couples?
10. Do I miss some of my clients' problem behaviors because I am afraid to discuss their sexual orientation, sex life, or relationship status?

Note. From Martell, Safren, and Prince (2004, p. 204). Copyright 2004 by The Guilford Press. Reprinted by permission.

Additional questions that can be used to guide a therapist's self-exploration are listed in Table 14.2. Therapists at all levels of training are encouraged to reflect periodically on their thoughts and behaviors related to treating diverse clients. It is essential to consider these and other questions deeply and honestly, avoiding superficial or socially desirable responding. Given the strong social pressure in the mental health community to remain unbiased, we suspect that many practitioners will deny these errors. However, the ongoing self-evaluation and admission of blind spots will ultimately help practitioners to function optimally when dealing with individuals of diverse backgrounds.

Furthermore, it is necessary to become knowledgeable about the sociocultural groups in which your clients are members. Such education should come from a combination of reading books, articles in professional journals, and the popular press; taking courses; traveling; and taking part in cultural events or informal discussions with friends or peers. Remember to use the information gleaned as a guide rather than to treat it as a rigid absolute. Within-group differences can be significant, and it is helpful to use newly discovered knowledge to help generate hypotheses or to demonstrate interest in, and connection with, the client. Information about a sociocultural group cannot substitute for thorough, idiographic assessment of an individual client's experience of the world.

Do Competent Cognitive-Behavioral Therapy

Do CBT as you know it. Given the countless empirical studies that demonstrate support for the learning theory substrate of CBT, there is a strong likeli-

TABLE 14.2. Additional Questions to Consider When Working with "Diverse" Clients

1. How do I understand the impact of cultural and economic privilege, and of cultural disadvantage and poverty, in the lives of my clients? How do I assess directly, or make inferences about, these constructs?

2. How willing am I to seek consultation to avoid issues that may arise from my own unacknowledged or unrecognized privilege—based on racial, ethnic, geographic, cultural and other advantages I may have? How often have I done this in the past?
   - What are some potential sources of consultation in my professional and personal networks? What people or organizations could I call upon? If areas of diversity are not represented in my own networks, how can I go about obtaining the necessary training, either through continuing education efforts or otherwise?
   - What are the personal or institutional barriers to seek such consultation? How might I address them to serve my clients competently?

3. What assumptions do I make about others' racial or ethnic identities based on their physical characteristics?
   - Do I feel comfortable asking about the background/heritage of others? What do I notice (thoughts, feelings) happening when I ask such questions? How is their experience similar or different across racial or ethnic groups?
   - What words/terms do I typically use to assess a client's diverse sociodemographic background? How have clients responded when I ask these questions? What do I seem to be doing well that I ought to keep doing? What are techniques or language that might be useful to change?
   - How can I remind myself to explicitly assess "diverse" aspects of identity when I meet new clients? What mechanisms can I put in place in my practices to ensure that I minimize a reliance on stereotypes and maximize a true idiographic assessment?

4. How do I conceptualize the complexities of the intersections of multiple identities—including cultural, racial, socioeconomic class, sexual orientation, physical ability, and others?
   - How do I discuss these issues with clients? Do I ever initiate discussion with diverse clients about the potential difficulty they face in managing multiple identities? Why or why not? What factors influence the likelihood of my discussing these issues with clients? If a client alludes to struggles with conflicting identity elements in session, how do I respond?

5. How flexible am I about who I allow to participate in treatment, so as not to invalidate a client's culturally congruent desire to involve extended support networks or others?
   - "Best practices" for therapy may work well for some clients but are culturally incompatible for others. What allowances do I make, in accommodating clients from different backgrounds, to make therapy more acceptable and or applicable to them? What allowances have clients asked for that I declined? What rationale did I use to explain my decisions? On what data are they based?

(cont.)

TABLE 14.2. *(cont.)*

6. In session, how do I acknowledge or highlight cultural, ethnic, sexual orientation, or other differences between myself and clients?
   - CBT therapists typically strive to be warm and genuine, while maintaining a task orientation. Given these goals, comments about similarities or differences between therapist and client can facilitate alliance building. How/when/with whom do I highlight these similarities or differences? How/when/with whom do I shy away for this type of comment?
   - A high degree of heterogeneity exists within many identity groups. Thus, even if I have some experience with, or insight into, a given group, those experiences may or may not be similar to the experiences of any given client. How can I communicate and demonstrate my understanding of this fact to clients?

7. How frequently do I inquire about specific, negative consequences that occur in my clients' lives because of their "diverse" identity or identities?
   - In what ways can I inquire about experiences of racism, sexism, heterosexism/homophobia, and so forth, that validate clients' experience? How do I best portray my genuine understanding of the struggles they may face?
   - What kinds of language would I use? How can I remember to assess these important experiences, in my intake, as well as during ongoing therapeutic work?

hood that the basic tenets of CBT treatment will be upheld for clients in many subgroups. The specific techniques employed, as far as we can tell, should remain the same. Given our beliefs that all behavior is caused, that all behavior is learned and therefore can be unlearned, and our focus on the interrelations of thoughts, feelings, and behaviors, these principles do and ought to guide all of our clinical endeavors. We still are problem-focused, oriented toward meeting the client's collaboratively determined goals, use functional analyses, and routinely give and review homework to strengthen skills development and generalization. On its face, therapy might not look all that different with clients of diverse backgrounds than with those having no or fewer marginalized identities.

THEMATIC ISSUES THAT VARY ACROSS CULTURAL SUBGROUPS

While considering clients' diverse group memberships, consider the following thematic areas that drive some differences in client behavior. For some subgroups, such as ethnic and racial minorities and LGBT individuals, guidelines for competent treatment have been promulgated by professional associations (American Psychological Association, 2000, 2003). Given the collective expertise of the authors and the extensive peer review process of scientists, as well as practitioners, these documents serve as an important starting point for treatment planning. For other groups, if established treatment guidelines are unavailable, look critically to the extant literature for any published information that may be helpful in case conceptualization or treatment planning. Seek peer support and supervisory consultation, as available.

Rather than suggesting specific considerations for specific groups, which can lead to overgeneralizations, we instead consider thematic differences that vary somewhat reliably across groups, and that tend to be overlooked in the clinical outcome literature. The following section provides just a few examples of the issues to which therapists should attend when providing clinical services to culturally diverse group members. The list is by no means exhaustive. Our goal is merely to provide a foundation for researchers and clinicians to recognize the many diverse facets and qualities of the people we encounter and with whom we work. The following themes are presented in no particular order:

Health Beliefs

The notion that beliefs about the underlying causes of illness and disease influence one's physical and mental health is not new. Indeed, the work of Kleinman, Eisenberg, and Good (2006) highlights how important it is to understand the client's perceptions and beliefs, because these *explanatory models of illness* affect a patient's compliance to treatment recommendations. Health beliefs influence not only who a client contacts but also receptivity to treatment (see, e.g., Ebreo, Shiraishi, Leung, & Yi, 2007, on the role of traditional Asian beliefs about physical ailments and disability). Beliefs that involve fate or inevitability can result in delaying or, worse, not pursuing intervention at all. However, if the therapist is knowledgeable about some of a client's health beliefs, it is possible to initiate treatment successfully, as well as keep the client engaged. Hinton and Otto's (2006) summary of *symptom meaning* among Cambodian refugees who have experienced significant trauma is an excellent review of how such knowledge can be used to benefit those whose health beliefs differ from beliefs in the traditional American health care system.

Self-Identification

Self-identification is an area of huge variation among ethnically diverse groups. Some individuals see themselves—and identify themselves outwardly—primarily through their ethnicity, whereas others view their ethnicity as secondary to other important identity components, such as sexual orientation or religious affiliation. For some people, ethnic identity also varies depending on the context. An individual with multiple stigmatized identities, such as an African American gay man, may emphasize his racial heritage in family settings but his sexual identity in social settings where peers predominate. The clinician needs to remain aware of the client's self-identification and how it may vary by context, to be comfortable discussing how varied identities might affect the client's presenting problems or primary therapeutic issues. Awareness of clients' level of acculturation, regardless of their generation, ethnic, racial identity, and activation of other identities, is important in assessing and evaluating clients' cognitions. Although a thorough discussion of these concepts is clearly beyond the scope of this chapter, we suggest that readers review Iwamasa, Hsia, and Hinton's (2006) summary of these and other terms. The essential element is for the therapist to understand that these concepts are fluid rather than static, and are thus likely to vary depending on the context, including the therapy setting.

Individualism and Collectivism

People from collectivist cultures may not relate to the individualistic assumptions of most psychotherapeutic practices. McDonald and Gonzalez (2006) note that the collectivist worldview of Native Americans, for example, considers the well-being of the group to supersede that of the individual, and that their understanding of "personhood" is not a unitary construct, as it is in individualistic cultures. Thus, to conduct culturally responsive CBT with clients from collectivist cultures, individuals' family structures and backgrounds need to be investigated. Similarly, European American notions of individuality separate individual therapy from family therapy, but it may be that entire families from some cultures (e.g., traditional Latino families) may arrive for a therapy session despite the fact that only one member of the family is identified as the patient by the CBT therapist. Understanding that the well-being of a given individual may make more sense in Latino culture, for example, when discussed in terms of caring for the family rather than taking care of the self (Organista, 2006), can lead to a more valid, culturally sensitive CBT.

Communication Styles

People's communication styles differ as much as their personality styles. The typical, dominant, culturally "acceptable" communication style in conversation between two people in the United States usually involves direct eye contact, an open body stance, and direct questioning and answering, because the culture values assertiveness and direct expression of thoughts. Most graduate training programs teach novice therapists such "foundational skills." Therapists in training are also often taught certain "rules" of therapy, such as not accepting gifts from clients and not engaging in self-disclosure.

In our experience, gift giving means different things to people of different cultures. In some cultures, bearing gifts demonstrates respect and is often viewed as a courtesy. For example, *omiyage* is a traditional gift-giving practice of Japanese when visiting someone's home for the first time. Also, bringing food items (usually homemade) is often a sign of gratitude among Latinos and African Americans. Thus, to decline accepting such gifts can be hurtful, viewed as disrespectful, and potentially may damage the therapeutic relationship. Similarly, being unwilling to disclose personal information, yet expecting clients to divulge any number of personal and intimate details about themselves, highlights a hierarchical stance that for some subgroup members may be experienced as disrespectful and generate distrust.

We often find that clients are curious about us, and if they do not ask questions directly, we often provide information about ourselves based on what we think they want to know (our age, our training, our family, etc.). Such self-disclosure often relaxes clients and can serve as a model for how to discuss personal details from their own lives comfortably. For some clients from Asian cultures, for example, focusing on themselves can be viewed culturally as being selfish or grandiose, so they are often reluctant to do so without prompting—or even with prompting. Among many collectivistic cultural groups, direct communication is viewed as disrespectful, and more subtle forms of communication, such as nonverbal and indirect behavioral communication, are valued. Iwamasa et al. (2006) and Organista (2006) provide a number of culture-specific examples of communication styles, and discuss therapists' ability to communicate skillfully given those differences.

Therapy Goals

Developing a realistic set of therapy goals is essential in CBT. As illustrated elsewhere in this volume, the ability to break down long-term goals into short-term goals maintains therapy progress and keeps clients focused on a larger goal and moving in their preferred direction. The ability to collaborate with clients to develop realistic goals may be a challenge to those therapists whose beliefs dictate that there is one "right" thing to do. Some clients may be less interested in behavioral or cognitive change, but may benefit from accepting certain aspects of their lives, and choosing to develop coping skills and patience. For many, the concept of faith or balance their lives may more effectively help them to find satisfaction in life (Iwamasa et al., 2006; Kelly, 2006; Organista, 2006).

Along with a focus on acceptance and change, a therapist may be challenged by a client's desire to "please" others or to rely on other members of his or her social network for assistance. Indeed, CBT therapists often believe that helping clients become more self-sufficient and independent will help them function better, and for many that is likely true. However, the ability to ask for help and to get along with others strengthens some clients' role in their cultural context, and improves social support and functioning (Iwamasa et al., 2006; Kelly, 2006; Organista, 2006).

Immigrant or Refugee Status

The 2000 U.S. Census result indicated that 1 in 10 people was an immigrant or refugee, and that 20% of the population had at least one parent born in another country. Although a large proportion of Asian and Latino populations comprise immigrants and refugees, the number of immigrants and refugees coming to the United States from Eastern European countries—

especially from countries that were a part of the former Soviet Union—has also increased. Most immigrants and refugees share some similar experiences in terms of adapting to the U.S. environment; however, significant differences distinguish refugees from immigrants.

Whereas immigrants voluntarily migrate, with goals such as improved economic, political, or educational opportunities, refugees leave their country involuntarily, often as a result of war, political persecution, or disaster. Typically, immigrants are more prepared to migrate, may have family or other contacts who have already established themselves in the new country, and may have some command of the language and understanding of the culture, and a plan of what activities they intend to pursue, such as attending school or establishing a business, once they arrive. On the other hand, refugees often have been economically and educationally deprived in their home country. They often have experienced significant trauma prior to migration, with no time to prepare to leave and little to no familiarity with the host culture or language. Indeed, they may be illiterate in their native language. For a specific example of psychological issues pertaining to immigrants and refugees, readers are encouraged to review Chung and Bemak (2007).

Given these issues, conducting CBT with immigrants and refugees requires not only knowledge about the client's experiences but also a willingness to anticipate and strategically develop and deliver CBT in a way to increase the client's active involvement in treatment in order to provide the most benefit. Fortunately, the field has some success in the delivery of CBT to immigrant and refugees populations. Clinicians would benefit from reviewing specific examples of using CBT with these individuals (e.g., Hinton & Otto, 2006; Hinton, Safran, Pollack, & Tran, 2006; Iwamasa et al., 2006; Otto & Hinton, 2006; Schulz, Huber, & Resick, 2006; Schulz, Resick, Huber, & Griffen, 2006).

Family Structure

The term "family" includes not only the nuclear family but also extended family members and even family friends in many cultural groups. Such a broad definition of "family" and "kinship networks" provides many members of culturally diverse groups with a large social support system. McCubbin, McCubbin, Thompson, and Thompson (1998) provide a model of resilience for ethnic/minority families. The model incorporates development, culture, values, interpersonal skills, and systems as variables that affect family functioning over time. The researchers suggest that all families have a unique blend of fluid risk and protective factors, and that resilient families are those that are able to use effectively the various protective factors throughout life. On the other hand, an individual's role within a family tends to be enduring, and efforts to move outside one's ascribed role in the family are often viewed unfavorably. Yee, DeBaryshe, Yuen, Kim, and McCubbin (2007) provide an excellent summary of traditional family values and themes among Asian American families, including collectivism, "relational orientation (defining self within the context of family relationships), "familialism" (which emphasizes the set hierarchy of the family), and obligation. They also review other family structures and roles, such as the structure of the marital relationship, parenting styles, sibling relationships, gender roles, language spoken in the home, and generational differences, among family members.

A clinical consideration in CBT is to understand how the client's beliefs about his or her behaviors may reflect on family members, as well as on him- or herself. It is important in situations that involve a conflict between personal desires and family obligations not to pathologize, critique, or dissuade a client's beliefs about his or her family, but to assist the client to anticipate the potential social consequences of making certain choices. The type of intervention may help the client be able to use problem-solving skills in situations that involve differences of opinions. Although the therapist may believe that one choice (e.g., asserting one's independence) is preferable to another (e.g., doing what one's parents prefer), the therapist should accept the complexity inherent in making such choices.

CONCLUSIONS

CBT and other evidence-based psychotherapy techniques with cognitive and behavioral principles have been rigorously studied for efficacy and effectiveness. One drawback of the extant research is its lack of focus on adapting CBT techniques to characteristics of individuals who come from diverse backgrounds, including ethnicity, race, age, sexual orientation, and disability, among other areas of human diversity of background and experience. Little research has investigated empirically *how* CBT interventions ought to be structured to maximize their relevance, acceptability, and effectiveness with diverse group members (e.g., Lau, 2006). This type of investigation is essential, because provision of culturally competent treatment for all people is an ethical imperative, as well as a clinical reality, given the number of people who present for therapy with one or more "diverse" identities.

Despite the lack of specific evidence about how to employ CBT techniques for culturally diverse individuals, we have used the available evidence, as well as clinical judgment, to make suggestions on this topic. As detailed earlier, we suggest an iterative process of learning about the sociocultural groups in which our clients are members, doing competent and theoretically consistent CBT, and devoting significant attention to some of the crosscutting themes that we discuss—including assessment and integration into the treatment plan of a client's health beliefs, relationship with family and the ways in which that relationship is constrained by pervasive cultural norms, immigration status, and so forth. The more knowledgeable, flexible, and open a therapist is to a culturally informed idiographic assessment and case conceptualization, the more likely he or she is to build a strong relationship with a client and achieve a successful treatment outcome.

REFERENCES

American Psychiatric Association. (1980). *Diagnostic and statistical manual of mental disorders* (3rd ed.). Washington, DC: Author.

American Psychological Association. (1992). Ethical principles and code of conduct. *American Psychologist, 48,* 1597–1611.

American Psychological Association. (2003). Guidelines on multicultural education, training, research, practice, and organizational change for psychologists. *American Psychologist, 58*(5), 377–402.

American Psychological Association. (2000). Guidelines for psychotherapy with lesbian, gay, and bisexual clients. *American Psychologist, 55*(12), 1440–1451.

American Psychological Association Presidential Task Force on Evidence-Based Practice. (2006). Evidence-based practice in psychology. *American Psychologist, 61*(4), 271–285.

Anderson, N. B., & Nickerson, K. J. (2005). Genes, race, and psychology in the genome era: An introduction. *American Psychologist, 60*(1), 5–8.

Chung, R. C., & Bemak, F. (2007). Asian immigrants and refugees. In F. Leong, A. G. Inman, A. Ebreo, L. H. Yang, L. Kinoshita, & M. Fu (Eds.), *Handbook of Asian American psychology* (2nd ed., pp. 227–244). Thousand Oaks, CA: Sage.

Dobson, K. S. (Ed.). (2001). *Handbook of cognitive-behavioral therapies.* New York: Guilford Press.

Ebreo, A., Shiraishi, Y., Leung, P., & Yi, J. K. (2007). Health psychology and Asian Pacific Islanders: Learning from cardiovascular disease. In F. Leong, A. G. Inman, A. Ebreo, L. H. Yang, L., Kinoshita, & M. Fu (Eds.), *Handbook of Asian American psychology* (2nd ed., pp. 303–322). Thousand Oaks, CA: Sage.

Ellis, A., & Cory, D. (1965). *Homosexuality: Its causes and cure.* New York: Lyle Stuart.

Gist, Y. J., & Hetzel, L. I. (2004). *We the people: Aging in the United States.* Washington, DC: U.S. Department of Commerce, Economics and Statistics Administration, U.S. Census Bureau.

Hall, C. C. I. (1997). Cultural malpractice: The growing obsolescence of psychology with the changing U.S. population. *American Psychologist, 52*(6), 642–651.

Hall, G. C. N. (2001). Psychotherapy with ethnic minorities: Empirical, ethical, and conceptual issues. *Journal of Consulting and Clinical Psychology, 69,* 502–510.

Haynes, S. N., & O'Brien, W. O. (2000). *Principles of behavioral assessment: A functional approach to psychological assessment.* New York: Kluwer Academic/Plenum Press.

Hays, P. A. (2006). Introduction: Developing culturally responsive cognitive-behavioral therapies. In P. A. Hayes & G. Y. Iwamasa (Eds.), *Culturally responsive cognitive-behavioral therapy* (pp. 3–19). Washington, DC: American Psychological Association.

Hinton, D. E., & Otto, M. W. (2006). Symptom presentation and symptom meaning among traumatized Cambodian refugees: Relevance to a somatically focused cognitive-behavior therapy. *Cognitive and Behavioral Practice, 13*(4), 249–260.

Hinton, D. E., Safren, S. A., Pollack, M. H., & Tran, M. (2006). Cognitive-behavioral therapy for Vietnamese refugees with PTSD and comorbid panic attacks. *Cognitive and Behavioral Practice, 13*(4), 271–281.

Hobbs, F., & Stoops, N. (2002). *Census 2000 Special Reports, Series CENSR-4: Demographic trends in the 20th century.* Washington, DC: U.S. Government Printing Office.

Iwamasa, G. Y., Hsia, C., & Hinton, D. (2006). Cognitive-behavioral therapy with Asian Americans. In P. A. Hayes & G. Y. Iwamasa (Eds.), *Culturally responsive cognitive-behavioral therapy* (pp. 117–140). Washington, DC: American Psychological Association.

Jones, J. H. (1981). *Bad blood: The Tuskegee Syphilis Experiment.* New York: Free Press.

Katz, R. V., Green, B. L., Kressin, N. R., Claudio, C., Wang, M. Q., & Russell, S. L. (2007). Willingness of minorities to participate in biomedical studies: Confirmatory findings from a follow-up study using the Tuskegee Legacy Project Questionnaire. *Journal of the National Medical Association, 99,* 1052–1060.

Kelly, S. (2006). Cognitive-behavioral therapy with African Americans. In P. A. Hayes & G. Y. Iwamasa (Eds.), *Culturally responsive cognitive-behavioral therapy* (pp. 97–116). Washington, DC: American Psychological Association.

Kim, W. (2006). Diversity among Southeast Asian ethnic groups: A study of mental health disorders among Cambodians, Laotians, Miens, and Vietnamese. *Journal of Ethnic and Cultural Diversity in Social Work, 15*(3/4), 83–100.

Kite, M. E., Russo, N. F., Brehm, S. S., Fouad, N. A., Hall, C. C., Hyde, J. S., et al. (2001). Women psychologists in academe: Mixed progress, unwarranted complacency. *American Psychologist, 56,* 1080–1098.

Kleinman, A., Eisenberg, L., & Good, B. (2006). Culture, illness, and care: Clinical lessons from anthropologic and cross-cultural research. *Focus, 4,* 140–149.

Korman, M. (1974). National conference on levels and patterns of professional training in psychology. *American Psychologist, 29,* 441–449.

Lau, A. S. (2006). Making the case for selective and directed cultural adaptations of evidence-based treatments: Examples from parent training. *Clinical Psychology: Science and Practice, 13,* 295–310.

Martell, C. R., Safren, S. A., & Prince, S. E. (2004). *Cognitive-behavioral therapies with lesbian, gay, and bisexual clients.* New York: Guilford Press.

McCubbin, H. I., McCubbin, M. A., Thompson, A. I., & Thompson, E. A. (1998). Resilience in ethnic families: A conceptual model for predicting family adjustment and adaptation. In H. I. McCubbin, E. A. Thompson, A. I. Thompson, & J. E. Fromer (Eds.), *Resilience in Native American and immigrant families* (pp. 3–48). Thousand Oaks, CA: Sage.

McDonald, J. D., & Gonzalez, J. (2006). Cognitive-behavioral therapy with American Indians. In P. A. Hayes & G. Y. Iwamasa (Eds.), *Culturally responsive cognitive-behavioral therapy* (pp. 73–96). Washington, DC: American Psychological Association.

Meyer, I. H. (2003). Prejudice, social stress, and mental health in lesbian, gay, and bisexual populations: Conceptual issues and research evidence. *Psychological Bulletin, 129*(5), 674–697.

Norcross, J. C., Hedges, M., & Prochaska, J. O. (2002). The face of 2010: A Delphi Poll on the future of psychotherapy. *Professional Psychology: Research and Practice, 33,* 316–322.

Norcross, J. C., Karg, R., & Prochaska, J. O. (1997). Clinical psychologists in the 1990's, Part II. *Clinical Psychologist, 50,* 4–11.

Organista, K. C. (2006). Cognitive-behavioral therapy with Latinos and Latinas. In P. A. Hayes & G. Y. Iwamasa (Eds.), *Culturally responsive cognitive-behavioral therapy* (pp. 73–96). Washington, DC: American Psychological Association.

Otto, M. W., & Hinton, D. E. (2006). Modifying exposure-based CBT for Cambodian refugees with posttraumatic stress disorder. *Cognitive and Behavioral Practice, 13*(4), 261–270.

Ridley, C. R. (1985). Imperatives for ethnic and cultural relevance in psychology training programs. *Professional Psychology: Research and Practice, 16,* 611–622.

Schulz, P. M., Huber, C., & Resick, P. A. (2006). Practical adaptations of cognitive processing therapy with Bosnian refugees: Implications for adapting practice to a multicultural clientele. *Cognitive and Behavioral Practice, 13*(4), 310–321.

Schulz, P. M., Resick, P. A., Huber, C., & Griffen, M. G. (2006). The effectiveness of cognitive processing therapy for PTSD with refugees in a community setting. *Cognitive and Behavioral Practice, 13*(4), 322—331.

Snyder, D. K., Castellani, A. M., & Whisman, M. A. (2006). Current status and future directions in couple therapy. *Annual Review of Psychology, 57,* 317–344.

Sue, D. W. (2001). Multidimensional facets of cultural competence. *Counseling Psychologist, 29,* 790–821.

Sue, S. (2006). Cultural competency: From philosophy to research and practice. *Journal of Community Psychology, 34*(2), 237–245.

Sue, S., & Zane, N. (1987). The role of culture and cultural techniques in psychotherapy: A critique and reformulation. *American Psychologist, 42,* 37–45.

U.S. Census Bureau. (2001). *U.S. Census 2000, Summary Files 1 and 2.* Retrieved January 7, 2008, from *www.census.gov/main/www/cen2000.html.*

U.S. Department of Health and Human Services. (1999). *Mental health: A report of the Surgeon General—Executive Summary.* Rockville, MD: Author.

Whaley, A. L., & Davis, K. E. (2007). Cultural competence and evidence-based practice in mental health services: A complementary perspective. *American Psychologist, 62*(6), 563–574.

Yee, B. W. K., DeBaryshe, B. D., Yuen, S., Kim, S. Y., & McCubbin, H. I. (2007). Asian American and Pacific Islander families: Resiliency and life-span socialization in a cultural context. In F. Leong, A. G. Inman, A. Ebreo, L. H. Yang, L. Kinoshita, & M. Fu (Eds.), *Handbook of Asian American psychology* (2nd ed., pp. 69–86). Thousand Oaks, CA: Sage.

Zweig, M. (2004). *What's class got to do with it?: American society in the twenty-first century.* Ithaca, NY: ILR Press.

Index

Self-statements. *see also* Self-reporting
   CBTs and, 28
   stress inoculation training and, 19–20
SEMG. *see* Surface electromyography
Sensitization, internalization and, 116
Set, PST and, 21
Sexual offending, efficacy of CBTs for,
   55–56, 60t
Sexual orientation, 454t, 455–456t. *see also*
   Diverse populations
SFT. *see* Schema-focused therapy
Shame, schema development and, 322–325t,
   327–328t, 336–343t
Shame-attacking exercises, REBT and, 13
Shaping, PST and, 211
Shoulds, as distortion/error, 280t
SISST. *see* Social Interaction Self-Statement
   Test
SIT. *see* Self-instructional training
Skills training
   mindfulness/acceptance and, 362–364
   REBT and, 13, 255–256
   self-control treatments and, 17
Skills-based therapies
   CBCT and, 424–427
   CT as, 279
Sleep difficulties, efficacy of CBTs for, 58–59,
   60t
SMI. *see* Schema Mode Inventory
Social anxiety disorder
   cognitive assessment and, 141
   efficacy of CBTs for, 44–45
Social Avoidance and Distress Scale, 140
Social cognition research, CBCT and,
   413–414
Social context of treatment, youth and,
   378–379
Social Interaction Self-Statement Test, 142
Social interest, REBT and, 228, 237
Social learning theory
   behavior therapy and, 105
   CBCT and, 412
Social problem-solving, aggression and,
   391
Social Problem-Solving Inventory, 200,
   201–202
Social problem-solving model, 198–200
Social Thoughts and Beliefs Scale, 146–147
Sociotropy, 120
Sociotropy-Autonomy scale, 120
Socratic questioning
   CBCT and, 428–429
   CT and, 288
   patient resistance and, 113

Solution
   defining, 199
   problem-solving process and, 388t
   PST and, 200, 209–210t
Somatoform disorders, efficacy of CBTs for,
   58, 60t, 65
Specificity, CT and, 303
Spirituality, CBTs and, 103
Spontaneity, schema development and, 320
SPSI. *see* Social Problem-Solving Inventory
SRET. *see* Self-Referent Encoding Task
SRR. *see* Systematic rational restructuring
STABS. *see* Social Thoughts and Beliefs Scale
Standards
   CBCT and, 427
   schema development and, 322–325t,
      327–328t, 336–343t
Static personality dimension, 232–233f
Stimulus-response models, 7
Stoicism, REBT and, 226
STOP & THINK technique, PST and,
   209–210t
Strategic eclecticism, 96, 99–100. *see also*
   Eclectic psychotherapy
Stream of consciousness, CBTs and, 28
Stress inoculation training, as type of CBT,
   19–20
Stress management
   case formulation and, 179–180
   cognitive assessment and, 135–136
   couples and, 415
   MBSR and, 354–355
   PST and, 21, 197, 202–206
Stroop color-naming task, 158–160
Structural dimensions of cognitive
   assessment, 134f
Structural psychotherapy, as type of CBT,
   22–24
Subjective personality dimension, 232–233f
Subjective units of distress, 187–188
Subjugation, schema development and,
   322–325t, 327–328t, 336–343t
Substance Abuse and Mental Health Services
   Administration, 397
Substance use disorders
   common factors eclecticism and, 97
   CT and, 14
   efficacy of CBTs for, 60t, 65
   efficacy of CT for, 108
   PST and, 198, 206
   recent developments in CBT for, 104
Substitutions, CT and, 14
Succorance, relationship quality and, 416
SUDS. *see* Subjective units of distress